Handbook of
FORENSIC ANALYTICAL TOXICOLOGY

Handbook of
FORENSIC ANALYTICAL TOXICOLOGY

Second Edition

AK Jaiswal MSc PhD FIC FASAW FISCA FISROSET
Chemist
Department of Forensic Medicine and Toxicology
All India Institute of Medical Sciences
New Delhi, India

Tabin Millo MBBS MD DNB MHR MNAMS FIMSA
Professor
Department of Forensic Medicine and Toxicology
All India Institute of Medical Sciences
New Delhi, India

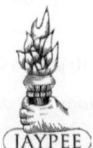

JAYPEE BROTHERS MEDICAL PUBLISHERS
The Health Sciences Publisher
New Delhi | London

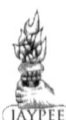 **Jaypee Brothers Medical Publishers (P) Ltd**

Headquarters
EMCA House
23/23-B, Ansari Road, Daryaganj
New Delhi 110 002, India
Landline: +91-11-23272143, +91-11-23272703
+91-11-23282021, +91-11-23245672
E-mail: jaypee@jaypeebrothers.com

Corporate Office
Jaypee Brothers Medical Publishers (P) Ltd.
4838/24, Ansari Road, Daryaganj
New Delhi 110 002, India
Phone: +91-11-43574357
Fax: +91-11-43574314
E-mail: jaypee@jaypeebrothers.com

Overseas Office
JP Medical Ltd.
83, Victoria Street, London
SW1H 0HW (UK)
Phone: +44-20 3170 8910
Fax: +44(0)20 3008 6180
E-mail: info@jpmedpub.com

Website: www.jaypeebrothers.com
Website: www.jaypeedigital.com

© 2022, Jaypee Brothers Medical Publishers

The views and opinions expressed in this book are solely those of the original contributor(s)/author(s) and do not necessarily represent those of editor(s) of the book.

All rights reserved by the author. No part of this publication may be reproduced, stored or transmitted in any form or by any means, electronic, mechanical, photocopying, recording or otherwise, without the prior permission in writing of the publishers.

All brand names and product names used in this book are trade names, service marks, trademarks or registered trademarks of their respective owners. The publisher is not associated with any product or vendor mentioned in this book.

Medical knowledge and practice change constantly. This book is designed to provide accurate, authoritative information about the subject matter in question. However, readers are advised to check the most current information available on procedures included and check information from the manufacturer of each product to be administered, to verify the recommended dose, formula, method and duration of administration, adverse effects and contraindications. It is the responsibility of the practitioner to take all appropriate safety precautions. Neither the publisher nor the author(s)/editor(s) assume any liability for any injury and/or damage to persons or property arising from or related to use of material in this book.

This book is sold on the understanding that the publisher is not engaged in providing professional medical services. If such advice or services are required, the services of a competent medical professional should be sought.

Every effort has been made where necessary to contact holders of copyright to obtain permission to reproduce copyright material. If any have been inadvertently overlooked, the publisher will be pleased to make the necessary arrangements at the first opportunity. The **CD/DVD-ROM** (if any) provided in the sealed envelope with this book is complimentary and free of cost. **It is Not meant for sale.**

Inquiries for bulk sales may be solicited at: jaypee@jaypeebrothers.com

Handbook of Forensic Analytical Toxicology / AK Jaiswal, Tabin Millo
First Edition: 2014
Second Edition: **2022**
ISBN: 978-93-90595-38-9
Printed at:

Preface to the Second Edition

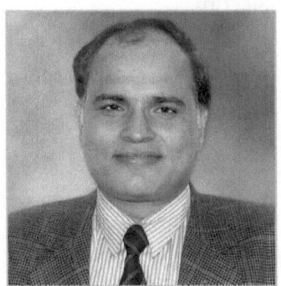

AK Jaiswal

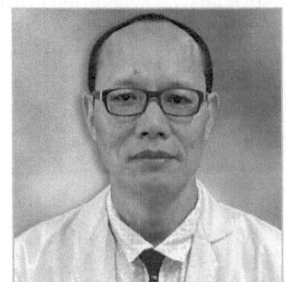

Tabin Millo

We are pleased to bring out the Second Edition of the book. The first edition was received with overwhelming response by the reader. All the printed copies were sold out. The second edition includes many new chapters and all the previous chapters have been thoroughly revised and updated with the latest research findings. *Handbook of Forensic Analytical Toxicology* is aimed at reaching out to the needs of student audience, studying BSc, MSc of forensic science and PhD students (forensic toxicology). It will also help the MD students of forensic medicine and toxicology to understand the basic principles of sample collection, preservation, analysis and reporting in forensic toxicology. Reliable and authentic analysis report of forensic samples in crime investigation forms a huge contribution to the investigating agency and the court of law. But, we need good infrastructure and qualified forensic scientists for good results. In the book, we have tried to cover all the main aspects of forensic analytical toxicology techniques. Chapter 1 covers the designing of modern toxicology laboratory with real photographs of the laboratory. Chapter 2 discusses in detail the collection, preservation, and forwarding of biological sample for toxicological analysis. Chapter 3 covers the extraction/isolation analysis of exhaustive list of poisons such as pesticides, volatile poisons, tranquilizers, barbiturates, alkaloids, metallic poisons, etc., with flow diagrams which will be easy to understand and guide the analytical work. It also has the detail on screening tests of all different poisons in Chapter 4. The details of major analytical equipment such as high-performance liquid chromatography (HPLC), gas liquid chromatography (GLC), thin layer chromatography (TLC), atomic absorption spectroscopy (AAS), voltammetry/polarography, UV-visible spectroscopy, etc., with photographs have been covered in different chapters, which is the special feature of this book, generally not available in other books. It also covers the do's and don'ts of each equipment with troubleshooting

PREFACE

tips. The safety measures and standard operating procedures (SOP) have been covered in the end chapters along with a special chapter on toxicology reporting. We hope the book will be of immense benefit for those people who are in the field of forensic toxicology and medicine. We invite your constructive suggestions for the improvement of the book in in the email Id: ashokjaiswal72@gmail.com/tabinmillo2003@rediffmail.com.

AK Jaiswal
Tabin Millo

Preface to the First Edition

Handbook of Forensic Analytical Toxicology is aimed at reaching out to the needs of student audience, studying BSc, MSc of Forensic Science, and PhD students. It will also help the MD students of Forensic Medicine and Toxicology to understand the basic principles of sample collection, preservation, analysis, and reporting in forensic toxicology. Reliable and authentic analysis report of forensic samples in crime investigation forms a huge contribution to the investigating agency and the court of law. But, we need good infrastructure and qualified forensic scientists for good results. In the book, we have tried to cover all the main aspects of forensic analytical toxicology techniques. Chapter 1 covers the designing of modern toxicology laboratory with real photographs of the laboratory. Chapter 2 discusses in detail the collection, preservation, and forwarding of biological sample for toxicological analysis. Chapter 3 covers the extraction/isolation analysis of exhaustive list of poisons such as pesticides, volatile poisons, tranquilizers, barbiturates, alkaloids, and metallic poisons with flow diagrams, which will be easy to understand and guide the analytical work. It also has the detail on screening tests of all different poisons in Chapter 4. The details of major analytical equipment such as high-performance liquid chromatography (HPLC), gas-liquid chromatography (GLC), thin-layer chromatography (TLC), atomic absorption spectroscopy (AAS), voltammetry/polarography, and ultraviolet (UV)-visible spectroscopy with photographs have been covered in different chapters, which are the special feature of this book, generally not available in other books. It also covers the Do's and Don'ts of each equipment with troubleshooting tips. The safety measures and standard operating procedures (SOP) have been covered in the end chapters along with a special chapter on toxicology reporting. We hope that this book will be of immense benefit for those people who are in the field of forensic toxicology and medicine. We invite your constructive suggestions for the improvement of the book in the subsequent edition.

AK Jaiswal
Tabin Millo

Acknowledgments

During our profession journey, we are sometimes motivated to take up certain tasks guided by the need of the time. It was the same motivation which led us to take up the assignment of writing this book. We felt that there is need for a simplified book in Forensic Analytical Toxicology to reach out to the students of forensic science, analytical chemistry and forensic medicine.

As we started the journey to author this book, there were many special people who encouraged us and gave valuable suggestions and support. We would like to especially thank Professor Sudhir K Gupta, Professor and Head, Department of Forensic Medicine and Toxicology, AIIMS, New Delhi, India for encouraging us and providing the latest facilities in the forensic toxicology laboratory. We would also like to express our heartfelt gratitude to our colleagues Professor DN Bhardwaj, Professor OP Murty, Professor Sanjeev Lalwani, Professor Adarsh Kumar, Dr Chittaranjan Behera, Dr Kulbhushan Prasad, Dr Abhishek Yadav and Laboratory technical staff Sunil and Kapil for their cordial support and suggestions. We especially thank our students for their valuable inputs in this journey.

We are indebted to our family members for their moral support and sacrificing their valuable time. We also thank the Forensic Scientific Community for providing us motivation and scientific inputs for the book. We express our thanks to the entire staff of M/s Jaypee Brothers Medical Publishers (P) Ltd., New Delhi, India, for their commitment to bringing out the highest standard of quality and state-of-the-art presentation of the book with their excellence in the art of publication. Lastly, we would like to acknowledge almighty God for his grace which helped us to complete this book.

A K Jaiswal
Tabin Millo

CONTENTS

1. **Modern Toxicology Laboratory**   1
   Human Resource *1*
   Location *3*
   Physical Facility, Area, and Space Requirement *3*
   Engineering Specifications *10*
   Requirements *12*
   Security *29*

2. **Procedure for Collection, Preservation, and Forwarding of Biological Sample for Toxicological Analysis**   39
   Biological Fluids *39*
   Urine *40*
   Biological Tissues *44*
   Containers *48*
   Sample Preservation and Storage *48*
   Packaging and Forwarding of Samples *48*

3. **Extraction/Isolation and Clean-up Methods**   52
   Extraction/Isolation Methods for Pesticides/Insecticides *52*
   Extraction/Isolation Methods for Volatile Poisons *57*
   Extraction/Isolation Method for Cyanide *60*
   Extraction/Isolation Methods for Tranquilizers *61*
   Extraction/Isolation Methods for Barbiturates *65*
   Extraction/Isolation Methods for Alkaloids *69*
   Extraction/Isolation Methods for Metallic Poisons *75*
   Extraction/Isolation Methods for Miscellaneous Poisons *78*

4. **Screening/Spot/Color Tests for Different Poisons**   90
   Screening/Spot/Color Tests for Pesticides/Insecticides *90*
   Test for Some Individual Pesticides *92*
   Screening/Spot/Color Tests for Volatile Poisons *98*
   Screening/Spot/Color Tests for Tranquilizers *106*
   Screening/Spot/Color Tests for Barbiturates *116*
   Screening/Spot/Color Tests for Alkaloids *120*
   Screening/Spot/Color Tests for Metallic Poisons *128*
   Screening/Spot/Color Tests for Antibiotics *139*
   Screening/Spot/Color Tests for Drug of Abuse *146*
   Screening/Spot/Color Tests for Acids and Bases *155*
   Screening/Spot/Color Tests for Toxic Anions *163*
   Screening/Spot/Color Tests for Plant Poisons *174*

5. **Thin Layer Chromatography and its Applications**   186
   Basic Requirement of Thin Layer Chromatography *187*
   Types of Thin Layer Chromatography Plates *195*
   Preparation of Thin Layer Chromatography Plates *197*
   Solvents/Mobile Phase used for Thin Layer Chromatography *198*
   Applying the Substance on Thin Layer Chromatography

CONTENTS

Plate/Loading of Sample and Standard *201*
Operation/Development of Chromatogram *202*
Detection Reagents/Spraying Reagents for Visualizing the Chromatogram *202*
Retention Factor *203*
Standard Operating Procedure for Thin Layer Chromatography (SOP for TLC) *217*
Safety Precautions Related to Thin Layer Chromatography *220*
Do's and Don'ts for Thin Layer Chromatography *220*
Forensic Applications of TLC *221*
Medicolegal Aspects *224*

6. Gas Chromatography and its Applications 228

Gas Chromatography *228*
Techniques of Gas-liquid Chromatography *229*
Terms used in Gas-liquid Chromatography *251*
Separation of Mixture *256*
Gas Chromatography Derivatization *257*
Accessories and Spares used in Gas-liquid Chromatography *258*
Do's and Don'ts for Gas-liquid Chromatography *261*
Headspace Gas Chromatography *263*
Technical Specifications for Gas-liquid Chromatography *265*
Forensic Applications of Gas-liquid Chromatography *267*
Comparison of Gas-liquid Chromatography with
High-performance Liquid Chromatography *276*
Troubleshooting in Gas Chromatography *276*

7. High-performance Liquid Chromatography and its Applications 287

Theory of High-performance Liquid Chromatography *288*
Terms used in High-performance Liquid Chromatography *288*
Types of High-performance Liquid Chromatography *294*
Elution Techniques in High-performance Liquid Chromatography *295*
Instrumentation *296*
Combination of High-performance Liquid Chromatography
with Other Techniques *315*
Regeneration of Analytical Column *316*
Effect of Temperature in High-performance Liquid Chromatography *317*
Technical Specifications for High-performance Liquid Chromatography System *317*
Derivatization Techniques in High-performance Liquid Chromatography *319*
Biological Sample Preparation for High-performance
Liquid Chromatography Analysis *319*
Qualitative and Quantitative Analysis in High-performance
Liquid Chromatography *320*
Method Validation *321*
Recent Development in High-performance Liquid
Chromatography is Ultra-performance Liquid Chromatography *322*
Performance of High-performance Liquid Chromatography *323*
Do's and Don'ts for High-performance Liquid Chromatography *323*
Troubleshooting in High-performance Liquid Chromatography *328*
Relevance of High-performance Liquid Chromatography
Over Gas-liquid Chromatography *331*
Forensic Applications of High-performance Liquid Chromatography *332*

8. Ultraviolet-visible Spectroscopy and its Applications 340

Spectroscopy *341*
Ultraviolet-visible Spectroscopy *342*

CONTENTS

Chromophore *350*
Auxochrome *351*
Absorption and Intensity Shifts *351*
Basis of Color in Organic Compounds *353*
Various Types of Double in Conjugation *354*
Woodward–Fieser Rules for Calculating λ_{max} for Conjugated Dienes and Trienes *355*
Woodward–Fieser Rules for Calculating Absorption Maximum in α, β-Unsaturated Carbonyl Compounds *357*
Rules for Calculating Absorption Maximum for Derivatives of Acyl Benzenes *361*
Instrumentation *362*
Calibration of Ultraviolet-visible Spectrophotometer *368*
Do's and Don'ts of Ultraviolet-visible Spectrophotometer *374*
Technical Specifications of Double-beam Ultraviolet-visible Spectrophotometer *375*
Solvents for Ultraviolet-visible Spectroscopy *376*
General Applications of Ultraviolet-visible Spectroscopy *376*
Forensic Applications of Ultraviolet-visible Spectrophotometer *379*

9. Atomic Absorption Spectroscopy and its Applications 383
Principle of Atomic Absorption Spectroscopy *383*
Instrumentation *386*
Sensitivity, Detection Limit and Working Range *393*
Interference in Atomic Absorption *394*
Techniques for Optimization *396*
Applications of the Atomic Absorption Spectroscopy *396*
Do's and Don'ts for Atomic Absorption Spectrometry *399*
Technical Specifications for Purchase Of Double Beam Atomic Absorption Spectrophotometer (AAS) *400*

10. Voltammetry/Polarography Trace Metal Analyzer and its Applications 405
Principle of Trace Metal Analyzer *405*
Stripping Methods *406*
Instrumentation *409*
Do's and Don'ts for Voltammetric Trace Metal Analysis *415*
Characteristics of Voltammetric Trace Metal Analyzer *415*
Basic Steps Involved in the Analysis of Different Metals *416*
Detection Limit of Voltammetric Trace Metal Analyzer *417*
Advantages of Voltammetric Trace Metal Analyzer Over Other Techniques *418*
Limitations of Voltammetric Trace Metal Analyzer *418*
Technical Specifications of Trace Metal Analyzer *419*
Standard Operating Procedure for Voltammetric Trace Metal Analyzer (797 VA Computrace) *419*
Forensic Applications of Voltammetric/Polarographic Trace Metal Analyzer *425*

11. Microwave Digestion System and its Applications 476
Principles of Microwave Technology *477*
Characteristics of Microwaves *477*
Material Behavior of Microwave *477*
Advantages of Microwave Technology Over Thermal Convection *479*
Microwave Decomposition/Digestion *479*
Instrumentation *480*
Do's and Don'ts for Handling Microwave Digestor *484*
Technical Specifications for Microwave Digestor *484*

CONTENTS

Comparison of Open and Closed Decomposition/Digestion *485*
Basic Procedure for Sample Digestion in the Microwave Digestor *485*
Forensic Applications of Microwave Digestor *488*

12. Breath Alcohol Analyzer and its Applications — 494
Types of Breathalyzers *494*
Principle of Breath Alcohol Testing *495*
Precautions *496*
Legal Status *497*
Legal Defense Challenges in Drunken Driving *498*

13. Laboratory Accreditation: A Tool for Quality Management System — 503
History of Accreditation *503*
Terms and Definitions *503*
Quality Management System *506*
International Organization for Standardization Quality Management Principles *506*
Quality Audit *509*
Managing an Audit Program *510*
Establishing Audit Program Objectives *511*
Implementing Audit Program *512*
Managing Audit Program Results *513*
Managing and Maintaining Audit Program Records *513*
Monitoring Audit Program *513*
Reviewing and Improving Audit Program *514*
Accreditation *514*
Identification, Classification, and Expression of Nonconformity *520*
Preassessment Visit *520*
On-site Assessment *520*
ISO/IEC 17025: 2017: Summary at a Glance *524*

14. Forensic Toxicology Reporting and Interpretation — 532
Classification of Poisons *532*
General Steps in Toxicological Examination *533*
Objectives of Toxicology Reporting *533*
Ways of Expressing Report *533*
Legal Standing of the Toxicology Report *535*
Interpretation of Results *535*
Causes of False-negative Report *538*
Causes of False-positive Report *540*

15. Do's and Don'ts for Different Personnel Involved in Crime Investigation of Poisoning Deaths — 547
General Instructions for Examining Scene of Crime *547*
Do's and Don'ts for Collection and Preservation of Samples *549*
Do's and Don'ts for Packing/Labeling the Samples *550*
Do's and Don'ts for Dispatch and Forwarding the Samples *551*
Do's and Don'ts for Police Investigating Officers *552*
Do's and Don'ts for Medical Officers *553*
Do's and Don'ts for Forensic Toxicologists/Scientists *554*

16. Safety Measures in the Laboratory — 556
Common Safety and Health Measurements in the Laboratory *556*
Safety Measurements to Chemical Exposure *559*
Waste Disposal Procedures for Biological Material *560*

Biomedical Waste Management Rules, 2016 *560*
First Aid Emergency Treatment in the Laboratory Accidents *562*

17. The Indian Laws Relating to Drugs and Poisons — 566
The Poisons Act, 1919 *567*
The Drugs and Cosmetics Act, 1940 *567*
The Drugs and Cosmetics Rules, 1945 *567*
The Pharmacy Act, 1948 *568*
The Drugs Control Act, 1950 *568*
The Drugs and Magic Remedies (Objectionable Advertisements) Act, 1954 *568*
The Narcotic Drugs and Psychotropic Substances Act, 1985 *569*
The Drugs (Price Control) Order, 1995 *569*
The Indian Penal Code, 1860 *570*
The Code of Criminal Procedure, 1973 *570*
The Indian Evidence Act, 1872 *571*
Recent Amendments of Indian Penal Code Dealing with
Acid Attack Case, 2013 *571*
Supreme Court Guidelines to Prevent Acid Attacks *572*

Appendix — 575
Appendix 1 *575*
Appendix 2 *578*
Appendix 3 *585*
Appendix 4 *586*
Appendix 5 *590*
Appendix 6 *591*
Appendix 7 *636*

Index — 655

Abbreviations

AAS	: Atomic absorption spectroscopy		GLC	: Gas liquid chromatoraphy
ASV	: Anodic stripping voltammetry		GSC	: Gas solid chromatography
			HDME	: Hanging drop mercury electrode
BHC	: Benzene hexa chloride		HEEP	: Height equivalent to an effective plate
CLND	: Chemical luminescence nitrogen detector		HETP	: Height equivalent to theoretical plate
CNS	: Central nervous system			
CPE	: Carbon paste electrode		HID	: Helium ionization detector
CSV	: Cathodic stripping voltammetry		HPLC	: High performance liquid chromatography
CVS	: Cyclic voltammetric stripping		HS	: Head space
			HSS	: High strength silica
DDT	: Dichloro diethyl trichloroethane		ICP	: Inductively coupled plasma
DDVP	: 2,2-Dichlorovinyl dimethyl phosphate		ICP-MS	: Inductively coupled plasma-mass spectrometry
DME	: Dropping mercury electrode		LC-FTIR	: Liquid chromatography fourier transform infrared spectroscopy
ECD	: Electrochemical detector		LC-MS	: Liquid chromatography-mass spectroscopy
EDL	: Electro discharge lamp			
ELSD	: Evaporative light-scattering detector		LLSD	: Laser light scattering detector
FID	: Flame ionization detector		LOD	: Limit of detection
FPD	: Flame photometric detector		LOQ	: Limit of quantitation
			LSD	: Lysergic acid diethylamide
FTIR	: Fourier transform infrared spectroscopy		MAD	: Micro argon detector
			MD	: Mass detector
GCE	: Glass carbon electrode		MDS	: Microwave digestion system
GC-MS	: Gas chromatography-mass spectroscopy			
			MME	: Multimode electrode
GDS	: General drug screen		OC	: Organochloro compound

ABBREVIATIONS

OP	:	Organophosphorus compound	**TCD**	:	Thermal conductivity detector
PDA	:	Photodiode array	**TLC**	:	Thin layer chromatography
PID	:	Photo ionization detector	**TMA**	:	Trace metal analyser
PVC	:	Polyvinyl chloride	**TMFE**	:	Thin mercury film electrode
RI	:	Refractive index	**UV**	:	Ultraviolet
SDME	:	Static mercury drop electrode			

Chapter 1

Modern Toxicology Laboratory

■ INTRODUCTION

A forensic toxicology laboratory is mainly provided with preserved viscera, body fluids, and other biological samples for the determination of presence or absence of toxic substances and their metabolites and to evaluate their role as a determinant or contributory factor in the cause and manner of death or suspect case of poisoning. A forensic toxicology laboratory also plays an integral role in human performance by determining the absence or presence of poisons and chemicals in blood, breath, or other appropriate specimens. A hospital medical toxicology laboratory has to conduct routine biochemical analysis of patients for therapeutic and academic purpose. It has no responsibility to criminal justice process, but a crime laboratory or forensic toxicology laboratory has responsibility to the prosecution, the victim, the suspect, the society, the police, and judiciary.

■ HUMAN RESOURCE

Human resource constitutes the backbone of any system. The personnel employed should be efficient, competent, and technically sound. The number of staff members will depend on the workload of the laboratory and can be segregated in three different levels—(1) administrative, (2) technical, and (3) nontechnical.

Director/Chief Scientist/Chief Toxicologist/Chief Chemist

A forensic toxicology laboratory should be directed by a person who is qualified by a reason of appropriate education (Master's degree in Chemistry/Forensic Science/Toxicology) and Doctorate in the field of Chemistry/Toxicology and experience to assume the required professional, organizational, educational, managerial, and administrative responsibilities. The director should have minimum 10 years of full-time laboratory experience in forensic toxicology laboratory. The director should also have a documented training and experience in the forensic application of analytical toxicology (such as court testimony, research, participation in continuing education programs, including knowledge of evidentiary procedures) that apply when toxicological samples are received, stored, processed, and analyzed and toxicological data/reports are submitted as a part of legal proceeding.

Responsibilities of Chief Scientist/Chief Toxicologist/Chief Chemist/Director

The responsibilities of chief scientist/chief toxicologist/chief chemist/director are:
1. Maintain and update the standard manual of the laboratory
2. Monitor laboratory practices to verify continuing compliance with policies and procedures
3. Evaluate instrument calibration and the maintenance of records
4. Periodically assess the adequacy of the report and review the activities
5. Maintain training records of laboratory personnel
6. Recommend training to improve the quality of laboratory staff, etc.

Forensic Scientists

A forensic toxicology laboratory should have a series of forensic scientists as scientist grade III, scientist grade II, and scientist grade I. The grades of scientists are based on their experience and expertise. Senior scientist should be looked upon as an individual with considerable expertise and may serve as a training coordinator for new analysts. He should be skilled in demonstration of competency and allowed to report and testify to the caseworks in the court of law.

Laboratory Technicians

A laboratory technician should have a minimum of Bachelor's degree in Natural Science/Forensic Science/Chemistry with hands on experience in Analytical Chemistry/Toxicology and capable of performing variety of test procedures for drugs, alcohol, and other chemicals.

Laboratory Assistants

A laboratory assistant should have Bachelor's degree in Natural Science. He should be capable of performing various test procedures and maintaining proper laboratory records.

Laboratory Attendants

A laboratory attendant should have an intermediate (10+2) in Science. The responsibility of laboratory attendant is to clean the laboratory equipment and arrange the chemicals and glasswares, etc.

Nontechnical Staff

The nontechnical staff consists of clerk, librarian, storekeeper, accountant, viscera cutter, peon, and sweeper. The number of nontechnical staff should be decided as per the requirement.

■ LOCATION

The forensic toxicology laboratory should be near the mortuary and must have rapid facility for sample transportation. The building should be in area with ample natural light through windows. The laboratory premises should be well connected by road transport network. It should have sufficient number of vehicles for transportation and travel of laboratory personnel from time to time. The area for the functional purpose in forensic toxicology laboratory can be divided into various segments.

■ PHYSICAL FACILITY, AREA, AND SPACE REQUIREMENT

Availability of adequate space and area is one of the prime factors, as it provides the foundation for all further planning and development of the laboratory. The space acquired should be sufficient enough to accommodate all the laboratory buildings, including open area for parking, waste disposal or incineration, etc. The laboratory premises should be well connected with road or with convenient transport network. The area in the main building can be divided into various segments as follows.

Reception and Visitor Room (Size 150 sq ft)

Visitor room should always be outside the second security gate.

Administrative or Office Room (Size According to Requirement)

It is a place required for all official works.

Laboratory Director/Chief Scientist Room (180 sq ft)

Director room should be situated inside the second security gate for the safety purpose.

Scientists Room (450 sq ft, Three Cabins of 15 × 10 sq ft each)

It is the room for the scientists to perform works such as documentation, report writing, etc. The room can be divided into cabins according to the number of scientists.

Library (360 sq ft)

The scientists and trainees regularly require consultation of reference books, journals, and other literatures during routine casework and for research purpose. To meet the needs, there must be a library in the laboratory premises, with computer facility and internet connection. It should be fully air conditioned with proper lighting.

Conference or Seminar Room (700 sq ft)

There should be a seminar or conference room for seminars, presentations, conferences, meetings, lectures, etc. It should be well equipped with a computer and a projector.

Stores (1,500 sq ft)

Proper storage facility is required for chemicals and reagents. Stores of glasswares and stationary items should be moisture free and rodent free.

Chemical Store (200 sq ft)

All chemicals which are used for laboratory working should be present in chemical store. The chemical store should consist of racks divided into blocks to store separate chemicals. This room should be air conditioned with proper ventilation.

Store for Sample or Parcel (900 sq ft)

It is a place to store samples. Store for exhibits should be divided into two portions, one for incoming (450 sq ft) case parcels and the other for outgoing (450 sq ft) case parcels. A cold chamber should be present in sample store. It should be divided into parts to store samples to prevent contamination. An ultraviolet (UV) lamp should be present inside the room for sterilization that destroys the microorganisms. The switch of UV lamp should always be outside the door of the storeroom. The sample store should always be near the isolation and extraction unit.

Glasswares and Other Consumables (200 sq ft)

It is a place for storing glasswares, gowns, aprons, rubber gloves, gumboots, towels, masks, and other consumables.

Stationary Store (200 sq ft)

Most frequently required stationaries in forensic toxicology laboratory are case files, registers, working sheets, pen and pencils, packing envelopes, boxes, packing cloths, reporting sheets, papers, carbon sheets, marker pens, etc. All stationary articles should be stored in moisture-free room.

Document Record Room (180 sq ft)

It is a room to maintain all records related to laboratory work, for example, old case files, training records. Regulation policy statement (the laboratory should maintain procedures to control that form the part of regulatory system) controls the data related to testing and calibration memoranda, related software, etc. The entire document forms the part of management system control in various media, whether hard copy or soft copy. Procedure manuals should be reviewed and approved for the authorized personnel and authorized edition of appropriate document should be available at all locations, as required for effective functioning of laboratory. These include specialization calibration charts, case file reporting proforma, analysis of records, books, literature, journals, memorandum, operation manuals, laboratory manuals, safety measurements, photographs, visitor records, employee's attendance records, reviews, requests, tenders and contract records, technical records, etc.

Case Opening Room (225 sq ft)

It is necessary to have a separate case opening room for the purpose of opening the case, parcel. It should be adjacent to the parcel store or preferably in between the parcel store and isolation/extraction room. It should have proper ventilation and exhaust fans.

Toxicology Museum (240 sq ft)

It is useful to have a toxicology museum for academic purpose. It should have all the poison samples properly preserved and labeled with brief facts about the poison. It can be obtained from the authorized supplier. List of items to be placed in toxicology museum has been listed in **Table 1.1**. Pictorial view of the museum is shown in **Figure 1.1**.

Table 1.1: List of poison samples for toxicology museum.

S. No.	Scientific name	Common name
1.	Arsenic oxide	Somalkhar sankhya
2.	Copper acetoarsenite	Hirwa Paris green
3.	Iodine	Iodine
4.	Oxazepam	Serepax
5.	Arsenic trisulfide	Hartal
6.	Mercuric sulfide	Ras-Sindoor
7.	Sulfuric acid	Gandhak ka Tezaab
8.	*Jatropha curcas*	Ratanjot, jangli, and arandi
9.	Dichlorodiphenyltrichloroethane	DDT
10.	Aloe vera	Elio
11.	*Helleborus niger*	Kali Kutki
12.	Mercury	Para
13.	*Capsicum annuum*	Lal Mirch pisi
14.	Croton tiglium	Jamalgota seed or Nepala
15.	Camphor—*Cinnamomum camphora*	Kapoor
16.	*Physostigma venenosum*	Sem ka key/Sem ka beej

Continued

MODERN TOXICOLOGY LABORATORY

Continued

S. No.	Scientific name	Common name
17.	Sodium carbonate	Washing soda
18.	*Sapindus trifoliatus*	Ritha
19.	Betel nut	Supari
20.	Calcium hydroxide	Slaked lime
21.	Lead sulfide	Surma
22.	Tobacco	Tambaku
23.	*Taxus baccata*	Yew
24.	Terpene oil	Terpene oil
25.	Sulfur powder	Sulfur powder, gandhak
26.	Arsenious oxide	Sankhya
27.	Sodium nitrate	Sodium nitrate
28.	Zinc sulfate	Safed tutiya
29.	Ammonium carbonate	Sal volatile
30.	Argemone seed	Prickly poppy
31.	Salicylic acid	Aspirin
32.	Borax	Suhaga tankankhar
33.	Boric acid	Boric acid
34.	Barium carbonate	Rat poison
35.	Acetic acid	Vinegar
36.	Paraffin wax	Paraffin wax
37.	Potassium permanganate	Lal dawa
38.	Ant poison	Ant poison
39.	Cuscuta	Akashbel
40.	Calcium oxychloride	Bleaching powder
41.	Benzene	Benzene
42.	Baygon	Baygon
43.	Bumoel	Bumoel
44.	Barium nitrate	Barium nitrate
45.	*Cannabis sativa*	Bhang
46.	*Abrus precatorius*	Rati or gunja
47.	Alum	Phitkari
48.	Quinine	Quinine
49.	Phenol	Phenol
50.	Nitrobenzene	Nitrobenzene
51.	Potassium dichromate	Potassium dichromate
52.	Plaster of Paris	POP
53.	Pearl ash	Pearl ash

Continued

Continued

S. No.	Scientific name	Common name
54.	Powdered glass	Powdered glass
55.	Diamond	Heera
56.	*Daucus carota*	Gajar ka beej
57.	*Hyoscyamus niger*	Ajwain khurasani
58.	Trichloromethane	Chloroform
59.	Carica papaya seed	Papaya ka beej
60.	Barbitone	Barbitone
61.	Hydrocyanic acid	Karwa badam
62.	Naphthalene balls	Phenyl ki goli
63.	Methaqualone and diphasyoramy	Mandrax-Drimoolis
64.	Amphetamine	Jagne ki goli
65.	*Myristica fragrans*	Jaiphal-nutmeg
66.	Acetylsalicylic acid	Aspirin
67.	Chloral hydrate	Chloral hydrate
68.	Mercuric chloride	Ras kapoor
69.	*Datura fastuosa* seed	Datura ka beej
70.	*Plumbago rosea*	Lal chitra
71.	*Ipomoea purga*	Jalap
72.	Ethyl alcohol	Sharab, daru, and wine
73.	*Papaver somniferum*	Afim (opium)
74.	Catfish	Catfish
75.	Aloes/Eilo	Elwa
76.	*Centipede*	Kankhajura
77.	*Calotropis gigantea*	Madar/Akdo
78.	Copper sulfate	Nila tutia
79.	Sodium hydroxide	Caustic soda
80.	Castor	Arandi seeds
81.	Formalin	Formol
82.	Eucalyptol	Eucalyptus oil
83.	*Datura fastuosa*	Datura
84.	Methyl alcohol	Methanol
85.	Hydrochloric acid	Hydrochloric acid
86.	Nitric acid	Nitric acid
87.	Potassium sulfate	Potassium sulfate
88.	Ferrous sulfate	Ferrous sulfate
89.	Ergotoxine and ergotamine	Ergotamine
90.	Areca	Betel nuts

Continued

MODERN TOXICOLOGY LABORATORY

Continued

S. No.	Scientific name	Common name
91.	Sapindus trifoliatus	Ritha
92.	Scorpion	Bichoo
93.	Red lead	Sindoor
94.	Hydrogen sulfide	Sulfur gandhak
95.	Strychnos nux-vomica seeds	Kuchila
96.	Potassium nitrate	Kalmi shora
97.	Semecarpus anacardium	Marking nut (Bhilawa)
98.	Lead carbonate	White lead and spheda
99.	Malathion	Malathion
100.	Lead acetate	Lead acetate
101.	Lead metal	Lead metal
102.	Magnesium carbonate	Magnesium carbonate

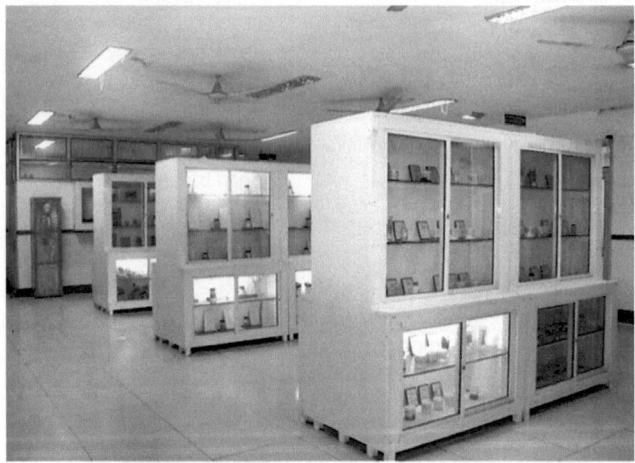

Fig. 1.1: Pictorial view of the museum.

Area of Sample Analysis

Area of sample analysis can be divided into several sections, such as extraction and isolation unit, screening test unit, sophisticated instrumental unit, washing room, etc.

Extraction and Isolation Unit (525 sq ft)

This room is used for extraction and isolation procedure of samples. The extraction and isolation of poison from postmortem samples and other body fluids are a challenging task and the initial step of isolation and purification of compounds are vital for proper analysis and reliable results. The room

should have proper ventilation with at least two exhaust fans and fume hood each. The following instruments are essential in this unit:
1. Glasswares
2. Tissue homogenizer
3. Steam distillation unit
4. Ice bath
5. Ice making machine
6. Muffle furnace
7. Oven
8. Water distillation unit
9. Hot plate
10. Microwave digester
11. Vortex mixer
12. Desiccators
13. Centrifuge machine
14. Water bath
15. Fume hood
16. Washbasin with continuous water supply
17. Room should be nonair conditioned
18. Electronic balance
19. Top-loading balance
20. Incubator

Screening Test Unit (300 sq ft)

Screening test is required to individualize a specific group of compounds. It can be done by various spot tests, microcrystal test, thin-layer chromatography (TLC), etc. The essential requirements for screening tests are listed as follows:
1. Chemicals
2. Refrigerators
3. Standard reference sample
4. pH meter
5. Vortex mixer
6. Gutzeit apparatus
7. Breath alcohol analyzer
8. Thin-layer chromatography preparation system
9. Ultraviolet cabinet
10. Immunoassay kits and reagents
11. Sink with continuous water supply
12. Kits for rapid screening of drugs
13. Conductivity meter
14. Melting point apparatus

Sophisticated Analytical Instrumental Unit (950 sq ft)

This unit should contain all sophisticated analytical instruments required for qualitative and quantitative estimation of toxic substances in the case samples and research work. The instruments used in forensic toxicology

laboratory should be highly sensitive because the quantity of material involved is extremely small, often in micro- and nanogram level. For a sample material to be identified positively, the techniques should be highly specific and rapid. We have listed the instruments, which are required for proper analysis of samples of routine work, research, and development activities and which require separate room for each instrument:
1. Ultraviolet and visible spectroscopy
2. Fourier-transform infrared spectroscopy (FTIR). It must be placed in separate cabin, which must be moisture free and fitted with dehumidifier
3. High-performance thin-layer chromatography (HPTLC)
4. Gas-liquid chromatography (GLC)
5. High-performance liquid chromatography (HPLC)
6. Gas chromatography-mass spectroscopy (GC-MS)
7. Liquid chromatography-mass spectroscopy (LC-MS)
8. Atomic absorption spectrometry (AAS)
9. Inductively coupled plasma (ICP)
10. Gas chromatography-headspace (GC-HS)
11. Inductively coupled plasma-mass spectrometry (ICP-MS)
12. Accelerated solvent extractor
13. Total organic halogen (TOX) analyzer
14. Voltammetric trace metal analyzer
15. Microwave digester
16. Ion chromatography

Instrumental unit should be fully air conditioned and dust free. All the gas cylinders must be placed in separate cabins outside the instrument rooms. Each instrument should be arranged in separate cabin, if possible.

Washing Room (150 sq ft)

There should be a separate room to clean and wash the used laboratory glasswares, etc. The washing room must have continuous source of water supply, geyser, and oven. It should have sufficient space in order to have separate area for chromic acid washing and normal washing. It should have proper ventilation with exhaust fan.

■ ENGINEERING SPECIFICATIONS

Floors

Laboratory work means long hours of standing and walking. It is desirable to have a resilient floor. This reduces breakage. However, the floor should be of a material which is acid, alkali, and salt resistant and can be easily cleaned and disinfected. In washing and sterilizing rooms, moisture-resistant floors are preferable.

Walls

The walls of the laboratory should be of the permanent, durable construction, but the partitions should be temporary, so that they can be taken out or replaced easily, if need arises or activities expand. Finish of the walls must be hard, impermeable, chemically resistant, and washable. Tiles, as wall finish, are desirable only in washing and sterilization rooms.

Ceiling
The ceilings should be made up of materials that are easily washable and disinfected, so as to reduce airborne contamination. The height of ceilings should be 2.5–2.8 m, so as to allow for wall-mounted racks and other equipment.

Doors
Width of the doors should not be <1 m wide to allow easy access of equipment. All the doors should open toward the corridor.

Lightning
As far as possible, sitting of laboratory should be such to allow natural light by providing square windows. Windows should be as tall as possible and should be at least 90 cm above the floor, so that benches can be put below them. Illumination of the laboratory needs to be carefully planned. Artificial light may be of fluorescent type. On the working benches, the intensity of light may be 250–500 lux.

Work Benches
Benching should be so designed that work with microscope can be done on benches running at right angle to the windows and walls. The top of the benches used for seating workers should be 80 cm above floor level and those of where workers stand should be 90 cm.

Sanitary Fittings
Basins for washing hands are essential in all laboratories and should have elbow-type taps. Waste pipes should be acid resistant. It is advisable to use polyvinyl chloride (PVC) piping between sink outlet and connection to the main drainage. Hot water connections are required only at the basins for washing hands and at washup sinks. Filtered soft water supply for biochemical investigations is a prerequisite. Sinks may be of porcelain.

Refrigeration
Refrigeration is to be provided in the laboratory. A minimum of two 165 L capacity is necessary. Refrigeration for storing standards and samples with −40°C must be available.

Communication
Intercom facilities should be provided within the laboratory sections and outside stations. Moreover, a dedicated telephone line is required for information of the callers.

Ventilation

A mechanical ventilator system is required in the laboratory areas. In the laboratory where fumes are expected, 10–15 air changes per hour are recommended. In other areas, 4–6 air changes per hour are sufficient.

Air Conditioning

A system that does not recirculate air is recommended, as laboratory procedures may involve working with an infectious agent.

Noise Control

Due consideration should be given to muffling of the sound produced by running of the equipment. Noise level in the laboratory should not exceed 40–50 dB.

Coloring

The coloring of the laboratory areas should preferably be lily white or apple, so as to give adequate light as laboratories involve direct observation of many procedures involved.

Fire Protection, Detection, and Fighting System

As laboratories are very vulnerable to fire hazards, fire fighting system should be installed in all the laboratory areas.
- Fire hydrants and fire extinguishers should be provided
- Fire exit routes are to be clearly identified and earmarked with red paint and well illuminated

Water Supply

Besides normal supply, separate reserve emergency overhead tank should be provided for toxicology laboratory services. Filtered soft water supply for biochemical investigations is a prerequisite for accurate estimations.

Electric Supply

Besides providing continuous electricity supply, provision of emergency light and stand by generators for laboratory is to be insured for its smooth functioning.

■ REQUIREMENTS

Glasswares

The glassware requirement in forensic toxicology laboratory varies widely. A wide range of glasswares are required in a forensic toxicology laboratory. These have to be purchased according to the requirement. Only those glasswares that are of certain significance related to analytical procedure are listed in **Table 1.2** and shown in **Figure 1.2**.

Table 1.2: List of glasswares.

S. No.	Name of glasswares	Quantity
1.	Burettes	
	• 10 mL cap	1
	• 25 mL cap	1
	• 50 mL cap	1
	• 100 mL cap	1
2.	Column chromatography	
	• 200 mm	1
	• 300 mm	1
3.	Graduated test tubes	
	• 15 mL	100
	• 20 mL	100
4.	Crucible	
	• 25 mL	5
	• 50 mL	5
5.	Lids for crucible	
	• 25 mL	5
	• 50 mL	5
6.	Bottle reagent amber	
	• 100 mL	1
	• 250 mL	1
	• 500 mL	1
	• 1,000 mL	1
	• 2,000 mL	1
	• 5,000 mL	1
7.	Tubes gas sampling	
	• 125 mL	2
	• 250 mL	2
	• 500 mL	2
8.	Water distillation system	1
9.	Beakers graduated	
	• 50 mL	10
	• 100 mL	10
	• 250 mL	10
	• 500 mL	10
	• 1,000 mL	10
10.	Bottle aspirator	
	• 250 mL	10
	• 500 mL	10
	• 1,000 mL	10
11.	Reagent bottle wide mouth with screw cap	
	• 100 mL	10
	• 250 mL	10
	• 500 mL	10
	• 1,000 mL	10
	• 2,000 mL	10
	• 5,000 mL	10

Continued

Continued

S. No.	Name of glasswares	Quantity
12.	Relative density bottle • 10 mL • 25 mL • 50 mL	 10 10 10
13.	Weighing bottle • 20 mL • 25 mL • 40 mL	 10 10 5
14.	Wash bottle • 250 mL • 500 mL • 1,000 mL	 5 5 5
15.	Stoppers for wash bottle • 250 mL • 500 mL • 1,000 mL	 5 5 5
16.	Wash bottle squeeze type • 500 mL	 5
17.	Condenser • 200 mm • 300 mm	 2 2
18.	Condenser interchangeable inner joint	2
19.	Cylinder graduated with penny head • 10 mL • 25 mL • 50 mL • 100 mL • 250 mL	 5 5 5 5 5
20.	Cylinder graduated single metric scale • 50 mL • 100 mL • 250 mL • 500 mL	 5 5 5 5
21.	Desiccators	5
22.	Tray drying • 1,500 mL • 1,200 mL	 10 10
23.	Dishes evaporating • 80 × 45 mm • 150 × 80 mm	 5 5
24.	Extractors interchangeable • 100 mL • 200 mL	 2 2
25.	Flask boiling • 100 mL • 250 mL	 2 2

Continued

Continued

S. No.	Name of glasswares	Quantity
26.	Flask boiling flat bottom • 150 mL • 250 mL • 500 mL	2 2 2
27.	Flask boiling round bottom • 150 mL • 250 mL • 500 mL	2 2 2
28.	Flask distilling • 125 mL • 250 mL • 500 mL	2 2 2
29.	Kjeldahl flask • 100 mL • 300 mL • 500 mL	5 5 5
30.	Flask iodine determination • 100 mL • 250 mL • 500 mL	5 5 5
31.	Volumetric flask • 25 mL • 50 mL • 100 mL • 250 mL • 500 mL	50 50 100 10 10
32.	Funnel plain • 25 mm • 50 mm • 100 mm	5 5 5
33.	Separating funnel globe shaped • 250 mL • 500 mL	10 10
34.	Separating funnel pear shaped • 250 mL • 500 mL	5 5
35.	Pipettes measuring • 0.1 mL • 1 mL • 2 mL • 5 mL • 10 mL	5 5 5 5 5
36.	Pipettes transfer volumetric • 5 mL • 10 mL • 20 mL	5 5 5

Continued

MODERN TOXICOLOGY LABORATORY

Continued

S. No.	Name of glasswares	Quantity
37.	Stopcocks straight bore • 2 mm • 4 mm • 6 mm	5 5 5
38.	Stopcocks high vacuum • 2 mm • 4 mm	2 2
39.	Stopper interchangeable ground joint • 24/29 • 29/32 • 45/40	10 10 10
40.	Centrifuge tubes graduated • 15 mL • 50 mL	20 20
41.	Test tubes with rim • 10 × 75 mm • 12 × 75 mm • 12 × 100 mm • 38 × 200 mm	5 5 5 5
42.	Watch glasses • 75 mm • 100 mm • 125 mm	5 5 5
43.	Funnel Büchner type • 35 mL • 80 mL • 200 mL	2 2 2
44.	Steam distillation unit	2
45.	Gutzeit apparatus	6

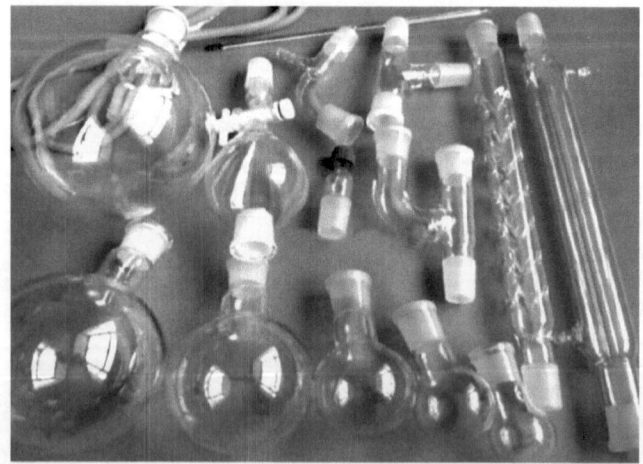

Fig. 1.2: Glasswares.

Chemicals/Reagents/Solvents

Chemicals are required to perform extraction and isolation of poisons, spot tests, solvent systems, and chromogenic reagents. Particular attention should be given for insuring a reliable supply of such chemicals. Availability of consumables for chromatographic and other techniques must be guaranteed, if equipment is to be used to full advantage. List of minimum required chemicals is given in **Table 1.3** and shown in **Figure 1.3**.

Table 1.3: List of chemicals/reagents/solvents.

S. No.	Name of chemicals	Grade	Minimum quantity
1.	Acetone	AR	500 mL
2.	Ammonium oxalate purified	AR	500 g
3.	1-amino-2-naphthol-4-sulfonic acid	AR	100 g
4.	Ammonium chloride	AR	500 g
5.	Ammonium sulfate	AR	500 g
6.	Ammonium thiosulfate	AR	500 g
7.	Ferrous ammonium sulfate (Mohr's salt)	AR	500 g
8.	Aniline	AR	500 mL
9.	Acetonitrile	AR	500 mL
10.	Ammonium heptamolybdate	AR	500 mL
11.	Aluminum oxide	AR	500 g
12.	Ammonium acetate	AR	500 mL
13.	Amyl alcohol	AR	500 mL
14.	Ammonium oxalate	AR	500 g
15.	Ammonium molybdate	AR	500 g
16.	Antimony(III) oxide	AR	100 g
17.	Aluminum foil	AR	Five packets
18.	Ammonium persulfate	AR	500 g
19.	Ammonium hydroxide	AR	500 mL
20.	Ascorbic acid	AR	500 g
21.	Arsenic trioxide	AR	100 g
22.	Arsenic pentoxide	AR	100 g
23.	Acetic acid	AR	1,000 mL
24.	Acetaldehyde	AR	1,000 mL
25.	Boric acid	AR	500 g
26.	Bromophenol blue	AR	25 g
27.	Benzene	AR	500 mL
28.	Bismuth nitrate	AR	500 g
29.	Barium sulfate purified	AR	500 g

Continued

MODERN TOXICOLOGY LABORATORY

Continued

S. No.	Name of chemicals	Grade	Minimum quantity
30.	Barium chloride dihydrate crystal pure	AR	500 g
31.	Barium chloride anhydrous	AR	500 g
32.	Bismuth(III) nitrate pentahydrate	AR	100 g
33.	Bromocresol green	AR	25 g
34.	Bromoform	AR	100 mL
35.	n-butanol for synthesis	AR	500 mL
36.	Buffer capsule for calibration of pH meter	AR	Two packets of each
37.	Barium carbonate	AR	500 g
38.	Chloroform	AR	500 mL
39.	Cyclohexane	AR	500 mL
40.	Cobalt acetate	AR	500 g
41.	Charcoal activated	AR	500 g
42.	Chromotropic acid	AR	500 mL
43.	Calcium acetate dried	AR	500 g
44.	Calcium chloride dehydrate	AR	500 g
45.	Calcium chloride	AR	500 g
46.	Cupric sulfate	AR	100 g
47.	Copper(II) sykoqate 5-hydride	AR	500 g
48.	Cadmium chloride	AR	100 g
49.	Cobaltous acetate tetrahydrate	AR	100 g
50.	Carbon tetrachloride	AR	1 L/1,000 mL
51.	Copper metal powder	AR	500 g
52.	Copper foil	AR	100 g
53.	m-cresol	AR	100 g
54.	Copper(II) sulfate pentahydrate	AR	500 g
55.	Congo red indicator paper	AR	One packet
56.	Chlorobenzene	AR	500 mL
57.	1,4-dinitrobenzene	AR	500 mL
58.	Dipotassium hydrogen orthophosphate	AR	500 mL
59.	Diphenylamine	AR	100 g
60.	Diethylamine	AR	500 mL
61.	1,4-Dioxane	AR	500 mL
62.	Dichloromethane	AR	500 mL
63.	Dextrose anhydrous	AR	100 g
64.	5,5-diethylbarbiturate	AR	100 g
65.	1,5-diphenylcarbazide	AR	100 g
66.	Diphenylcarbazone	AR	100 g

Continued

Continued

S. No.	Name of chemicals	Grade	Minimum quantity
67.	Dimethyl sulfate	AR	500 g
68.	Dimethylformamide	AR	500 mL
69.	Diethyl ether	AR	1,000 mL
70.	Dithizone	AR	100 mL
71.	4,4-diethylaminobenzaldehyde	AR	500 mL
72.	Ethanol	AR	2,000 mL
73.	Ethyl acetate	AR	500 mL
74.	Ethylenediaminetetraacetic acid (EDTA)	AR	100 g
75.	Ferrous sulfate	AR	500 g
76.	Furfural	AR	500 g
77.	Ferric sulfate	AR	500 g
78.	Basic Fuchsin for microscope	AR	100 g
79.	Florisil	AR	100 g
80.	Formaldehyde solution	AR	1,000 mL
81.	Hydroquinone	AR	100 g
82.	Hydrogen peroxide	AR	500 mL
83.	Glycerol about 98% purified	AR	500 mL
84.	Hydrochloric acid	AR	10 L
85.	n-hexane	AR	1,000 mL
86.	Fehling's solution	AR	500 mL
87.	Iron(III) chloride anhydrous purified	AR	500 g
88.	Iron(II) sulfide	AR	500 g
89.	Isoamyl alcohol	AR	500 mL
90.	Isoamyl acetate	AR	500 mL
91.	Iodine solid	AR	100 g
92.	Isopropylamine	AR	500 mL
93.	Iron(II) sulfate anhydrous	AR	500 g
94.	Iron chloride crystal purified	AR	500 g
95.	Iron(III) sulfate anhydrous	AR	500 g
96.	Iodine resublimed	AR	100 g
97.	Lead acetate	AR	100 g
98.	Lead acetate dihydrate	AR	100 g
99.	Lead acetate trihydrate	AR	100 g
100.	Mercuric bromide	AR	100 g
101.	Magnesium oxide	AR	500 g
102.	Mercuric sulfate	AR	500 g
103.	Magnesium chloride crystal	AR	500 g

Continued

MODERN TOXICOLOGY LABORATORY

Continued

S. No.	Name of chemicals	Grade	Minimum quantity
104.	Mercury(II) oxide red purified	AR	500 g
105.	Methyl blue	AR	100 mL
106.	Methanol	AR	1,000 mL
107.	Mercury(II) chloride	AR	500 mL
108.	Molybdic acid	AR	100 mL
109.	Methyl tert-butyl acid	AR	100 mL
110.	Mercurous nitrate	AR	500 g
111.	Mercuric acid nitrate	AR	500 g
112.	Mercuric iodide	AR	100 mL
113.	Mercuric oxide red	AR	100 g
114.	Methylene blue	AR	100 g
115.	Nitrobenzene	AR	500 mL
116.	Nitric acid	AR	5,000 mL
117.	Nickel sulfate	AR	100 g
118.	Neutral red chloride	AR	100 g
119.	p-nitrobenzylpyridine	AR	100 g
120.	α-naphthol	AR	100 g
121.	Ninhydrin	AR	100 g
122.	Oxalic acid	AR	500 g
123.	m-phosphoric acid	AR	100 mL
124.	o-phosphoric acid	AR	100 mL
125.	Phenobarbital sodium	AR	100 g
126.	Potassium dichromate	AR	500 g
127.	Potassium hydroxide	AR	500 g
128.	Potassium metabisulfite	AR	100 mL
129.	Propanol	AR	500 mL
130.	Phenol	AR	500 mL
131.	Potassium chromate	AR	500 g
132.	Picric acid	AR	500 g
133.	Potassium bicarbonate	AR	500 g
134.	2-propanol	AR	500 g
135.	Potassium carbonate anhydrous	AR	500 g
136.	Potassium perchloric acid	AR	500 g
137.	Potassium chloride	AR	1,000 g
138.	Potassium permanganate	AR	500 g
139.	Potassium iodide	AR	500 g
140.	Paraffin liquid	AR	One packet

Continued

Continued

S. No.	Name of chemicals	Grade	Minimum quantity
141.	Phenolphthalein indicator	AR	100 g
142.	Potassium ferrocyanide	AR	100 g
143.	Petroleum ether	AR	500 mL
144.	Pyrogallol	AR	500 mL
145.	Potassium bromide	AR	500 g
146.	Palladium chloride	AR	5 g
147.	Perchloric acid	AR	500 g
148.	Platinic chloride/platinum(III)	AR	1 g
149.	Petroleum benzene	AR	500 mL
150.	Potassium hexacyanoferrate(II) trihydrate	AR	100 g
151.	Potassium hexacyanoferrate(III)	AR	100 g
152.	Potassium sulfate	AR	500 mL
153.	Potassium nitrate	AR	500 g
154.	Pyridine	AR	500 mL
155.	pH indicator paper	AR	One packet
156.	Rhodamine B	AR	100 g
157.	Resorcinol crystal	AR	500 g
158.	Sulfuric acid	AR	5,000 mL
159.	Sodium chloride	AR	5,000 g
160.	Sucrose	AR	100 g
161.	Silica gel	AR	500 g
162.	Sodium carbonate	AR	500 g
163.	Sodium hydroxide	AR	500 mL
164.	Silicic acid	AR	500 g
165.	Sodium nitrate	AR	500 g
166.	Sodium sulfate	AR	500 g
167.	Sodium dihydrogen phosphate	AR	500 g
168.	Sodium fluoride	AR	100 g
169.	Sodium disulfide	AR	500 g
170.	Sodium potassium tartrate	AR	500 g
171.	Stannous dioxide	AR	500 g
172.	Selenium dioxide	AR	500 g
173.	Sodium dihydrogen orthophosphate	AR	500 g
174.	Sodium hydroxide pellet	AR	500 g
175.	Sodium hydrogen carbonate	AR	500 g
176.	Sodium diethyldithiocarbamate	AR	100 g
177.	Sodium dithionate	AR	100 g

Continued

MODERN TOXICOLOGY LABORATORY

Continued

S. No.	Name of chemicals	Grade	Minimum quantity
178.	Sodium oxide	AR	500 g
179.	Silver diethyldithiocarbamate	AR	500 g
180.	Sodium molybdate	AR	500 g
181.	Sodium metal	AR	500 g
182.	Sodium diorthophosphate	AR	100 g
183.	Starch	AR	1 kg
184.	Sodium borohydrate	AR	500 g
185.	Sodium thiosulfate	AR	500 g
186.	Sodium thiosulfate pentahydrate	AR	100 g
187.	Sodium acetate anhydrous pure	AR	100 g
188.	Silver nitrate	AR	10 g
189.	Sodium sulfite anhydrous pure	AR	500 g
190.	Selenous acid	AR	100 g
191.	Disodium oxalate	AR	100 g
192.	Sodium tungstate	AR	10 g
193.	Succinic acid	AR	100 g
194.	Thallium chloride	AR	100 g
195.	Toluene	AR	500 mL
196.	Tin(II) chloride	AR	100 g
197.	Tetraethylenepentamine	AR	100 g
198.	Tetrahydrofuran	AR	100 g
199.	Urea	AR	1 kg
200.	Uranyl acetate	AR	500 g
201.	Universal indicator pH paper	AR	One packet
202.	Xylene	AR	100 mL
203.	Zinc (metal) powder	AR	500 g
204.	Zinc (metal) dust	AR	500 g
205.	Zinc chloride	AR	500 g
206.	Zinc phosphide	AR	500 g
207.	Zinc acetate	AR	500 g
208.	Zinc oxide	AR	500 g
209.	Zinc sulfate	AR	500 g

Plasticware

Large number of plasticwares are also required for toxicology laboratory. It has to be purchased according to the demands. List of minimum required plasticware is given in **Table 1.4** and shown in **Figure 1.4**.

MODERN TOXICOLOGY LABORATORY

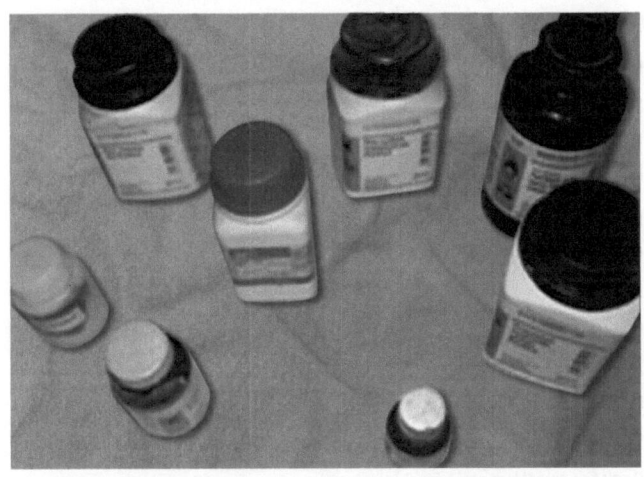

Fig. 1.3: Chemicals/reagents/solvents.

Table 1.4: List of plasticwares.

S. No.	Name of items	Quantity (in Pc/Pcs)
1.	Pipette bulb	2
2.	Drying rock	1
3.	Pasteur pipette	2
4.	Hand protector grip	2
5.	Safety goggles	2
6.	Safety eyewear box	1
7.	Wide mouth bottle with capacity of 1,000 mL	6
8.	Aspirator bottle with stopcock of capacity (20 L)	3
9.	Wash bottles of capacity 250 mL	3
10.	New type wash bottles of capacity 250 mL	3
11.	New type wash bottles of capacity 500 mL	3
12.	Conical flask of capacity 250 mL	6
13.	Measuring beaker of capacity 2,000 mL	4
14.	Beaker of capacity 1,000 mL	4
15.	Measuring cylinder of capacity 250 mL	6
16.	Funnel of capacity 100 mL	12
17.	Large funnel of capacity 200 mL	2
18.	Büchner funnel 70 mm	2
19.	Separatory funnel 250 mL	2
20.	Pipette rack horizontal	2
21.	Retort stand 22 × 15 central	2
22.	Burette clamp (single)	3

Continued

MODERN TOXICOLOGY LABORATORY

Continued

S. No.	Name of items	Quantity (in Pc/Pcs)
23.	Separatory funnel holder (single)	2
24.	Funnel holder (single)	2
25.	Pipette stand vertical (28 places)	1
26.	Pipette stand vertical (94 places)	1
27.	Handypette pipette aid (10 mL)	2
28.	Pipette bulb (up to 100 mL)	2
29.	Utility tray (320 × 260 × 100 mm)	2
30.	Drying rack (20 pegs)	1
31.	Drying rack (30 pegs)	1
32.	Microcentrifuge tubes (1.5 mL)	500
33.	Rack for microtubes (1.5 mL)	2
34.	Centrifuge tube conical bottom (50 mL)	100
35.	Centrifuge bottle (250 mL)	3
36.	Cryo babies (32.5 × 12.7)	1,000
37.	Cryo tags (38 × 19)	1,000
38.	Ice bucket (4,500 mL)	1
39.	Cryo cube box (50 places, 1.8 mL)	4
40.	Test tube stand (31 places, 16 mm)	2
41.	SPINIX™ orbital shaker	1
42.	Pasteur pipette (3 mL)	500
43.	Hand protector grip	1
44.	Scoop (250 mL)	2
45.	Scoop (1,000 mL)	2
46.	Scoop (2,000 mL)	2
47.	SPINOT™ magnetic stirrer hot plate (10 × 10 cm)	1
48.	SPINOT™ magnetic stirrer hot plate (18 × 18 cm)	1
49.	Flask stand (160 mm)	2

Equipment and Machinery

We need sophisticated analytical instruments, which are sensitive and reliable for the analysis of poisons in the biological samples. The equipment and machinery can be further divided into two categories, i.e., major equipment and minor equipment.

Major Equipment

For quantitative analysis and trace analysis, we need sophisticated analytical instruments such as GLC, AAS, ICP, HPLC, etc. Complete list of major equipment is given in **Table 1.5** and shown in **Figures 1.5A** to **N**.

MODERN TOXICOLOGY LABORATORY

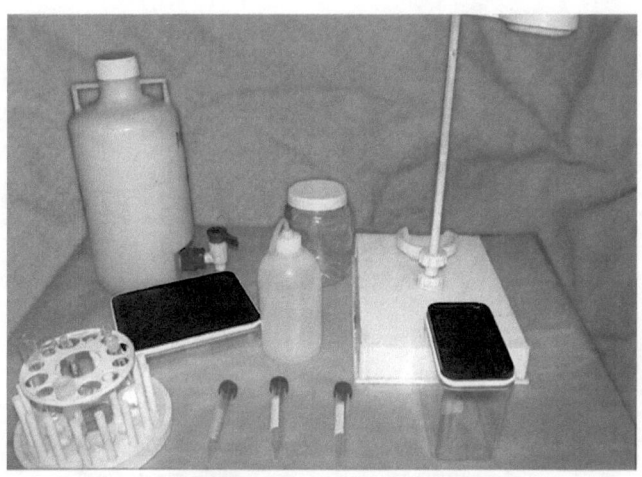

Fig. 1.4: Plasticwares.

Table 1.5: List of major equipment.

S. No.	List of equipment	Quantity
1.	Gas-liquid chromatography (GLC)	Two
2.	High-performance liquid chromatography (HPLC)	Two
3.	Inductively coupled plasma (ICP) spectrometry	One
4.	Ultraviolet (UV)-visible spectrophotometer	Two
5.	Gas chromatography-headspace (GC-HS)	One
6.	Atomic absorption spectrometry (AAS)	One
7.	Gas chromatography-mass spectroscopy (GC-MS)	One
8.	High-performance thin-layer chromatography (HPTLC)	One
9.	Fourier-transform infrared spectroscopy (FTIR)	One
10.	Voltammetric trace metal analyzer	One
	Inductively coupled plasma-mass spectrometry (ICP-MS)	
11.	Ion chromatography	One
12.	Pressurized solvent extraction/accelerated solvent extractor	One
13.	Liquid chromatography-mass spectroscopy (LC-MS)	One
14.	Microwave digester	One

Minor Equipment

For qualitative test, color/spot test is done by using some minor equipment. Complete list of minor equipment is given in **Table 1.6** and shown in **Figures 1.6A** to **J**.

Reference Material

Standards for chemicals, poisons, etc., are essential for standardization and calibration of instruments. A certified reference material (CRM), suitable

MODERN TOXICOLOGY LABORATORY

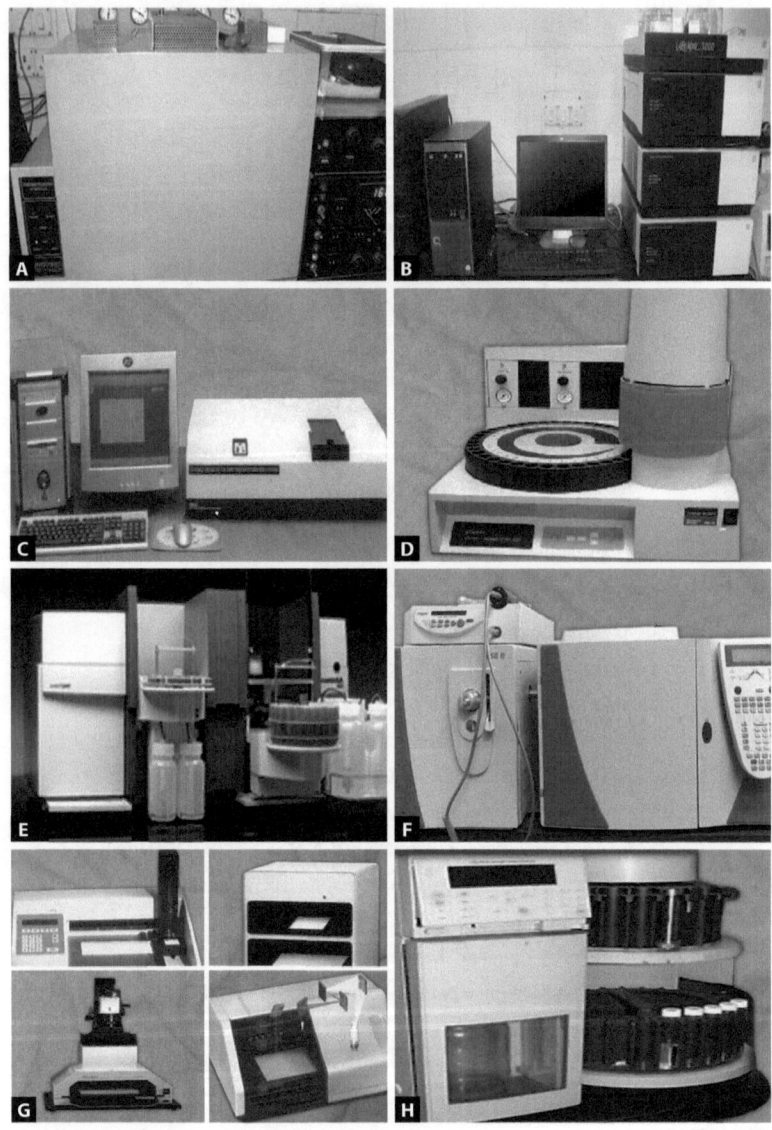

Figs. 1.5A to H: Major equipment used in laboratory. (A) Gas-liquid chromatography (Nucon); (B) High-performance liquid chromatography (Dionex Ultimate 3,000); (C) Ultraviolet (UV)-visible spectrophotometer (ECIL); (D) Gas chromatography with headspace (PerkinElmer); (E) Atomic absorption spectrometry (Analytik Jena); (F) Gas chromatography-mass spectrometry (PerkinElmer); (G) High-performance thin-layer chromatography (Desaga); and (H) Accelerated solvent extractor (Dionex).

for the preparation of a standard, to which calibration materials can be compared, must be certified by a method generally recognized by scientific community as one that validates the CRM for this purpose. Reference materials (RMs) should be stored at low temperature or protected from

MODERN TOXICOLOGY LABORATORY

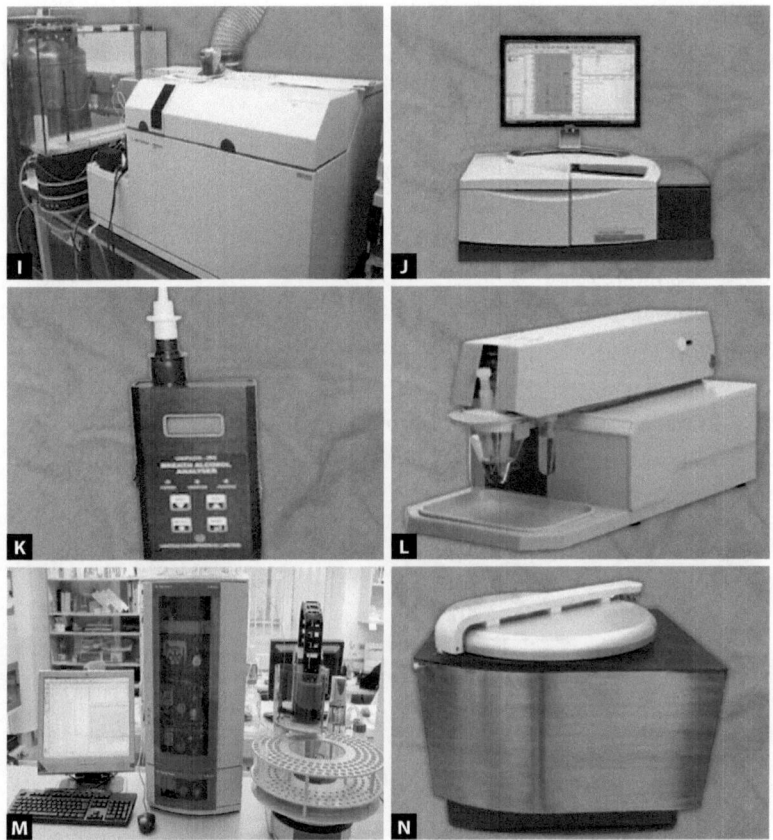

Figs. 1.5I to N: Major equipment used in laboratory. (I) Inductively coupled plasma mass spectrometry; (J) Fourier-transform infrared spectroscopy (Varian); (K) Voltammetric trace metal analyzer (Metrohm); (L) Breath analyzer (Uniphos); (M) Ion chromatography (Metrohm); and (N) Microwave digester (Aurora).

Table 1.6: List of minor equipment.

S. No.	List of equipment	Quantity
1.	Deep freezer (–20°C)	One
2.	Oven	Two
3.	pH meter	One
4.	Conductivity meter	One
5.	Double distilled glass apparatus	One
6.	Refrigerator	Two
7.	Tissue homogenizer	Two
8.	Gas purification panel for all gases	One
9.	Top loading balance	One
10.	Micropipette controller	Ten

Continued

MODERN TOXICOLOGY LABORATORY

Continued

S. No.	List of equipment	Quantity
11.	Micropipette (different range)	One
12.	Dispenser	Five
13.	Computer with printer for laboratory	Two
14.	Hot plates	Two
15.	Ultraviolet (UV)-viewing cabinet	One
16.	Analytical balance	One
17.	Water bath	Two
18.	Muffle furnace	One
19.	Fume hood	One
20.	Centrifuge machine (medico type) of capacity 6/4 tube of 10 mL each	One
21.	Microscope	Two
22.	Breath analyzer	Two

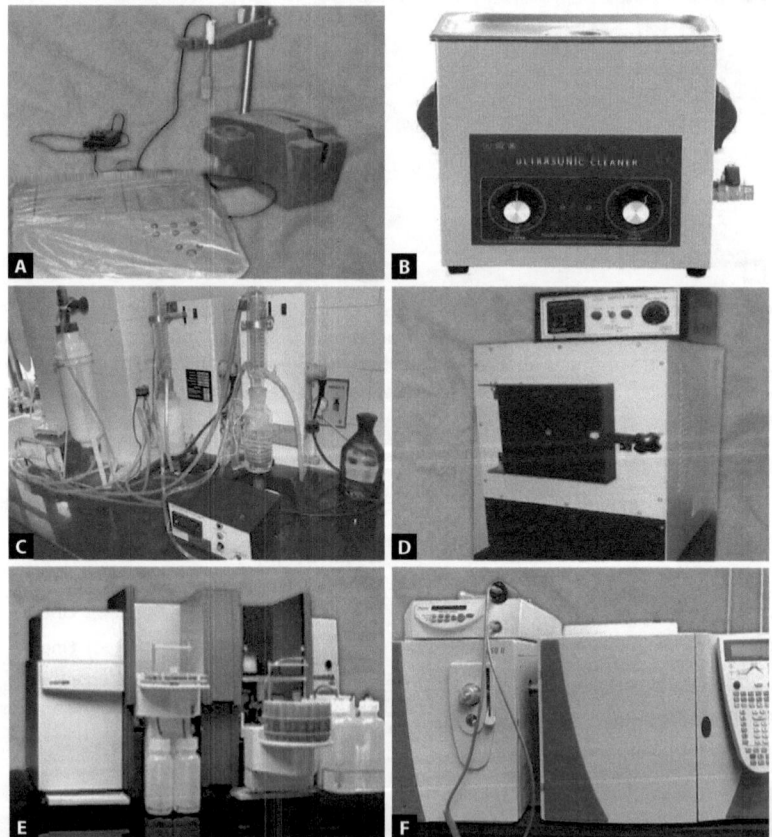

Figs. 1.6A to F: Minor equipment used in laboratory. (A) pH meter; (B) Ultrasonic bath; (C) Double distillation unit; (D) Muffle furnace; (E) Mini centrifuge; (F) Vortex mixer.

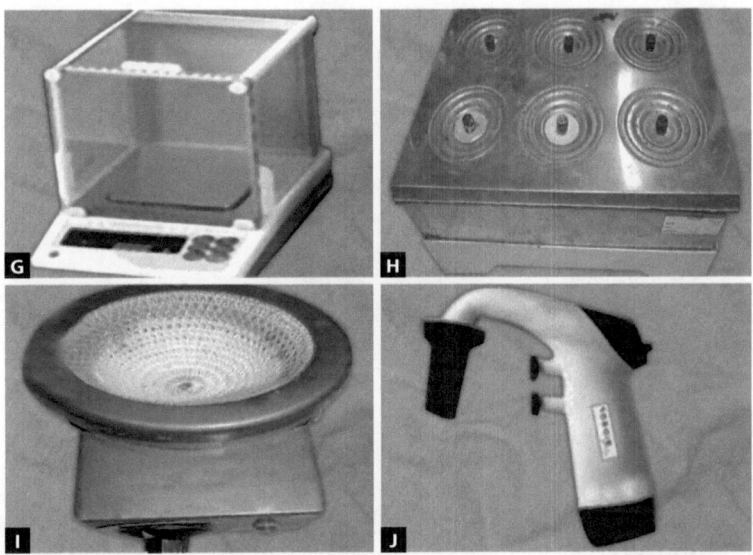

Figs. 1.6G and J: Minor equipment used in laboratory. (G) Electronic weighing balance; and (H) Water bath; (I) Heating mantle and (J) Micropipette controller (Biogene).

light and moisture. Lists of drugs standard, pesticides standard, metallic standard, AAS standard, and UV-visible spectrophotometer standard are given in **Tables 1.7** to **1.11**, respectively.

High-performance Liquid Chromatography Solvents

High-performance liquid chromatography instruments require special type of solvents called HPLC solvent. List of few HPLC solvents is given in **Table 1.12** and shown in **Figure 1.7**.

Miscellaneous Items

Several miscellaneous items are also required in the laboratory for different purposes, which are listed below in **Table 1.13** and shown in **Figure 1.8**.

Waste Disposal Procedures for Biological Material

The laboratory should have documented waste management policy. There must be a clear policy in place for the disposal of materials on completion of examination.

■ SECURITY

The entire laboratory should be secure and the document and exhibit store area should be strictly prohibited to unauthorized person. The area should be locked by biometric lock. The physical layout of the laboratory must be such that unauthorized person cannot enter without direction and unauthorized person should be escorted and may be required to sign a log

MODERN TOXICOLOGY LABORATORY

Table 1.7: List of drugs standard.

S. No.	Name	% purity	Quantity
1.	Morphine	90–100	1 g
2.	Diazepam	90–100	1 g
3.	Nitrazepam	90–100	1 g
4.	Allobarbital	90–100	1 g
5.	Barbital	90–100	1 g
6.	Phenobarbital	90–100	1 g
7.	Alprazolam	90–100	1 g
8.	Bromazepam	90–100	1 g
9.	Atropine sulfate	90–100	1 g
10.	Brucine	90–100	1 g
11.	Codeine	90–100	1 g
12.	Thebaine	90–100	1 g
13.	Papaverine	90–100	1 g
14.	Narcotine	90–100	1 g
15.	Amphetamine	90–100	1 g
16.	Ephedrine	90–100	1 g
17.	Nicotine	90–100	1 g
18.	Amphetamine HCl	90–100	1 q
19.	Heroin HCl	90–100	1 g
20.	Chlordiazepoxide	90–100	1 g
21.	Cocaine	90–100	1 g

(HCl: hydrochloride)

Table 1.8: List of pesticides standard.

S. No.	Name	Quantity
1.	BHC	1 g
2.	Zolone	1 g
3.	Chlordane	1 g
4.	Malathion	1 g
5.	Heptachlor	1 g
6.	Butachlor	1 g
7.	Cygon	1 g
8.	Naled (Dibrom)	1 g
9.	Dieldrin	1 g
10.	Strobane	1 g
11.	Toxaphene	1 g
12.	Chloropicrin	1 g

Continued

Continued

S. No.	Name	Quantity
13.	DDE	1 g
14.	Guthion	1 g
15.	Diazinon	1 g
16.	Phosdrin	1 g
17.	DDT	1 g
18.	2,4-D	1 g
19.	Fenvalerate	1 g
20.	Cypermethrin	1 g
21.	Carbofuran	1 g
22.	Chlorpyriphos	1 g
23.	Ethion	1 g
24.	Dimethoate	1 g
25.	Isoproturan	1 g
26.	Endosulfan	1 g
27.	Quinalphos	1 g
28.	Aluminum phosphide	1 g
29.	Zinc purified	1 g

(BHC: benzene hexachloride; DDT: dichlorodiphenyltrichloroethane)

Table 1. 9: List of metallic standard.

S. No.	Name	Quantity
1.	Arsenic trioxide	100 g
2.	Arsenic pentoxide	100 g
3.	Mercuric chloride	100 g
4.	Mercuric sulfate	100 g
5.	Zinc metal	100 g
6.	Antimony nitrate	100 g
7.	Bismuth nitrate	100 g
8.	Cadmium nitrate	100 g
9.	Chromium nitrate	100 g
10.	Cobalt nitrate	100 g
11.	Copper nitrate	100 g
12.	Iron nitrate	100 g
13.	Lead nitrate	100 g
14.	Molybdenum nitrate	100 g
15.	Nickel nitrate	100 g

Continued

MODERN TOXICOLOGY LABORATORY

Continued

S. No.	Name	Quantity
16.	Platinum nitrate	100 g
17.	Rhodium nitrate	100 g
18.	Selenium nitrate	100 g
19.	Thallium nitrate	100 g
20.	Tungsten nitrate	100 g
21.	Uranium nitrate	100 g

Table 1.10: List of AAS/ICP standard.

S. No.	List of standards	Concentration	Quantity
1.	Aluminum standard solution	1,000 ppm	100 mL
2.	Antimony standard solution	1,000 ppm	100 mL
3.	Arsenic standard solution	1,000 ppm	100 mL
4.	Barium standard solution	1,000 ppm	100 mL
5.	Beryllium standard solution	1,000 ppm	100 mL
6.	Bismuth standard solution	1,000 ppm	100 mL
7.	Boron standard solution	1000 ppm	100 mL
8.	Cadmium standard solution	1,000 ppm	100 mL
9.	Calcium standard solution	1,000 ppm	100 mL
10.	Cesium standard solution	1,000 ppm	100 mL
11.	Chromium standard solution	1,000 ppm	100 mL
12.	Cobalt standard solution	1,000 ppm	100 mL
13.	Copper standard solution	1,000 ppm	100 mL
14.	Germanium standard solution	1,000 ppm	100 mL
15.	Gold standard solution	1,000 ppm	100 mL
16.	Indium standard solution	1,000 ppm	100 mL
17.	Iron standard solution	1,000 ppm	100 mL
18.	Lead standard solution	1,000 ppm	100 mL
19.	Lithium standard solution	1,000 ppm	100 mL
20.	Magnesium standard solution	1,000 ppm	100 mL
21.	Manganese standard solution	1,000 ppm	100 mL
22.	Mercury standard solution	1,000 ppm	100 mL
23.	Molybdenum standard solution	1,000 ppm	100 mL
24.	Nickel standard solution	1,000 ppm	100 mL
25.	Palladium standard solution	1,000 ppm	100 mL
26.	Platinum standard solution	1,000 ppm	100 mL
27.	Potassium standard solution	1,000 ppm	100 mL

Continued

Continued

S. No.	List of standards	Concentration	Quantity
28.	Scandium standard solution	1,000 ppm	100 mL
29.	Selenium standard solution	1,000 ppm	100 mL
30.	Silicon standard solution	1,000 ppm	100 mL
31.	Silver standard solution	1,000 ppm	100 mL
32.	Sodium standard solution	1,000 ppm	100 mL
33.	Strontium standard solution	1,000 ppm	100 mL
34.	Tellurium standard solution	1,000 ppm	100 mL
35.	Thallium standard solution	1,000 ppm	100 mL
36.	Tin standard solution	1,000 ppm	100 mL
37.	Titanium standard solution	1,000 ppm	100 mL
38.	Tungsten standard solution	1,000 ppm	100 mL
39.	Vanadium standard solution	1,000 ppm	100 mL
40.	Zinc standard solution	1,000 ppm	100 mL
41.	Zirconium standard solution	1,000 ppm	100 mL

(AAS: atomic absorption spectrometry; ICP: inductively coupled plasma)

Table 1.11: List of ultraviolet (UV)-visible spectrophotometer standard.

S. No.	List of chemicals	Quantity
1.	UV-visible standard 1 potassium dichromate	1 unit
2.	UV-visible standard 1a potassium dichromate	1 unit
3.	UV-visible standard 2 sodium nitrite solution	1 unit
4.	UV-visible standard 3 sodium iodide solution	1 unit
5.	UV-visible standard 4 potassium chloride	1 unit
6.	UV-visible standard 5 toluene	1 unit
7.	UV-visible standard 6 holmium oxide	1 unit

Table 1.12: List of high-performance liquid chromatography (HPLC) solvents.

S. No.	List of HPLC solvents	Quantity
1.	Acetone	5 × 1 L
2.	Acetonitrile	5 × 1 L
3.	Carbon tetrachloride	5 × 1 L
4.	Chloroform	5 × 1 L
5.	Cyclohexane	5 × 1 L
6.	Dichloromethane	5 × 1 L
7.	Ethyl acetate	5 × 1 L

Continued

MODERN TOXICOLOGY LABORATORY

Continued

S. No.	List of HPLC solvents	Quantity
8.	n-hexane	5 × 1 L
9.	Hexane	5 × 1 L
10.	Isooctane	5 × 1 L
11.	Methanol	5 × 1 L
12.	2-propanol	5 × 1 L
13.	Tetrahydrofuran	5 × 1 L
14.	Toluene	5 × 1 L
15.	Distilled water	5 × 1 L

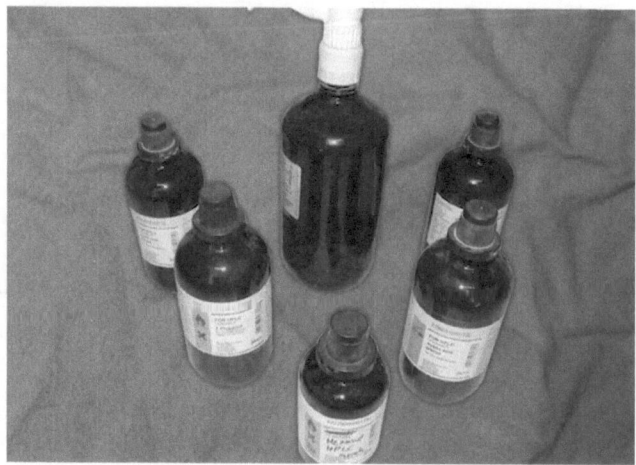

Fig. 1.7: High-performance liquid chromatography (HPLC) solvents.

Table 1.13: List of miscellaneous items.

S. No.	Name of items	Quantity
1.	Filter paper Whatman No-40	5 packets
2.	Filter paper Whatman No-41	5 packets
3.	Filter paper Whatman No-42	5 packets
4.	Ordinary filter paper sheet	1 packet
5.	Glass marker	1 packet
6.	Stickers of different sizes	1 packet
7.	Burners	5 numbers
8.	Tongs	3 numbers
9.	Tripod stand	6 numbers
10.	Scissor	2 nos.
11.	Gloves	2 packets
12.	Masks	2 packets

MODERN TOXICOLOGY LABORATORY

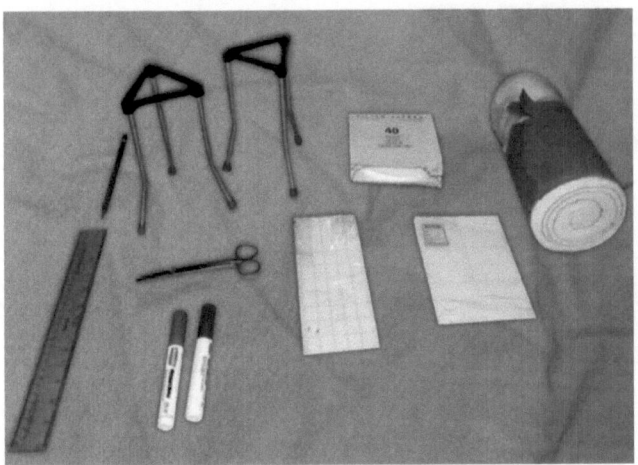

Fig. 1.8: Miscellaneous items.

book upon entry and exit from the laboratory, recording the full name and address, name of the person to whom the visitor will meet, and time, date, and purpose of the visit.

■ CONCLUSION

In the field of crime investigation, forensic toxicology has a significant role. The deaths due to poisoning are on increase every year with economic advancement and development in science and technology. The poisoning deaths may be due to acute or chronic poisoning. It involves wide range of poisons such as agricultural poisons, pharmaceutical drugs, drugs of abuse, household poisons, food poisons, mass disaster due to leakage of chemicals and gases from industries, occupational and environmental hazards, etc. In India, there are about 35 forensic science laboratories in various states. These laboratories are overburdened with analytical samples due to increasing crimes related to poisoning and the court of law expects authentic scientific reports as evidence. The government needs to setup well-planned and equipped forensic toxicology laboratory to deal with poisoning cases. Layout of forensic toxicology laboratory is given in **Figure 1.9**. We have tried to describe in detail the manpower requirement, area requirement, and equipment, glassware, and chemical requirements, along with a clear layout diagram of the laboratory. This chapter provides a detailed guideline for setting up a well-planned modern forensic toxicology laboratory.

MODERN TOXICOLOGY LABORATORY

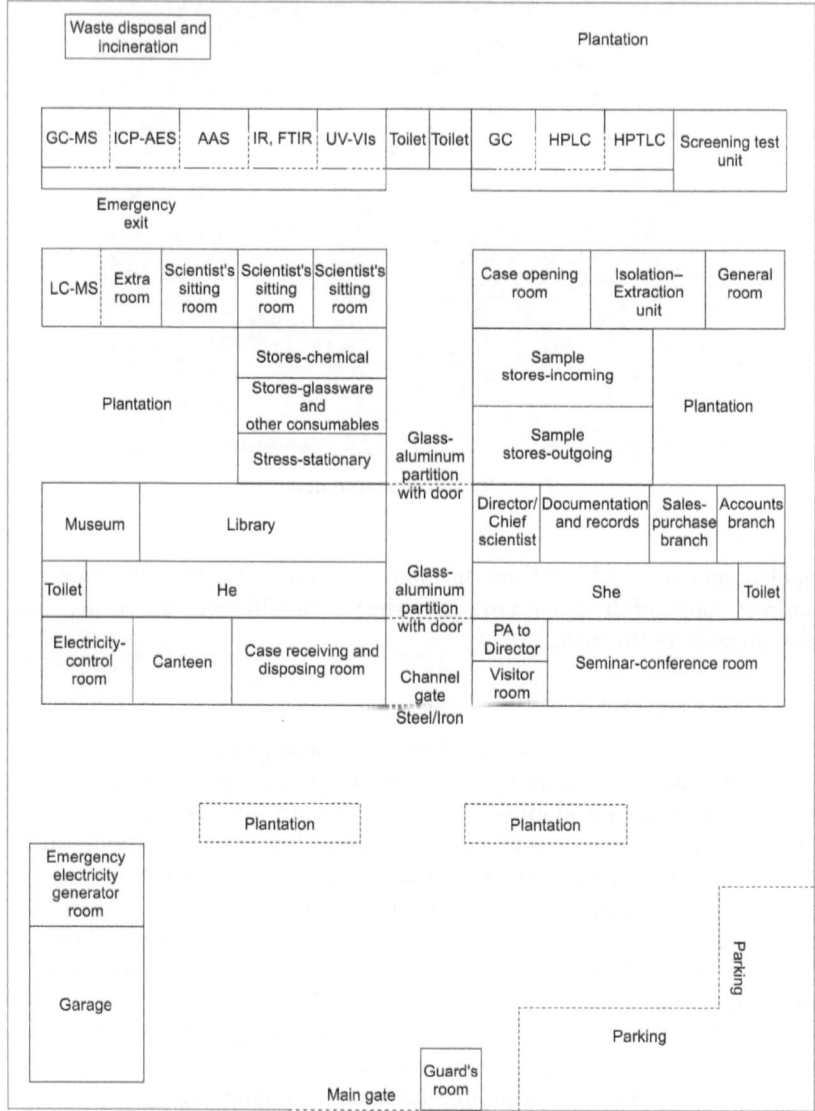

(AES: atomic emission spectroscopy; FTIR: Fourier-transform infrared spectroscopy; GC-MS: gas chromatography-mass spectroscopy; HPLC: high-performance liquid chromatography; HPTLC: high-performance thin-layer chromatography; ICP: inductively coupled plasma; LC-MS: liquid chromatography-mass spectrometry; UV: ultraviolet)

Fig. 1.9: Layout of forensic toxicology laboratory.

■ FURTHER READINGS

1. Bapuly AK. Forensic Science: Its Application in Crime Investigation, 1st edition. New Delhi: Paras Medical Publishers; 2006.
2. Borosil Scientific and Laboratory Glassware; 2007.
3. Borosil Scientific and Laboratory Ware Catalogue; 2006.
4. Burnett D. A Practical Guide to Accreditation in Laboratory Medicine. London: ACB Venture Publications; 2002.
5. Clarke EGC, Moffat AC. Clarke's Isolation and Identification of Drugs, 2nd edition. London: Pharmaceutical Press; 1986.
6. Curry AS. Analytical Methods in Human Toxicology, 1st edition. London: Macmillan Press Ltd; 1985.
7. Gray DJP. Davidson's Principles and Practice of Medicine, 12th edition. London: Churchill Livingstone; 1997.
8. Kirk PL. DFS Manual of Toxicology, 1st edition. New Delhi: Selective and Scientific Publishers; 2005.
9. World Health Organization (WHO). (1997). Guidelines for poison control. [online] Available from https://www.who.int/publications/i/item/guidelines-for-poison-control. [Last accessed March, 2021].
10. Jaiswal AK, Millo T, Murty OP. Extraction, isolation and clean-up methods for pesticides/insecticides and alkaloids from biological material. Part-I. Int J Med Toxicol Legal Med. 2006;9:28-32.
11. Armour MA. Hazardous Laboratory Chemicals Disposal Guide, 3rd edition. Boca Raton: CRC Press; 2003.
12. Merck Chemical and Reagent Catalogue; 2002.
13. Merck Chemical and Reagent Catalogue; 2006–2007.
14. National Academy of Medical Sciences. (1998). CME Monograph: Proceedings of National Workshop on Practical and Emergency Medical Toxicology. [online] Available from https://www.researchgate.net/publication/282075188_CME_Monograph_-_proceedings_of_National_Workshop_on_Practical_and_Emergency_Medical_Toxicology_AIIMS_24-26th_February_1998_-_sponsored_by_national_Academy_of_Medical_Sciences_new_Delhi. [Last accessed March, 2021].
15. Sharma BR. Forensic Science in Criminal Investigation and Trials, 4th edition. New Delhi: Universal Law Publishing Co Ltd; 2004.

MODERN TOXICOLOGY LABORATORY

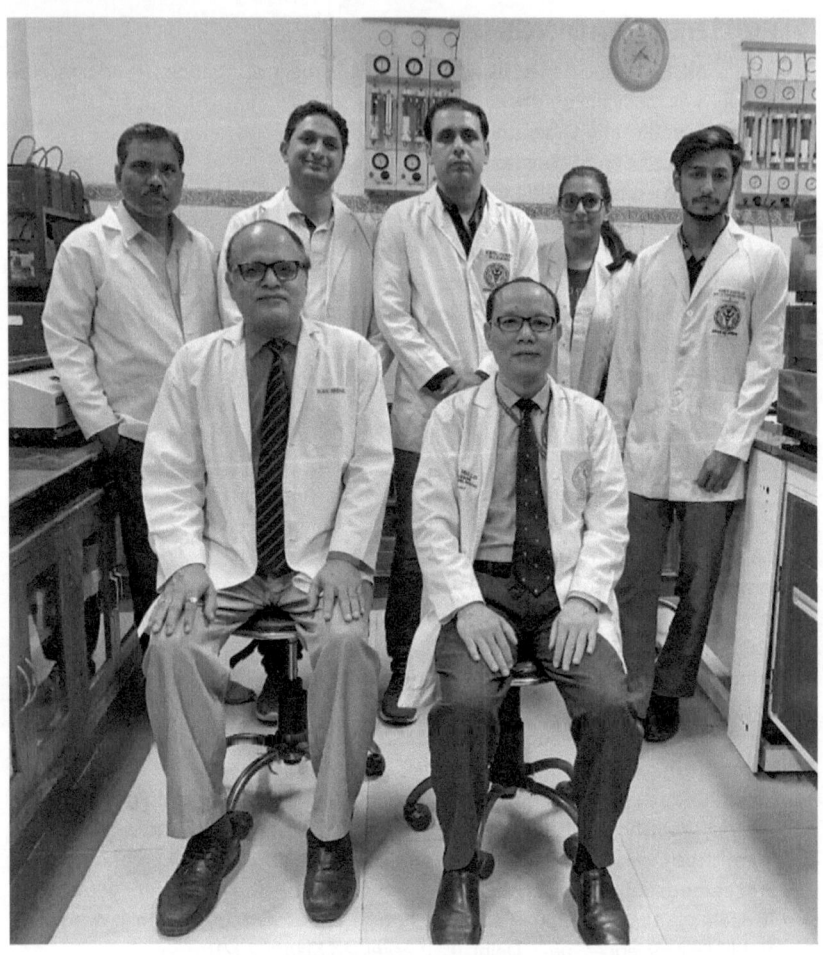

Team of Forensic Toxicology Laboratory, AIIMS Delhi
(It is all about team work).

Chapter 2

Procedure for Collection, Preservation, and Forwarding of Biological Sample for Toxicological Analysis

■ INTRODUCTION

Collection of proper biological samples in medicolegal autopsy cases is an essential step in the process of toxicology casework. Improper collection of samples can greatly alter or negate the toxicological analysis report. After death, there is a rapid change in the cellular level biochemistry due to autolysis. The drugs and other poisons may get released from the binding sites in tissues and major organs. The unabsorbed drug may diffuse from stomach. Therefore, care should be taken in selection of blood and tissue sampling sites. Many a times, the autopsy is conducted before all the circumstantial evidences are collected and investigated. Hence, it is vital to preserve all the necessary samples at the time of autopsy. Ideally, the samples for toxicological or biochemical analysis should be collected before the postmortem. However, it may not be possible for all the samples and there may be difficulty in sampling without opening the body.

■ BIOLOGICAL FLUIDS

Blood

In all postmortem cases, a blood specimen should be always obtained when blood is available. It is used as a reference sample for identification in unidentified cases by deoxyribonucleic acid (DNA) profiling and also for complete toxicological analysis. Peripheral blood concentration has been shown to be more reliable for toxicological analysis than the conventional heart blood. Therefore, in all suspected poisoning deaths or in all cases of unknown causes of deaths, a femoral or subclavian blood specimen should be collected. It is relatively isolated from internal organs of the chest and abdomen and hence less influenced by the postmortem redistribution phenomenon. It is the most useful biological fluid for quantitative analysis. But its analysis gives total fraction of the xenobiotics (free and bound xenobiotics to proteins). Quantitation of free fraction would be useful, but is not generally possible.

The most satisfactory way of obtaining a venous blood sample is venipuncture of the femoral vein by direct puncture in the groin before the autopsy begins. Before postmortem, it can be collected by inserting the needle at about two fingerbreadth below the inguinal ligament at middle point marked between the anterior superior iliac spine and the pubic symphysis. But it is best obtained by puncturing the femoral vein using a 30 mL syringe with wide bore needle, after exposing the vein by dissection and clamping or ligating it proximal to the collection site, near the inguinal ligament. The leg may be slightly elevated to obtain more blood and should not be massaged or shaken to increase flow. Generally, it is difficult to collect >5–10 mL blood from ligated femoral vein. For analysis of volatile xenobiotics, a gas syringe should be used.

Usually, 10 mL of blood is sufficient and it has to be preserved in sodium fluoride (10 mg/mL or 1–5%) and anticoagulant potassium oxalate (30 mg/10 mL of blood concentration). Sodium fluoride protects blood from postmortem changes such as bacterial production of ethanol or other alcohols. It should be collected in a fresh wide-mouthed plastic/glass container of 30 mL with screw cap. A portion of blood without preservative should be saved, namely in cases of suspicion of fluoride poisoning. Blood is the most useful sample for complete toxicological analysis.

The other sources of blood sample from postmortem cases are cardiac blood, blood clots from subdural, subarachnoid, or epidural spaces, and blood clots from thoracic or abdominal cavities. These samples are useful for qualitative or screening analysis. The cardiac blood should be preferably collected from right chamber (30 mL in screw-caped plastic container). It is useful for screening analysis, since large volume is available. It is important to mention the sampling site in the label for better interpretation.

The glass container should be made of amber glass to inhibit photodegeneration. It also helps to protect other labile drugs such as cocaine, nitrazepam, and clonazepam from degradation. The rubber or cork caps should be avoided.

■ URINE

Urine specimen is of great value even in small amount, especially in screening of an unknown drug or poison, particularly substance abuse, since the concentrations are generally higher than in blood and a number of metabolites may also be present. It has the advantage of a longer detection period. Drugs can be detected in urine for a longer period than in blood. It contains >99% water and contains relatively less endogenous substances that can interfere with chromatography or immunoassay.

However, there are also few disadvantages. Many a times, urine is not available in postmortem case as it might have been evacuated during the dying process. Many drugs are metabolized so extensively that the drug is not detected in urine. However, if the metabolites are searched for, urine can be a useful fluid. The urinary concentrations are difficult to interpret and correlation between the concentration of drug in urine and blood is very poor. Urine specimens can be of valuable in the quantitative analysis of alcohol, where there is uncertainty over the validity of a blood specimen.

Before conducting the autopsy, urine can be collected by urethral catheterization or suprapubic puncture with 5–10 mL syringe and needle (22 gauge 3 inches). With the body in supine position, palpate the bladder and identify the insertion site at midline and 2 cm above the pubic bone. At the insertion site, introduce the 22 gauge 3 inch needle attached to the 10 mL syringe. Direct the needle below (the bladder is a peritoneal organ in adults) at a 10–20° angle from the perpendicular at midline. Gently aspirate while introducing the needle. If no urine is aspirated, withdraw the needle to the subcutaneous space and readvance in a slightly different direction, 10° upward or downward and aspirate again. But it can be best obtained during autopsy after exposing the abdomen by puncturing the fundus of the bladder with syringe and needle. If bladder contains only little amount of urine, it may be necessary to open bladder to collect any residual quantity. If urine is not available, the bladder could be washed with a saline solution in order to obtain any sample. For ethanol analysis, it has to be preserved in sodium fluoride (10 mg/mL) in a 30-mL glass/plastic container with a screw cap. A sample of 20 mL without preservative is sufficient for toxicological analysis. It is difficult to correlate the blood and the urine level. Generally, urine has higher concentrations compared to other samples and acquires great value, if obtained up to 96 hours after intoxication. There exists no correlation with toxic effects at the time of collection. Bladder is primarily a reservoir and unlike blood, it is not in equilibrium with tissues.

Vitreous Humor

The vitreous humor specimen is particularly useful for ethanol estimation. It is a useful fluid to detect hyperglycemia and acetone in diabetes and insulin-related deaths. It is especially very useful for toxicological screening where the body has decomposed. The eye is an organ distant from the major thoracic and abdominal organs and it is a closed space. It is less influenced by contamination, putrefaction, and postmortem redistribution. Therefore, fluid in the eye resists putrefaction longer than other body fluids as it is sterile and remains well protected in eye. It is useful for certain biochemical tests such as urea, creatinine, glucose, lactose, and alcohol.

Vitreous humor must be collected from both eyes in separate vials of 10 mL. It is preserved with sodium fluoride (10 mg/mL). A puncture should be made through the sclera at the outer canthus with a fine 19 gauge needle in 5 mL syringe. It should be placed laterally as far as possible, pulling the lid out, so that when released, it returns to cover the puncture mark for cosmetic reasons. The sclera should be punctured at a latitude of about 60° taking the pupil as the north pole. The needle should be directed toward the center of the eyeball. The fluid comes out slowly because of its viscosity.

Gentle aspiration will usually yield 2–3 mL of vitreous humor. Once the sample has been collected, the syringe should be detached from the needle, leaving the needle in place. A volume of water or physiological saline, equal to the amount of vitreous humor removed, should be slowly injected into the eye to achieve cosmetic restoration. Vitreous humor is easy to collect and remains clear and sterile for up to 3 days or so after death. It becomes cloudy and brown with decomposition.

There exists good correlation with the blood-free xenobiotics concentration. Xenobiotics with high binding percentages to serum proteins will present in much lower concentrations than blood (e.g., tricyclic antidepressants). The concentrations lag behind blood levels by approximately 1–2 hours. It is useful for interpretation of blood alcohol results or when blood is not available. If positive, it is useful to prove antemortem ethanol ingestion and, therefore, discarding postmortem ethanol production by fermentation. If it is negative for ethanol, but blood samples are positive, ethanol production in blood should be suspected due to postmortem putrefaction. It may not become contaminated by embalming process and can be of use to screen even in embalmed bodies. In these cases, it is important that a sample of embalming fluid should be submitted for analysis as control. It has a high water and low lipid content in comparison to blood. Therefore, concentration of highly lipophilic xenobiotics in vitreous humor will be lower (e.g., benzodiazepines). Presence of high postmortem glucose concentrations suggests perimortem hyperglycemia and if combined with elevated acetone level, it suggests diabetic ketoacidosis. Due to the rapid postmortem decrease of normal glucose concentrations, low or even zero levels may erroneously suggest hypoglycemia. Vitreous humor lacks esterase that hydrolyzes and, therefore, reduces the blood concentrations of certain xenobiotics (e.g., cocaine, heroin, 6-monoacetylmorphine).

The main disadvantage of vitreous humor is its relatively small volume (about 3 mL in each eye). Also, there is relatively little information in the literature on the concentrations expected after therapeutic doses of most drugs. While the vitreous:blood ratio for some drugs is close to unity, it is considerably less than unity for many drugs. Therefore, there is difficulty of interpretation of the results for many drugs.

Bile

Bile is helpful in estimating drugs conjugates, which are concentrated by liver and excreted into the gallbladder, such as opiates, benzodiazepines, colchicine, buprenorphine, and acetaminophen. These drugs undergo enterohepatic circulation (i.e., those extremely conjugated with glucuronic acid, glutathione, or sulfate). Detection of these drugs is more likely in the bile than in the blood. The concentrations of these drugs may be 1,000 times lower in blood. With better and sensitive screening techniques such as immunoassays, bile is no more a routine sample for toxicology analysis.

It is preserved only in selected cases. It is also a useful sample for chronic exposure of drugs such as opioids, cannabinoids, benzodiazepines, etc. It is particularly useful when urine is absent and in cases of long survival after last administration. Like urine, bile is a waste fluid and with possible exception of ethanol, the correlation between blood and bile concentration of drugs is generally poor. It is relatively a dirty fluid, containing high concentrations of bile salts and other substances that may interfere with toxicological analysis. It can be collected by aspiration or directly after incising the gallbladder into a glass/plastic container with screw cap. It can be collected directly from common bile duct, if cholecystectomy was performed. It should be always collected prior to liver sample. It is a viscous fluid, which makes it difficult to be sucked by needle and syringe. The gallbladder should be tied to reduce contamination. Collect all the available bile in a 10 mL plastic screw-capped container without preservative. A 10 mL of bile is adequate for toxicological analysis. The concentrations may be altered by postmortem diffusion from the liver and stomach and it is useful for qualitative analysis only.

Cerebrospinal Fluid

The cerebrospinal fluid (CSF) sample is rarely required for toxicological analysis. If needed, it should be collected by cisternal puncture. It is difficult to collect CSF at postmortem by conventional lumbar puncture. It is relatively easier to obtain by cisternal puncture. With the neck flexed, palpate the atlanto-occipital membrane in the midline and, using a needle and syringe, gently introduce a disposable spinal needle through the skin at that point, directing the needle toward the bridge of the nose. As the atlanto-occipital membrane is punctured at a depth of ~2 cm, loss of resistance will be felt, following which CSF can be aspirated. The lack of any intrathecal pressure may make this collection very difficult or even impossible. Alternatively, it can be obtained from the posterior fossa after the brain has been removed, but this procedure may lead to blood contamination. Clear CSF may sometimes be obtained from the lateral ventricles either by needle puncture reflecting the dura and parting the cerebral spheres or cutting down through the cortex. Collect all available CSF in a 10 mL screw-capped plastic container without preservative, except for ethanol analysis. It presents in a similar composition to plasma, except that high-molecular weight proteins are absent. The drug concentrations are generally higher in blood. Its correlation with blood is poor and, therefore, useful for qualitative analysis only.

Other Body Fluids

In cases where blood and urine are not available, other available body fluids such as pericardial and synovial fluids can be used for toxicological analysis, like alcohol.

BIOLOGICAL TISSUES

Liver

Many tissues are often used for toxicological analysis. Liver is the most useful tissue for toxicological analysis. There are many advantages of liver tissue. Firstly, large amount of tissue is available. Secondly, its relative ease of collection. Thirdly, its relative ease of sample preparation compared with other tissues. Fourthly, there is also a relatively large database of liver drug concentrations available in the literature compared to the amount of data for other tissues. Fifthly, because it concentrates many substances, concentration of many basic drugs is higher in liver compared to blood, making detection easier. It is the major organ and an important depot, making at least the qualitative analysis for certain drugs easier than in blood, in some cases such as tricyclic antidepressant (e.g., concentrations of the tricyclic antidepressant are roughly 10–50 times higher in the liver than the blood, partly because of absorption of drug from the small intestine by hepatic portal system). It can contain large amount of drugs and metabolites and in some difficult cases may help establish, whether acute or chronic toxicity has occurred. Although very difficult to become routine, if quantitative analysis is required, this is the most promising solid tissue, since more data exist for liver drug concentrations than for any other organ. But quantitative relationships between liver and blood concentrations for most drugs are not available. Since concentrations of drugs in liver do not change markedly postmortem at least in the early period, ratios for peripheral blood have been proposed either as markers of postmortem redistribution and to establish correlations. Ratios lower than 5 suggest low or even none propensity for postmortem redistribution. Ratios exceeding 20–30 suggest significant postmortem redistribution. The only disadvantage of liver as a specimen is that it tends to be fatty and can putrefy faster than blood. The high lipid and protein content may cause interference in toxicological analysis. Ideally, the part of the liver retained should be fresh unfixed, taken from the deep right lobe of liver from the periphery region, away from the stomach, major vessels, and gallbladder. It avoids contamination with diffusion of drugs from gastric content into the left lobe. A minimum of 30 g in a plastic container with screw cap without preservative is sufficient for toxicological analysis. But in India, it is advisable to preserve minimum of 100 g, as enough tissue may be needed for repeat test or for re-evaluation in the other laboratory, if needed, as all laboratories do not have sophisticated equipment.

Stomach Contents

The other commonly preserved viscera samples are stomach and small intestine with its contents. The sample is useful when drugs have been taken orally as the concentrations will be many times higher than in other fluids. The advantage of gastric content is that drug concentration may be quite high after drug overdose even after the majority of the drug has passed into the small intestine. The stomach content is uncomplicated by metabolism. Analysis of drugs that are metabolized extensively in the body may be detected unchanged. In the same way, drugs that may be difficult to detect in the blood because of extensive distribution in the body might be detected readily in the stomach. Sometimes, in cases where death has occurred shortly after drug ingestion, it may be possible to see remains of tablets or capsules and identified. The sample of the tablet may be analyzed to identify the drug. It can also be helpful to determine the amount of drug present in stomach, if blood concentration is difficult to interpret. The disadvantage of stomach content is its composition which varies from a thin fluid to a semisolid to solid, depending on the amount and type of food content. Stomach contents are rarely homogeneous and, therefore, difficult to measure accurately the representative concentration of drugs in the volume of stomach received, unless the contents are homogenized. The accurate estimation of a dose in the gastric content is difficult, as the total stomach content is often not sent to the laboratory. But sending the whole stomach with its contents becomes voluminous, especially if the stomach is full. In such cases, we can collect 30 mL portion of the total homogenized stomach content in a plastic container with screw cap. But it is important to note down the total volume in the container's label. Therefore, the results should be reported as the amount of drug present in the volume or mass of stomach content received. If the stomach content is absent, we can collect 30 g of the stomach wall. The stomach should be ligated on both ends (distal esophagus and pylorus) and dissected out. Then the greater curvature should be opened up, so that the contents can be directly poured onto the wide-mouthed jar. About 30 cm of small intestine is preserved with its contents is also useful for testing. The macroscopic findings (e.g., tablets and capsules) should be rapidly separated, dried, and stored in a separate container. Any characteristic odor should be noted down. But caution should be taken, if cyanide or phosphide gases are suspected to have been ingested, to avoid inhalation. The analysis of stomach can be useful to guide blood analysis. But we should be careful about the misinterpretation of drug concentration in the stomach. Firstly, the concentration of drug concentration of a substance in the stomach is practically meaningless by itself. Shortly, after a therapeutic dose, the concentration of a substance in the stomach may be very high even if the total amount is not. Secondly, the absence of a large amount of residual drug in the stomach does not necessarily rule out an oral overdose. It may take several hours to die from a drug overdose, during which most or all of the drug could have passed from the stomach to the small intestine or even have been largely absorbed. High concentrations of some drugs can delay gastric emptying. Therefore, the gastric drug concentrations should never be on the same basis as those for blood. The presence of a drug or metabolite in the gastric content does not necessarily prove oral administration, especially if the concentration is low. Indeed, drugs distributed by the extracellular fluid will be present in the fluid that ultimately forms the gastric secretions. The gastric juice may contain significant amount of basis drugs and metabolites circulating in the blood. In practical situation, many drug overdose patients undergo gastric lavage procedure and are administered activated oral charcoal in the hospital. This large amount of charcoal in the stomach leads to an underestimation of the total amount of drug present. Therefore, the toxicologist should also review the antemortem clinical record of the patient for correct information.

Other Tissues

Other body tissue can also be useful for investigation of deaths due to poisons. Brain, fat tissue, lung, spleen, and kidney have been used for drug analysis. Ideally, a wet unfixed tissue of 50 g should be collected into separate plastic container with screw cap. Brain can be helpful for drugs that act on the central nervous system and lipophilic drugs (e.g., drug of abuse, organochlorated insecticides) and volatile drugs. Brain is relatively isolated organ and not affected by postmortem redistribution from stomach or by the putrefaction of thorax and abdominal organs. High lipid content may cause analytical problems. In case of lung, the sample has to be preferably collected from the apex of the right lung. The basal lobes of the lung are prone to postmortem redistribution from gastric contents due to proximity to stomach. The whole lung may have to be preserved in case of solvent abuse or volatile substance poisoning. After opening the thorax, the lung is mobilized and the main bronchus tied off tightly with a string ligature. The hilum is then divided and the lung is placed immediately into a glass container and sealed with polytetrafluoroethylene (Teflon) or aluminum foil-lined lids and immediately sent for analysis (prevents the volatile in the sample from escaping). The spleen can be helpful when blood is not available such as in fire-related deaths and for toxins that accumulate in erythrocytes such as carbon monoxide and cyanide. The kidney specimen can be helpful for heavy metal poisons that tend to concentrate in kidney or ethylene glycol analysis. Capsule should be removed while sending the sample. Fat tissues are rarely used for toxicology analysis. It can be used for analyzing lipophilic drugs. Samples from abdominal subcutis are commonly taken. Poison detected in fat reflects antemortem accumulation and not the result of postmortem redistribution. All these tissues are only useful for qualitative analysis and for assessment of the overall body burden of a toxin.

Bone and Muscle Tissue

In case of decomposed, exhumed, burnt, or skeletonized body, it becomes difficult and challenging to collect samples for drug analysis due to absence of blood or scarcity of solid tissues. But, whatever remains, is available, we have to collect all the relevant samples though it may not be the preferred sample. If bones are available, the whole long bone should be collected and preserved. It has to be dried in normal temperature and sealed in plastic bag. If we feel sufficient to preserve a small sample, we can preserve 50 g of long bones such as femur. It should be cut into small pieces (e.g., femur ring) or crushed. There are no data to suggest that one anatomic region is better than another. Larger bones are certainly easier to work/extract analytes than smaller bones. Bone marrow samples may be useful in drug identification (qualitative and also quantitative) in case where all the soft tissues have degenerated. The skeletal muscle is useful for toxicological analysis in advanced decomposition cases, since it is resistant to autolysis. A 50 g muscle tissue (preferably quadriceps muscle) is collected in a plastic container with screw cap.

Hair and Nail

Hair and nails are useful samples for analyzing chronic poison (heavy metals) or drug of abuse (opioid). These should be sent if chronic poisoning is suspected, particularly to distinguish between episodic or continuous exposure or for those poisons, which may have already been eliminated from the body by the time of death. Hair should be plucked from the scalp with the entire root, shaft, and tip. About 150–200 hairs should be collected and laid aligned by rolling into a clean plastic or foil sheet with an indication of the scalp ends on the attached label. It is plucked in postmortem cases prior to autopsy. The hair should be collected from the posterior vertex region of the scalp, which presents the least growth variation in comparison to other region of the scalp and other body hair types. Collection from multiple sites within the vertex region is acceptable to avoid a visible bald patch that may cause some discomfort. The whole nail from one toe or finger can be lifted and collected in a plastic packet.

Maggots

In decomposed body, if maggots are present, 20 g of maggots can be collected in a plastic or glass container with saturated common salt as the preservative. If drugs or intoxicants are detected, they could only have originated from tissues upon which the larvae were feeding. However, the correlation between the level in the larvae and the human has not been established. It only provides qualitative information about the drug used.

Injection Sites or Snakebite

In case of death due to injection of drugs or suspected snakebite, the sample from the injection site has to be preserved. The skin sample, with the underneath muscle tissue around the injection site area, must be preserved along with a control sample of similar composition from the opposite normal site in saturated solution of common salt.

Tablets, Powders, and Syringes

These samples should be packed with care and any needle protected by a suitable shield to avoid injury. These items may be particularly useful in deaths of medical personnel or drug addicts who may use agents which are difficult to detect once they have entered the body.

CONTAINERS

The use of disposables, hard plastics (**Fig. 2.1A**), or glass containers is recommended for preservation. The plastic containers with screw caps (especially of polypropylene) are increasingly used and have the advantage of not smashing when dropped or frozen and also much lighter. The container should be new and preferably rinsed with distilled water and sterilized before use, unless the manufacturer's states it unnecessary. If volatile poisons (solvents, ethanol, anesthetic gases, etc.) are to be analyzed, samples should be promptly collected and glass containers sealed with polytetrafluoroethylene (Teflon) or aluminum foil-lined lids are preferable to avoid greater loss by diffusion registered through plastic container. The containers should be filled (but not overfilled) to minimize headspace and, therefore, losses due to evaporation. It should be opened at the time of analysis and only when cold at 4°C.

SAMPLE PRESERVATION AND STORAGE

The ideal samples are best sent in their original state without adding any preservative in a refrigerated storage (4°C) within few hours. But generally it is not possible to send in this ideal state, due to lack of good autopsy facilities, cold storage facilities, quick transport arrangements, legal formalities, and quick forensic laboratory services. It usually gets delayed. Therefore, sample has to be kept in ideal preservatives to provide optimal conditions, till they reach the laboratory. The specimen is generally preserved at 4°C for short term until they are analyzed. For long-term storage, it has to be kept in freezer (–20°C) until analyzed and disposed off. Exception is the hair and nail samples, which are stable at room temperature. If plasma or serum is needed for analysis, these are separated before frozen. In India, the most commonly used preservative for viscera tissues is saturated solution of common salt (**Fig. 2.1B**). It is easily available, cheap, and effective preservative. It is important that the solution should be prepared using pure sodium chloride in distilled water to avoid any contaminants. The other option is rectified spirit (90% ethanol), except in cases of poisoning due to alcohol, chloral hydrate, chloroform, phenol, formaldehyde, ether, and phosphorus. In acid or alkali poisoning, rectified spirit is the prescribed preservative. The blood for toxicological analysis has to be preserved in sodium or potassium fluoride at the concentration of 10 mg/mL of blood and potassium oxalate (if blood not clotted) at the concentration of 30 mg/10 mL of blood. Sodium or potassium fluoride should be also added to urine and vitreous humor, especially if alcohol estimations are required. It prevents decomposition of the sample.

PACKAGING AND FORWARDING OF SAMPLES

All samples should be properly sealed and labeled with the deceased's name, postmortem number or institutional case number, nature of sample, collection site, preservative used, and date and time of collection. Particular

PROCEDURE FOR COLLECTION, PRESERVATION, AND FORWARDING OF BIOLOGICAL SAMPLE FOR ...

attention should be paid to the packaging of samples (**Figs. 2.1C** to **E**) to avoid loss during transport and to comply with health and safety regulations. It should be protected by the use of tamper-evident seals around the lids and accompanied by an intact chain of custody record. A self-adhesive, tamper-resistant stickers should be placed over the container lids to assure that samples were not adulterated. It should be handed over to the investigating officer after obtaining proper receipt. Avoid mix-up of samples. Avoid contamination. Use different dress suit for each case. Clear the dissection table of all biological tissue or fluids. Communication between toxicologist and pathologist is required whenever needed.

The following documents should be enclosed along with the samples. The toxicological request forms, filled as complete as possible with details mentioned below, placed with samples inside a sealed plastic opaque bags and submitted to the laboratory for analysis.

1. Name, address, and phone number of forensic pathologist and investigating officer
2. Circumstances of death and details of drugs thought to be implicated

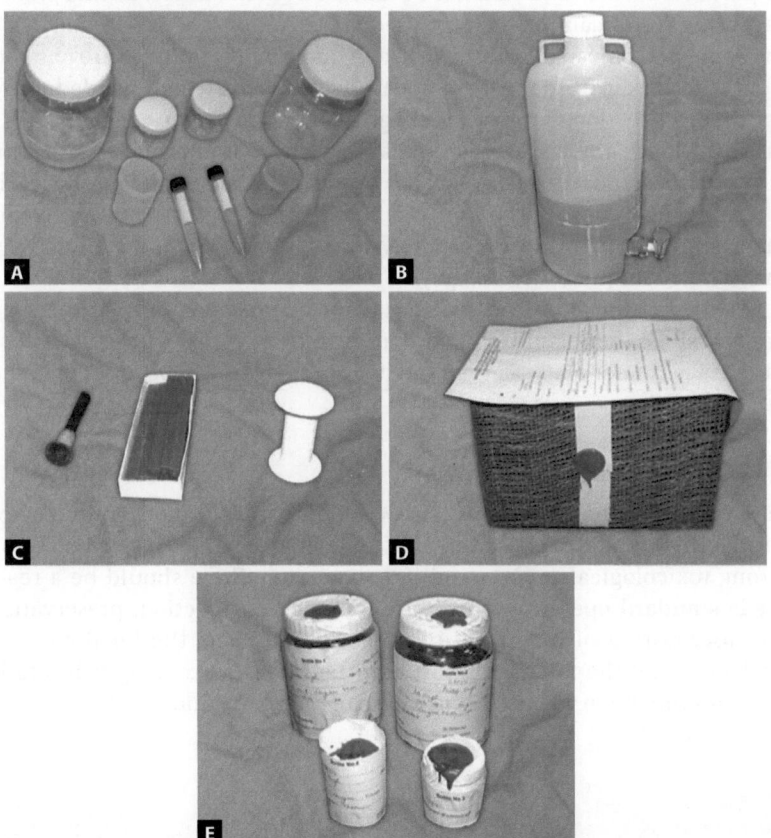

Figs. 2.1A to E: (A) Plastic containers; (B) Container with saturated solution of common salt; (C) Sealing materials; (D) Sealed viscera box; and (E) Sealed viscera bottles.

3. Past medical history including current or recent prescription medication
4. Details of emergency hospital treatment and medication given
5. Copy of forensic pathologist report, if available

In India, it is usually forwarded by the police officer (Assistant Commissioner of Police and above rank) along with the copy of postmortem report to the forensic science laboratory. It is important that the abovementioned details are also provided to the forensic toxicologist. A chain of custody report should be completed and signed to evidence sample integrity.

The samples collected during the autopsy may not yield the expected normal results. However, much useful information can be obtained by the thoughtful analysis of samples obtained at the autopsy and the interpretation of results obtained. Most drugs and poisons including alcohol show variation in concentration in blood according to the time of specimen collected after death, choice of specimen site, methods of sampling, and the volume of blood collected. The blood specimens taken from central sites, e.g., heart tend to give particularly high value for most of the analysts. It is particularly important that blood should not be milked from the limbs, as this process can bring significant changes in the concentration of critical analytes in the expressed blood. The most consistent quantitative findings are obtained from blood taken from the femoral vein, which is the recommended site for specimen collection. Because of very great variations in the concentration of drugs in blood samples taken from different sites, it is important that sample collection is standardized, so that the results obtained can be meaningfully interpreted by comparison with the databases that are being developed incorporating the results of the analysis of samples of blood collected by a uniform technique at the autopsy.

Proper collection and preservation of postmortem samples are crucial, since there is usually no opportunity to go back for collection of samples at a later stage as the body will probably have been cremated or buried.

■ CONCLUSION

Forensic expert has to exercise his wisdom to collect the right biological sample by standard procedure for toxicological analysis. It will avoid wrong toxicological reports and interpretation. There should be a ready made standard operating procedure for sample collection, preservation, and forwarding of biological samples maintaining the legal chain of evidence. And the forensic expert and the forensic toxicologist has to be in communication for better toxicological analysis and interpretation of the result.

FURTHER READINGS

1. Baker RC, Cravey RH, Baselt RC. Introduction to Forensic Toxicology, 1st edition. California: Biomedical Publication; 1981.
2. Ballantyne B, Marrs T, Syversen T. General and Applied Toxicology, 2nd edition. London: Macmillan Press; 1999.
3. Burton J, Rutty G. The Hospital Autopsy, 2nd edition. New Delhi: Arnold Publishers; 2001.
4. Goff ML, Lord WD. Entomotoxicology. A new area for forensic investigation. Am J Forensic Med Pathol. 1994;15:51-7.
5. World Health Organization (WHO). (1997). Guidelines for poison control. [online] Available from https://www.who.int/publications/i/item/guidelines-for-poison-control. [Last accessed March, 2021].
6. Jones GR, Pounder DJ. Site dependence of drug concentrations in postmortem blood—a case study. J Anal Toxicol. 1987;11:186-90.
7. Flanagan RJ. (2005). Developing Analytical Toxicology Services: Principles and Guidance. [online] Available from https://www.who.int/ipcs/publications/training_poisons/hospital_analytical_toxicology.pdf. [Last accessed March, 2021].
8. McCurdy WC. Postmortem specimen collection. Forensic Sci Int. 1987;35:61-5.
9. Moriya F, Hashimoto Y. Pericardial fluid as an alternative specimen to blood for postmortem toxicological analyses. Leg Med (Tokyo). 1999;1:86-94.
10. Noguchi TT, Nakamma GR, Griesemer EC. Drug analysis of skeletonizing remains. J Forensic Sci. 1978;23:490-2.
11. O'Neal CL, Poklis A. Postmortem production of ethanol and factors which influence interpretation: a critical review. Am J Forensic Med Path. 1996;17:8-20.
12. Ohshima T, Kondo T, Sato Y, Takayasu T. Postmortem alcohol analysis of the synovial fluid and its availability in medico-legal practices. Forensic Sci Int. 1997;90:131-8.
13. White PC. Crime Scene to Court: The Essentials of Forensic Sciences, 1st edition. Cambridge: Royal Society of Chemistry; 1998.
14. Plueckhahn VD. The evaluation of autopsy blood alcohol levels. Med Sci Law. 1968;8:168-76.
15. Pounder DJ. Forensic entomo-toxicology. J Forensic Sci. 1991;31:469-72.
16. Prouty RW, Anderson WH. The forensic science implications of site and temporal influences on postmortem blood-drug concentrations. J Forensic Sci. 1990;35:243-70.
17. Dinis-Oliveira RJ, Vieira DN, Magalhães T. Guidelines for Collection of Biological Samples for Clinical and Forensic Toxicological Analysis. Forensic Sci Res. 2016;1:42-51.
18. Dinis-Oliveira RJ, Carvalho F, Duarte JA, Remião F, Marques A, Santos A, et al. Collection of biological samples in forensic toxicology. Toxicol Mech Methods. 2010;20:363-414.
19. NHS Trust. (2017). Guidance for Obtaining Postmortem Samples for Toxicology Analysis. [online] Available from https://www.nbt.nhs.uk/severn-pathology/pathology-services/clinical-biochemistry/toxicology. [Last accessed March, 2021].

Chapter 3

Extraction/Isolation and Clean-up Methods

■ EXTRACTION/ISOLATION METHODS FOR PESTICIDES/INSECTICIDES

Pesticides/insecticides are extensively used in agriculture and household remedies for the control of insects and pests. Due to their easy availability, inadvertent knowledge, and quick action, these pesticides are being largely used for suicidal purposes. Basically, all these pesticides/insecticides are broadly classified as organophosphorus (OP) compound, organochlorine (OC) compound, carbamates, and pyrethroids.

Organophosphorus compounds are the derivatives of the oxoacids of phosphorus or thiophosphoric acid. The different acids from which organophosphates are being derived are phosphoric acid, thiophosphoric acid, dithiophosphoric acid, and miscellaneous OP compound. The important derivatives of the phosphoric acid having insecticidal activity are dichlorvos, naked, phosphamidon, phosphinon, phosdrin, bidrin, birlane, gardona, dimefox, mipafox, avenin, and cyolane. The replacement of one of the oxygen atoms by sulfur in the derivatives of phosphoric acid decreases the toxicity of the compounds related to mammals without substantial changes in the insecticidal or acaricidal activity. Thiophosphoric acid derivatives are more toxic to mammals compared to thiono derivatives. The common thiophosphoric acid are parathion, methyl parathion, paraoxon, thiophos ME, fenitrothion, chlorthion, dicapthon, ronnel, bromophos, fenthion, dasanit, diazinon, demeton, methyldemeton, dursban, potasan, vamidothion, acetophos, chlorpyrifos, etc. Derivatives of dithiophosphoric acid under the class are more stable but less toxic than the corresponding compound of thiophosphoric acid. These derivatives are found effective as insecticide in agricultural applications. The list of some important compounds are malathion, dimethoate, morphothion, formothion, thimet, ethion, ekatin, disyston, tetrathion, phosalone, imidan, guthion, menazon, edifenphos, etc. Other miscellaneous OP compound includes trichlorfon, O-ethyl O-(4-nitrophenyl) phenylphosphonothioate (EPN), etc.

Organochlorine insecticides such as dichlorodiphenyltrichloroacetic acid (DDT), benzene hexachloride (BHC), lindane, endrin, dieldrin, endosulfan, heptox, chlordan, toxaphene, kelthane, heptachlor, methoxychlor, etc., are being extensively used in agriculture and are also familiar in domestic applications. New varieties of these insecticides are emerging every year. Owing to easy availability, these insecticides are frequently used in suicidal cases. Accidental poisoning cases are also known. Carbamates such as propoxur, carbaryl, carbofuran, zineb, etc., are also used for homicidal/suicidal cases. The mechanism of toxic manifestation in mammalian system is similar to OP insecticides, but the toxicity of the former is comparatively lesser. The pyrethroids have also emerged as a major class of synthetic organic insecticides from the time of its use for agricultural applications. Commonly used pyrethroids are fenvalerate, permethrin, dichlorovinyl, cyfluthrin, deltamethrin, fenpropathrin, bifenthrin, etc. These compounds are comparatively less toxic than other classes in respect of mammalian toxicity. Owing to their availability, these compounds are misused in criminal poisoning cases.

The procedures for extraction, isolation, and clean-up for analysis of pesticides in different biological materials have been shown in flowchart manner, which can be of handy reference for student/analyst/scientist/forensic toxicologist. Solvent extraction procedure is the most frequent method of choice, which is simple and easily available. It serves a threefold purpose, namely as a concentration step, as a clean-up procedure, and to render the sample in a form suitable for analysis.

From Tissues

Up to 50 g tissues + anhydrous sodium sulfate (Na_2SO_4) + 50 mL n-hexane is taken in a round bottom or in a conical flask fitted with air condenser and heated in water bath for 2–3 hours. The contents are filtered.

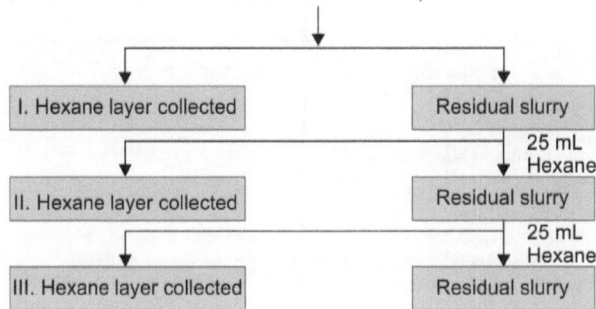

Three hexane layers I, II, and III are pooled + 15 mL of acetonitrile saturated with n-hexane is taken in a separating funnel and shaken vigorously for 2–3 minutes.

EXTRACTION/ISOLATION AND CLEAN-UP METHODS

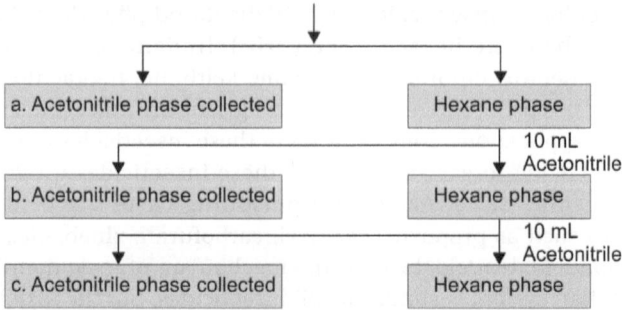

Acetonitrile phases a, b, and c are pooled + 50 mL water + 15 mL hexane is taken in a separating funnel and shaken vigorously for 2–3 minutes.

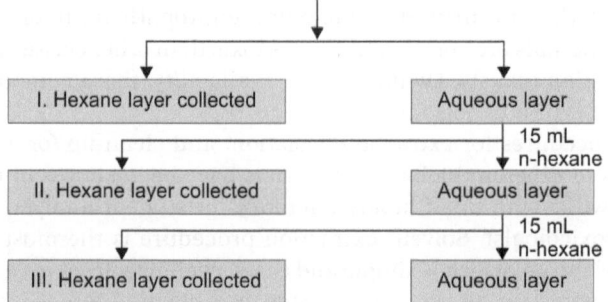

Hexane layer is pooled and concentrated to 1 mL either by nitrogen or in water bath.

Clean-up Process

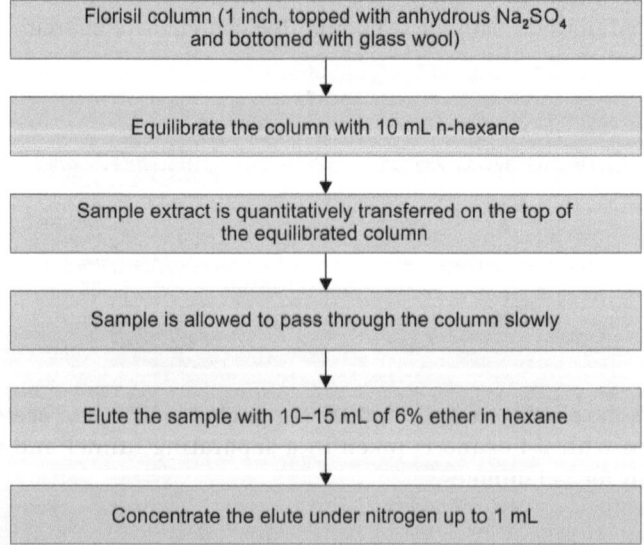

From Stomach Wash, Urine, Vomit, Etc.

20 mL of biological fluid (stomach wash, urine, vomit, etc.) + 50 mL of n-hexane is taken in a round bottom flask fitted with air condenser and heated in a water bath for half an hour. The contents are cooled, filtered, and mixed with 20 mL of hexane and taken in a separating funnel.

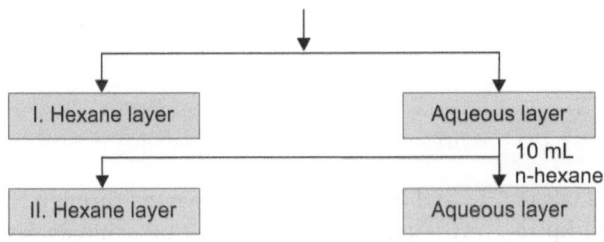

Hexane layer is collected, passed through anhydrous Na_2SO_4, and evaporated up to 1 mL. Loaded on a column of florisil already equilibrated with 10 mL n-hexane, sample allowed to percolate down the column and then eluting with 10 mL n-hexane:ether mixture (2:1) in a graduated tube and again concentrated up to 1 mL.

From Blood

Method I

10 mL blood + 10 mL of 10% sodium tungstate solution + 15 mL of 0.1 N sulfuric acid (H_2SO_4) and shaken for 2 minutes.

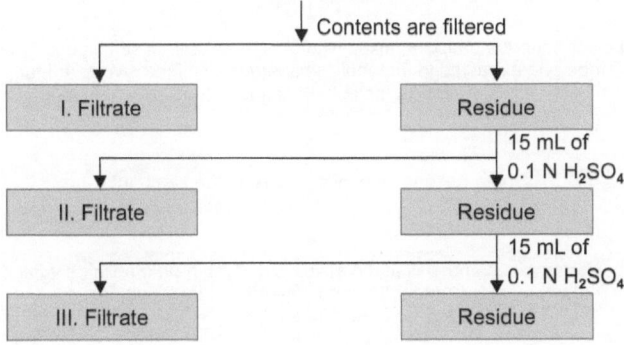

(H_2SO_4: sulfuric acid)

Filtrates I, II, and III are pooled + 20 mL of n-hexane is taken in a separating funnel and shaken for 2 minutes.

EXTRACTION/ISOLATION AND CLEAN-UP METHODS

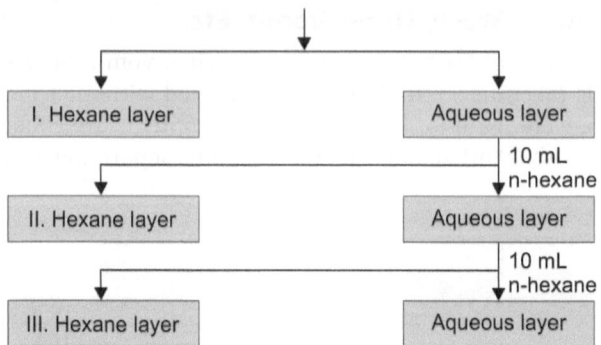

Hexane layers I, II, and III are pooled and passed through Na_2SO_4 and evaporated up to 1 mL. Clean-up process will be same as discussed in tissues.

Method II

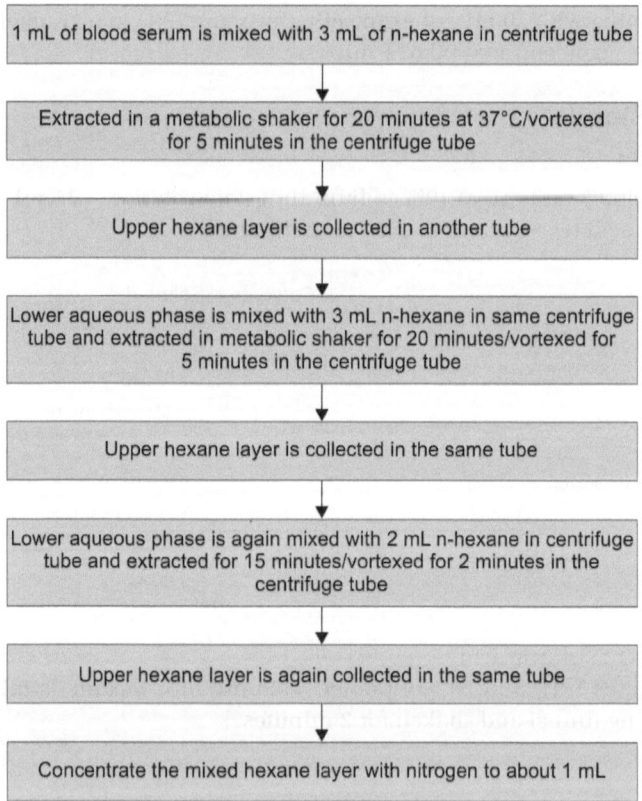

■ EXTRACTION/ISOLATION METHODS FOR VOLATILE POISONS

Poisons, which are volatile in nature, are called as volatile poisons such as acetaldehyde, acetone, aniline, benzene, benzyl alcohol, carbon disulfide, carbon tetrachloride, chloral hydrate, chloroform, cresols, ethyl alcohol, hydrocyanic acid, formaldehyde, isopropyl alcohol, methyl alcohol, naphthalene, paraldehyde, phenol, nitrobenzene, etc. But mainly ethanol and methanol are the most commonly used volatile poisons.

Acetaldehyde: It is colorless, inflammable liquid with boiling point (bp) 20.2°C. It is miscible in water, ether, and ethanol and obtained as byproduct of alcoholic fermentation.

Acetone: It is a clear colorless volatile inflammable liquid with bp 56°C. It is miscible in water, ether, chloroform, and ethanol and obtained as a product of destructive distillation of wood/byproduct of starch fermentation.

Aniline: It is colorless but with time turns to brown color due to nitroso compound formation with bp 184°C. It is miscible in alcohol, benzene, chloroform, and other organic solvents, but insoluble in water and forms salts with mineral acids.

Benzene: It is a clear colorless, inflammable liquid with characteristic aromatic smell with bp 80°C. It is partially miscible in water, miscible in alcohol, acetone, ether, and glacial acetic acid, and obtained in light oil fraction of coal tar distillation.

Benzyl alcohol: It is a colorless liquid with faint aromatic odor with bp 203°C. It is soluble in water, methanol, chloroform, and ether and obtained as ester of cinnamic acid and benzoic acid in Balsam of Tolu and Peru.

Carbon disulfide: It is a colorless liquid with faint aromatic odor with bp 203–208°C and inflammable liquid with characteristic aromatic smell with bp 80°C. It is soluble in water, miscible in ethanol, ether, and chloroform, and obtained from coal tar.

Carbon tetrachloride: It is a heavy clear colorless liquid with chloroform-like odor and is volatile. It is almost insoluble in water, miscible in dehydrated alcohol, chloroform, and ether, and synthesized by chlorination of hydrocarbon.

Chloral hydrate: It is colorless/white crystal, which liquefies between 50°C and boils at 98°C. It is soluble in ether and chloroform and partially soluble in water and it is a synthetic compound.

Chloroform: It is colorless volatile liquid with bp 61°C. It is insoluble in water and miscible with dehydrated alcohol and ether.

EXTRACTION/ISOLATION AND CLEAN-UP METHODS

Cresols: They are almost colorless to pale brownish-yellow liquid, which becomes darker with age/light exposure. It is soluble in water, miscible in ethanol, ether, and chloroform, and occurs in coal tar and in pine and bleached wood tar.

Ethyl alcohol: It is transparent, colorless, and volatile liquid having spirituous odor and burning taste with bp 78.4°C. It is hygroscopic and found as free alcohol in some fruit juices/as ester in some eucalyptus oil and produced by starch, molasses, and grapes fermentation.

Formaldehyde: It is colorless, inflammable gas. It is soluble in water and slightly soluble in ethanol and ether.

Hydrocyanic acid: This smells like bitter almonds. Salts are highly soluble in water and alkaline in nature and are obtained naturally from cherry, apricot, peach, pears, and bitter almond.

Isopropyl alcohol: It is a clear colorless, inflammable, and volatile liquid with bp 81–83°C. It is miscible in water, ethanol, chloroform, and ether and obtained by fermentation.

Kerosene: It is an inflammable oily liquid of characteristic odor with boiling range of 150–300°C. It is obtained by petroleum fractionation.

Methyl alcohol: It is a colorless extremely poisonous liquid of peculiar odor with bp of 67°C. It is soluble in water and organic solvents and synthesized commercially/obtained from the liquid fraction pyroligneous acid in the destructive distillation of wood.

Naphthalene: It is a colorless with melting point of 80°C and bp of 208°C. It is practically insoluble in water, miscible in ethanol and chloroform and highly soluble in ether, and obtained in middle oil fraction of coal tar distillation.

Nitrobenzene: It is a pale yellow oily liquid with bp of 206°C, having odor of bitter almonds. It is practically insoluble in water, miscible in ether and methanol, and produced by nitration of benzene.

Paraldehyde: It is a clear colorless or pale yellow liquid with bp of 123–126°C. It is soluble in water, miscible in ethanol, chloroform, and ether, and produced by polymerization of acetaldehyde.

Phenol: It is a colorless or faintly pink, deliquescent crystals, or crystalline mass with bp of 181°C. It is partially soluble in water, soluble in ethanol, chloroform, and ether, and obtained in light oil fraction of coal tar distillation.

Extraction/isolation of volatile poison is done by distillation, which may be acidic, basic, or neutral.

The procedures for extraction/isolation for analysis of volatile poisons in different biological materials have been shown in a flowchart manner, which can be of handy reference for student/analyst/scientist/forensic toxicologist.

EXTRACTION/ISOLATION AND CLEAN-UP METHODS

Neutral and Acid Distillation
From Viscera

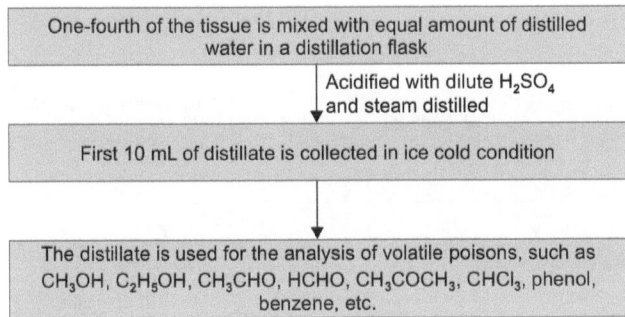

From Blood

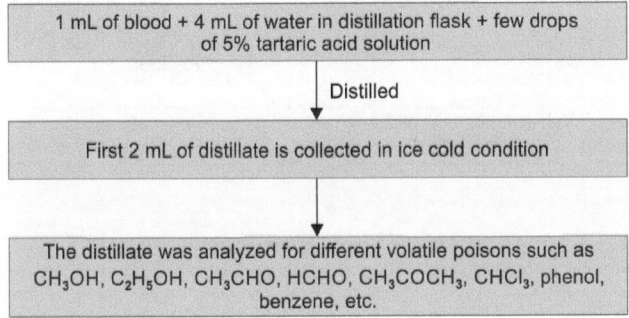

From Urine

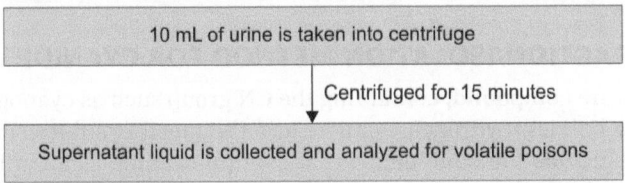

Alkaline Distillation
Method I

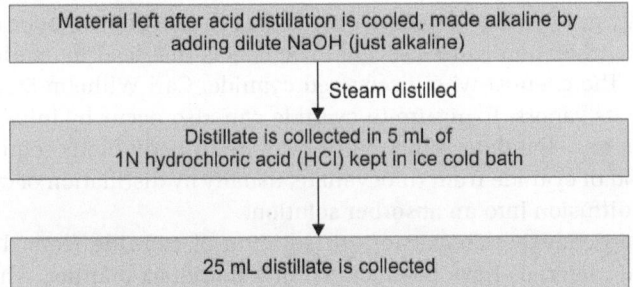

Method II

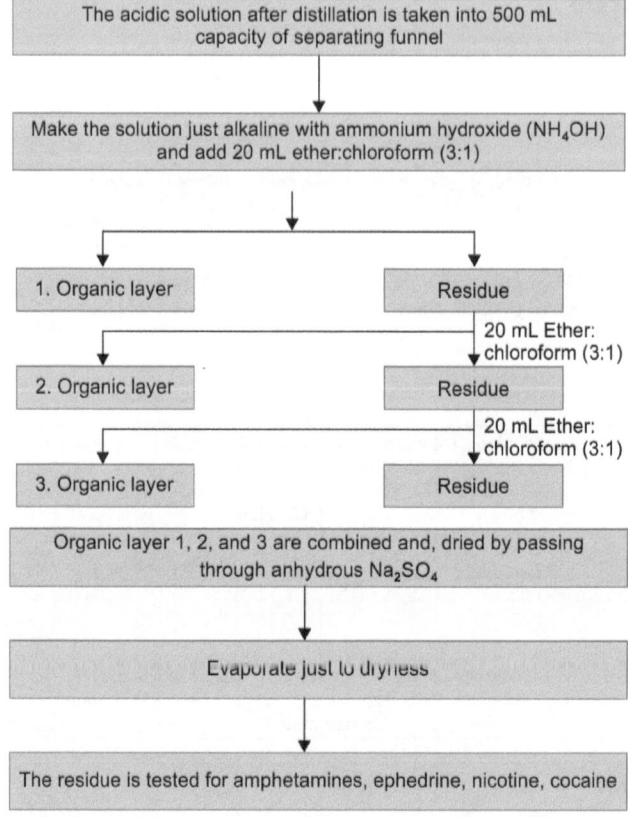

■ EXTRACTION/ISOLATION METHOD FOR CYANIDE

Cyanides are compound, containing the CN group such as cyanogens, the cyanogen halides, hydrogen cyanide, and the metal cyanides. The metal cyanides include the compounds that contain cyanide as an anion such as KCN and compounds in which cyanide is complexed to a metal as a ligand. Cyanide is one of the most rapidly acting of all poisons and in the form of the hydrocyanic acid and its sodium and potassium salts, it is one of the most deadly. The hydrocyanic acid is extremely volatile producing the deadly gas hydrogen cyanide, which has the distinctive odor of bitter almonds. Inhalation causes severe toxic effects that lead to death within minutes. The chemist who discovered cyanide, Carl Wilhelm Steele, was killed by its vapors. Exposure to cyanide can also occur by inhalation of cyanogen gas. The determination of cyanide in body fluids requires the separation of cyanide from thiocyanate, usually by distillation of cyanides or microdiffusion into an absorber solution.

The procedures for extraction/isolation of cyanide from different biological materials have been shown in a flowchart manner, which can be used by student/analyst/scientist/forensic toxicologist.

From Tissues

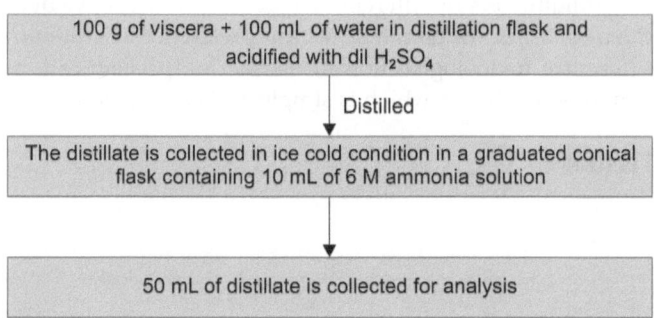

From Blood

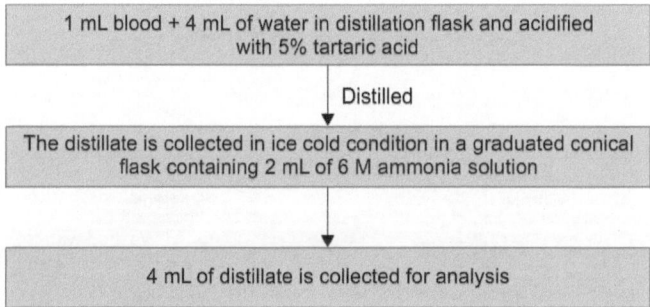

■ EXTRACTION/ISOLATION METHODS FOR TRANQUILIZERS

Tranquilizer is an old term that means a drug which reduces mental tension and produces calmness without inducing sleep or depressing mental faculties. Common tranquilizers are chlorpromazine, promazine, promethazine, prochlorperazine, mepazine, ethopropazine, trimeprazine, perphenazine, thiopropazate, triflupromazine, trifluoperazine, fluphenazine, methoxypromazine, thioridazine, reserpine, benactyzine, azacyclonol, hydroxyzine, imipramine, etc. Tranquilizers are divided into major tranquilizer and minor tranquilizer groups. Major tranquilizers include phenothiazines, indoles, thioxanthenes, butyrophenones, piperazine, and piperidine compounds. Minor tranquilizers are more common of the tranquilizers. These include benzodiazepines, which are very commonly prescribed as antianxiety drugs or anxiolytics. They are often referred to as sedatives/hypnotics. They are central nervous system (CNS) depressants with specific sites of action. The primary route of administration for these medications is oral, swallowed as a tablet, capsule, or liquid. They are also available in solution form for intravenous use. Tranquilizers are the most widely prescribed psychotherapeutic agents in the world and are most involved in suicide attempts and accidental overdoses.

EXTRACTION/ISOLATION AND CLEAN-UP METHODS

The procedures for extraction/isolation and clean-up procedures for analysis of tranquilizers in different biological materials have been shown in a flowchart manner, which can be of handy reference for student/analyst/scientist/forensic toxicologist. Solvent extraction procedure is the most frequent method of choice, which is simple and easily available.

From Tissues
Step 1

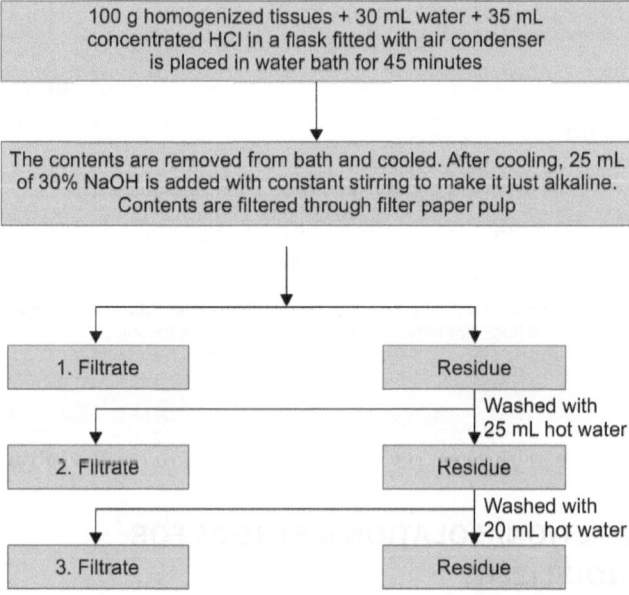

Step 2

The filtrates 1, 2, and 3 are combined, taken into a separating funnel. Up to 40 mL of ether is taken into a separating funnel and shaken for 5 minutes.

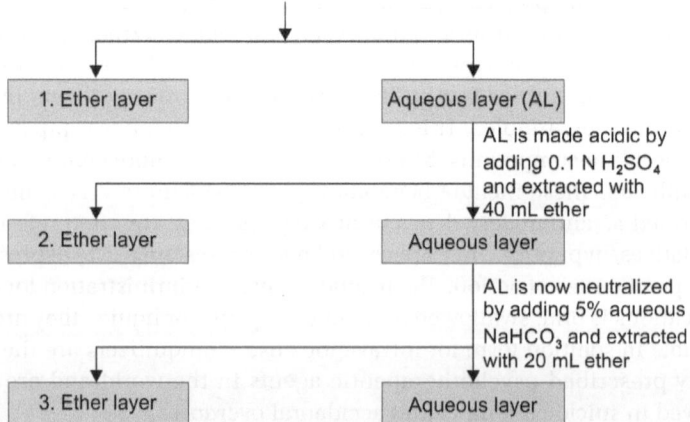

EXTRACTION/ISOLATION AND CLEAN-UP METHODS

The entire three ether layers 1, 2, and 3 are combined and taken into a separating funnel and washed with 25 mL portion of water.

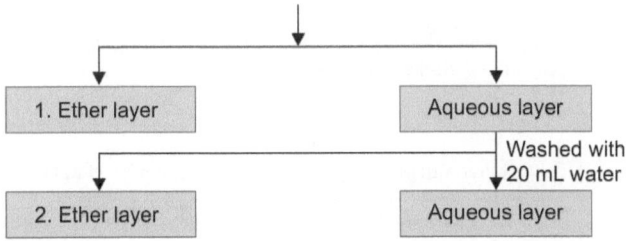

Ether layer is combined and passed through anhydrous Na_2SO_4 and evaporated to dryness. The residue contains tranquilizers.

From Stomach Wash/Vomit/Urine
Step 1

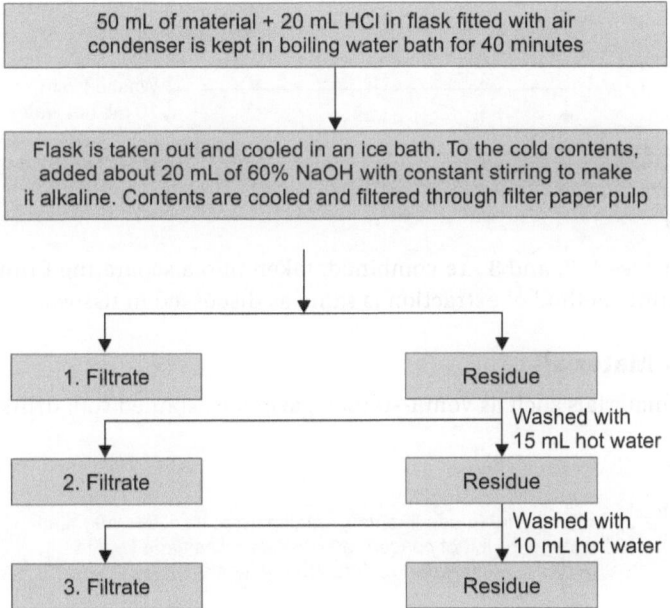

Step 2

The filtrates 1, 2, and 3 are combined and remaining method of extraction is same as discussed in tissues.

From Blood
Step 1

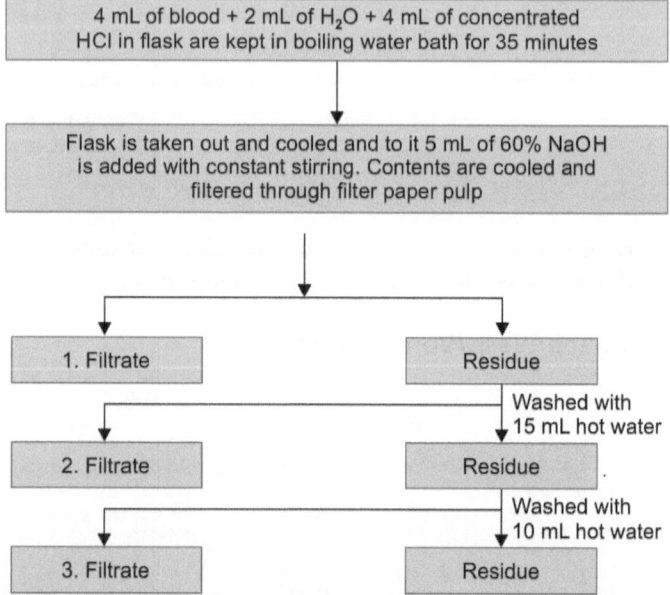

Step 2
The filtrates 1, 2, and 3 are combined, taken into a separating funnel and remaining method of extraction is same as discussed in tissues.

Other Materials
Other materials such as vomit-stained garments, stained soil, drinks, etc.

Step 1

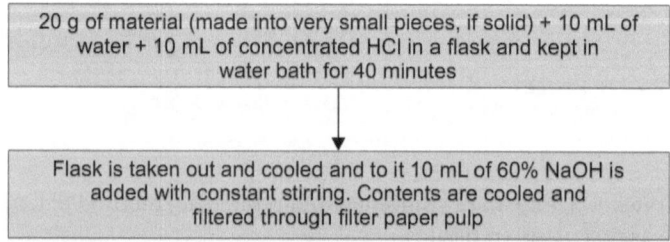

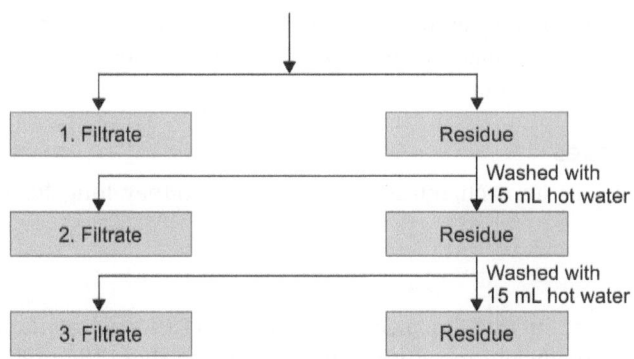

The remaining step of extraction is similar as described for tissues.

■ EXTRACTION/ISOLATION METHODS FOR BARBITURATES

Barbiturates are white, crystalline, and odorless powders, with a bitter taste. It is a group of drugs known as sedative-hypnotics, which were generally prescribed for their sleep inducing and anxiety decreasing effects. It acts as depressant on the CNS. They are basically derived from malonic acid and urea. Common barbiturates are barbitone, phenobarbitone, butobarbitone, amobarbitone, pentobarbitone, heptabarbitone, allobarbitone, secobarbitone, methylphenobarbitone, thiopentone, talbutal, aprobarbitone, nealbarbitone, cyclobarbitone, vesparex, etc. They have been largely replaced with drugs such as benzodiazepine due to their propensity for addiction and reduced effect over extended use. They are classified into four major groups depending on their mode of action:

1. Long-acting barbiturates (duration of action 6–12 h), e.g., phenobarbitone
2. Intermediate-acting barbiturates (duration of action 3–6 h), e.g., amobarbitone
3. Short-acting barbiturates (duration of action <3 h), e.g., pentobarbitone
4. Ultrashort-acting barbiturates (duration of action <15–20 min), e.g., thiopentone

Barbiturates mainly act in CNS, though they may indirectly affect the organ systems. Direct effects include sedation and hypnosis at lower dosages. It can cause a depression of the medullary respiratory center and induce a respiratory depression. Chronic poisoning may occur due to prolonged use of barbiturates in epilepsy. It is characterized by apathy, loss of power of concentration, along with hallucination. Physical effects commonly encountered are sleepiness, nausea, breathing disorders, slurred speech, and coma. Symptoms of acute barbiturate intoxication include altered level of consciousness, difficulty in thinking, drowsiness or coma, incoordination, sluggishness, and staggering. It can be detected for up to 5 days after ingestion in serum and urine. In case of overdose, hypothermia, hypotension, and respiratory depression are usually encountered.

EXTRACTION/ISOLATION AND CLEAN-UP METHODS

The procedures for extraction/isolation for analysis of barbiturates in different biological materials have been shown in a flowchart manner by using solvent extraction procedure.

From Tissues

Tissues such as stomach, intestine, liver, spleen, kidney, lung, heart, brain, etc.

Step 1

50 g tissues are cut into fine pieces + 100 mL 20% HCl + ammonium sulfate [$(NH_4)_2SO_4$] (sufficient to saturate the solution, so that little of it remains at the bottom) is taken in a round bottom flask fitted with air condenser and heated in water bath for 4 hours. The contents are filtered off through a sintered glass funnel containing filter paper pulp.

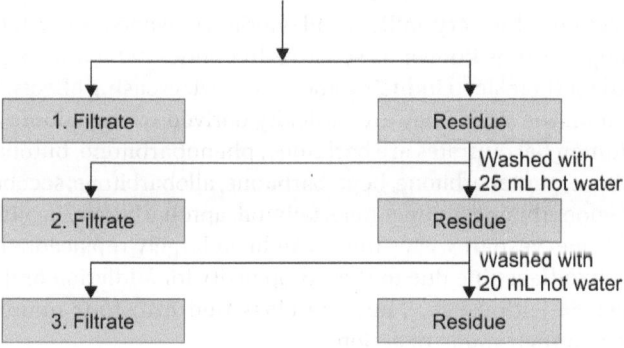

Step 2

Three filtrates 1, 2, and 3 are pooled + 50 mL ether is taken in a separating funnel and shaken for 5 minutes.

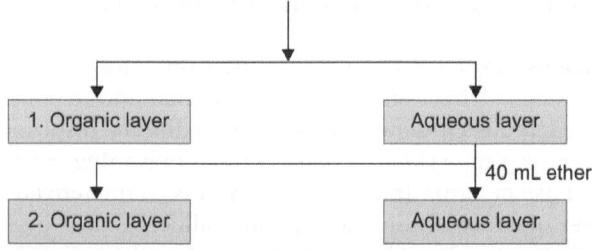

The organic layers 1 and 2 are combined and washed with 15 mL of saturated sodium bicarbonate solution.

EXTRACTION/ISOLATION AND CLEAN-UP METHODS

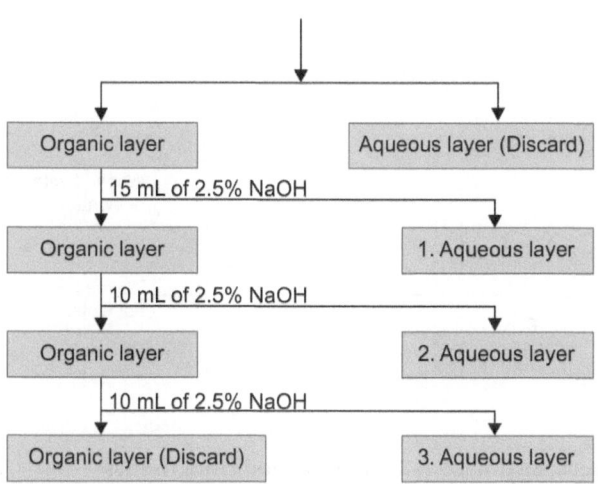

The aqueous layers 1, 2, and 3 are pooled and acidified with dilute H_2SO_4 and then extracted with 20 mL ether.

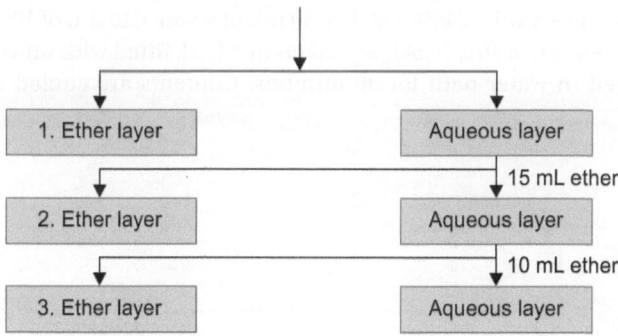

The ether layers 1, 2, and 3 are combined and dried by passing through anhydrous Na_2SO_4. The ether is evaporated to dryness and the residue containing barbiturate in crystalline form is obtained.

Cleanup process is same as for pesticides.

From Stomach Wash/Vomit/Urine, Etc.

Step 1

Up to 25 mL material + 10 mL 5% HCl + $(NH_4)_2SO_4$ is taken in a beaker and heated in water bath for 30 minutes. The contents are filtered through a sintered funnel containing paper pulp.

EXTRACTION/ISOLATION AND CLEAN-UP METHODS

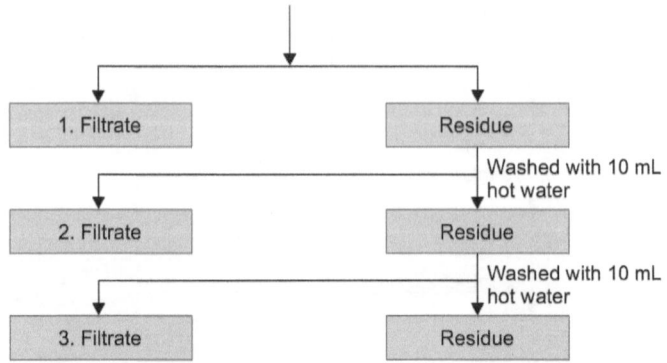

Step 2
Same as described in step 2 for extraction from tissues.

From Blood
Step 1
5 mL of blood + 1 mL of 10% NaOH + 30 mL of water + 10 mL of 10% sodium tungstate + 4 mL of 10% H_2SO_4 are taken in a flask fitted with air condenser and heated in water bath for 30 minutes. Contents are cooled and then filtered.

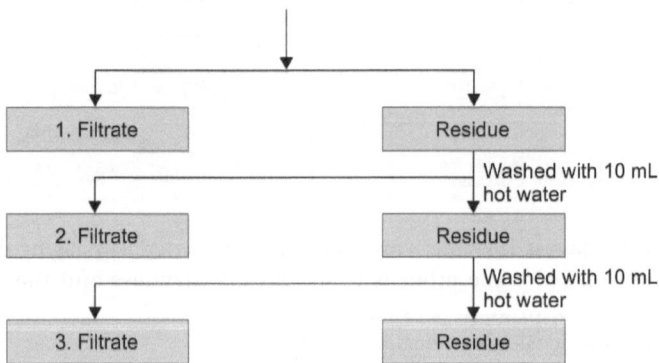

Step 2
Same as described in step 2 for extraction from tissues.

From Other Materials (Vomit-stained Garments, Soil, Suspected Drink, Tea, Coffee, Etc.)
Step 1
10 g material + 25 mL of water + 100 mL of 5% HCl in a flask fitted with air condenser is placed in boiling water bath for 40 minutes. Contents are filtered through sintered glass funnel containing the filter paper pulp.

EXTRACTION/ISOLATION AND CLEAN-UP METHODS

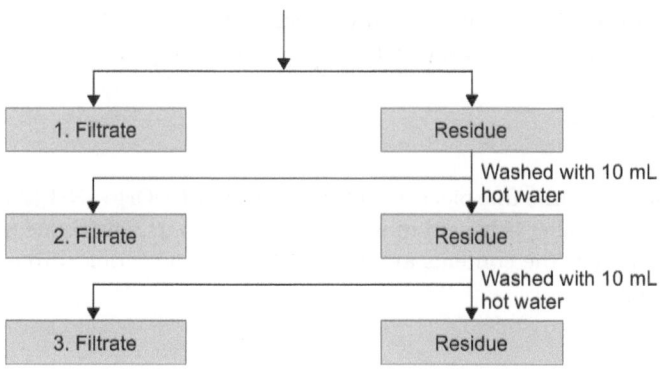

Step 2
Same as described in step 2 for extraction from tissues.

■ EXTRACTION/ISOLATION METHODS FOR ALKALOIDS

Alkaloids are the plants-derived alkali containing nitrogen atom. Alkaloids are basic and form water-soluble salts. They are white solids with well-defined crystalline substances, which unite with acids to form salts. In plants, they may exist in free state or as salts. Opium, a dark brown-colored semisolid mass, is obtained by incision of the unripe capsules of *Papaver somniferum linn*. It contains about 28 alkaloids, which do not exist as free bases, but in combination with acids. The important alkaloids being are morphine, codeine, thebaine, narcotine, and papaverine. Morphine is also used to synthesize heroin by acetylation. Morphine is one of the most common drugs used for suicidal purpose, primarily because the death is painless. For homicidal purpose, opium is rarely used because of the bad taste. In rural areas, opium has been used to commit infanticide by breastfeeding of an infant by women with nipple smeared with lincture of opium. Accidental poisoning is more frequent in children. Morphine is also used as cattle poison and for doping race horses. The poison acts on CNS. Besides these, other alkaloids are atropine, hyoscine, hyoscyamine, scopolamine, tropine, homatropine, apoatropine, nicotine, cocaine, novocaine, procaine, quinine, cinchonine, arecoline, berberine, yohimbine, atrocin, dionine, sparteine, pethidine, ephedrine HCl, flaxedil, solanine, physostigmine, gelsemium, ecgonine, coramine, coniine, etc. In case of alkaloid poisoning, the extraction and isolation are most important step. Extractions are based on the basicity of alkaloids and normally occur in plants as salts. All methods of alkaloid extraction yield impure compounds; hence, thin-layer chromatography (TLC) and high-performance liquid chromatography (HPLC) are the techniques commonly used for the isolation. The procedures for extraction, isolation, and cleanup procedures for analysis of alkaloids in different biological material have been shown in a flowchart manner, which can be of handy reference for student/analyst/

scientist/forensic toxicologist. Solvent extraction procedure is the most frequent method of choice, which is simple and easily available.

From Tissues

Step 1

50 g tissues (cut into fine pieces) + 100 mL of 5% CH_3COOH + $(NH_4)_2SO_4$ solid in a 500 mL beaker is heated in water bath for 4 hours. The tissue proteins are coagulated. The contents are filtered off without suction through filter paper pulp.

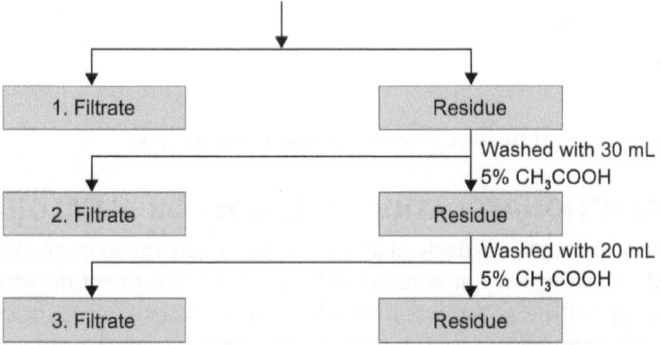

Step 2

Three filtrates 1, 2, and 3 are pooled + NH_4OH (to make it alkaline) + 50 mL mixture of ether:chloroform (3:1) taken in a separating funnel and shaken for few minutes.

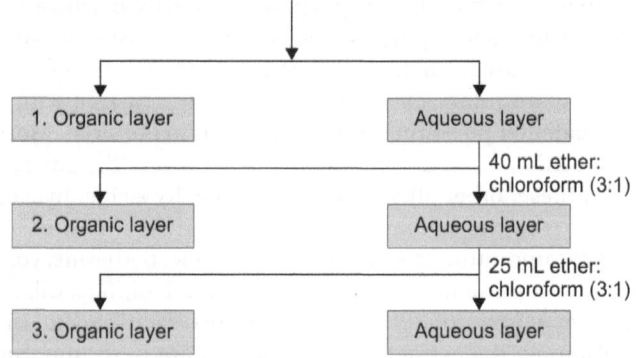

Organic layer is combined (say A)
Aqueous layer is combined (say B)
Combined organic layers (A) + 50 mL portion of 0.1 N H_2SO_4 is taken in a separating funnel.

EXTRACTION/ISOLATION AND CLEAN-UP METHODS

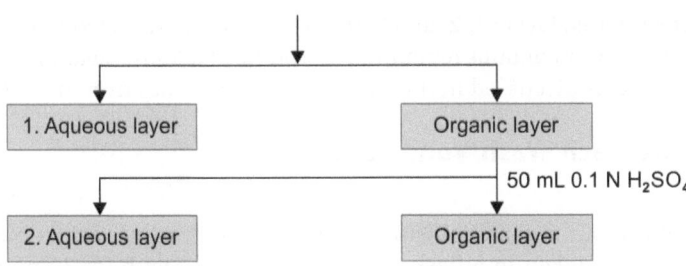

Pooled aqueous layer + NH_4OH (to make it alkaline) + 100 mL ether:chloroform (3:1) mixture.

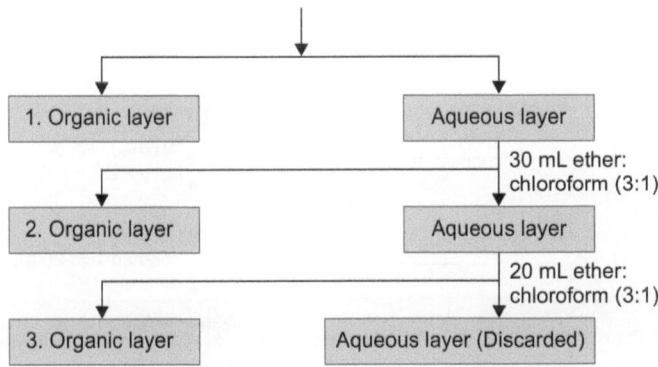

The organic layers 1, 2, and 3 are pooled, passed through Na_2SO_4, and evaporating to dryness, which contain most of the alkaloids and bulk of morphine.

Step 3

Aqueous layer (B) + 50 mL chloroform:isopropanol (isopropyl alcohol) (4:1)

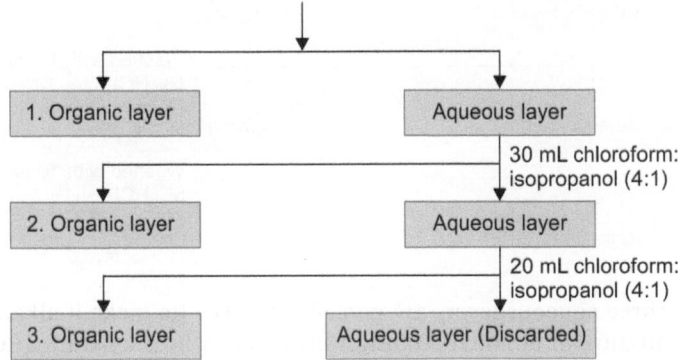

EXTRACTION/ISOLATION AND CLEAN-UP METHODS

Three organic layers 1, 2, and 3 are pooled and evaporated to dryness. This organic layer contains remaining morphine alkaloids. Cleanup process will be same as discussed in the extraction of pesticides from tissues.

From Stomach Wash/Vomit/Urine

Step 1

Up to 50 mL of the material (stomach wash, vomit, urine, etc.) + 5% HCl + $(NH_4)_2SO_4$ is taken in a flask and heated in water bath for 30 minutes. The contents are filtered off through a sintered glass Buchner funnel using filter paper pulp.

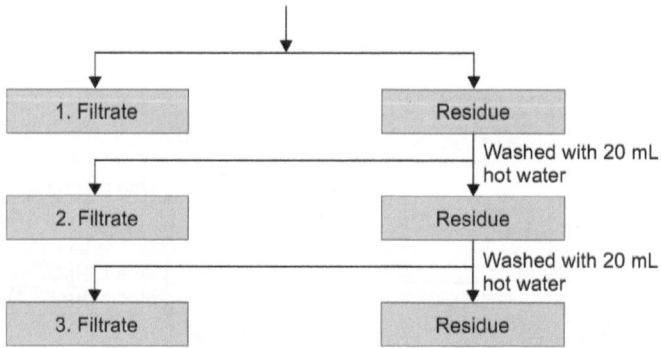

Step 2

Three filtrates 1, 2, and 3 are pooled + 50 mL of ether is taken in a separating funnel and shaken for 5 minutes.

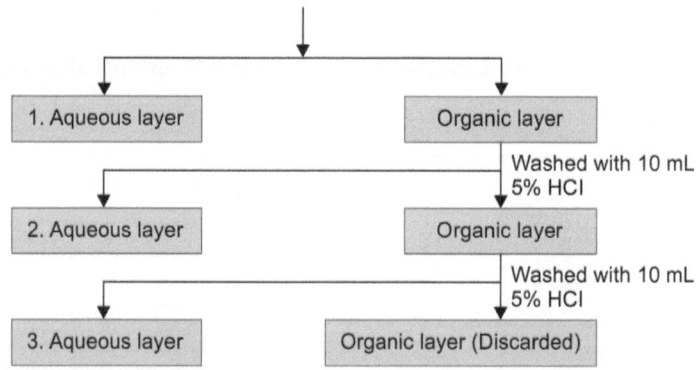

The three aqueous layers are pooled + NH_4OH (to make it alkaline) + 25 mL mixture of ether:chloroform (3:1) is taken in a separating funnel and shaken.

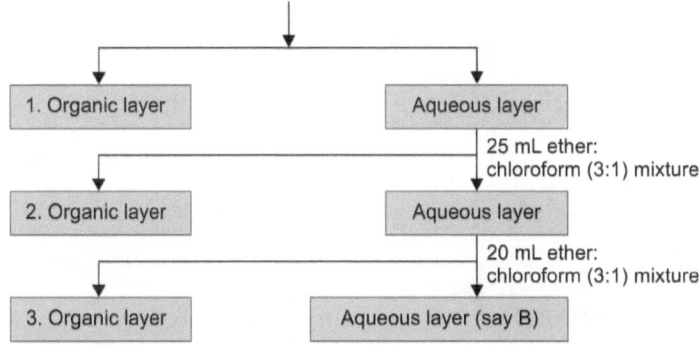

Organic layers 1, 2, and 3 are combined (say A) and aqueous layers are combined (say B).

The organic layer (A) is passed through anhydrous Na_2SO_4 and then evaporated to dryness with nitrogen or on water bath.

Step 3

Similar to tissues as discussed earlier.

From Blood

Step 1

Up to 5 mL of blood + 1 mL of 10% NaOH + 30.5 mL of water + 10 mL of 10% sodium tungstate + 3.5 mL of 10% H_2SO_4 is taken in a flask and contents are stirred well. The flask is heated in water bath for 15 minutes, after which precipitated protein and fat is filtered off through a sintered glass Buchner funnel using filter paper pulp.

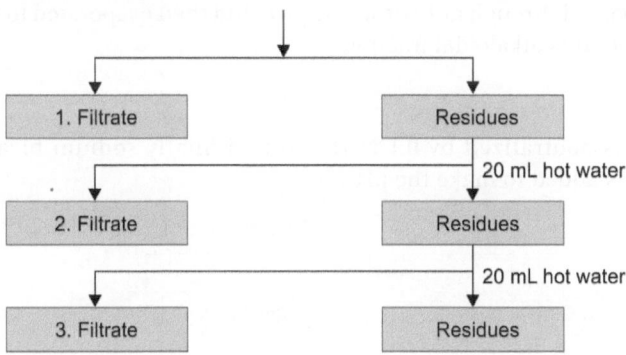

Step 2

Three filtrates 1, 2, and 3 are pooled + 50 mL ether is taken in a separating funnel and shaken for 5 minutes.

EXTRACTION/ISOLATION AND CLEAN-UP METHODS

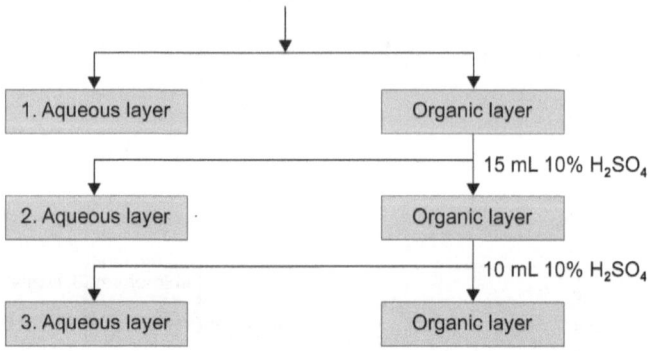

Aqueous layer is pooled + NH_4OH (just to make alkaline) + 25 mL chloroform:ether (1:3) mixture is taken in a separating funnel and shaken.

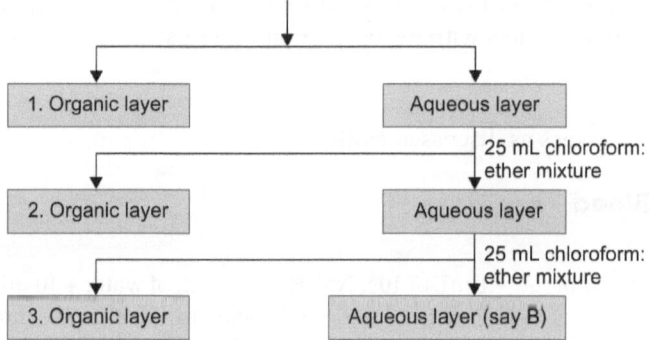

Organic layers 1, 2, and 3 are combined (say A) and aqueous layer is combined (say B).

A is passed through anhydrous Na_2SO_4 and then evaporated to dryness, which contains alkaloidal fraction.

Step 3

Layer B is neutralized by 0.1 N H_2SO_4 and finally sodium bicarbonate solution is added to make the pH 7.5.

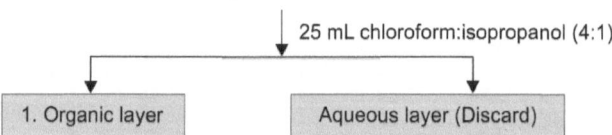

Organic layer is evaporated up to dryness and the residue contains morphine alkaloids.

From Other Materials

Other materials such as vomit-stained garments, soil, suspected food materials, etc.

Step 1

Up to 25 g material + 20 mL water +10 mL of 5% HCl is taken in a flask and heated in water bath for 30 minutes. The contents are filtered off through a sintered glass Buchner funnel containing filter paper pulp.

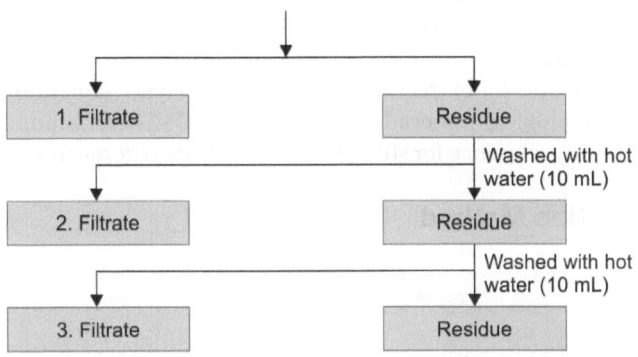

Step 2

Similar to step 2 and step 3 for extraction of alkaloids from tissues.

■ EXTRACTION/ISOLATION METHODS FOR METALLIC POISONS

Heavy metals are chemical elements with a specific gravity that is at least five times the specific gravity of water. Some well-known toxic metallic elements with specific gravity more than water are arsenic (5.7), cadmium (8.65), iron (7.9), lead (11.34), mercury (13.546), etc. In small amount, these metals are necessary for normal body growth and are present in food stuffs, fruits and vegetables, and multivitamin products. Heavy metals become toxic when they are not metabolized in the body and start accumulating in the body. They enter the body through various ways such as food, air, water, ingestion, absorption through skin, and industrial exposure. The Agency for Toxic Substances and Disease Registry (ATSDR) provides the necessary information regarding the commonly encountered toxic heavy metals. Heavy metals are an expression often used for elements, not necessarily "true" metals, with a specific gravity exceeding 5 mg ± 1. Poisoning due to heavy metals is not uncommon in our country due to rapid industrialization and water contamination. The term "toxic metal" is applied to those elements shown to be disruptive of enzymatic processes. Arsenic, antimony, bismuth, cadmium, lead, thallium, and mercury are termed as toxic metals. Metal concentration in biological materials can be measured by colorimetry, fluorimetry, spectrography, polarography, neutron activation analysis, chromatography, X-ray fluorescence, and atomic emission and atomic absorption spectrometry. The atomic absorption spectrometry, both

EXTRACTION/ISOLATION AND CLEAN-UP METHODS

flame and flameless, is the most commonly utilized techniques for metal analysis. Flameless atomization is about 10 times more efficient than flame atomization. All biological samples require some sort of pretreatment prior to instrumental analysis such as dilution with deionized water or addition of certain salt solution or precipitation of proteins with trichloroacetic acid for serum, plasma, and urine. Hair nails and tissues must be solubilized by wet or dry ashing.

The procedures for extraction/isolation for analysis of metallic poisons in different biological materials are shown in a flowchart manner, which can be of handy reference for student/analyst/scientist/forensic toxicologist.

Wet Digestion Method

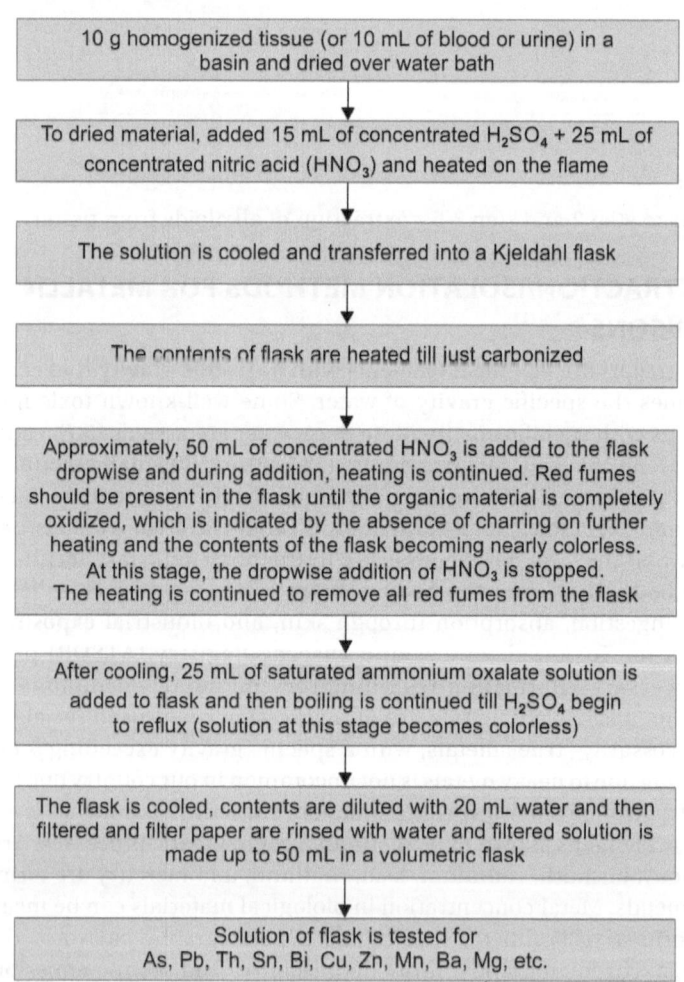

Dry Ashing Method

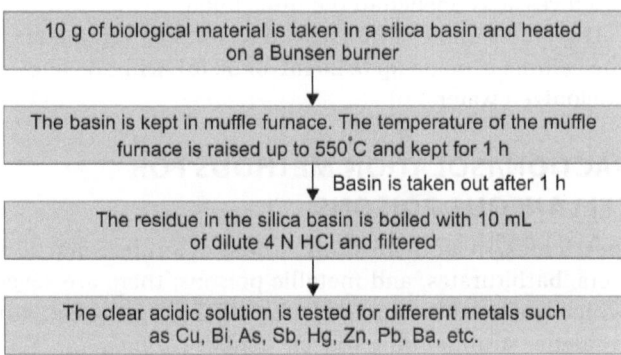

Microwave Digestion Method

Digestion of sample in microwave is very easy. The steps in this process are:
- *Step 1*: Vessels are cleaned with 1:1 HNO_3: water mixture and dried
- *Step 2*: The sample is taken into the liner vessel
- *Step 3*: 15 mL HNO_3 (concentration depending on the sample) is added to each vessel inside the fume hood to allow the sample to outgas and then the vessels are sealed
- *Step 4*: In the reference vessel, 1 mL of water (instead of sample) is added along with 15 mL HNO_3 for sample blank
- *Step 5*: Vessel carrousels are loaded in the microwave digestion oven and the microwave is run with various programs specific for different substances as mentioned in **Table 3.1**

Table 3.1: Temperature program for digestion of biological sample with microwave digester.

Samples	Concentration of nitric acid (HNO_3) required (%)	Sample required	Step	Time required (seconds)	Starting temperature (°C)	Ending temperature (°C)
Blood	50	1 mL	1	210	28	100
			2	600	100	160
			3	600	160	170
Tissue	50	1 g	1	200	28	120
			2	600	120	180
			3	600	180	200
Urine	50	5 mL	1	200	28	100
			2	400	100	160
			3	400	160	170
Hair	70	0.1 g	1	300	28	100
			2	700	100	160
			3	700	160	170
Nail	70	0.1 g	1	300	28	100
			2	700	100	160
			3	700	160	170

- *Step 6*: After digestion, the liner vessels are allowed to cool down and then, each vessel is opened in the fume hood
- *Step 7*: Digested sample is transferred to suitable volumetric flask and then the volume is made up to 20 mL or 50 mL with the help of milli-Q water/deionized water

■ EXTRACTION/ISOLATION METHODS FOR MISCELLANEOUS POISONS

Besides pesticides/insecticides, alkaloids, cyanide, volatile poisons, tranquilizers, barbiturates, and metallic poisons, there are several other poisons which are used for homicidal/suicidal purpose, e.g., turpentine oil, naphthalene, sulfonamide, *Croton tiglium (Jamalgota)*, *Semecarpus anacardium* (Bhilawa or marking nut), oduvan (*Cleistanthus collinus*), colocynth (indrayani or bitter apple), ergot, *Calotropis gigantica* and *Calotropis procera* (madar, akdo), mushrooms, nicotine, antibiotics, kaner, cresol, nitrobenzene, aniline, and kerosene oil. In any toxicological analysis, the most important step is the sample preparation. Procedures for extraction/isolation of the miscellaneous compounds in different biological materials are given in a flowchart manner, which can be of handy reference for student/analyst/scientist/forensic toxicologist.

Extraction/Isolation of Turpentine Oil

Turpentine oil is colorless oily liquid having a peculiar odor. It is insoluble in water but soluble in organic solvents such as alcohol, ether, and chloroform. It is largely used in varnish and paints. It is extracted from biological material as follows:

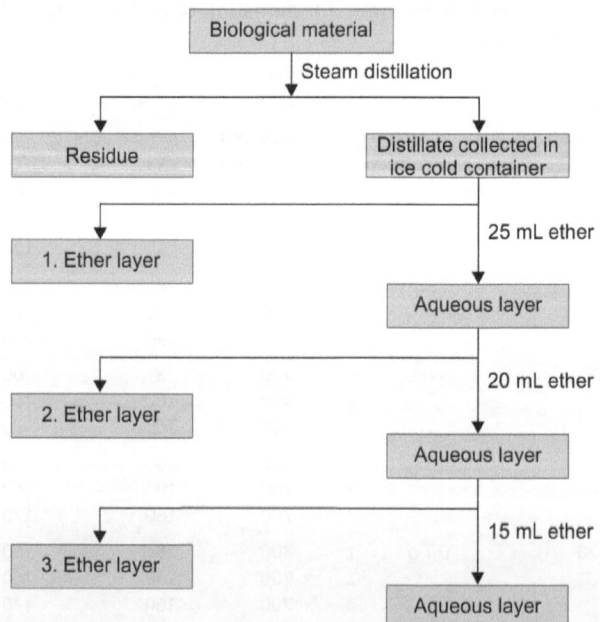

Ether layers 1, 2, and 3 are pooled and evaporated at room temperature leaving oil of turpentine. The clear active extract is concentrated in a boiling water bath or by nitrogen gas.

Extraction/Isolation of Naphthalene

It is isolated by distillation. The distillate is extracted with ether or other organic solvent and solvent is removed by evaporation. Extraction process will be same as isolation of turpentine oil.

Extraction/Isolation of Sulfonamides

Sulfonamides are commonly used in medicines due to their bacteriostatic or bactericidal action. The use of sulfonamide for a prolonged period or its use in large dose produces toxic effects and may also cause death. In some cases, due to idiosyncrasy, the administration of even small doses for a short period may produce toxicity.

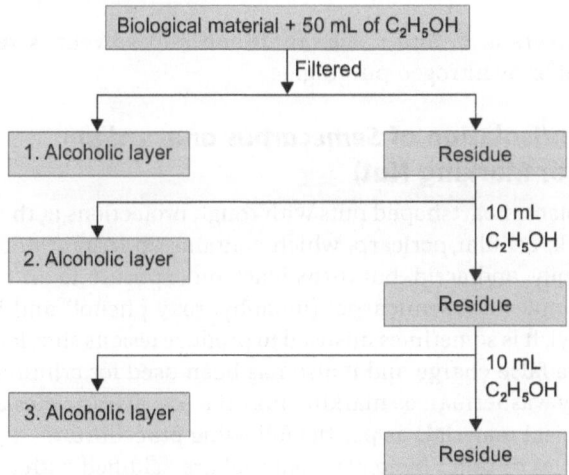

Alcoholic layers 1, 2, and 3 are pooled and dried up to dryness. Add 25 mL of acetone and concentrated, which is ready for analysis.

Extraction/Isolation of *Croton tiglium (Jamalgota)*

The seeds of *Croton* contain crotin, a toxalbumin which is not expressed with the oil. The seeds as well as oil are highly poisonous. The oil is brown, viscous, has unpleasant odor and acrid, and has burning taste. Seeds are oval, dark brown with longitudinal lines. Crotonoside, a glycoside, which is less poisonous, is also present. The oil contains a powerful vesicating resin composed of crotonic acid, methylcrotonic acid, and several other fatty acids. Poisoning is usually accidental. The root and oil are sometimes taken internally as an abortifacient. The seeds are mostly used in the indigenous system of medicine. In case of poisoning by seed, active principle crotin is isolated by ether from the aqueous acidic solution as for barbiturates. Alternatively, it is extracted as shown below.

EXTRACTION/ISOLATION AND CLEAN-UP METHODS

Biological material acidified with tartaric acid and 50 mL of ether, stirred slowly for 2 minutes

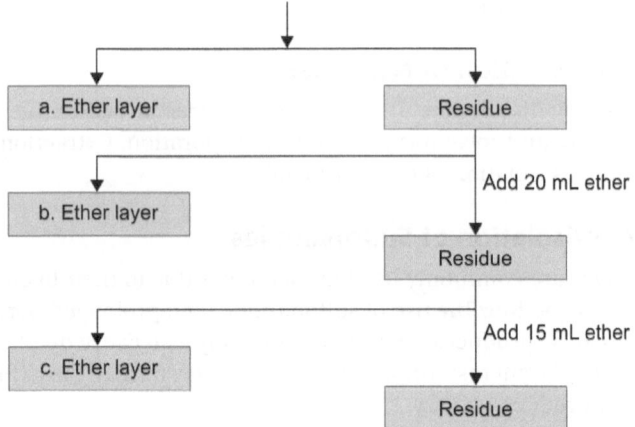

Ether layers a, b, and c are combined and solvent is removed by evaporation or by nitrogen purging.

Extraction/Isolation of *Semecarpus anacardium* (Bhilawa or Marking Nut)

These are black, heartshaped nuts with rough projections at the base. They have a thick, cellular pericarp, which contains an irritant juice, which is brownish, oily, and acrid, but turns black on exposure to air or lime. The active principles are semicarpol (monohydroxy phenol) and bhilawanol (odihydroxy). It is sometimes misused to produce lesions simulating bruises to support a false charge and it also has been used for criminal abortion. It is used by washerman as marking ink. The active principles are isolated from biological materials as per the following procedure.

The tissues or other biological material are acidified with acetic acid + 50 mL C_2H_5OH and shaken well.

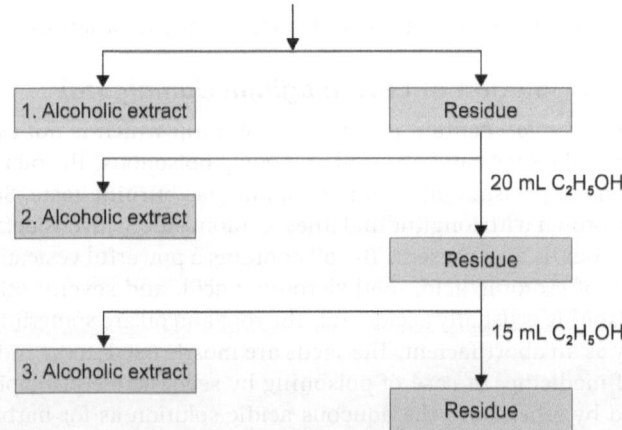

Alcoholic extracts 1, 2, and 3 are combined and evaporated till dryness + 25 mL 1 N H_2SO_4 + 25 mL petroleum ether.

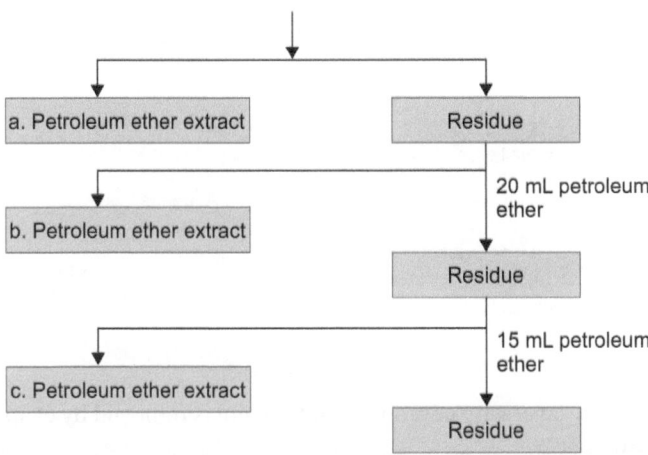

The petroleum ether extracts are combined and concentrated.

Extraction/Isolation of Oduvan *(Cleistanthus collinus)*

The leaves and barks of this plant are commonly used for the purpose of homicide or suicide. The active principle of this plant, which owes its poisonous properties, is a glycoside oduvan. It is also known as fish poison. It is isolated by the following procedure.

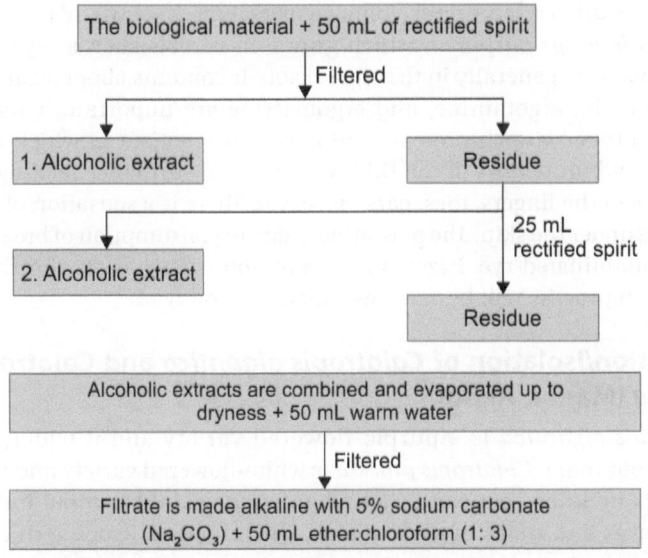

EXTRACTION/ISOLATION AND CLEAN-UP METHODS

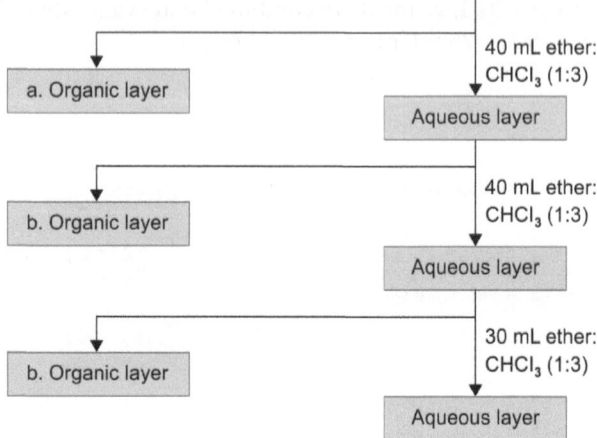

The organic layers are combined and solvent is removed by evaporation and tested.

Extraction/Isolation of Colocynth (Indrayani or Bitter Apple)

The root and the fruit of the plant *Citrullus colocynthis* contain a poisonous glycoside colocynthin. It is a purgative and acts as a powerful irritant to the alimentary canal, when ingested in a large dose. Extraction process will be same as isolation of oduvan.

Extraction/Isolation of Ergot

Ergot is the dried sclerotinum (compact mycelium or spawn) of the parasitic fungus *Claviceps purpurea*, which grows on cereals such as rye, barley, wheat, oat, etc., generally in the wet season. It contains about 30 alkaloids, but ergotoxin, ergotamine, and ergometrine are important, which owe its toxic properties. Chronic poisoning causes ergotism in which there is tingling and numbness of the skin; vasomotor disturbance leading to dry gangrene of the fingers, toes, ears, nose, etc. There is a sensation of insects creeping under the skin. The poisoning is due to consumption of bread made with contaminated rye. Ergot is also commonly used as an abortifacient. Extraction process will be same as isolation of oduvan.

Extraction/Isolation of *Calotropis gigantica* and *Calotropis procera* (Madar, Akdo)

Calotropis gigantica is a purple-flowered variety and it widely grows throughout India. *Calotropis procera* is white-flowered variety and it grows generally in desert, but can be found growing wild throughout India. The fresh leaves and stalks of these plants, when incised, exude a thick acrid milky juice, which is a powerful irritant and is highly toxic. It is used as cattle poison, for criminal abortion, and rarely for infanticide. Extraction process will be same as isolation of oduvan.

Extraction/Isolation of Mushrooms

Amanita phalloides and *Amanita muscaria* are the common varieties of poisonous fungi. *Amanita muscaria* grows singly in sandy soil and is of large size. It contains an alkaloid *muscarine*, the action of which resembles stimulation of parasympathetic postganglionic nerves. *Amanita phalloides* is also called the deadly agaric or dead cap. It grows in woody places to a height of 15–20 cm. The fungus is a powerful poison and contains phalloidin, phallon, and bamnatin, which are cyclopeptides. These polypeptides are heat stable and insoluble in water. They are cyclotoxic. Poisoning is usually accidental.

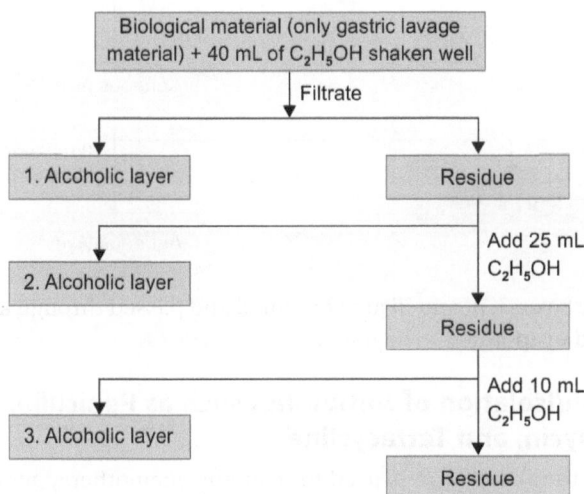

Alcoholic layers 1, 2, and 3 are pooled and dried up to dryness. The residue is dissolved in acetone and tested.

Extraction/Isolation of Nicotine

Nicotine is cardiac poison. It exists in all parts of tobacco plant, mainly in leaves which contain 0.6–8% of nicotine in combination with malic and citric acid. It is colorless, volatile, and hygroscopic alkaloid and turns brown on exposure to air. It has burning acrid taste and a penetrating disagreeable odor. It is soluble in water, alcohol, and ether. It is a common drug of abuse through smoking or chewing. It first stimulates and then paralyzes the cerebral and spinal centers. In smaller doses, it contracts the pupil, but when toxic symptoms develop it dilates them.

EXTRACTION/ISOLATION AND CLEAN-UP METHODS

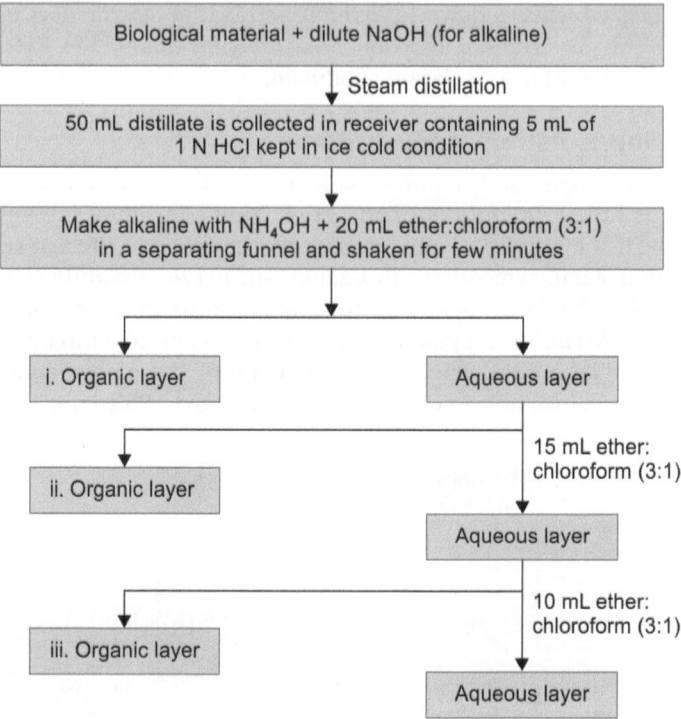

Organic layers i, ii, and iii are combined and passed through anhydrous Na_2SO_4 and evaporated to dryness.

Extraction/Isolation of Antibiotics such as Penicillin, Streptomycin, and Tetracycline

In modern time, this term is used to refer any chemotherapeutic agent or antimicrobial agent with activity against microorganisms such as bacteria, fungi, and protozoa. For example, penicillin class is produced by fungi from genus *Penicillium* or streptomycin from bacteria of genus *Streptomyces*. It can be classified as bactericidal or bacteriostatic. Bactericidal kills bacteria directly, while bacteriostatic prevents them from dividing. Its adverse effects can range from fever and nausea to major allergic reactions including photodermatitis. Commonly, it causes diarrhea. Streptomycin was the first antibiotic remedy for tuberculosis. It kills sensitive microbes by hurting cell membranes and inhibiting protein synthesis. This prevents initiation of protein synthesis and leads to death of microbial cells.

Macerated tissues + 5 mL of 0.1 N NaOH in a beaker and left for 24 hours

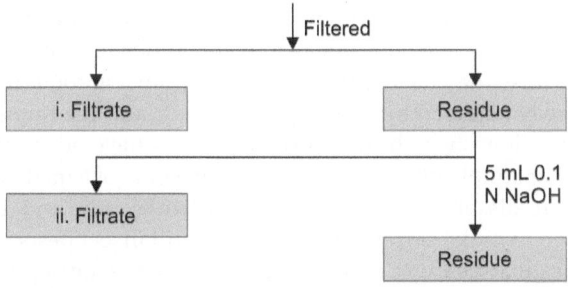

Filtrates are pooled and evaporated up to 1 mL and tested.

Extraction/Isolation of Kaner

There are two types of kaner namely white oleander and yellow oleander whose biological names are *Nerium odorum* and *Cerebera thevetia*, respectively. These are cardiotoxic poisons. Yellow oleander grows in temperate region throughout the world. These grow in larger shrubs usually 2.5–3.5 m tall. These contain chemicals called cardiac glycosides. The flowers are sweet perfumed, funnel shaped, bright yellow, or peach in color, 5.5–7 cm long. Leaves are glossy green, strap-like, and 5.5–15 cm long. Fruit is angular, green when immature and black after ripening.

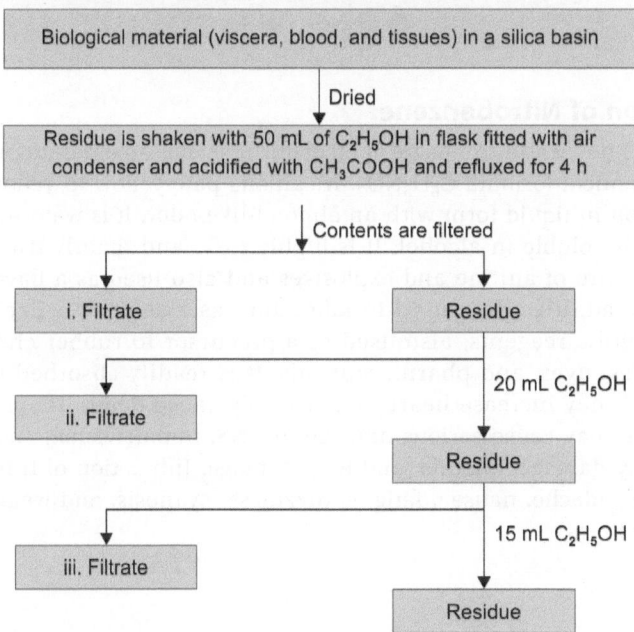

Filtrates i, ii, and iii are pooled and evaporated up to 1 mL.

Extraction/Isolation of Cresol

It is an organic compound which is methylphenol. It has methyl group substituted onto the benzene ring of a phenol molecule. They can be solid or liquid because they have different melting points at room temperature. They are slowly oxidized by long exposure to air and the impurities often give them a yellowish- to brownishred tint. They have odor characteristic to that of other simple phenols, reminiscent to some of a medicine smell. It can be used to dissolve other chemicals as disinfectants and deodorizers. They are used to make certain chemicals that kill insect pests and are also used as household cleaners. Its solution is also used as antiseptic in surgery. They are found in many foods and in wood and tobacco smoke, crude oil, coal tar, etc. Low level exposure to cresols is not harmful, but at high level, it induces irritation and burning of eyes, skin, mouth and throat, abdominal pain and vomiting, heart damage, anemia, liver and kidney damage, facial paralysis, coma, and death.

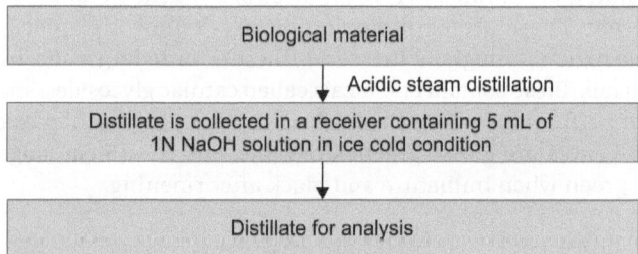

Isolation of Nitrobenzene

It is also known as nitrobenzol or oil of mirbane. It is an organic compound with chemical formula $C_6H_5NO_2$. It exhibits pale yellow to yellowbrown coloration in liquid form with an almond-like odor. It is water-insoluble oil, but is soluble in alcohol. It is highly toxic and mainly used in the manufacture of aniline and explosives and also used as a flavoring or perfume additive. It is used in laboratory as a solvent, especially for electrophilic reagents, also used as a precursor to rubber chemicals, pesticides, dyes, and pharmaceuticals. It is readily absorbed through skin and may increase heart rate or rarely cause death. Its prolonged exposure may cause serious damage to CNS, impair vision, cause liver or kidney damage, anemia, and lung damage. Inhalation of fumes may induce headache, nausea, fatigue, dizziness, cyanosis, and weakness in arms and legs.

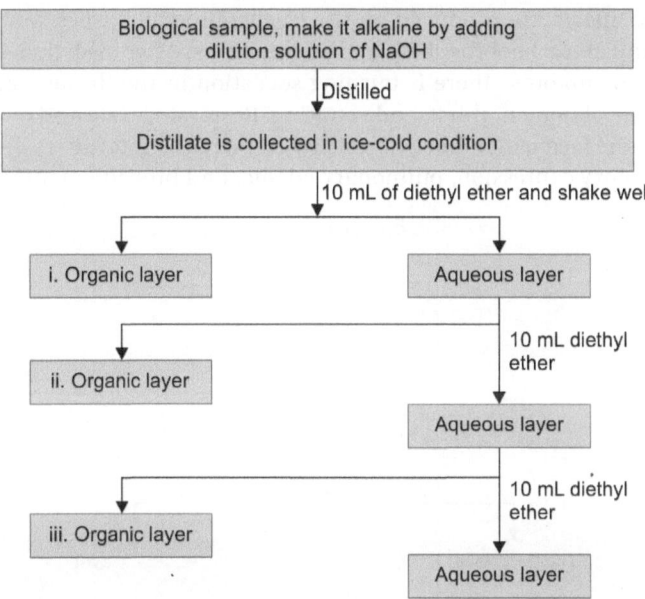

Organic layers i, ii, and iii are combined and passed through anhydrous Na_2SO_4 which is preserved for analysis.

Isolation of Aniline

Aniline, phenylamine, or aminobenzene is an organic compound with the formula C_6H_7N. It is a coal tar derivative and is prepared by nitrobenzene by means of nascent hydrogen. Its main application is in the manufacturing of polyurethane. It possesses unpleasant odor of rotten fish and also has a burning taste; it is highly acrid poison. It ignites readily and burn with smoky flame. It hardly dissolves in water, but dissolves freely in alcohol, ether, and chloroform. It is used for marking aniline dyes for printing and cloth making inks and also in rubber industry. In addition to this, it is also a starting product for the manufacture of many drugs such as paracetamol. It is toxic by inhalation of vapor and absorption through the skin or swallowing. It causes headache, drowsiness, cyanosis, and mental confusion and in severe cases can cause convulsions. Prolonged exposure to the vapor or slight skin exposure over a period of time affects the nervous system and the blood, causing tiredness, loss of appetite, headache, and dizziness.

Isolation method is same as for nitrobenzene.

Isolation of Kerosene Oil

It is a refined product of petroleum oil, prepared by fractionation of crude petroleum oil. It contains aromatic, aliphatic, and variety of branched and unsaturated hydrocarbons. It is used as illuminating fuel, heating fuel, motor fuel, and vehicle for many pesticides and cleaning agents. When it is inhaled, the toxic effects are produced on the tracheobronchial trees resulting in the chemical tracheobronchitis and pneumonitis. After ingestion, it shows irritative symptoms. There is burning sensation in the throat along with pain in the abdomen, thirst, and vomiting. Respiratory rate and pulse slow down as the face pallor and cyanosis go on increasing. It causes death due to respiratory expression, pulmonary edema, and bronchopneumonia.

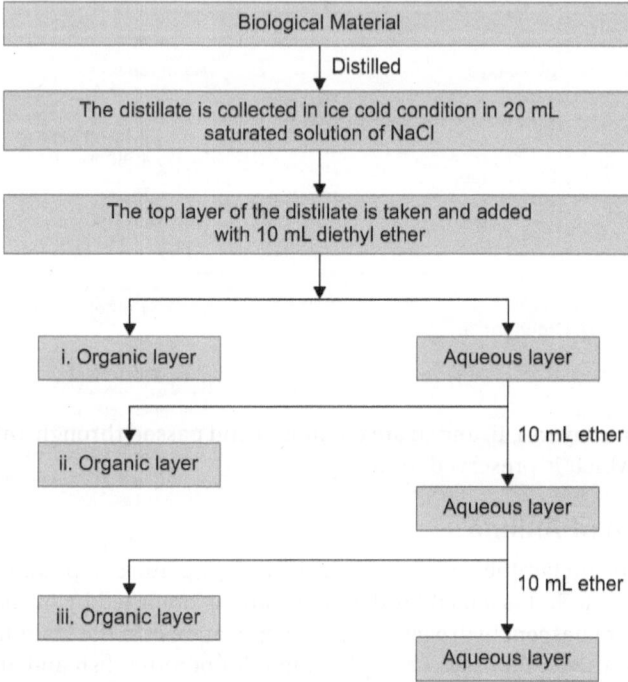

Organic layers i, ii, and iii are pooled and passed through anhydrous Na_2SO_4, evaporated at room temperature, and preserved for test.

■ CONCLUSION

In any analysis of poison/chemicals, sample preparation is the most vital step. The result of the analytical methods depends on the amount and purity of the sample extracted/isolated. There is no single extraction method applicable to all poisons/chemicals. Every poison has to be extracted using the best suitable extraction method. It is important for the forensic toxicologists/scientists to know the best available method and help to detect the poison/chemicals in the crime investigation. In this chapter the procedure of extraction/isolation for pesticides/insecticides, volatile poisons, tranquilizers, barbiturates, alkaloids, metallic poisons, etc., from biological material has been discussed in a flow chart manner which can be handy reference for student/analyst/scientist/toxicologist in day today work. The extraction techniques have been developed after repeated trial and testing. The techniques are being improved every time.

FURTHER READINGS

1. Ballantyne B, Marrs TC, Syversen T. General and Applied Toxicology, 2nd edition. London: Macmillan Press Ltd.; 2000. pp. 214553.
2. Bamford E. Poisons, Their Isolation and Identification, 1st edition. London: J and A Churchill; 1947.
3. Brookes VJ, Alyea HN. Poisons Identification and Treatment. New York: D. Van Nostrand Company, Inc.; 1946.
4. Chevers N. Manual of Medical Jurisprudence for India, 1st edition. Philadelphia: Saunders; 1902.
5. Clarke EGC, Moffat AC. Clarke's Isolation and Identification of Drugs: In Pharmaceuticals, Body Fluids and Post Mortem Material, 2nd edition. London: Pharmaceutical Press; 1986.
6. Curry AS. Analytical Methods in Human Toxicology, 1st edition. London: Macmillan Press Ltd.; 1985. pp. 24950.
7. Kakani SL. DFS Manual of Toxicology, 1st edition. New Delhi: Selective and Scientific Publishers; 2005. pp. 5990.
8. Frear DEH. Chemistry of Insecticides, Fungicides and Herbicides. New York: D. Van Nostrand Company, Inc.; 1948.
9. Jaiswal AK, Kashyap SK, Gupta M, Mewar SK, Rana SVS. Analysis of dimethoate in viscera sample using HPTLC plates. Amity J Behav Forensic Sci. 2006;2(2):8590.
10. Jaiswal AK, Millo T, Murthy OP. Toxicology Manual Series: Article–I, Extraction/Isolation and Cleanup methods for Pesticides/Insecticides and Alkaloids. Int J Med Tox Leg Med. 2006;9(1):2832.
11. Jaiswal AK, Millo T, Murthy OP. Toxicology Manual Series: Article–II, Extraction/Isolation and Cleanup Methods for Barbiturates and Tranquilizers from Biological Material. Int J Med Tox Leg Med. 2007;9(2):1721.
12. Jaiswal AK, Millo T, Murthy OP. Toxicology Manual Series: Article–III Extraction/Isolation methods for Metallic, Volatile and Cyanide poisons from Biological Samples. Int J Med Tox Leg Med. 2007;10(1):302.
13. Jaiswal AK, Millo T, Murthy OP. Toxicology Manual Series: Article–IV Extraction/Isolation methods for miscellaneous poisons from Biological Samples. Int J Med Tox Leg Med. 2008;10(2):225.
14. Jaiswal AK, Millo T, Murthy OP. Toxicology Manual Series: Article–V Extraction/Isolation methods for miscellaneous poisons from Biological Samples. Int J Med Tox Leg Med. 2008;11(1):4852.
15. Jickells S, Negrusz A. Clark's Analytical Toxicology, 1st edition. London: Pharmaceutical Press; 2008. pp. 1908.
16. Lesche EM. Clinical Toxicology, 1st edition. London: J and A Churchill; 1934.
17. Mathiharan K, Patnaik AK. Modi's Medical Jurisprudence and Toxicology, 23rd edition. New Delhi: Lexis Nexis; 2005. pp. 107216.
18. Reddy NKS, Murty OP. The Essentials of Forensic Medicine and Toxicology, 17th edition. New Delhi: Jaypee Brothers Medical Publishers (P) Ltd.; 1997. pp. 449-51.
19. Patty FA. Industrial Hygiene and Toxicology. New York: Interscience Publisher Inc.; 1948.
20. Pillay VV. Comprehensive Medical Toxicology, 2nd edition. Hyderabad: Paras Medical Publishers; 2008. pp. 4378.
21. Proceedings of National Workshop on Practical and Emergency Medical Toxicology. New Delhi: All India Institute of Medical Sciences; 1998.
22. Tiwari SN. Manual of Toxicology, 1st edition. Agra: Forensic Science Laboratory; 1976.
23. Withaus RA. Manual of Toxicology, 1st edition. London: Bailliere, Tindall & Cox; 1911.

Chapter 4

Screening/Spot/Color Tests for Different Poisons

■ SCREENING/SPOT/COLOR TESTS FOR PESTICIDES/INSECTICIDES

Organophosphorus compounds (OP) such as dichlorvos, naled, phosphamidon, phosphinon, phosdrin, bidrin, birlane, gardona, dimefox, mipafox, avenin, cyolane, parathion, methyl parathion, paraoxon, thiophos ME, fenitrothion, chlorothion, dicapthon, ronnel, bromophos, fenthion, dasanit, diazinon, demeton, methyldemeton, dursban, potasan, vamidothion, acetophos, chlorpyrifos, malathion, dimethoate, morphothion, formothion, thimet, ethion, ekatin, disyston, tetrathion, phosalone, imidan, guthion, monazon, edifenphos, trichlorfon, EPN, etc. *Organochloro compound (OC)* such as dichlorodiphenyltrichloroethane (DDT), benzene hexachloride (BHC), lindane, endrin, dieldrin, endosulfan, heptox, chlordane, toxaphene, kelthane, heptachlor, methoxychlor, etc. *Carbamates* such as propoxur, carbaryl, *carbofuran* and zineb, etc. and *pyrethroids* such as fenvalerate, permethrin, cyfluthrin, deltamethrin, fenpropathrin, bifenthrin, etc., are isolated from biological materials by solvent extraction method. Detailed method for isolation/extraction from different biological samples has been discussed in Chapter 3. After extraction/isolation, the next step is screening/color test of individual poisons. Therefore, in the present section of the chapter, an attempt has been made to set out standard procedure for screening/spot/color test for *organophosphorus compound (OP), organochloro compound (OC), carbamates, pyrethroids* and some individual pesticides such as DDT, BHC, endrin, dieldrin, aldrin endosulfan, carbaryl, deltamethrin, malathion, *parathion*, mevinphos, sumithion, dimethyldichlorovinylphosphate (DDVP), clofenotane, diazinon/dimethoate, methoxychlor, aluminum/zinc phosphide, etc., in a stepwise manner which can be of handy reference to student/analyst/scientist/forensic toxicologist.

Organophosphorus Pesticides/Insecticides
Ammonium Molybdate Test
1. A portion of the acetone extract is taken into a test tube and the solvent is evaporated completely by immersing the tube in a water bath.

2. 2 mL of 6% freshly prepared ammonium persulfate solution is added into the tube and heated in a water bath for 10 minutes.
3. The tube is cooled rapidly in an ice bath, and 3 mL of 1.5% aqueous solution of urea is added and the tube is again kept in the water bath for 5 minutes.
4. After cooling, 1 mL of 5% ammonium molybdate in 10 N sulfuric acid is added.
5. The mixture is shaken well and 1 mL of 2% aqueous solution of ascorbic acid is added to the mixture and the tube is kept in the water bath for 1 minute.
6. Blue color indicates the presence of phosphorus.

Potassium Hydroxide Test
1. A fraction of extracted residue is taken in 1 mL of ethanol in a micro crucible.
2. 1 mL of 10% potassium hydroxide solution is added and heated.
3. Formation of bright yellow color indicates the presence of some p-nitrophenyl derivative such as ethyl parathion, methyl parathion, sunithion, paraoxon or chlorthion.

Organochloro Insecticides
Sulfuric Acid Test
1. A portion of extracted residue is taken in a minimum volume of toluene.
2. Two drops of fuming sulfuric acid reagent are added to it.
3. Red color is observed, which indicates the presence of organochlorine pesticides.

Carbamates Pesticides
Hydrochloric Acid Test
1. The extracted residue is dissolved in a few drops of ethyl alcohol.
2. A portion of it is applied as a spot on a piece of Whatman® No. 41 paper.
3. After drying, one drop of furfural is poured over it and dried again.
4. The spotted paper is then exposed to the vapors of hydrochloric acid.
5. A steel blue-colored spot is produced, which shows the presence of carbamate.

Pyrethroids
2-(2-aminoethylamino) Ethanol Test
1. A portion of residue is taken in a test tube.
2. 2-(2-aminoethylamino) ethanol in ethanol is added to it.
3. Equal volume of alcoholic potassium hydroxide is added to it.
4. Sulfur red color is obtained, which shows the presence of pyrethroids.

TEST FOR SOME INDIVIDUAL PESTICIDES

Parathion

Silver Nitrate–Naphthylethylenediamine Dihydrochloride Test

1. A portion of extracted residue is placed in a micro crucible with 5 mL of alcohol in it.
2. 10 mL of water and 2 g of paraffin wax followed by 2 mL of 5N hydrochloric acid are added to it.
3. 0.5 g of zinc powder is added to it.
4. The contents are heated under condenser on a water bath for 10 minutes.
5. Contents are cooled in an ice bath to solidify the paraffin and filtered.
6. Residual zinc dust and wax are washed three times with 5 mL of distilled water and the filtrate and washings are combined.
7. Clear combined liquid is cooled in an ice bath and to it is added 1 mL of 0.25% sodium nitrite solution.
8. After 10 minutes, 2 mL of 1% aqueous N-1-naphthylethylenediamine dihydrochloride is added.
9. Magenta dye is formed, which shows the presence of parathion.

O-Cresol Test

1. A portion of extracted residue is heated with 1 mL of 5N sodium hydroxide solution in a micro crucible.
2. Yellow color is obtained due to the hydrolysis of parathion to p-nitrophenol.
3. Solution is acidified with 2 mL of 5N hydrochloric acid.
4. 0.5 g of zinc dust is added and heated for 10 minutes.
5. Contents are cooled and made alkaline with excess of 5N sodium hydroxide and few drops of ammonium hydroxide are added to it.
6. After cooling, 1 mL of o-cresol is added to it.
7. A blue-colored dye is formed, which shows the presence of parathion.

Palladium Chloride Test

1. A portion of extracted residue is taken in a micro crucible.
2. 5 mL of alcohol is added to it.
3. 1 mL of palladium chloride is added to it.
4. Contents are heated in a water bath for 2 minutes.
5. Brown color is obtained which shows the presence of parathion.

Ammonium Molybdate Test

1. A portion of extracted residue is taken in a micro crucible.
2. 0.5 mL of nitric and 0.2 mL of sulfuric acid is added to it.
3. Contents are heated in water bath for 30 minutes.
4. 1 mL of 10% ammonium molybdate is added to it.
5. Contents are heated for another 5 minutes.
6. Yellow color is obtained, which shows the presence of parathion.

Malathion
Carbon Tetrachloride Test
1. 1 mL of extract is taken in a test tube.
2. 2 mL of carbon tetrachloride is added to it.
3. 1 mL of 10% ethanolic potassium hydroxide solution is added to it.
4. 1 mL of 1% copper sulfate solution is added to it and shaken for 1 minute.
5. Yellow color is formed in the carbon tetrachloride layer which shows the presence of malathion.

Palladium Chloride Test
Same as discussed for parathion.

Ammonium Molybdate Test
Same as discussed for parathion.

Sodium Nitroprusside Test
1. A portion of extracted residue is taken in a micro crucible.
2. Minimum volume of 2M sodium hydroxide is added to it.
3. Solution is evaporated to dryness.
4. Two drops of water are added to it.
5. 0.5 mL of sodium nitroprusside reagent is added to it.
6. Violet color is observed, which shows the presence of malathion.

Sumithion
Sodium Hydroxide Test
1. A portion of extracted residue is taken in a micro crucible.
2. 1 mL of alcohol is added to it.
3. Few drops of 10% sodium hydroxide solution are added and heated for a minute.
4. Yellow color is obtained, which shows the presence of sumithion.

DDVP
Carbon Tetrachloride–Carbon Disulfide Test
1. A portion of extracted residue is taken in a test tube and 1 mL of alcohol is added to it.
2. 1 mL of 5% aqueous sodium hydroxide solution is added.
3. Keep it in the ice bath for 30 minutes and shake the solution for 3 minutes.
4. 25 mL of carbon tetrachloride and 15 mL of ethanol are added.
5. 25 mL of distilled water is added followed by 5 mL of carbon disulfide.
6. Yellow color is obtained in the aqueous layer which shows the presence of DDVP.

SCREENING/SPOT/COLOR TESTS FOR DIFFERENT POISONS

Dinitrophenyl Hydrazine Test
1. A portion of extracted residue is taken in 1 mL of water in a test tube.
2. 3.5 mL of borate barbiturate buffer solution (pH = 9) is added to it.
3. 0.5 mL of 0.05 M glycine is added to it.
4. Transfer the solution in a hard glass tube having loosely fitted stopper.
5. Tube is kept in a water bath for 3 hours.
6. 1 mL of 6 N hydrochloric acid and 1.5 mL of saturated solution of 2, 4-dinitro phenyl-hydrazine in methanol is added.
7. The solution is kept in a boiling water bath for 5 min and cooled.
8. 2.5 mL of 10% methanolic potassium hydroxide is added.
9. Violet color is obtained, which confirms the presence of DDVP.

Clofenotane
Liebermann's Test
1. A portion of residue is taken on white tile.
2. 2–3 drops of Liebermann's reagent are added to it.
3. Brown color is obtained which shows the presence of clofenotane.

Potassium Hydroxide Test
1. A fraction of extracted residue is taken in 1 mL of ethanol in a micro crucible.
2. A pellet of potassium hydroxide is added to it and evaporated to dryness.
3. 0.5 mL of water and 1 mL of carbon tetrachloride are added to the residue.
4. Solution is shaken well and allowed for separation of the layers.
5. Lower layer of carbon tetrachloride is decanted.
6. 1 mL of Erdmann's reagent is added to it.
7. Play-of-color is observed from red to orange, and finally to green in the acid layer, which shows the presence of clofenotane.

Diazinon/Dimethoate
Silver Nitrate–Naphthylethylenediamine Hydrochloride Test
1. A portion of extracted residue is taken in a micro crucible.
2. 5 mL of alcohol is added to it.
3. 10 mL of water and 2 g of paraffin wax followed by 2 mL of 5 N HCl are added to it.
4. 0.5 g of zinc powder is added to it.
5. The contents are heated under condenser on water bath for 5–10 minutes.
6. The contents are cooled in an ice bath to solidify the paraffin and filtered.
7. Residual zinc dust and wax are washed three times with 5 mL of distilled water, and the filtrate washing is combined.
8. Clear combined liquid is cooled in an ice bath and 1 mL of 0.25% sodium nitrite solution is added to it.

9. After 5–10 min, 2 mL of 1% aqueous N-1-naphthylethylenediamine dihydrochloride is added to it.
10. Magenta dye is formed, which shows the presence of diazinon.

Ammonium Molybdate Test
Same as discussed for Parathion.

DDT
Hydroquinone Test
1. A portion of residue is taken in a test tube.
2. 1 mL of 0.5% solution of hydroquinone acid is added to it.
3. A wine red color obtained shows the presence of DDT.

Xanthydrol Test
1. An area of about 12 square inches of the surface thought to contain DDT is thoroughly scrubbed with the oil-impregnated swab.
2. A test tube is then inserted into the hydroxide bottle and two pellets are picked up on the lip and allowed to slide to the bottom.
3. The bottle is immediately recapped to avoid absorption of moisture.
4. 2 mL of 0.4% xanthydrol in pyrimidine are added to the tube with the help of a pipette.
5. Tube is heated on a water bath.
6. When the contents turn green, the swab is inserted and the tube is again heated for a few seconds.
7. Red color is obtained which shows the presence of DDT.

Potassium Hydroxide Test
1. A portion of extracted residue suspected to contain DDT is taken in 1 mL of n-hexane and transferred into a hard glass tube.
2. Tube is kept in a boiling water bath for 10 minutes.
3. Dried residue in the tube is then cooled in an ice bath.
4. 10 mL of chilled nitrating mixture consisting of concentrated nitric acid and sulfuric acid is added to it.
5. Tube is then placed in a hot water bath and heating is continued for 1 hour.
6. After cooling, the liquid is diluted with 50 mL of ice cold water and transferred to a separating funnel.
7. It is extracted thrice with 10 mL portions of chloroform.
8. Chloroform layers are combined and washed with 50 mL of 1% potassium hydroxide solution and three times with 50 mL portions of distilled water.
9. Chloroform layer is then passed through anhydrous sodium sulfate and the contents are evaporated upto dryness.
10. Residue is taken with few drops of chloroform and transferred into two separate spots on a white tile and chloroform is evaporated off.

11. To one spot, one drop of a 20% alcoholic potassium hydroxide solution is added.
12. A play-of-colors from rose to bright blue to green to yellow is observed, which shows the presence of DDT.

Aluminum Chloride Test
1. A small portion of extracted residue is taken in a test tube.
2. 5 mL of chlorobenzene is added to it.
3. Warm the test tube gently and filtered the solution.
4. 0.1 g of anhydrous aluminum chloride is added to it.
5. A red to deep violet color is obtained depending upon the concentration of DDT.

Endrin
Sulfuric Acid Test
1. Extracted residue is taken in a test tube and few drops of n-hexane are added to it.
2. Few drops of concentrated sulfuric acid are added.
3. A red-color is obtained, which shows the presence of endrin.

Phenyl Azide-sulfanilic Acid Test
1. Extracted residue is taken in a test tube and treated with sodium metal in the presence of isopropyl alcohol.
2. The product is taken into methyl alcohol and then treated with phenyl azide.
3. After the reaction the mixture is treated with diazotized sulfanilic acid in acidic medium.
4. A red colored complex is obtained, which shows the presence of endrin.

Potassium Hydroxide Test
1. A portion of the extracted residue is nitrated with nitrating mixture.
2. The product is then extracted with chloroform.
3. Solution is evaporated till dryness.
4. Residue is taken in a few drops of cyclohexane.
5. A few drops of 1% alcoholic potassium hydroxide are added to it.
6. A violet color slowly changing to brown, and finally to yellow, shows the presence of endrin.

BHC/Lindane
Vanadium Reagent Test
1. The extracted residue is taken in 1 mL of petroleum ether and transferred to a flask and solvent is removed by evaporation.
2. 2 mL of purified aniline is added and refluxed for 1–2 hours vigorously on a boiling water bath, then cooled at room temperature and transferred to 250 mL separating funnel.

3. 50 mL of 3 N HCl is added, followed by 50 mL of distilled water addition.
4. 20 mL of ether is added to it and extracted.
5. Ether layer is combined and passed through anhydrous sodium sulfate and evaporated to about 1 mL and finally upto dryness.
6. 4–5 drops of pentane are added to dissolve the residue.
7. 10 mL of sulfuric acid is added followed by Vanadium reagent.
8. Violet color is produced which shows the presence of BHC.

Ethylmethyl Ketone Test

1. The extracted residue containing BHC is treated with dichloromethane dissolved in acetic acid.
2. 0.5 g of zinc powder is added to it.
3. The dichlorination takes place forming free benzene, which is nitrated with nitrating mixture.
4. The mixture is cooled and diluted with ice cold water.
5. Extracted thrice with 10 mL portions of chloroform.
6. Chloroform extracts are evaporated to dryness.
7. Residue is taken into 5 mL of ethyl methyl ketone.
8. 5 mL of 10% NaOH is added to it.
9. Red color is formed which shows the presence of BHC.

Methoxychlor

Liebermann's Test

1. A portion of residue is taken on a white tile.
2. 2–3 drops of Liebermann's reagent are added to it.
3. Black-violet color is obtained which shows the presence of methoxychlor.

Dieldrin/Aldrin

Carbon Tetrachloride Test

1. A fraction of extracted residue is taken in 1 mL of ethanol in a micro crucible.
2. A pellet of potassium hydroxide is added to it and evaporated to dryness.
3. 0.5 mL of water and 1 mL of carbon tetrachloride are added to the residue.
4. Solution is shaken well and allowed for separating of the layers.
5. Lower layer of carbon tetrachloride is decanted.
6. 1 mL of Erdmann's reagent is added to it.
7. Formation of pink color in acid layer shows the presence of dieldrin.

Sulfuric Acid Test

1. A portion of extracted residue is taken in a minimum volume of toluene.
2. Two drops of fuming sulfuric acid reagent are added to it.
3. Red color is observed, which shows the presence of dieldrin.

SCREENING/SPOT/COLOR TESTS FOR DIFFERENT POISONS

Aluminum Phosphide/Zinc Phosphide

1. Extracted residue is taken in a conical flask filled with a guard tube containing lead acetate-soaked cotton.
2. 1 mL of cadmium sulfate solution is added.
3. Solution is acidified with 1 mL of dilute sulfuric acid.
4. The mixture is gently heated in a water bath at 40–60°C.
5. The gas evolved during the process is allowed to come in contact with silver nitrate paper.
6. Silver nitrate paper turns gray or black, which shows the presence of phosphine.
7. The paper is then dried and cut into pieces.
8. Pieces of paper are then dissolved in dilute nitric acid.
9. The extract is evaporated to dryness for 2–3 times.
10. The residue is then taken in a few drops of concentrated nitric acid.
11. 1 mL of ammonium molybdate solution is added and warmed.
12. The formation of a canary yellow precipitate, confirms the presence of phosphine.

■ SCREENING/SPOT/COLOR TESTS FOR VOLATILE POISONS

The volatile poisons such as acetaldehyde, acetone, aniline, benzene, benzyl alcohol, carbon disulfide, carbon tetrachloride, chloral hydrate, chloroform, cresols, ethyl alcohol, hydrocyanic acid, formaldehyde, isopropyl alcohol, methyl alcohol, naphthalene, paraldehyde, phenol and nitrobenzene, etc., are isolated from biological materials by distillation method. Among the volatile poisons ethyl alcohol, methyl alcohol, formaldehyde, and chloroform are common. Hydrocyanic acid is an extremely volatile and fatal substance. The militants have used it for committing suicide because it causes rapid death. Detailed method for isolation/extraction has been discussed in Chapter 3. After extraction/isolation, the next step is screening/color test of individual poisons. Therefore, in the present section of the chapter, an attempt has been made to set out standard procedure for screening/spot/color test for volatile poisons in a stepwise manner, which can be of handy reference to student/analyst/scientist/forensic toxicologist.

Ethyl Alcohol

Dichromate Test

1. 1 mL of distillate is taken in a clean and dry test tube.
2. 0.2 mL of 2% potassium dichromate is added to it.
3. 1 mL of concentrated sulfuric acid is added.
4. The yellow color of the dichromate changes to green or blue, indicating the presence of ethyl alcohol.

Iodoform Test

1. A few drops of 10% sodium hydroxide are added to 1 mL of the distillate.
2. Iodine solution is added dropwise till the solution becomes brown.

3. The contents are warmed on a low flame.
4. Few drops of sodium hydroxide solution are added to change the color of the solution from brown to yellow.
5. If after warming, the solution becomes colorless, a few drops of iodine solution are added.
6. The tube is kept overnight and the precipitate is observed under microscope.
7. Characteristic hexagonal crystals of iodoform are seen, which confirms the presence of ethyl alcohol.
8. Acetone, aldehyde, and amyl alcohol if present will also give this test.

Ester Test

1. 0.5 g of sodium acetate is added to 0.5 mL of the distillate in a test tube.
2. 1 mL of sulfuric acid is added.
3. The test tube is warmed on a low flame and finally cooled.
4. 5 mL of sodium carbonate solution is added and again cooled.
5. Fruity odor of ethyl acetate is observed, which confirms the presence of ethyl alcohol.

Methyl Alcohol

Potassium Permanganate—Oxalic Acid—Schiff's Reagent Test

1. 0.5 mL of ethyl alcohol is added in 4.5 mL of the distillate in a test tube.
2. 2 mL of 3% $KMnO_4$ solution and 0.2 mL of phosphoric acid are added in the test tube.
3. The test tube is kept for 10 minutes and 1 mL of 10% oxalic acid is added in the test tube, followed by 1 mL of concentrated sulfuric acid.
4. The contents are cooled at room temperature and 5 mL of Schiff's reagent is added and the color is noticed after 30 minutes.
5. Purple color is observed, which confirms the presence of methyl alcohol.
6. A positive control and a blank control with 5 mL of distilled water are also performed sidewise.
7. The color developed in the sample is matched with that of the control sample, confirming the presence of methyl alcohol.

Phosphoric Acid—Potassium Permanganate Chromotropic Acid Test

1. 0.2 mL of 5% phosphoric acid is added in 0.5 mL of the distillate in a hard glass test tube.
2. 0.2 mL of 5% potassium permanganate solution is added to it.
3. After 5 minutes, saturated solution of sodium bisulfite is added until brownish color persists.
4. One drop of phosphoric acid is added to it, followed by a drop of sodium bisulfite solution.
5. 5 mL of freshly prepared chromotropic acid solution is added to this colorless solution.
6. Violet color is obtained, which confirms the presence of methyl alcohol.

Formaldehyde
Schiff's Reagent Test
1. 1 mL of the distillate is taken in a clean and dry test tube.
2. 2 mL of Schiff's reagent is added to it.
3. Test tube is kept for 30 minutes at room temperature.
4. Purple color formation indicates the presence of formaldehyde.
5. The color persists even after addition of 0.5 mL of concentrated sulfuric acid.

Chromotropic Acid Test
1. 0.5 mL of distillate is taken in a clean and dry test tube.
2. 5 mL of chromotropic acid solution is added to it.
3. The contents are heated on a hot water bath at 60°C for 30 minutes.
4. The test tube is kept for cooling for 10 minutes.
5. Violet color is observed, which confirms the presence of formaldehyde.

Tollen's Reagent Test
1. 1 mL of the distillate is taken in a clean and dry test tube.
2. 1 mL of Tollen's reagent is added to it.
3. Test tube is kept in a hot water bath for 10 minutes.
4. Gray precipitate or a silver mirror indicates the presence of formaldehyde.

Phenylhydrazine Potassium Ferricyanide Test
1. 0.5 mL of freshly prepared 10% aqueous solution of phenylhydrazine hydrochloride is added in 2 mL of the distillate in a test tube.
2. Five drops of freshly prepared 5% solution of potassium ferricyanide are added.
3. 1 mL of concentrated hydrochloric acid is added to it.
4. A brilliant pink or magenta color is obtained which indicates the presence of formaldehyde.

Phenylhydrazine-Sodium Nitroprusside Test
1. 2 mL of the distillate is taken in a clean and dry test tube.
2. 1.0 mL of freshly prepared 1.0% aqueous solution of phenylhydrazine hydrochloride is added to it.
3. 1 mL of freshly prepared solution of sodium nitroprusside is added.
4. The mixture is made alkaline by adding excess of dilute sodium hydroxide solution.
5. An intense blue color is obtained which indicates the presence of formaldehyde.

Acetaldehyde
Schiff's Reagent Test
1. 2 mL of Schiff's reagent is added to 1 mL of the distillate in a test tube.

2. The test tube is kept for 30 minutes at room temperature.
3. A purple color indicates acetaldehyde but formaldehyde also gives a purple color.
4. 0.5 mL concentrated sulfuric acid is added to develop the purple color.
5. The purple color disappeared, which is due to acetaldehyde. In the presence of formaldehyde the purple color persists.

Caustic Potash Test

1. A few drops of aqueous caustic potash solution are added to 0.5 mL distillate in a test tube.
2. The solution is boiled for a few seconds.
3. In presence of acetaldehyde the solution turns to yellow.
4. In excess of acetaldehyde, yellow precipitate is obtained, which changes from yellow to orange and then to brown.

Sodium Nitroprusside Test

1. 1 mL of distillate is taken in a clean and dry test tube.
2. 1 mL of 0.5% aqueous sodium nitroprusside solution is added to it.
3. Five drops of aqueous sodium hydroxide solution are added.
4. Wine-red color indicates the presence of acetaldehyde.

Tollen's Reagent Test

Same as discussed for formaldehyde.

Ammonium Hydroxide Test

1. 1 mL of distillate is taken in a test tube.
2. A few drops of ammonium hydroxide are added to it.
3. Test tube is kept for few minutes at room temperature.
4. A white crystalline compound of aldehyde ammons indicates the presence of aldehyde.

Sodium Bisulfate Test

1. 1 mL of distillate is taken in a clean and dry test tube.
2. 0.5 mL of aqueous sodium bisulfite solution is added to it.
3. Test tube is kept for 10 minutes at room temperature.
4. A white crystalline compound (aldehyde bisulfate) indicates the presence of aldehyde.

Acetone

Legal's Test

1. Two drops of freshly prepared saturated aqueous solution of sodium nitroprusside are added to 1 mL of the distillate in a test tube.
2. One drop of 10% sodium hydroxide is added to it.
3. Red or yellowish-red color is produced.

SCREENING/SPOT/COLOR TESTS FOR DIFFERENT POISONS

4. Few drops of glacial acetic acid are added to acidify the solution.
5. The color is carmine or purplish-red that indicates the presence of acetone.

Iodoform Test
Same as described in ethyl alcohol.

Chloroform
Fujiwara Test
1. 1 mL of pyridine is added to 1 mL of the distillate in a test tube.
2. 2 mL of 20% sodium hydroxide solution is added in the above test tube.
3. Test tube is kept on water bath for 1 minute.
4. A pink to red color indicates the presence of chloroform.
5. Chloral hydrate and other polyhalogenated compounds can also give a positive test.

Potassium Hydroxide Test
1. 1 mL of 10% alcoholic solution of potassium hydroxide is mixed with 1 mL of the distillate in a test tube.
2. One drop of aniline is added to it.
3. The test tube is heated on water bath for a few minutes.
4. An intolerable odor of phenyl isocyanide indicates the presence of chloroform.

Nessler's Reagent Test
1. 1 mL of distillate is taken in a clean and dry test tube.
2. 1 mL of Nessler's reagent is added to it.
3. The test tube is kept for 20 minutes at room temperature.
4. No brown color or precipitate confirms the presence of chloroform.

Beta-naphthol Test
1. 1 mL of distillate is taken in a clean and dry test tube.
2. 1 mL of strongly alkaline solution of beta-naphthol is added to it.
3. Test tube is heated in water bath for a few minutes.
4. A blue color turning to green, and finally brown indicates the presence of chloroform.

Benzene
Nitrating Mixture Reagent Test
1. Chilled nitrating mixture is added to about 0.05 g (or one drop) of the residue obtained after evaporation of the ether extract from the steam distillate.
2. The contents are transferred to a hard glass tube and then heated by keeping the tube in a hot water bath.

3. The contents are cooled and diluted with water.
4. Bitter almond-like odor due to the formation of nitrobenzene is observed, which confirms the presence of benzene.

Sodium Hydroxide—Ethyl Methyl Ketone Reagent Test
1. One drop of the chilled nitrating mixture is added to one drop of the residue of ether extract of the distillate.
2. The contents are mixed thoroughly and allowed to stand for half an hour.
3. The mixture is cooled in an ice bath.
4. 2 mL of cold water is added to the mixture.
5. 40% sodium hydroxide solution is added dropwise, till the acid is neutralized and then two drops of alkali are added in excess.
6. 10 mL of ethyl methyl ketone is added and shaken.
7. After 10 minutes, 5 mL of ethyl methyl ketone layer is separated.
8. 10 mL of 10% alcoholic potassium hydroxide solution is added.
9. A red color indicates the presence of benzene.

Chloral Hydrate
Fujiwara Test
1. 1 mL of distillate is taken in a clean and dry test tube.
2. 1 mL of pyridine is added to it.
3. 2 mL of 20% sodium hydroxide is added.
4. The test tube is kept on water bath for 1 minute.
5. A pink to red color indicates the presence of chloral hydrate.

Nessler's Reagent Test
1. 1 mL of the distillate is taken in a clean and dry test tube.
2. 1 mL of Nessler's reagent is added to it.
3. The test tube is kept in water bath for 1 minute.
4. A yellow to reddish-brown color indicates the presence of chloral hydrate.

Resorcinol Test
1. 0.5 mL of 20% aqueous sodium hydroxide solution is added to 1 mL of the distillate in a test tube.
2. 0.5 mL of saturated aqueous resorcinol solution is added.
3. The mixture is boiled for few minutes.
4. A red color indicates the presence of chloral hydrate.

Carbon Disulfide
Lead Acetate Test
1. One or two drops of lead acetate solution are added to the solution to be tested.
2. An excess of potassium hydroxide solution is added.

3. The test tube is kept in the water bath and boiled for some time.
4. A black precipitate will appear if carbon disulfide is present.

Thiocyanate Test
1. A portion of the distillate is boiled for 5 minutes with 1 mL each of ammonium hydroxide and ethyl alcohol.
2. The solution is concentrated to 1 mL.
3. The solution is acidified with dilute hydrochloric acid and a drop of ferric chloride solution is added.
4. The red color of thiocyanate indicates the presence of carbon disulfide.

Castiglioni's Test
1. 1 mL of the distillate is taken in a clean and dry test tube.
2. 2 mL of alcoholic solution of piperazine is added to it.
3. Solution is kept for two minutes.
4. The yellow precipitate indicates the presence of carbon disulfide.

Cyanide

Prussian Blue Test
1. Sodium hydroxide is added to a portion of the distillate to make it alkaline.
2. The solution is concentrated over a hot water bath to 2 mL.
3. 0.5 mL of freshly prepared ferrous hydroxide solution is added along with one drop of ferric chloride solution.
4. The mixture is heated just to boiling and then dilute sulfuric acid is added to it dropwise to make the solution just acidic.
5. The contents are warmed on water bath.
6. A Prussian blue color indicates the presence of hydrocyanic acid.
7. If cyanide is present in traces, the Prussian blue color or the precipitate is observed on keeping the contents in a test tube overnight.

Nitroprusside Test (Vortman's Test)
1. A few drops of a freshly prepared aqueous potassium nitrite solution are added to 5 mL of the distillate.
2. Four drops of ferric chloride solution are added followed by dropwise addition of dilute sulfuric acid with shaking till the mixture assumes a bright yellow color.
3. The mixture is heated in boiling water for a few minutes.
4. After cooling, dilute ammonium hydroxide solution is added to precipitate out the excess of iron and then it is filtered.
5. A few drops of dilute solution of ammonium sulfide are added to the clear filtrate.
6. Violet color is obtained which changes gradually to blue-green and finally to yellow.
7. In presence of very small amount of HCN, violet color is not noticed, instead a bluish-green color is obtained.

Crystal Test

1. Few drops of dilute sulfuric acid are added to the distillate in a conical flask.
2. A drop of silver nitrate solution is placed on a microscopic slide and is inverted immediately over the mouth of the flask, just after adding the acid into the flask.
3. The flask is then gently heated in a boiling water bath.
4. The silver nitrate solution assumes white turbidity, which when examined under a microscope, needle-shaped crystals are seen.

Sulfocyanate Test

1. 1 mL of yellow ammonium sulfide is added in 2 mL of the concentrated distillate in a porcelain basin.
2. The liquid in porcelain basin is evaporated to dryness, in a boiling water bath.
3. The residue is dissolved in 1 mL of water containing two drops of dilute hydrochloric acid which is then warmed and filtered.
4. Few drops of very dilute ferric chloride solution are added to the clear filtrate.
5. A blood-red color is obtained in the presence of HCN.
6. On adding few drops of mercuric chloride solution, the red color is discharged.

Guaiacum Copper Sulfate Paper Test

1. Guaiacum copper sulfate test paper strips are prepared by dipping strips of Whatman® No. 41 filter paper first in 0.1% aqueous solution of copper sulfate and then into a tincture of guaiacum (10% solution).
2. Guaiacum copper sulfate test paper is suspended in the jar containing the tissue/blood/urine/biological sample.
3. The paper is kept in the jar for 30 minutes.
4. A blue color confirms the presence of cyanide.

Picric Acid Paper Test

1. The picric acid test paper is prepared by dipping strips of Whatman® No. 41 filter paper into a solution containing 1 g of picric acid in 10% sodium carbonate solution.
2. Place the picric acid test paper near the sample.
3. In the presence of hydrocyanic acid, the strip turns yellow or brown within 5 minutes.
4. This yellow color confirms the presence of cyanide.

Ferrous Hydroxide Paper Test

1. Ferrous hydroxide test paper is suspended in the jar containing the tissues suspected to contain hydrocyanic acid.
2. Paper is taken out after 30 minutes from the jar.

3. Paper is then kept in a porcelain basin containing 5 mL of dilute sulfuric acid.
4. Blue color on test paper confirms the presence of cyanide.

Turpentine Oil
Sulfuric Acid Test
1. The distillate is collected in an ice-cold container and extracted with ether which on evaporation at room temperature leaves oil of turpentine.
2. To one drop of the oil is added one drop of strong sulfuric acid on a spotting tile.
3. A deep reddish-brown color confirms the presence of turpentine oil.

Hydrochloric Acid Test
1. The distillate is collected in an ice-cold container and extracted with ether which on evaporation at room temperature leaves oil of turpentine
2. Few drops of concentrated HCl followed by few drops of ferric chloride solution are added to it.
3. A rose color confirms the presence of turpentine oil.

■ SCREENING/SPOT/COLOR TESTS FOR TRANQUILIZERS

The tranquilizers such as acepromazine, acetophenazine, chlordiazepoxide azacyclonol, benzoctamine, bromazepam, butaperazine, carfenazine, chlordiazepoxide, chlorpromazine, clobazam, clopenthiol, diazepam, ethomoxane, fluanisone, levomepromazine, lorazepam, loxapine, mebutamate, medazepam, meprobamate, oxypertine, pecazine, pericyazine, perphenazine, piperacetazine, petrabenazine, thioridazine, tiotixene, nitrazepam, trimetozim and thioproperazine, etc., are isolated from biological materials by solvent extraction method. Detailed method for isolation/extraction has been discussed in Chapter 3. After extraction/isolation, the next step is screening/color test of individual poisons. Therefore, in the present section of the chapter, an attempt has been made to set out standard procedure for screening/spot/color test for tranquilizers in a stepwise manner.

Acepromazine
Liebermann's Test
1. 1–2 mL of extract is taken in a test tube.
2. Few drops of Liebermann's reagent are added to it.
3. Brown color is observed, which indicates the presence of acepromazine.

Marquis Test
1. 1–2 mL of extract is taken in a test tube.
2. Few drops of Marquis reagent are added to it.
3. Color from yellow to green to red is observed, which indicates the presence of acepromazine.

Forrest Test
1. 1–2 mL of extract is taken in a test tube.
2. Few drops of Forrest reagent are added to it.
3. Red color is observed, which indicates the presence of acepromazine.

FPN Test
1. 1–2 mL of extract is taken in a test tube.
2. Few drops of FPN reagent are added to it.
3. Color changes from brown to orange which indicates the presence of acepromazine.

Acetophenazine
Forrest Test
1. 1–2 mL of extract is taken in a test tube.
2. Few drops of Forrest reagent are added to it.
3. Color changes from pink to orange which indicates the presence of acetophenazine.

FPN Test
1. 1–2 mL of extract is taken in a test tube.
2. Few drops of FPN reagent are added to it.
3. Orange color is observed, which indicates the presence of acetophenazine.

Marquis Test
1. 1–2 mL of extract is taken in a test tube.
2. Few drops of Marquis reagent are added to it.
3. Color changes from red to violet which indicates the presence of acetophenazine.

Azacyclonol
Liebermann's Test
1. 1–2 mL of extract is taken in a test tube.
2. Few drops of Liebermann's reagent are added to it.
3. Brown color is observed, which indicates the presence of azacyclonol.

Marquis Test
1. 1–2 mL of extract is taken in a test tube.
2. Few drops of Marquis reagent are added to it.
3. Yellow color is observed, which indicates the presence of azacyclonol.

Mandelin's Test
1. 1–2 mL of extract is taken in a test tube.
2. Few drops of Mandelin's reagent are added to it.
3. Red color is observed, which indicates the presence of azacyclonol.

Benzoctamine

Marquis Test
1. 1–2 mL of extract is taken in a test tube.
2. Few drops of Marquis reagent are added to it.
3. Reddish-violet color is observed, which indicates the presence of benzoctamine.

Mandelin's Test
1. 1–2 mL of extract is taken in a test tube.
2. Few drops of Mandelin's reagent are added to it.
3. Color changes from blue to green, which indicates the presence of benzoctamine.

Bromazepam

Formaldehyde–Sulfuric Acid Test
1. 1–2 mL of extract is taken in a test tube.
2. Few drops of formaldehyde–sulfuric acid reagent are added to it.
3. Yellow color is observed, which indicates the presence of bromazepam.

Butaperazine

Marquis Test
1. 1–2 mL of extract is taken in a test tube.
2. Few drops of Marquis reagent are added to it.
3. Brownish-violet color is observed, which indicates the presence of butaperazine.

Mandelin's Test
1. 1–2 mL of extract is taken in a test tube.
2. Few drops of Mandelin's reagent are added to it.
3. Brownish-violet color is observed, which indicates the presence of butaperazine.

Carfenazine

Formaldehyde–Sulfuric Acid Test
1. 1–2 mL of extract is taken in a test tube.
2. Few drops of formaldehyde–sulfuric acid (6 drops: 4 drops) reagent are added to it.
3. Blue color is observed, which indicates the presence of carfenazine.

Forrest Test
1. 1–2 mL of extract is taken in a test tube.
2. Few drops of Forrest reagent are added to it.
3. Red color is observed, which indicates the presence of carfenazine.

Mandelin's Test

1. 1–2 mL of extract is taken in a test tube.
2. Few drops of Mandelin's reagent are added to it.
3. Color changes from orange to reddish and observed as violet which indicates the presence of carfenazine.

Chlordiazepoxide
Marquis Test

1. 1–2 mL of extract is taken in a test tube.
2. Few drops of Marquis reagent are added to it.
3. Yellow color is observed, which indicates the presence of chlordiazepoxide.

Chlorpromazine
Formaldehyde–Sulfuric Acid Test

1. 1–2 mL of extract is taken in a test tube.
2. Few drops of formaldehyde-sulfuric acid reagent are added to it.
3. Reddish-violet color is observed, which indicates the presence of chlorpromazine.

Mandelin's Test

1. 1–2 mL of extract is taken in a test tube.
2. Few drops of Mandelin's reagent are added to it.
3. Color changes from green to violet, which indicates the presence of chlorpromazine.

Marquis Test

1. 1–2 mL of extract is taken in a test tube.
2. Few drops of Marquis reagent are added to it.
3. Violet color is observed, which indicates the presence of chlorpromazine.

Clobazam

1. 1–2 mL of extract is taken in a test tube.
2. Few drops of nitric acid are added to it.
3. Solution is heated in water bath at 100°C for a minute.
4. Mixture is cooled and diluted with water.
5. 2 mL of 40% sodium hydroxide solution is added to it, till a colorless solution is obtained and solution is heated for 2–3 minutes.
6. Red color is observed, which indicates the presence of clobazam.

Clopenthiol
Formaldehyde–Sulfuric Acid Test

1. 1–2 mL of extract is taken in a test tube.
2. Few drops of formaldehyde-sulfuric acid reagent are added to it.
3. Red color is observed, which indicates the presence of clopenthiol.

SCREENING/SPOT/COLOR TESTS FOR DIFFERENT POISONS

Liebermann's Test
1. 1–2 mL of extract is taken in a test tube.
2. Few drops of Liebermann's reagent are added to it.
3. Red color is observed, which indicates the presence of clopenthiol.

Sulfuric Acid Test
1. Few drops of extract are taken on a white tile or test tube.
2. Few drops of sulfuric acid are added to it.
3. Orange color is observed, which indicates the presence of clopenthiol.

Diazepam
Formaldehyde–Sulfuric Acid Test
1. 1–2 mL of extract is taken in a test tube.
2. Few drops of formaldehyde–sulfuric acid reagent are added to it.
3. Orange color is observed, which indicates the presence of diazepam.

Ethomoxane
Mandelin's Test
1. 1–2 mL of extract is taken in a test tube.
2. Few drops of Mandelin's reagent are added to it.
3. Reddish-brown color is observed, which indicates the presence of ethomoxane.

Marquis Test
1. 1–2 mL of extract is taken in a test tube.
2. Few drops of Marquis reagent are added to it.
3. Violet color is observed, which indicates the presence of ethomoxane.

Fluanisone
Mandelin's Test
1. 1–2 mL of extract is taken in a test tube.
2. Few drops of Mandelin's reagent are added to it.
3. Brown color is observed, which indicates the presence of fluanisone.

Levomepromazine
Formaldehyde–Sulfuric Acid Test
1. 1–2 mL of extract is taken in a test tube.
2. Few drops of formaldehyde–sulfuric acid reagent are added to it.
3. Blue color is observed, which indicates the presence of levomepromazine.

Mandelin's Test
1. 1–2 mL of extract is taken in a test tube.
2. Few drops of Mandelin's reagent are added to it.
3. Bluish violet color is observed, which indicates the presence of levomepromazine.

Forrest Test

1. 1–2 mL of extract is taken in a test tube.
2. Few drops of Forrest reagent are added to it.
3. Violet color is observed, which indicates the presence of levomepromazine.

Lorazepam
Sulfuric Acid Test

1. Few drops of extract are taken on a white tile.
2. Few drops of sulfuric acid are added to it.
3. Yellow color is observed, which indicates the presence of lorazepam.

Marquis Test

1. 1–2 mL of extract is taken in a test tube.
2. Few drops of Marquis reagent are added to it.
3. Yellow color is observed, which indicates the presence of lorazepam.

Loxapine
Liebermann's Test

1. 1–2 mL of extract is taken in a test tube.
2. Few drops of Liebermann's reagent are added to it.
3. Solution is heated with few drops of nitric acid for 2–3 minutes.
4. Solution is diluted with distilled water.
5. Yellow color precipitate is obtained which indicates the presence of loxapine.

Mebutamate
Nessler's Test

1. Two to three drops of extract are taken in a porcelain basin.
2. Two to three drops of Nessler's reagent are added to it.
3. Mixture is agitated and heated at 100°C in water bath.
4. A brown color is observed, which indicates the presence of mebutamate.

Furfuraldehyde

1. One to two drops of extract are taken on a filter paper.
2. One drop of furfuraldehyde reagent is added to it.
3. Filter paper is exposed to hydrochloric acid fumes for 2–3 minutes.
4. BLACK color is observed, which indicates the presence of mebutamate.

Medazepam
Formaldehyde–Sulfuric Acid Test

1. 1–2 mL of extract is taken in a test tube.
2. Few drops of formaldehyde–sulfuric acid reagent are added to it.
3. 1 mL of distilled water and cold nitric acid is added to it.
4. Red color is observed, which shows the presence of medazepam.

Meprobamate

Nessler's Test
1. Two to three drops of extract are taken in a porcelain basin.
2. Two to three drops of Nessler's reagent are added to it.
3. The mixture is agitated and heated to 100°C in a water bath.
4. Grayish-black color is observed, which indicates the presence of meprobamate.

Furfuraldehyde
1. One to two drops of extract are taken on a filter paper.
2. One drop of furfuraldehyde reagent is added to it.
3. Filter paper is exposed to hydrochloric acid fumes for 2–3 minutes.
4. Gray to black color is observed, which indicates the presence of meprobamate.

Nitrazepam

Formaldehyde–Sulfuric Acid Test
1. 1–2 mL of extract is taken in a test tube.
2. Few drops of formaldehyde–sulfuric acid reagent are added to it.
3. Orange color is observed, which shows the presence of nitrazepam.

Oxypertine

Liebermann's Test
1. 1–2 mL of extract is taken in a test tube.
2. Few drops of Liebermann's reagent are added to it.
3. Blue color is observed, which indicates the presence of oxypertine.

Marquis Test
1. 1–2 mL of extract is taken in a test tube.
2. Few drops of Marquis reagent are added to it.
3. Grayish-green is observed, which indicates the presence of oxypertine.

Mandelin's Test
1. 1–2 mL of extract is taken in a test tube.
2. Few drops of Mandelin's reagent are added to it.
3. Gray color is observed, which indicates the presence of oxypertine.

Pecazine

Marquis Test
1. 1–2 mL of extract is taken in a test tube.
2. Few drops of Marquis reagent are added to it.
3. Color changes from green to violet, which indicates the presence of pecazine.

Mandelin's Test

1. 1–2 mL of extract is taken in a test tube.
2. Few drops of Mandelin's reagent are added to it.
3. Violet color is observed, which indicates the presence of pecazine.

Pericyazine

Formaldehyde–Sulfuric Acid Test

1. 1–2 mL of extract is taken in a test tube.
2. Few drops of formaldehyde–sulfuric acid reagent are added to it.
3. Red color is observed, which indicates the presence of pericyazine.

Mandelin's Test

1. 1–2 mL of extract is taken in a test tube.
2. Few drops of Mandelin's reagent are added to it.
3. Red color is observed, which indicates the presence of pericyazine.

FPN Test

1. 1–2 mL of extract is taken in a test tube.
2. Few drops of FPN reagent are added to it.
3. Orange color is observed, which indicates the presence of pericyazine.

Perphenazine

Formaldehyde–Sulfuric Acid Test

1. 1–2 mL of extract is taken in a test tube.
2. Few drops of formaldehyde–sulfuric acid (6 drops:4 drops) reagent are added to it.
3. Violet color is observed, which indicates the presence of perphenazine.

Liebermann's Test

1. 1–2 mL of extract is taken in a test tube.
2. Few drops of Liebermann's reagent are added to it.
3. Reddish-brown color is observed, which indicates the presence of perphenazine.

Marquis Test

1. 1–2 mL of extract is taken in a test tube.
2. Few drops of Marquis reagent are added to it.
3. Violet is observed, which indicates the presence of perphenazine.

Forrest Test

1. 1–2 mL of extract is taken in a test tube.
2. Few drops of Forrest reagent are added to it.
3. Reddish-violet color is observed, which indicates the presence of perphenazine.

Piperacetazine

Formaldehyde–Sulfuric Acid Test
1. 1–2 mL of extract is taken in a test tube.
2. Few drops of formaldehyde–sulfuric acid (6 drops:4 drops) reagent are added to it.
3. Bluish-violet color is observed, which indicates the presence of piperacetazine.

FPN Test
1. 1–2 mL of extract is taken in a test tube.
2. Few drops of FPN reagent are added to it.
3. Color changes from brown to orange, which indicates the presence of piperacetazine.

Sulfuric Acid Test
1. Few drops of extract are taken on a white tile.
2. Few drops of sulfuric acid are added to it.
3. Color changes from yellow to red, which indicates the presence of piperacetazine.

Mandelin's Test
1. 1–2 mL of extract is taken in a test tube.
2. Few drops of Mandelin's reagent are added to it.
3. Play-of-color from green to red to violet is observed, which indicates the presence of piperacetazine.

Tetrabenazine

Liebermann's Test
1. 1–2 mL of extract is taken in a test tube.
2. Few drops of Liebermann's reagent are added to it.
3. Black color is observed, which indicates the presence of tetrabenazine.

Marquis Test
1. 1–2 mL of extract is taken in a test tube.
2. Few drops of Marquis reagent are added to it.
3. Yellow color is observed, which indicates the presence of tetrabenazine.

Mandelin's Test
1. 1–2 mL of extract is taken in a test tube.
2. Few drops of Mandelin's reagent are added to it.
3. Brown color is observed, which indicates the presence of tetrabenazine.

Thioridazine
Formaldehyde-Sulfuric Acid Test
1. 1–2 mL of extract is taken in a test tube.
2. Few drops of formaldehyde-sulfuric acid reagent are added to it.
3. Blue color is observed, which indicates the presence of thioridazine.

Marquis Test
1. 1–2 mL of extract is taken in a test tube.
2. Few drops of Marquis reagent are added to it.
3. Color changes from violet to blue, which indicates the presence of thioridazine.

Forrest Test
1. 1–2 mL of extract is taken in a test tube.
2. Few drops of Forrest reagent are added to it.
3. Blue color is observed, which indicates the presence of thioridazine.

Tiotixene
Formaldehyde-Sulfuric Acid Test
1. 1–2 mL of extract is taken in a test tube.
2. Few drops of formaldehyde-sulfuric acid reagent are added to it.
3. Red color is observed, which indicates the presence of tiotixene.

Liebermann's Test
1. 1–2 mL of extract is taken in a test tube.
2. Few drops of Liebermann's reagent are added to it.
3. Reddish-brown color is observed, which indicates the presence of tiotixene.

Sulfuric Acid Test
1. Few drops of extract are taken on a white tile.
2. Few drops of sulfuric acid are added to it.
3. Orange color is observed, which indicates the presence of tiotixene.

Trimetozim
Liebermann's Test
1. 1–2 mL of extract is taken in a test tube.
2. Few drops of Liebermann's reagent are added to it.
3. Black color is observed, which indicates the presence of trimetozim.

Marquis Test
1. 1–2 mL of extract is taken in a test tube.
2. Few drops of Marquis reagent are added to it.
3. Reddish-brown color is observed, which indicates the presence of trimetozim.

Thioperazine

Formaldehyde–Sulfuric Acid Test
1. 1–2 mL of extract is taken in a test tube.
2. Few drops of formaldehyde–sulfuric acid reagent are added to it.
3. Pink color is observed, which indicates the presence of thioperazine.

Marquis Test
1. 1–2 mL of extract is taken in a test tube.
2. Few drops of Marquis reagent are added to it.
3. Red color is observed, which indicates the presence of thioperazine.

Mandelin's Test
1. 1–2 mL of extract is taken in a test tube.
2. Few drops of Mandelin's reagent are added to it.
3. Play of color from brown to green to violet is observed, which indicates the presence of thioperazine.

Forrest Test
1. 1–2 mL of extract is taken in a test tube.
2. Few drops of Forrest reagent are added to it.
3. Red color is observed, which indicates the presence of thioperazine.

■ SCREENING/SPOT/COLOR TESTS FOR BARBITURATES

Barbiturates are drugs that act as central nervous system depressants and by virtue of this, they produce a wide spectrum of effects, from mild sedation to total anesthesia. They are also effective as anxiolytics, as hypnotics, and as anticonvulsants. They have addiction potential, both physical and psychological. Benzodiazepine is a psychoactive drug. Benzodiazepine enhances the effect of the neurotransmitter gamma-aminobutyric acid, which results in sedative, hypnotic (sleep-inducing), anxiolytic (anti-anxiety), anticonvulsant, muscle relaxant, and amnesic action. These properties make benzodiazepine useful in treating anxiety, insomnia, agitation, seizures, muscle spasms, alcohol withdrawal and as a premedication for medical or dental procedures. Amphetamine is a psychostimulant drug that is known to produce increased wakefulness and focus in association with decreased fatigue and appetite. Amphetamine is related to drugs such as methamphetamine and lisdexamfetamine, which is a group of potent drugs that act by increasing levels of dopamine and norepinephrine in the brain, inducing euphoria. Initially, amphetamine was more popularly used to diminish the appetite and to control weight. The drug is also used recreationally and as a performance enhancer. Recreational users of amphetamine have coined numerous euphemisms for amphetamine, such as speed and Crank.

The barbiturates such as barbitone, phenol-barbitone, buto-barbitone, amobarbitone, pento-barbitone, hepta-barbitone, allo-barbitone, seco-barbitone, methyl-pheno-barbitone, thiopentone, talbutal, aprobarbitone, neal-barbitone, cyclo-barbitone, vesparex, etc., are isolated from biological materials by liquid-liquid extraction method. Detailed method for isolation/extraction has been discussed in Chapter 3. After extraction/isolation, the next step is screening/color test of individual poisons. In the present section of the chapter, an attempt has been made to set out standard procedure for screening/spot/color test for barbiturates in a stepwise manner.

Barbiturate
Koppanyi-Zwikker Test
1. 2 mL of extract is taken in a test tube.
2. Few drops of Koppanyi–Zwikker reagent are added to it.
3. Violet color is observed, which shows the presence of barbiturates.

Cobalt-acetate Test
1. 2 mL of extract dissolved in methanol is taken in a test tube.
2. Few drops of 1% solution of dry cobalt acetate are added to it.
3. Few drops of 5% solution of isopropylamine are added to it.
4. Violet color is observed, which shows the presence of barbiturates.

Mercuric Sulfate Test
1. 2 mL of extract dissolved in chloroform is taken in a test tube.
2. 0.5 mL of 0.5% solution of mercuric sulfate is added to it.
3. 0.5 mL of 0.1% solution of diphenyl carbazone is added to it.
4. Violet color is observed, which shows the presence of barbiturates.

Test for Some Individual Barbiturates
Allobarbital
Mercurous Nitrate Test
1. 2 mL of extract is taken in a test tube.
2. Few drops of mercurous nitrate solution are added to it.
3. Black color is observed, which indicates the presence of allobarbital.

Vanillin Test
1. 2 mL of extract is taken in a test tube.
2. Few drops of vanillin reagent are added to it.
3. Brown color is observed, which indicates the presence of allobarbital.

Amobarbital
Mercurous Nitrate Test
1. 2 mL of extract is taken in a test tube.
2. Few drops of mercurous nitrate solution are added to it.
3. Grayish-black color is observed, which indicates the presence of amobarbital.

SCREENING/SPOT/COLOR TESTS FOR DIFFERENT POISONS

Brallobarbital
Vanillin Test
1. 2 mL of extract is taken in a test tube.
2. Few drops of vanillin reagent are added to it.
3. Brownish to orange color is observed, which indicates the presence of brallobarbital.

Butalbital
Vanillin Test
1. 2 mL of extract is taken in a test tube.
2. Few drops of vanillin reagent are added to it.
3. Colorless solution is observed, which indicates the presence of butalbital.

Cyclobarbital
Vanillin Test
1. 2 mL of extract is taken in a test tube.
2. Few drops of vanillin reagent are added to it.
3. Green color is observed, which indicates the presence of cyclobarbital.

Koppanyi–Zwikker Test
1. 2 mL of extract is taken in a test tube.
2. Few drops of Koppanyi-Zwikker reagent are added to it.
3. Violet color is observed, which shows the presence of cyclobarbital.

Mercuric Sulfate Test
1. 2 mL of extract dissolved in chloroform is taken in a test tube.
2. 0.5 mL of 0.5% solution of mercuric sulfate is added to it.
3. 0.5 mL of 0.1% solution of diphenyl carbazone is added to it.
4. Violet color is observed, which shows the presence of cyclobarbital.

Cyclopentobarbital
Vanillin Test
1. 2 mL of extract is taken in a test tube.
2. Few drops of vanillin reagent are added to it.
3. Brick red color is observed, which indicates the presence of cyclopentobarbital.

Methohexital
Vanillin Test
1. 2 mL of extract is taken in a test tube.
2. Few drops of vanillin reagent are added to it.
3. Colorless solution is observed, which indicates the presence of methohexital.

Methylphenobarbital
Liebermann's Test
1. 2 mL of extract is taken in a test tube.
2. Few drops of Liebermann's reagent are added to it.
3. Reddish-orange color is observed, which indicates the presence of methylphenobarbital.

Mercurous Nitrate Test
1. 2 mL of extract is taken in a test tube.
2. Few drops of mercurous nitrate solution are added to it.
3. Black color is observed, which indicates the presence of methylphenobarbital.

Pentobarbital
Vanillin Test
1. 2 mL of extract is taken in a test tube.
2. Few drops of vanillin reagent are added to it.
3. Violet color is observed, which indicates the presence of pentobarbital.

Mercurous Nitrate Test
1. 2 mL of extract is taken in a test tube.
2. Few drops of mercurous nitrate solution are added to it.
3. Gray color is observed, which indicates the presence of pentobarbital.

Phenobarbital
Liebermann's Test
1. 2 mL of extract is taken in a test tube.
2. Few drops of Liebermann's reagent are added to it.
3. Red to orange color is observed, which indicates the presence of phenobarbital.

Mercuric Sulfate Test
1. 2 mL of extract dissolved in chloroform is taken in a test tube.
2. 0.5 mL of 0.5% solution of mercuric sulfate is added to it.
3. 0.5 mL of 0.1% solution of diphenylcarbazone is added to it.
4. Bluish-violet color is observed, which shows the presence of phenobarbital.

Secbutabarbital
Vanillin Test
1. 2 mL of extract is taken in a test tube.
2. Few drops of vanillin reagent are added to it.
3. Orange color is observed, which indicates the presence of secbutabarbital.

Thialbarbital

Vanillin Test
1. 2 mL of extract is taken in a test tube.
2. Few drops of vanillin reagent are added to it.
3. Brown to orange color is observed, which indicates the presence of thialbarbital.

Palladium Chloride Test
1. 2 mL of extract is taken in a test tube.
2. 1 mL of palladium chloride solution is added to it.
3. Solution is heated for 2 minutes.
4. Orange to yellow color is observed, which indicates the presence of thialbarbital.

Thiopental

Vanillin Test
1. 2 mL of extract is taken in a test tube.
2. Few drops of vanillin reagent are added to it.
3. Brown color is observed, which indicates the presence of thiopental.

Palladium Chloride Test
Same as discussed for thialbarbital.

■ SCREENING/SPOT/COLOR TESTS FOR ALKALOIDS

The main purpose of alkaloids in plants is that they act as a protective shield against insects and as a source of nitrogen and growth regulators in metabolic system. The alkaloids such as aconitine, brucine, berberine, codeine, chelidonine, ergometrine, ergotamine, harman, heroin, hydrastine, hydrastinine, hydroquinine, ibogaine, monocrotaline, morphine, neopine, nicotine, narceine, solanidine, solanine, strychnine, thebaine and yohimbine, etc., are isolated from biological materials by solvent extraction method. Alkaloids are nitrogenous bases in plants, which frequently cause physiological responses when administered to animals.

Detailed method for isolation/extraction has been discussed in Chapter 3. After extraction/isolation, the next step is screening/color test of individual poison. Therefore, in present section of the chapter, an attempt has been made to set out standard procedure for screening/spot/color test for alkaloids in a stepwise manner which can be of handy reference to student/ analyst/scientist/forensic toxicologist.

Aconitine

Palets Reaction Test
1. 1 mL of extract made in acetic acid is taken in a porcelain basin.
2. Solution is heated and evaporated to dryness.

3. Few drops of a mixture of phosphoric acid and sodium molybdate (25:1) are added.
4. Contents are heated over a flame until vapor appears.
5. Violet color is observed, which shows the presence of aconitine.

Alverex Reaction Test
1. 1 mL of extract made in acetic acid solution is taken in a porcelain basin.
2. Solution is heated and evaporated to dryness.
3. Few drops of bromine are added and evaporated to dryness on hot water bath.
4. Added 0.5 mL of alcoholic saturated solution of sodium hydroxide and again evaporated to dryness.
5. Red color is obtained after the cooling.
6. Few drops of copper sulfate solution are added to it.
7. Green color is observed, which shows the presence of aconitine.

Brucine
Nitric Acid Test
1. Dried residue of extract is taken on a spot tile.
2. One drop of nitric acid is added to it.
3. Play of color from blood red to reddish yellow, and finally to yellow color is obtained.
4. Few drops of stannous chloride solution are added to it.
5. Intense purple color is observed, which disappears on addition of concentrated nitric acid, which shows the presence of brucine.

Vitalis Test
1. Dried residue of extract is taken in a porcelain basin.
2. One to two drops of nitric acid are added to it.
3. It is evaporated to dryness on water bath.
4. Few drops of alcoholic caustic potash solution are added to it.
5. Violet color is observed, which changes to red and then disappears.
6. Violet color appears on addition of alcoholic caustic potash solution, which shows the presence of brucine.

Crystal Test
1. Two drops of acetic acid are added to dried residue of the extract.
2. The acetic acid solution of extract is taken into the cavity slide and evaporated to dryness.
3. The dried residue is dissolved in one drop of alcohol by rubbing with the help of a small glass rod and one drop of methyl iodide is added to it.
4. It is then examined under a microscope after 10 minutes.
5. Formation of these rosette-shaped crystals confirms the presence of brucine.

Berberine
Marquis Test
1. 2 mL of extract is taken in a test tube.
2. Few drops of Marquis reagent are added to it.
3. Green color is observed, which indicates the presence of berberine.

Mandelin's Test
1. 2 mL of extract is taken in a test tube.
2. Few drops of Mandelin's reagent are added to it.
3. Color changes from blue green to brown, which indicates the presence of berberine.

Codeine
Discussed in Screening/Spot/Color test for drug of abuse.

Chelidonine
Marquis Test
Same as discussed for Barberine.

Mandelin's Test
1. 2 mL of extract is taken in a test tube.
2. Few drops of Mandelin's reagent are added to it.
3. Color changes from yellow to green which indicates the presence of chelidonine.

Sulfuric Acid Test
1. Few drops of extract are taken on a white tile.
2. Few drops of sulfuric acid are added to it.
3. Brown color is observed, which indicates the presence of chelidonine.

Ergometrine
p-Dimethylaminobenzaldehyde Test
1. 2 mL of extract is taken in a test tube.
2. Few drops of p-dimethylaminobenzaldehyde reagent are added to it.
3. Violet color is observed, which indicates the presence of ergometrine.

Marquis Test
1. 2 mL of extract is taken in a test tube.
2. Few drops of Marquis reagent are added to it.
3. Brown color is observed, which indicates the presence of ergometrine.

Ergotamine
Marquis Test
1. 2 mL of extract is taken in a test tube.
2. Few drops of Marquis reagent are added to it.
3. Brown color is observed, which indicates the presence of ergotamine.

Mandelin's Test
1. 2 mL of extract is taken in a test tube.
2. Few drops of Mandelin's reagent are added to it.
3. Color changes from violet to brown, which indicates the presence of ergotamine.

Harman
Marquis Test
1. 2 mL of extract is taken in a test tube.
2. Few drops of Marquis reagent are added to it.
3. Green color is observed, which indicates the presence of harman.

Mandelin's Test
1. 2 mL of extract is taken in a test tube.
2. Few drops of Mandelin's reagent are added to it.
3. Green color is observed, which indicates the presence of harman.

Heroin
Discussed in Screening/Spot/Color test for drug of abuse.

Hydrastine
Liebermann's Test
1. 2 mL of extract is taken in a test tube.
2. Few drops of Liebermann's reagent are added to it.
3. Green color is observed, which indicates the presence of hydrastine.

Mandelin's Test
1. 2 mL of extract is taken in a test tube.
2. Few drops of Mandelin's reagent are added to it.
3. Color changes from red to reddish-brown, which indicates the presence of hydrastine.

Hydrastinine
Mandelin's Test
1. 2 mL of extract is taken in a test tube.
2. Few drops of Mandelin's reagent are added to it.
3. Color changes from orange to green, which indicates the presence of hydrastinine.

Hydroquinine

Thalleioquin Test
1. Few drops of extract are taken on a filter paper.
2. One to two drops of thalleioquin reagent are added to it.
3. Green color is observed, which indicates the presence of hydroquinine.

Froehde's Test
1. One drop of extract is taken in a porcelain basin.
2. Few drops of Froehde's reagent are added to it.
3. Play of color is observed from yellow to greenish-yellow and finally to greenish-blue, indicating the presence of hydroquinine.

Ibogaine

Liebermann's Test
1. 2 mL of extract is taken in a test tube.
2. Few drops of Liebermann's reagent are added to it.
3. Black color is observed, which indicates the presence of ibogaine.

Marquis Test
1. 2 mL of extract is taken in a test tube.
2. Few drops of Marquis reagent are added to it.
3. Gray to orange color is observed, indicating the presence of ibogaine.

Mandelin's Test
1. 2 mL of extract is taken in a test tube.
2. Few drops of Mandelin's reagent are added to it.
3. Color change from gray to violet, indicates the presence of ibogaine.

Monocrotaline

Mandelin's Test
1. 2 mL of extract is taken in a test tube.
2. Few drops of Mandelin's reagent are added to it.
3. Green color is observed, which indicates the presence of monocrotaline.

Morphine

Marquis Test
1. A small amount of suspected material/residue of extract is taken on the spotted tiles.
2. A few drops of water are added and the sample is smeared against the spotted tile with a glass rod or spatula.
3. A drop of the liquid is transferred to another spotted tile.
4. One drop of Marquis reagent is added.
5. Purple-red color is produced, which gradually changes to violet and finally to blue. This indicates the presence of morphine.

SCREENING/SPOT/COLOR TESTS FOR DIFFERENT POISONS

Mecke's Test
1. A small amount of residue of the extract of suspected material is taken on the spotted tiles.
2. A drop of Mecke's reagent is added.
3. Blue to green color is formed, which indicates the possible presence of morphine.

Nitric Acid Test
1. A small amount of residue of the extract of suspected material is taken on the spotted tiles/test tube.
2. One drop of concentrated nitric acid is added.
3. Orange color changes rapidly to red, and then slowly to yellow indicating the presence of morphine.

Froehde's Test
1. One drop of the extract is taken in a porcelain basin and dried.
2. One drop of Froehde's reagent is added to the above porcelain basin.
3. A violet color changes to green color and finally to pink. This indicates the presence of morphine.

Husemann's Test
1. A portion of the extracted residue is taken in a porcelain basin.
2. 1 mL of concentrated sulfuric acid is added to the above porcelain basin and heated on water bath for 2 hours.
3. After cooling, a line is drawn in the solution (in porcelain basin) with a thick platinum wire dipped in fuming nitric acid.
4. Violet colored lines appear immediately, which change to blood red and then to reddish-yellow and finally fades away, indicating the presence of morphine.

Denigès-Oliver's Test
1. Two drops of the acetic acid solution are taken into the porcelain basin.
2. To the above porcelain basin one drop of ammonium hydroxide is added followed by two drops of hydrogen peroxide (20% volume).
3. The solution is then rubbed gently with the small clean foil of copper.
4. The resulting effervescence ceases, a pink or wine red color is observed, which indicates the presence of morphine.

Porphyroxine Test
1. Two drops of acetic acid solution of the extracted residue are taken into a porcelain basin.
2. Two drops of dilute hydrochloric acid are added to the above basin and warmed over a low flame.
3. A pink or rose-red color is obtained, which confirms the presence of morphine.

Neopine

Marquis Test

1. 2 mL of extract is taken in a test tube.
2. Few drops of Marquis reagent are added to it.
3. Blue to violet color change is observed, which indicates the presence of neopine.

Nicotine

Mayer's Test

1. 2 mL of extract is taken in a test tube.
2. Few drops of Mayer's reagent are added to it.
3. Yellowish-white color is observed, which indicates the presence of nicotine.

Dragendorff's Test

1. 2 mL of extract is taken in a test tube.
2. Few drops of Dragendorff's reagent are added to it.
3. Orange color is observed, which indicates the presence of nicotine.

Phosphomolybdic Test

1. 2 mL of extract is taken in a test tube.
2. Few drops of phosphomolybdic acid are added to it.
3. Yellowish white color is observed, which indicates the presence of nicotine.

Narceine

Liebermann's Test

1. 2 mL of extract is taken in a test tube.
2. Few drops of Liebermann's reagent are added to it.
3. Black color is observed, which indicates the presence of narceine.

Marquis Test

1. 2 mL of extract is taken in a test tube.
2. Few drops of Marquis reagent are added to it.
3. Color changes from brown to green, which indicates the presence of narceine.

Mandelin's Test

1. 2 mL of extract is taken in a test tube.
2. Few drops of Mandelin's reagent are added to it.
3. Color changes from green to brown, which indicates the presence of narceine.

Solanidine
Marquis Test
1. 2 mL of extract is taken in a test tube.
2. Few drops of Marquis reagent are added to it.
3. Violet color is observed, which indicates the presence of solanidine.

Mandelin's Test
1. 2 mL of extract is taken in a test tube.
2. Few drops of Mandelin's reagent are added to it.
3. Color changes from orange to violet and finally to blue, which indicates the presence of solanidine.

Solanine
Marquis Test
1. 2 mL of extract is taken in a test tube.
2. Few drops of Marquis reagent are added to it.
3. Yellow to violet color change is observed, which indicates the presence of solanine.

Mandelin's Test
1. 2 mL of extract is taken in a test tube.
2. Few drops of Mandelin's reagent are added to it.
3. Color changes from orange to violet and finally to blue, which indicates the presence of solanine.

Strychnine
Manganese Dioxide Test
1. Two drops of extract made in acetic acid are taken in a porcelain basin and dried.
2. Pinch of manganese dioxide is added to dried residue.
3. Lines are drawn with the help of glass rod dipped in manganese dioxide and sulfuric acid.
4. Play of color is observed from blue to violet, which changes to reddish-purple to red and finally to yellow, which shows the presence of strychnine.

Mandelin's Test
1. To the brucine-free residue, one drop of Mandelin's reagent is added.
2. A deep violet-blue or deep purple color appears, which finally changes to yellow on long standing.
3. This change in color indicates the presence of the strychnine.

SCREENING/SPOT/COLOR TESTS FOR DIFFERENT POISONS

Potassium Dichromate-sulfuric Acid Test
1. The brucine-free residue of extract is taken in a porcelain dish.
2. One drop of pure concentrated sulfuric acid is added to it.
3. No coloration is observed.
4. A crystal of potassium dichromate is drawn by a glass rod through sulfuric acid.
5. A play of colors is observed—first a momentary blue changing to a violet-color, which gradually changes to reddish-purple, red or orange and finally to yellow.
6. This play of color indicates the presence of strychnine.

Thebaine
Marquis Test
1. 2 mL of extract is taken in a test tube.
2. Few drops of Marquis reagent are added to it.
3. Reddish-orange color is observed, which indicates the presence of thebaine.

Mandelin's Test
1. 2 mL of extract is taken in a test tube.
2. Few drops of Mandelin's reagent are added to it.
3. Brown to orange color change is observed, which indicates the presence of thebaine.

Yohimbine
Liebermann's Test
1. 2 mL of extract is taken in a test tube.
2. Few drops of Liebermann's reagent are added to it.
3. Blue color is observed, which indicates the presence of yohimbine.

Mandelin's Test
1. 2 mL of extract is taken in a test tube.
2. Few drops of Mandelin's reagent are added to it.
3. Blue to green color is observed, which indicates the presence of yohimbine.

■ SCREENING/SPOT/COLOR TESTS FOR METALLIC POISONS

The metallic poisons such as thallium (Tl), magnesium (Mg), manganese (Mn), barium (Ba), nickel (Ni), aluminium (Al), chromium (Cr), cadmium (Cd), lead (Pb), copper (Cu), zinc (Zn), tin (Sn), bismuth (Bi), mercury (Hg), antimony (Sb), arsenic (As), etc., are isolated from biological materials by dry ashing/digestion method. Detailed method for isolation/extraction from biological material has been discussed in Chapter 3. In present section of the chapter, an attempt has been made to set out standard procedure for screening /spot/color test for metallic poisons in a stepwise manner which can be of handy reference.

Arsenic
Reinsch's Test
1. 5 mL of test solution is taken in a China crucible.
2. Few drops of HCl are added to it.
3. Small piece of cleaned copper strip is added to it and heated on water bath.
4. A black deposit on copper strip indicates the presence of arsenic.
5. The stained copper strip obtained by Reinsch's test is washed cautiously with water followed by alcohol and finally with ether to remove the adhering fat, etc.
6. The strip is then dried by keeping it between filter paper sheets, cut into small pieces of 2 × 2 mm size and taken in the Reinsch's tube.
7. The tube is heated slowly on the flame of spirit lamp.
8. The tube is cooled and viewed under microscope, characteristic octahedral crystals of arsenious oxide are seen, which confirms the presence of arsenic.

Gutzeit Test
1. The solution obtained from the wet digestion process is tested by this technique.
2. 1 mL of the solution is taken into a Gutzeit apparatus, two pellets of pure zinc metal are added to it, and 5 mL of dilute sulfuric acid are poured over the contents.
3. The evolved gas is purified by passing over lead acetate paper (to absorb sulfide gas) followed by mercuric chloride test paper.
4. A yellow stain is obtained on mercury chloride paper which indicates the presence of arsenic.

Silver Nitrate Solution Test
1. 2 mL of digested sample is taken in a test tube.
2. Few drops of silver nitrate solution are added to it.
3. Brownish-red precipitate is formed (distinction from arsenite and phosphate, which yield yellow precipitate).
4. The precipitate formed is soluble in acids and ammonia solution but insoluble in acetic acid.

Ammonium Molybdate Test
1. 2 mL of digested sample is taken in a test tube.
2. Few drops of ammonium molybdate are added to it.
3. Solution is boiled in a water bath for few minutes.
4. A yellow crystalline precipitate of ammonium arsenomolybdate is obtained (distinction from arsenites, which gives no precipitate, and

SCREENING/SPOT/COLOR TESTS FOR DIFFERENT POISONS

from phosphates, which yield a precipitate in the cold or upon gentle warming).
5. The precipitate obtained is insoluble in nitric acid but soluble in ammonia solution and in solutions of caustic alkalis.

Bettendorf's Test
1. A drop of test solution is mixed up with 1-2 drops of concentrated ammonia solution in a micro crucible.
2. Two drops of 10% (v/v) hydrogen peroxide and two drops of magnesium sulfate solution are added to it.
3. Above solution is evaporated slowly and heated until fumes ceases.
4. The residue is then treated with 1-2 drops of a solution of stannous chloride in concentrated hydrochloric acid and warmed slightly.
5. A brown or black precipitate or coloration is obtained which confirms the presence of arsenic.

Antimony
Reinsch's Test
1. 5 mL of test solution is taken in a China crucible.
2. Few drops of HCl are added to it.
3. Small piece of cleaned copper strip is added to it and heated on water bath.
4. Bluish black deposit on the copper strip indicates the presence of antimony.
5. The stained copper strip after necessary cleaning is heated in the Reinsch's tube.
6. Tube is viewed under the high power of the microscope.
7. Characteristic needle-shaped crystals of Sb_2O_3 are obtained, which confirms the presence of antimony.

Micro Test
1. A portion of the stained copper strip obtained from the Reinsch's test is taken into a spotted tile.
2. Few drops of dilute hydrochloric acid are added to it to dissolve the black deposit.
3. This solution is spotted on a piece of filter paper.
4. The paper is dried and exposed to hydrogen sulfide.
5. An orange spot shows the presence of antimony.

Rhodamine B Test Reagent
1. 1 mL of the digested sample is taken in a test tube.
2. Solution is made strongly acidic with hydrochloric acid.
3. A little amount of solid sodium nitrite is added to it.
4. 1 mL of 0.01% aqueous solution of Rhodamine B is added to it.
5. The bright red color of the reagent changes to blue indicating the presence of antimony.

Mercury
Reinsch's Test
1. 5 mL of test solution is taken in a China crucible.
2. Few drops of HCl are added to it.
3. Small piece of cleaned copper strip is added to it and heated on water bath.
4. A silvery shining deposit on the copper strip indicates the presence of mercury.
5. After necessary cleaning, the dried shining copper strip pieces are heated slowly in a Reinsch's tube.
6. The deposit on the copper side is viewed under a microscope.
7. Shining round globules of metallic mercury are observed, which confirms the presence of mercury.

Diphenylcarbazone Test
1. A filter paper impregnated with a freshly prepared 1% alcoholic solution of diphenylcarbazone is taken.
2. One drop of test solution is added on the filter paper.
3. Violet or blue fleck is obtained on the filter paper, which confirms the presence of mercury.

Cuprous Iodide Test
1. One drop of potassium-iodide-sodium-sulfite solution is placed on a spot plate or a filter paper.
2. A drop of copper sulfate solution is added to it.
3. A drop of test solution with the help of capillary is added to it.
4. Appearance of red or orange color, indicates the presence of mercury.

Stannous Chloride–Aniline Test
1. A drop of test solution is placed on the filter paper.
2. A drop of freshly prepared stannous chloride solution and a drop of aniline are added to it.
3. A black to brown color change indicates the presence of mercury.

Bismuth
Reinsch's Test
1. 5 mL of test solution is taken in a China crucible.
2. Few drops of HCl are added to it.
3. Small piece of cleaned copper strip is added to it and heated in a water bath.
4. A gray deposit on the copper strip indicates the presence of bismuth.
5. After necessary cleaning, the dried shining copper strip pieces are heated slowly in a Reinsch's tube.
6. Copper strip does not sublime on heating in Reinsch's tube, indicates the presence of bismuth.

Potassium Iodide–Cinchonine Test

1. A portion of the stained copper strip from the Reinsch's test is taken in a spotted tile.
2. A few drops of nitric acid are added to dissolve the deposit.
3. The solution is then evaporated and the residue is divided into two portions.
4. One drop of potassium iodide solution, is added in one portion followed by a drop of acidified aqueous cinchonine solution.
5. Orange color is obtained, which indicates the presence of bismuth.

Tin

Flame Test

1. 2 mL of the test solution is taken in a porcelain dish.
2. A pellet of pure zinc metal and 2 mL of concentrated hydrochloric acid are added to it.
3. The contents are stirred with a test tube full of cold water.
4. The bottom end of the test tube is brought into the nonluminous flame of the burner.
5. A characteristic blue flame mantle is observed around the bottom of the test tube, which indicates the presence of tin.

Zinc

Hydrogen Sulfide Test

1. To one portion of the ammonical solution of digested sample, hydrogen sulfide gas is passed, white precipitate is obtained.
2. The precipitate is filtered, washed thrice with 10 mL boiled water and dissolved in dilute hydrochloric acid.
3. The solution is again boiled to remove any traces of remaining hydrogen sulfide gas.
4. Saturated caustic soda solution is added dropwise to it.
5. A white precipitate is obtained. On adding excess of alkali and boiling, the precipitate dissolves.
6. To this clear solution, hydrogen sulfite gas is again passed.
7. A white precipitate is obtained, which confirms the presence of zinc.

Potassium Ferrocyanide Test

1. A portion of the ammonical solution of digested sample is acidified with acetic acid.
2. 0.5 mL of potassium ferrocyanide solution is added to it.
3. A white gelatinous precipitate is obtained.
4. Few drops of bromine water are added to the precipitate, which produces yellow color and boiled.
5. A bluish green precipitate is obtained, which confirms the presence of zinc.

Ammonium Mercuric Thiocyanate—Copper Sulfate Test
1. Few drops of test solution are placed on a spot plate.
2. Solution is acidified with sulfuric acid.
3. One drop of 0.25 M copper sulfate solution and one drop of ammonium mercuric thiocyanate solution are added to it.
4. A violet (or blackish purple) precipitate appears, which confirms the presence of zinc.

Copper
Group Test
1. The analysis of copper is done in the residue obtained after incineration of the organic material in the muffle furnace.
2. In presence of copper, the dry residue generally assumes a greenish-blue tinge.
3. The residue is dissolved in 5 mL of concentrated hydrochloric acid, boiled and filtered. The presence of copper is established by performing the following tests in the clear filtrate.
   - 0.5 mL of the acidic solution is diluted with 2 mL of water and warmed.
   - It is passed with hydrogen sulfide gas. A brownish-black precipitate is obtained.
   - The precipitate is filtered through Whatman® filter paper, washed thrice with boiling water and then dissolved in 2 mL of nitric acid.
   - The nitric acid is removed by evaporation and the residue is taken in 1 mL of water.
   - Two drops of the aqueous solution are taken in a spotted tile and a few drops of ammonium hydroxide are added to it.
   - A blue color is obtained.
   - The blue colored solution obtained is made acidic by adding few drops of acetic acid.
   - A few drops of potassium ferrocyanide solution are then added to it.
   - A chocolate brown color is obtained confirming the presence of copper.

Feigl's Test
1. Two drops of the aqueous solution are taken in a test tube.
2. Two drops of dilute zinc nitrate solution and two drops of mercury-ammonium thiocyanate reagent are added to it.
3. Pink to violet colored precipitate is obtained, which confirms the presence of copper.

Rubinic Acid Test
1. The aqueous solution is spotted on a piece of Whatman® No. 41 filter paper.
2. It is dried and sprayed with rubinic acid.

3. It is then exposed to ammonia vapors.
4. An olive-green colored spot is observed, which confirms the presence of copper.

2, 2´-Diquinolyl (Cuproin) Test
1. A drop of the test solution (pH above 3) is taken and placed on a spot plate.
2. Several crystals of hydroxylamine hydrochloride are added to it.
3. Three drops of a saturated ethanol solution of cuproin are added to it.
4. A purple to pink color change is obtained, which confirms the presence of copper.

Benzoinoxime Test
1. A drop of the weakly acidic test solution is treated on filter paper.
2. A drop of 5% alcoholic solution of benzoinoxime is added to it.
3. It is then exposed to ammonia vapors.
4. Green color is observed, which confirms the presence of copper.

Ammonium Thiocyanate and o-Tolidine or p-Phenylenediamine Test
1. A drop of the reagent solution is placed on filter paper.
2. A drop of neutral or slightly acidic test solution is added to it.
3. Light or dark blue stain is formed according to the amount of copper present.

Lead
Hydrochloric Acid Test
1. 1 mL of test solution is taken in a test tube.
2. 1 mL of dilute HCl is added to it.
3. A white precipitate is obtained, which dissolves on boiling and reappears on cooling indicating the presence of lead.

Potassium Iodide Test
1. 1 mL of test solution is taken in a test tube.
2. One drop of dilute nitric acid and 1 mL of potassium iodide solution is added to it.
3. A bright yellow precipitate is obtained.
4. On boiling the contents, the precipitate dissolves out, and on cooling, golden and yellow spangles are obtained. This indicates the presence of lead.

Bicarbonate Test
1. A portion of the solution suspected to contain lead is spotted on a piece of filter paper and dried.

2. To it, one drop each of dilute aqueous pyridine, and very dilute solution of sodium bicarbonate followed by one drop of 0.1% gallocyanine is added.
3. A violet colored spot is observed, which confirms the presence of lead.

Dithizone Test
1. Take 1 mL of extract (neutral or faintly alkaline) in a micro test tube.
2. Few crystals and then two drops of dithizone solution are added to it and shaken for 1 minute.
3. The green color of the reagent changes to red, indicating the presence of lead.

Cadmium
Hydrogen Sulfide Test
1. Hydrogen sulfide gas is passed through the acidic solution of the extract/test solution.
2. A yellow precipitate of cadmium sulfide is obtained.
3. Cadmium sulfide is soluble in hydrochloric acid, but insoluble in ammonia.

Potassium Cyanide Test
1. To 1 mL of extract, potassium cyanide solution is added dropwise.
2. A white precipitate is formed, which dissolves on adding excess of reagent.
3. Hydrogen gas is passed through it.
4. Yellow precipitate is obtained which confirms the presence of cadmium.

Dinitro-p-diphenyl Carbazide Test
1. One drop of acidic or neutral or ammonical is placed on a spot plate.
2. One drop of sodium hydroxide (2M) and one drop of potassium cyanide solution are added to it.
3. One drop of dinitro-p-diphenyl carbazite reagent and two drops of formaldehyde solution are added to it.
4. A brown precipitate is formed, which very rapidly becomes greenish-blue indicating the presence of cadmium.

Nitronaphthalene Test
1. A drop of the 4-nitronaphthalene reagent is placed on a drop reaction paper.
2. One drop of extract (which should be slightly acidified with 2M acetic acid containing a little sodium potassium tartrate) is added.
3. A drop of 2M potassium hydroxide solution is added.
4. A bright pink spot surrounded by a blue circle is obtained, which confirms the presence of cadmium.

Chromium

Diphenyl Carbazide Tests

1. One drop of acidified solution of extract is placed on a spot plate.
2. Two drops of 0.1 M peroxydisulfate solution and one drop of 0.1 M silver nitrate solution are added and allowed to stand for 2 min.
3. Then one drop of diphenyl carbazide is added.
4. A violet or red color is obtained which confirms the presence of chromium.

Chromotropic Acid Tests

1. One drop of extract is placed in a semi-micro test tube.
2. One drop of chromotropic acid solution and one drop of dilute nitric acid are added.
3. Red coloration is observed, which confirms the presence of chromium.

Aluminium

Aluminon Reagent Test

1. Ammonia solution is added to 1 mL of extract.
2. White gelatinous precipitate appears.
3. The precipitate is taken in a micro test tube and 2M HCl is added to dissolve it.
4. To this, 1 mL of 10 M ammonium acetate and 2 mL of 0.1% aqueous solution of the aluminon reagent is added.
5. Ammoniacal ammonium acetate solution is added in excess to decolorize the dyestuff and prevent interference of chromium, silica, etc.
6. A bright-red precipitate appears, which confirms the presence of aluminum.

Alizarin Reagent Test

1. 1 mL of the extract is placed on a spot plate.
2. One drop of the alizarin reagent is added.
3. Then acetic acid is added dropwise, until the violet color disappears.
4. One drop of acid is then added to it.
5. A red precipitate is observed indicating the presence of aluminum.

Nickel

α-Nitroso β-Naphthol Test

1. One drop of acidic solution extract is placed on drop reaction paper.
2. One drop of α-Nitroso β-Naphthol reagent is added.
3. A brown precipitate if formed confirms the presence of nickel.

Dimethyl Glyoxime Reagent Test

1. One drop of extract is placed on a drop reaction paper.

2. One drop of reagent is added and the paper is held over ammonia vapor.
3. Alternatively, one drop of extract is placed on a spot plate.
4. A drop of reagent and one drop of dilute ammonia solution are added.
5. A red spot or precipitate is produced, which confirms the presence of nickel.

Barium
Flame Test
A persistent apple green flame is observed.

Potassium Dichromate Test
1. The acidified test solution is boiled with few drops of concentrated nitric acid.
2. It is made alkaline by adding ammonium chloride and ammonium hydroxide.
3. Filter it and add excess of ammonium carbonate. White precipitate is obtained.
4. The precipitate is dissolved in acetic acid and is divided into three portions.
5. To one portion, add sulfuric acid it gives white precipitate, which is insoluble in nitric acid.
6. To the second portion, add few drops of potassium chromate, which gives yellow precipitate.
7. The third portion is evaporated to dryness and the residue is dissolved in water. A drop of it is spotted on the filter paper and dried. A drop of sodium rhodizonate is added on the spot. Red color spot is obtained, which confirms the presence of barium.

Manganese
Sodium Carbonate and Potassium Nitrate
1. Dry residue (obtained after incineration of organic matter) is fused with thrice its weight of mixture consisting of sodium carbonate and potassium nitrate.
2. A green mass is obtained.
3. It is dissolved in sufficient amount of water. Purple color is formed, which confirms the presence of manganese.

Sodium Bismuthate Test
1. A drop of extract is placed on a spot plate.
2. Add a drop of concentrated nitric acid and a little sodium bismuthate to it.
3. The purple color of permanganic acid appears, which confirms the presence of manganese.

SCREENING/SPOT/COLOR TESTS FOR DIFFERENT POISONS

Ammonium Peroxydisulfate Test
1. Five drops of extract are taken in a micro crucible.
2. A drop of 0.1 N silver nitrate solution is added to it and stirred.
3. Few milligram of solid ammonium peroxodisulfate is added and heated gently.
4. The characteristic color of permanganate appears, which confirms the presence of manganese.

Sodium Phosphate Test
1. 0.5 mL of test solution is taken in a test tube.
2. Few drops of sodium phosphate are added to it.
3. Pink color precipitate appears, which confirms the presence of manganese.

Magnesium
Sodium Hydrogen Phosphate Test (Group Analysis)
1. Magnesium is isolated from tissue, etc., by dry ashing method.
2. It is detected by usual group analysis with sodium hydrogen phosphate.
3. White precipitate is obtained with sodium hydrogen phosphate.

Cobalt Nitrate Test
1. A drop of test solution is mixed with cobalt nitrate on charcoal.
2. Rosy pink incrustation confirms the presence of magnesium.

Caustic Soda Test
1. A drop of test solution is taken in a test tube.
2. Titan yellow reagent and a drop of 0.1 N caustic soda solution are added to it.
3. Orange or red color is obtained, which confirms the presence of magnesium.

Thallium
Hydrochloric Acid Test
1. One drop of test solution is added on a microscopic slide.
2. Add a drop of hydrochloric acid.
3. White precipitate of irregular crosses and clusters of crystals are formed.

Uranyl Acetate
1. Few drops of test solution are taken in a test tube.
2. A drop of uranyl acetate solution is added to it.
3. Formation of needles and prisms shows the presence of thallium.

Potassium Chromate Solution Test
1. 1 mL of extract is taken in a test tube.
2. Potassium chromate solution is added to it.

SCREENING/SPOT/COLOR TESTS FOR DIFFERENT POISONS

3. The formation of a yellow precipitate indicates the presence of thallous ion.

Ammonium Sulfide Solution Test
1. 1 mL of extract is taken in a test tube.
2. Ammonium sulfide solution is added to it.
3. A black precipitate appears, which confirms the presence of thallium.

Potassium Ferrocyanide Test
1. 1 mL of extract is taken in a test tube and made alkaline.
2. Potassium ferrocyanide solution is added to it.
3. A brown precipitate appears, which confirms the presence of thallium.

■ SCREENING/SPOT/COLOR TESTS FOR ANTIBIOTICS

Ampicillin is a penicillin antibiotic and is used for bacterial infections. It is used for treating infections of the middle ear, sinuses, stomach and intestines, bladder and kidney caused by susceptible bacteria. Cefaloridine is a semisynthetic antibiotic produced by modifying cephalosporin, which is used in acute infections with rapidly proliferating bacteria. Chloramphenicol is an antibiotic used to treat a variety of bacterial infections such as typhoid, cholera, and meningitis. Chlortetracycline is a tetracycline antibiotic and is used in the form of the hydrochloride salt as an antibacterial drug. Clindamycin is a lincosamide antibiotic, which is used to treat infections with anaerobic bacteria. Clomocycline is a tetracycline antibiotic, which is used in prophylactic treatment for infection by *Bacillus anthracis* (anthrax).

It is also effective against *Yersinia pestis* and malaria. Demeclocycline is a tetracycline antibiotic. It is used in bacterial infections (acne, gonorrhea, pertussis, and urinary tract infections), caused by both gram-negative and gram-positive organisms. Doxycycline is a tetracycline antibiotic, it is used to treat many different bacterial infections, such as urinary tract infections, acne, gonorrhea, and *Chlamydia*, periodontitis (gum disease). Erythromycin is a macrolide antibiotic, it is used to treat several types of infections, upper/lower respiratory tract infections, skin infections, acute pelvic inflammatory disease, erythrasma, etc. Gentamicin is an aminoglycoside antibiotic; it is used to treat many types of bacterial infections, particularly those caused by gram-negative bacteria. Lymecycline is a tetracycline broad-spectrum antibiotic. It is used to treat various infections such as bronchitis, water infections, and stomach infections. Mafenide is a sulfonamide and is used to treat severe burns. Methacycline is a tetracycline antibiotic, it is used to treat respiratory tract, sexually transmitted, otitis media, and AIDS-related infections. Methenamine is used on a long-term basis to treat urinary tract infections, chronic infections and to prevent recurrence of infections. Nitrofurantoin is an antibiotic that fights bacteria in the body and is used to treat and prevent urinary tract infections. Nitrofurazone is bactericidal for most pathogens that commonly cause surface skin infections. Nitroxoline is an antibiotic used in the treatment of acute or recurrent urinary tract infections caused by *E. coli*. Phthalyl sulfacetamide and phthalylsulfathiazole are used for stomach infections. Rifamycin is a natural antibiotic produced by *Streptomyces mediterranei* and used to treat tuberculosis. Rolitetracycline is a tetracycline antibiotic and used to treat severe bacterial infections. Streptomycin is an aminoglycoside and is used for treating tuberculosis. Sulfadiazine is a sulfa derivative, and it is used to treat toxoplasmosis and urinary tract infections. Sulfamerazine is a sulfonamide antibacterial, and it is used to treat toxoplasmosis and urinary tract infections but generally used in combination with sulfadiazine and with sulfamethazine. Tetracycline is a group of broad-spectrum antibiotics, it is effective against *Haemophilus influenzae, Streptococcus pneumoniae, Mycoplasma pneumoniae, Chlamydia psittaci, Chlamydia trachomatis* and *Neisseria gonorrhoeae*. The above mentioned antibiotics are isolated from biological materials by solvent extraction method. Detailed method for isolation/extraction has been discussed in Chapter 3. After extraction/isolation, the next step is screening/color test of individual poisons. Therefore, in present section of the chapter, an attempt has been made to set out standard procedure for screening/spot/color test for antibiotics in a stepwise manner, which can be of handy reference for student/analyst/scientist/forensic toxicologist.

Ampicillin

Liebermann's Test

1. 2 mL of extract is taken in a test tube.
2. Few drops of Liebermann's reagent are added to it.
3. Orange color is observed, which indicates the presence of ampicillin.

Cefaloridine

Mandelin's Test

1. 2 mL of extract is taken in a test tube.
2. Few drops of Mandelin's reagent are added to it.
3. Violet color is observed, which indicates the presence of cefaloridine.

Marquis Test

1. 2 mL of extract is taken in a test tube.
2. Few drops of Marquis reagent are added to it.
3. Red-violet color is observed, which indicates the presence of cefaloridine.

Chloramphenicol

Fujiwara Test

1. 2 mL of extract is taken in a test tube.
2. 2 mL of freshly prepared 20% sodium hydroxide solution is added.
3. 1 mL of pyridine is added to it.
4. Heat the test tube in a water bath at 100°C for 2 minutes.
5. Red color is observed, which indicates the presence of chloramphenicol.

Nessler's Test
1. Two to three drops of extract are taken in a porcelain basin.
2. Two to three drops of Nessler's reagent are added to it.
3. The mixture is agitated and heated to 100°C in a water bath.
4. A brown-orange color is observed, which indicates the presence of chloramphenicol.

Chlortetracycline
Benedict's Test
1. 1 mL of extract is taken in a test tube.
2. 0.5 mL of Benedict's reagent is added to it.
3. Solution is heated at 100°C for 3 minutes.
4. Red color is observed, which indicates the presence of chlortetracycline.

Mandelin's Test
1. 2 mL of extract is taken in a test tube.
2. Few drops of Mandelin's reagent are added to it.
3. Brown to yellow color is observed, which indicates the presence of chlortetracycline.

Marquis Test
1. 2 mL of extract is taken in a test tube.
2. Few drops of Marquis reagent are added to it.
3. Yellow to green color is observed, which indicates the presence of chlortetracycline.

Clindamycin
Palladium Chloride Test
1. 2 mL of extract is taken in a test tube.
2. 1 mL of palladium chloride solution is added to it.
3. Solution is heated for 2 minutes
4. Yellow color is observed, which indicates the presence of clindamycin.

Sodium Nitroprusside Test
1. 1 mL of extract is taken in a porcelain basin.
2. Few drops of 2 M sodium hydroxide are added to it.
3. Evaporate the solution to dryness.
4. Residue obtained is dissolved in two drops of water.
5. 0.5 mL of sodium nitroprusside solution is added to it.
6. Violet color is observed, which indicates the presence of clindamycin.

Clomocycline
Liebermann's Test
1. 2 mL of extract is taken in a test tube.

2. Few drops of Liebermann's reagent are added to it.
3. Black color is observed, which indicates the presence of clomocycline.

Sulfuric Acid Test
1. Few drops of extract are taken on a white tile.
2. Few drops of sulfuric acid are added to it.
3. Blue-black color is observed, which indicates the presence of clomocycline.

Cycloserine
Sodium Nitroprusside Test
1. 1 mL of extract is taken in a porcelain basin.
2. Few drops of 2M sodium hydroxide are added to it.
3. Evaporate the solution to dryness.
4. Residue obtained is dissolved in two drops of water.
5. 0.5 mL of sodium nitroprusside solution is added to it.
6. Blue color is observed, which indicates the presence of cycloserine.

Demeclocycline
Nessler's Test
1. Two to three drops of extract are taken in a porcelain basin.
2. Two to three drops of Nessler's reagent are added to it.
3. Agitated and heated the mixture to 100°C in a water bath.
4. A brown color is observed, which indicates the presence of demeclocycline.

Sulfuric Acid Test
1. Few drops of extract are taken on a white tile.
2. Few drops of sulfuric acid are added to it.
3. Brown-blue color is observed, which indicates the presence of demeclocycline.

Doxycycline
Sulfuric Acid Test
1. Few drops of extract are taken on a white tile.
2. Few drops of sulfuric acid are added to it.
3. Yellow color is observed, which indicates the presence of doxycycline.

Erythromycin
Marquis Test
1. 2 mL of extract is taken in a test tube.
2. Few drops of Marquis reagent are added to it.
3. Brown color is observed, which indicates the presence of erythromycin.

Gentamicin
Nessler's Test
1. Two to three drops of extract are taken in a porcelain basin.
2. Two to three drops of Nessler's reagent are added to it.
3. Agitated and heated the mixture to 100°C in a water bath.
4. A black color is observed, which indicates the presence of gentamicin.

Ninhydrin Test
1. The residue is extracted in methanol.
2. One drop of extracted residue is taken on a filter paper.
3. One drop of ninhydrin reagent is added to it and air-dried in hot air.
4. Violet color is observed, which indicates the presence of gentamicin.

Lymecycline
Marquis Test
1. 2 mL of extract is taken in a test tube.
2. Few drops of Marquis reagent are added to it.
3. Orange color is observed, which indicates the presence of lymecycline.

Mafenide
Koppanyi–Zwikker Test
1. The residue is extracted in 1 mL ethanol in a test tube.
2. One drop of 1% solution of cobalt nitrate in ethanol is added to it.
3. 10 µL of pyrrolidine is added to it.
4. Mixture is agitated for 2 minutes.
5. Violet color is observed, which shows the presence of mafenide.

Methacycline
Sulfuric Acid Test
1. Few drops of extract are taken on a white tile.
2. Few drops of sulfuric acid are added to it.
3. Red color is observed, which indicates the presence of methacycline.

Mandelin's Test
1. 2 mL of extract is taken in a test tube.
2. Few drops of Mandelin's reagent are added to it.
3. Play of color is observed, which shows change in color from yellow to orange to violet, which indicates the presence of methacycline.

Methenamine
Salicylic Acid–Sulfuric Acid
1. 100 mg of sample is mixed with an equal amount of salicylic acid.
2. Solution is heated with 1 mL of sulfuric acid.
3. Red color is observed, which shows the presence of methenamine.

Nitrofurantoin

Potassium Hydroxide Test

1. 2 mL of extract is taken in a test tube.
2. Few drops of 20% solution of potassium hydroxide in methanol are added to it and heated.
3. Yellow-orange color indicates the presence of nitrofurantoin.

Nitrofurazone

Potassium Hydroxide Test

1. 2 mL of extract is taken in a test tube.
2. Few drops of 20% solution of potassium hydroxide in methanol are added to it.
3. Red color is observed on heating, which indicates the presence of nitrofurazone.

Nitroxoline

Mandelin's Test

1. 2 mL of extract is taken in a test tube.
2. Few drops of Mandelin's reagent are added to it.
3. Green color is observed, which indicates the presence of nitroxoline.

Phthalylsulfacetamide

Copper Sulfate Test

1. Sample is dissolved in a minimum volume of 0.1 M sodium hydroxide.
2. 1% solution of copper sulfate solution is added dropwise to it.
3. Blue color is observed, which indicates the presence of phthalylsulfacetamide.

Phthalylsulfathiazole

Copper Sulfate Test

1. Sample is dissolved in a minimum volume of 0.1 M sodium hydroxide.
2. Dropwise 1% solution of copper sulfate solution is added to it.
3. Green color is observed, which indicates the presence of phthalylsulfathiazole.

Pyrazinamide

Sodium Nitroprusside Test

1. 1 mL of extract is taken in a porcelain basin.
2. Few drops of 2 M sodium hydroxide are added to it.
3. Evaporate the solution to dryness.
4. Residue obtained is dissolved in two drops of water.

5. 0.5 mL of sodium nitroprusside solution is added to it.
6. Orange color is observed, which indicates the presence of pyrazinamide.

Rifamycin
Mandelin's Test
1. 2 mL of extract is taken in a test tube.
2. Few drops of Mandelin's reagent are added to it.
3. Yellow-brown color is observed, which indicates the presence of rifamycin.

Rolitetracycline
Mandelin's Test
1. 2 mL of extract is taken in a test tube.
2. Few drops of Mandelin's reagent are added to it.
3. Play of color is observed, which changes from violet to red to orange, indicating the presence of rolitetracycline.

Streptomycin
Benedict's Test
1. 1 mL of extract is taken in a test tube.
2. 0.5 mL of Benedict's reagent is added to it.
3. Solution is heated at 100°C for 3 minutes.
4. Orange to brown color change is observed, which indicates the presence of streptomycin.

Ferric Chloride Test
1. Small quantity of streptomycin sulfate with 1 M sodium hydroxide.
2. Excess of hydrochloric acid is added to it.
3. Few drops of ferric chloride are added to it.
4. Violet color is observed, which indicates the presence of streptomycin.

Sulfadiazine
Coniferyl Alcohol Test
1. Place a drop of extract of the sample in a test tube.
2. A drop of coniferyl alcohol is added to it.
3. Filter paper is exposed to hydrochloric acid fumes.
4. Orange color is observed, which indicates the presence of sulfadiazine.

Mercurous Nitrate Test
1. Sample is dissolved in a minimum amount of ethanol in a test tube.
2. A drop of mercurous nitrate is added to it.
3. Shake and examine it at intervals of 2 minutes.
4. Black color is observed, which indicates the presence of sulfadiazine.

Sulfamerazine

Koppanyi–Zwikker Test
1. The residue is extracted in 1 mL ethanol in a test tube.
2. One drop of 1% solution of cobalt nitrate in ethanol is added to it.
3. 10 µL of pyrrolidine is added to it.
4. Mixture is agitated for 2 minutes.
5. Pink color is observed, which shows the presence of sulfamerazine.

Tetracycline

Formaldehyde–Sulfuric Acid Test
1. 2 mL of extract is taken in a test tube.
2. Few drops of formaldehyde–sulfuric acid (6 drops:4 drops) reagent are added to it.
3. Green color is observed, which changes to yellow to brownish-yellow, indicating the presence of tetracycline.

■ SCREENING/SPOT/COLOR TESTS FOR DRUG OF ABUSE

Morphine is a compound that is used as a narcotic pain reliever. Morphine is used to treat moderate to severe pain. Short-acting formulations are taken as needed for pain. Extended-release formulations are used when round-the-clock pain relief is needed. Morphine acts directly on the central nervous system (CNS) to relieve pain. Heroin or diacetylmorphine is a semisynthetic opioid drug synthesized from morphine. It is the diacetyl ester of morphine. Heroin is an addictive drug that is processed from morphine and usually appears as a white or brown powder or as a black, sticky substance. It is injected, snorted, or smoked.

Codeine or methyl morphine is a natural alkaloid found in opium poppy. Codeine is an opiate used for its analgesic, antitussive, and antidiarrheal properties. Codeine is used to relieve mild to moderate pain. It is also used in combination with other medications, to reduce coughing. Cocaine is an alkaloid derived from coca, the dried leaves of the plant *Erythroxylum coca*. Cocaine first acts as a stimulant and then a depressant of the nervous system. Cocaine is said to reduce appetite and feeling of fatigue. It is commonly used as a pleasing intoxicant. Drug addicts use it as snuff, either alone or mixed with boric acid.

Methaqualone is a sedative-hypnotic drug that is similar in effect to barbiturates, as CNS depressant. Its use peaked in the 1960s and 1970s as a hypnotic, for the treatment of insomnia, and as a sedative and muscle relaxant. It has also been used illegally as a recreational drug, commonly known as Quaaludes or as Mandrax (methaqualone 250 mg combined with diphenhydramine 5 mg). South Africa is the largest abuser of Mandrax in the world. In South Africa, it is commonly referred to as "smarties", or "geluk-tablette's" (meaning happy tablets). Mescaline or 3,4,5-trimethoxyphenethylamine is a naturally occurring psychedelic alkaloid of the phenethylamine class. It is mainly used as an entheogen, and as a tool to supplement various practices for transcendence, including in meditation, psychonautics, art projects, and psychedelic psychotherapy. Psilocin and Psilocybin are the main psychoactive compounds in magic mushrooms. The active dose of psilocin is 2–20 mg. The effects are psychotomimetic and psilocin is considered a psychedelic drug. Chemically speaking, psilocin is a tryptamine and an alkaloid. Chemical name for psilocin is 4-hydroxy-dimethyltryptamine.

It is believed that after taking, psilocybin is easily converted into psilocin.

Atropine is a naturally occurring alkaloid of *Atropa belladonna*. It is a competitive antagonist of muscarinic cholinergic receptors. It is absorbed from the gastrointestinal tract and is excreted in the urine. Atropine undergoes hepatic metabolism and has a plasma half-life of 2–3 hours. Phenothiazine is a tranquilizing drug with antipsychotic actions thought to act by blocking dopaminergic transmission (messages sent using the substance dopamine) within the brain. This yellow tricyclic compound is soluble in acetic acid, benzene, and ether. The compound is related to the thiazine class of heterocyclic compounds. Derivatives of the parent compounds find wide use as drugs.

Lysergic acid diethylamide (LSD), also known as lysergide and colloquially as acid, is a semisynthetic psychedelic drug of the ergoline family. LSD was first synthesized by Albert Hofmann in 1938 from ergot, a grain fungus that typically grows on rye. The short form LSD comes from its early code name LSD-25. LSD is sensitive to oxygen, ultraviolet light, and chlorine, especially in solution, though its potency may last for years if it is stored away from light and moisture at low temperature. In pure form, it is a colorless, odorless, and mildly bitter solid. LSD is typically delivered orally, usually on a substrate such as absorbent blotter paper, a sugar cube, or gelatin. In its liquid form, it can also be administered by intramuscular or intravenous injection.

The drugs of abuse such as morphine, heroin, cocaine, barbiturate, benzodiazepines, amphetamines, methamphetamine, methaqualone, mescaline, psilocin, atropine, phenothiazine, LSD, etc., are isolated from biological materials by solvent extraction method. Detailed method for isolation/extraction has been discussed in Chapter 3. After extraction/isolation, the next step is screening/color test of individual poisons. Therefore, in present section of the chapter, an attempt has been made to set out standard procedure for screening/spot/color test for drug of abuse in a stepwise manner, which can be of handy reference for student/analyst/scientist/forensic toxicologist.

Morphine

Discussed in Screening/Spot/Color test for alkaloids.

Heroin/Smack/Brown Sugar/Diacetylmorphine
Marquis Test

1. A small amount of residue of the extract of suspected material is taken on the spotted tiles/test tube.

2. Few drops of Marquis reagent are added.
3. Purple violet color appears, which indicates the presence of heroin.

Mecke's Test
1. A small amount of residue of the extract of suspected material is taken on the spotted tiles/test tube.
2. Few drops of Mecke's reagent are added.
3. Green color appears, indicating the presence of heroin.

Froehde's Test
1. A small amount of residue of the extract of suspected material is taken on the spotted tiles/test tube.
2. Few drops of Froehde's reagent are added.
3. The appearance of purple becoming gray color indicates the presence of heroin.

Nitric Acid Test
1. A small amount of residue of the extract of suspected material is taken on the spotted tiles/test tube.
2. Few drops concentrated nitric acid are added.
3. Yellow color appears, which turns into green on standing, indicating the presence of heroin.

Mandelin's Test
1. A small amount of residue of the extract of suspected material is taken on the spotted tiles/test tube.
2. Few drops of Mandelin's reagent are added.
3. Reddish-brown color appears, indicating the presence of heroin.

Codeine

Marquis Test
Same as discussed in morphine.

Nitric Acid Test
1. Place a small amount of material/extract on the spotted tiles.
2. Few drops of concentrated nitric acid are added.
3. Greenish-yellow color appears, indicating the presence of codeine.

Mandelin's Test
1. A small amount of the residue of the extract of suspected material is taken on the spotted tiles/test tube.
2. Few drops of Mandelin's reagent are added.
3. Olive-green color appears, indicating the presence of codeine.

Cocaine

Scott Test

1. A small amount of residue of the extract of suspected material is taken on the spotted tiles/test tube.
2. Five drops of 2% cobalt thiocyanate solution are added and shaken well.
3. A blue color appears at once, which indicates the presence of cocaine.
4. One drop of concentrated hydrochloric acid is added and mixed.
5. Blue color disappears, and a clear pink color solution appears. If the blue color does not disappear, add one more drop of concentrated hydrochloric acid.
6. 8–10 drops of chloroform are added, and shaken.
7. Chloroform layer appears, which confirms the presence of cocaine.

Ethyl Benzoate Test

1. Place a small amount of material in the test tube.
2. One drop of nitric acid is added.
3. Solution is evaporated to dryness.
4. Few drops of alcoholic potash are added.
5. Odor of ethyl benzoate is observed, which confirms the presence of cocaine.

Gold Chloride Test

1. Small amount of material/extract is taken in a spotted tile.
2. One drop of 5% gold chloride solution in water is added to it.
3. A precipitate is formed, which appears as a delicate rosette or long rod-shaped crystal under microscope.
4. The precipitate remains insoluble even on the addition of a drop of dilute HCl.

Permanganate Crystal Test

1. The suspected material is dissolved in a few drops of saturated solution of alum.
2. One drop of the above solution is added with one drop of saturated $KMnO_4$ solution on a microscopic slide.
3. It is mixed gently for 2 minutes and covered with a cover slip and viewed under a microscope.
4. Characteristic rectangular pink colored crystals are seen, which confirms the presence of cocaine.

Chromic Acid Test

1. Extract of the suspected material is taken in a test tube.
2. 5% solution of chromic acid is added dropwise to the test tube.
3. A yellow color is first obtained, which gets dissolved on shaking.

5. 1 mL concentrated HCl is added to the above clear solution.
6. Orange crystalline precipitate is formed, which confirms the presence of cocaine.

Barbiturates

Dille-Koppanyi Test

1. Place a small amount of the suspected material on the spot plate.
2. Three to four drops of cobaltous acetate solution are added to it.
3. Three to four drops of 5% isopropylamine solution are also added to it.
4. A reddish purple or purple-violet color, indicates the possible presence of barbiturates.

Mercuric Sulfate-Diphenylcarbazone Test

1. A portion of the extracted residue is dissolved in 2 mL of chloroform and is taken into a test tube.
2. 0.5 mL of 0.5% solution of mercuric sulfate is added to it.
3. Then 0.5 mL of 0.1% diphenylcarbazone solution in chloroform is added to it.
4. A blue or dark violet color is obtained in case of barbiturate.
5. In the absence of barbiturate, only a pink color of diphenylcarbazone solution is observed.

Ring Test

1. The residue of the extract of the sample is dissolved in 1 mL of chloroform and taken in a test tube.
2. To the extract of sample, two drops of freshly prepared 1% cobalt acetate in methanol are added.
3. To the above solution, 1% lithium hydroxide in methanol is added dropwise.
4. A blue ring is formed at the junction, which indicates the presence of barbiturates.

Benzodiazepines

Dinitrobenzene Potassium Hydroxide Reagent Test

1. Small amount of the suspected material is taken on the spot plate.
2. One drop of dinitrobenzene reagent is added to it.
3. One drop of potassium hydroxide reagent is also added to it.
4. Reddish-purple or pink color is observed, which confirms the presence of benzodiazepines.

Hydrochloric Acid Test

1. A small amount of suspected material is placed on a spot plate.
2. Two drops of 2 N HCl are added to it.
3. Yellow color appears, indicating the possible presence of benzodiazepine derivatives.

Formaldehyde–Sulfuric Acid Reagent Test
1. 1 mL of suspected sample is taken in the test tube.
2. Few drops of formaldehyde–sulfuric acid reagent are added to it.
3. Red-violet or blue-violet color is observed, which confirms the presence of benzodiazepines.

Marquis Reagent Test
1. 1 mL of suspected sample is taken in the test tube.
2. Few drops of Marquis reagent are added to it.
3. Yellow or orange color is obtained that confirms the presence of benzodiazepines.

Amphetamine and Methamphetamine
Marquis Reagent
1. Small amount of the sample (1–2 mg of powder; one or two drops, if liquid) is taken in the depression of a spot plate.
2. Marquis reagent is added dropwise (not more than three drops) to the above spot plate.
3. An immediate orange color turning to brown develops, which confirms the presence of amphetamine and methamphetamine.

Ninhydrin Reagent
1. A small amount of the sample is dissolved (1–2 mg of powder) in methanol.
2. One drop of the solution is taken on a filter paper and one drop of ninhydrin reagent is added to it.
3. It is then, heated on a hot-plate at 110°C.
4. The color turns to pinkish-orange upon heating, this confirms the presence of amphetamine and methamphetamine.

Simon's Method
1. Small amount of the sample is taken on the spotting tile, and it is then mixed with a drop of 20% aqueous sodium carbonate solution.
2. Then, one drop of 50% ethanolic acetaldehyde solution is added to it, followed by few drops of 1% aqueous sodium nitroprusside solution.
3. Blue color is formed, which confirms the presence of methamphetamine.
4. Slow pink to cherry-red color confirms the presence of amphetamines.
5. This test may be used to distinguish methamphetamine from amphetamine.

Methaqualone
Cobalt Thiocyanate Test
1. A small/appropriate amount of suspected material is taken in a test tube.

2. One drop of 16% hydrochloric acid solution is added to it.
3. Then one drop of cobalt thiocyanate solution is added.
4. A blue color appears, which confirms a positive test for the presence of methaqualone.

Fischer–Morris Test

1. Place a small/appropriate amount of suspected material in a test tube.
2. Seven drops of concentrated formic acid (88%) and five drops of 5% aqueous sodium nitrite solution are added.
3. It is then allowed to stand for 1–2 minutes. Then 15 to 20 drops of chloroform are added. It is shaken well and allowed to stand.
4. In the water layer, methaqualone does not give any color, while it gives yellow color in chloroform layer.

Mescaline

Marquis Test

1. Place a small/appropriate amount of suspected material in a test tube/spot plate.
2. One drop of Marquis reagent is added to it, followed by two drops of concentrated sulfuric acid.
3. Orange to orange-red color appears, indicating the presence of mescaline.

Mecke's Reagent Test

1. Place a small/appropriate amount of suspected material in a test tube/spot plate.
2. Few drops of Mecke's reagent are added.
3. Orange color appears that changes to brown color, indicating the presence of mescaline.

Froehde's Reagent Test

1. Place a small/appropriate amount of suspected material in a test tube/spot plate.
2. Few drops of Froehde's reagent are added.
3. Brown color appears, which indicates the presence of mescaline.

Liebermann's Test

1. Place a small/appropriate amount of suspected material in a test tube spot plate.
2. Few drops of Liebermann's reagent are added.
3. Black color appears, which indicates the presence of mescaline.

Psilocin/Psilocybin
Ehrlich Reagent Test
1. Place a small/appropriate amount of suspected material in a test tube spot plate.
2. Two drops of Ehrlich's reagent are added.
3. Violet-gray color appears, which changes to violet color after sometime, indicating the presence of psilocin or psilocybin.

Marquis Test
1. Place a small/appropriate amount of suspected material in a test tube/spot plate.
2. One drop of Marquis reagent is added.
3. Two drops of concentrated sulfuric acid are added.
4. Green-brown color appears, indicating the presence of psilocin.
5. Orange color appears, indicating the presence of psilocybin.

Froehde's Reagent Test
1. Place a small/appropriate amount of suspected material in a test tube/spot plate.
2. Few drops of Froehde's reagent are added.
3. Green color changes to blue-gray color, which indicates the presence of psilocin.
4. Olive-green changes to yellow, indicating the presence of psilocybin.

Mecke's Reagent Test
1. Place a small/appropriate amount of the suspected material in the test tube/spot plate.
2. Few drops of Mecke's reagent are added.
3. Green color changes to greenish-black color, which indicates the presence of psilocin.
4. While the appearance of greenish-yellow, changing to brownish-green, indicates the presence of psilocybin.

Atropine (Atropa belladonna)
Vitali's Test
1. A portion of residue of the extract is treated with few drops of fuming nitric acid in a porcelain basin.
2. It is then allowed to evaporate to dryness.
3. The residue is then cooled and moistened with a few drops of freshly prepared alcoholic caustic potash solution.
4. Violet color is produced, which soon changes to red and finally disappears.
5. The color is made to reappear by adding more alcoholic caustic potash solution, which confirms the presence of atropine.

SCREENING/SPOT/COLOR TESTS FOR DIFFERENT POISONS

Gerrard's Test
1. 1 mL of 2% mercuric chloride solution in 50% alcohol is added to the residue of the extract.
2. Red color develops immediately, which confirms the presence of atropine.
3. Hyoscyamine produces a yellow color, which becomes red on burning, while hyoscyamine does not produce any change of color.

Phenothiazine Drugs
Formaldehyde–Sulfuric Acid Reagent Test
1. 1 mL of suspected sample is taken in a test tube.
2. Few drops of formaldehyde–sulfuric acid reagent are added to it.
3. Red-violet or blue-violet color is seen, which confirms the presence of phenothiazine.

FPN Reagent Test
1. Small portion of residue of the extract is taken in a test tube.
2. Few drops of FPN reagent are added to it.
3. Orange-red/violet-red/brown-red/pink/violet/blue confirms the presence of phenothiazine.

Forrest Reagent Test
1. Small portion of residue of the extract is taken in a test tube.
2. Few drops of Forrest reagent are added to it.
3. Red/violet-red/brown-red/orange/pink-orange/red-orange/brown, confirms the presence of phenothiazine.

LSD (Lysergide)
Ehrlich's Reagent
1. Place a small/appropriate amount of the suspected material in the spot plate.
2. Two drops of Ehrlich's reagent are added.
3. Blue to purple color appears, which indicates the presence of LSD.

Marquis Reagent Test
1. Place a small/appropriate amount of the suspected material in the test tube/spot plate.
2. Two drops of Marquis reagent are added.
3. Orange color changes to brown, which then changes to purple, indicating the presence of LSD.

Froehde's Reagent Test
1. Place a small/appropriate amount of suspected material in the test tube/spot plate.

Table 4.1: Classification of acids and bases.

Type	Strong	Weak
Acids	Perchloric acid	Acetic acid
	Hydroiodic acid	Formic acid
	Hydrobromic acid	Hydrocyanic acid
	Hydrochloric acid	Oxalic acid
	Nitric acid	Nitrous acid
	Sulfuric acid	Hydrofluoric acid
Bases	Sodium hydroxide	Ammonia
	Potassium hydroxide	Methylamine
	Barium hydroxide	Pyridine

2. Two drops of Froehde's reagent are added.
3. Olive-green color changes to blue, which then changes to green, indicating the presence of LSD.

Mecke's Reagent Test
1. Place a small/appropriate amount of suspected material in the test tube/spot plate.
2. Two drops of Mecke's reagent are added to it.
3. Olive-green color changes to blue-black, indicating the presence of LSD.

SCREENING/SPOT/COLOR TESTS FOR ACIDS AND BASES

An acid is defined as a substance which when dissolved in water, undergoes dissociation with the formation of hydrogen ions as the only positive ion. Degree of dissociation differs from acid to acid. Strong acids dissociate almost completely at medium dilutions, whereas weak acids dissociate only slightly at medium or low concentrations. Common acids are hydroiodic acid, hydrobromic acid, hydrochloric acid, nitric acid, sulfuric acid, acetic acid, formic acid, hydrocyanic acid, oxalic acid, nitrous acid. A base is defined as a substance which when dissolved in water undergoes dissociation with formation of hydroxyl ions as the negative ions, e.g., sodium hydroxide, potassium hydroxide, ammonia and pyridine, etc. Classification of acids and bases are given in **Table 4.1**. In the present section of the chapter, an attempt has been made to set out standard procedure for screening/spot/color test for acids and bases in a stepwise manner.

Acids

Litmus Paper Test
1. One drop of extract is taken on a blue litmus paper.
2. Blue litmus turns red, showing the presence of acid.

SCREENING/SPOT/COLOR TESTS FOR DIFFERENT POISONS

Congo Red Paper Test
1. One drop of extract is taken on a congo red paper.
2. Blue color is observed showing the presence of acids.

Test for Some Individual Acids
Perchloric Acid (HClO$_4$)
Methylene Blue Test
1. A drop of extract is taken on a filter paper impregnated with solution of zinc sulfate and potassium nitrate.
2. Few drops of methylene blue are added to it.
3. Violet color is observed, showing the presence of perchloric acid.

Zinc Uranyl Acetate Test
1. 2 mL of extract is taken in a test tube.
2. Few drops of zinc uranyl acetate reagent are added to it.
3. Lemon-yellow precipitate is observed, showing the presence of perchloric acid.

Diphenylamine Test
1. A drop of extract is taken on a spot tile.
2. A drop of 1% diphenylamine solution is added to it.
3. Black color is observed, showing the presence of perchloric acid.

Hydroiodic Acid (HI)
Silver Nitrate Test
1. 2 mL of extract is taken in a test tube.
2. Few drops of silver nitrate solution are added to it.
3. Yellow color is observed, showing the presence of hydroiodic acid.

Mercuric Nitrate Test
1. A strip of filter paper is first dipped into mercuric nitrate solution.
2. Few drops of extract are added to it.
3. Orange or vermilion color is observed on the test paper within 10 minutes of heating, showing the presence of hydroiodic acid.

Hydrobromic Acid (HBr)
Silver Nitrate Test
1. 2 mL of extract is taken in a test tube.
2. Few drops of silver nitrate solution are added to it.
3. Cream color is observed, showing the presence of hydrobromic acid.

Magnesium Peroxide Test
1. 2 mL of extract is taken in a test tube.
2. Pinch of magnesium peroxide is added to it.
3. Few drops of sulfuric acid are added to it.
4. Yellowish-red vapors are evolved.

5. Vapors evolved are brought in contact with starch paste.
6. Orange-yellow color is observed, showing the presence of hydrobromic acid.

Hydrochloric Acid
Gunzberg's Test
1. Few drops of Gunzberg reagent are taken in a porcelain basin.
2. Solution in basin is evaporated to dryness and cooled.
3. Few drops of extract are added to dried reagent in a porcelain basin.
4. Purplish-red color is observed, showing the presence of hydrochloric acid.

Silver Nitrate Test
1. 2 mL of extract is taken in a test tube.
2. Few drops of silver nitrate solution are added to it.
3. Curdy white precipitate is observed, which is soluble in ammonia and insoluble in nitric acid, indicating the presence of hydrochloric acid.

Nitric Acid (HNO_3)
Caustic Soda Test
1. 2 mL of extract is taken in a test tube.
2. Few drops of 1% caustic soda solution are added to it.
3. Orange color is observed, showing the presence of nitric acid.

Diphenylamine Test
1. Two drops of extract are taken on a spot tile.
2. One drop of 1% diphenylamine solution is added to it.
3. Blue color is obtained, showing the presence of nitric acid.

Brucine Test
1. Two drops of extract are taken on a spot tile.
2. One drop of 0.1% brucine solution is added to it.
3. Red color is obtained, showing the presence of nitric acid.

Antazoline Hydrochloride Test
1. Two drops of extract are taken on a spot tile.
2. One drop of 1% antazoline hydrochloride solution is added to it.
3. One drop of concentrated sulfuric acid is added to it.
4. Red color is obtained, showing the presence of nitric acid.

Ferrous-sulfate Test
1. 2 mL of extract is taken in a test tube.
2. 1 mL of ferrous sulfate solution is added to it.
3. 1 mL of concentrated sulfuric acid is slowly added by the side of the test tube.
4. Formation of a brown ring at the junction of liquid shows the presence of nitric acid.

Sulfuric Acid (H₂SO₄)

Barium Chloride Test
1. 2 mL of extract is taken in a test tube.
2. Few drops of nitric acid are added.
3. 1 mL of barium chloride solution is added to it.
4. White precipitate is observed, showing the presence of sulfuric acid.

Methyl Violet Test
1. 2 mL of extract is taken in a test tube.
2. Few drops of aqueous solution of 0.01% methyl violet are added to it.
3. A greenish-blue color is observed, showing the presence of sulfuric acid.

Copper Turning Test
1. 2 mL of concentrated extract is taken in a test tube.
2. Few pieces of copper turnings are added to it.
3. Solution in the test tube is again boiled.
4. Pink color of the solution is observed, which slowly fades out showing the presence of sulfuric acid.

Acetic Acid (CH₃COOH)

Ferric Chloride Test
1. 2 mL of extract is taken in a test tube.
2. Few drops of neutral ferric chloride solution are added to it.
3. Red color is observed, which disappears on addition of few drops of hydrochloric acid showing the presence of acetic acid.

Lanthanum Nitrate Test
1. One drop of extract is taken on a spot tile.
2. One drop of 5% solution of lanthanum nitrate is added to it.
3. One drop of 0.01 N iodine solution followed by a drop of 1 N ammonia solution is added.
4. Formation of blue or brown ring around the drop of ammonia in few minutes shows the presence of acetic acid.

Calcium Carbonate Test
1. 2 mL of extract is taken in a test tube.
2. Few drops of neutral calcium carbonate solution are added to it.
3. One drop of ferric chloride solution is added to it.
4. Red-brown color is observed, showing the presence of acetic acid.

Formic Acid (HCOOH)

Sulfuric Acid Test
1. 2 mL of extract is taken in a test tube.
2. 1 mL of sulfuric acid is added to it.
3. Solution is warmed for few minutes.
4. Carbon monoxide is evolved at the mouth of test tube.

5. Mouth of test tube is brought on flame, blue flame is observed at the mouth of the test tube, showing the presence of formic acid.

Ferric chloride test
1. 2 mL of extract is taken in a test tube.
2. 1 mL of sodium hydroxide solution is added to it.
3. 1 mL of ferric chloride solution is added to it.
4. Reddish-orange color is observed, showing the presence of formic acid.

Hydrocyanic Acid (HCN)
Guaiacum–Copper Sulfate Test
1. A strip of filter paper is first dipped into 0.1% aqueous solution of copper sulfate.
2. After that the filter paper is dipped in a 10% guaiacum solution.
3. Few drops of extract are added over filter paper.
4. Filter paper turns to blue color after 30 minutes, showing the presence of hydrocyanic acid.

Picric Acid Test
1. A strip of filter paper is first dipped into solution containing 1 g of picric acid in 10% sodium carbonate solution.
2. Few drops of extract are added over filter paper.
3. Filter paper turns yellow to brown within 5 minutes, showing the presence of hydrocyanic acid.

Prussian Blue Test
1. 2 mL of concentrated alkaline distillate is taken in a porcelain basin.
2. Few drops of freshly prepared 5% solution of ferrous sulfate followed by a drop of ferric chloride solution are added to it.
3. Mixture is heated till boiling, and few drops of sulfuric acid are added to it to make the solution acidic.
4. A Prussian blue color is observed, showing the presence of hydrocyanic acid.

Vortman's Test
1. 2 mL of concentrated alkaline distillate is taken in a porcelain basin.
2. Distillate is concentrated by heating it in a water bath.
3. Few drops of freshly prepared potassium nitrite solution followed by few drops of ferric chloride solution are added.
4. Few drops of sulfuric acid are added to it and a bright yellow color is observed.
5. Solution is boiled and 1 mL of ammonium hydroxide solution is added, after the solution is cooled.
6. Filter the solution to remove excess of iron.
7. To the filtrate, few drops of ammonium sulfide are added.
8. Violet color is obtained, which gradually changes to blue and finally to yellow, showing the presence of hydrocyanic acid.

SCREENING/SPOT/COLOR TESTS FOR DIFFERENT POISONS

Sulfocyanate Test
1. 2 mL of concentrated alkaline distillate is taken in a porcelain basin.
2. 1 mL of ammonium sulfide is added in a porcelain basin.
3. Solution is evaporated to dryness in a boiling water bath.
4. Residue obtained is dissolved in 1 mL of acidulated water (containing two drops of hydrochloric acid), warmed, and filtered.
5. To the filtrate, a few drops of very dilute ferric chloride solution are added.
6. A blood-red color is obtained.
7. On adding a few drops of mercuric chloride solution, the red color disappears, showing the presence of hydrocyanic acid.

Oxalic Acid ($C_2O_4H_2$)
Lime Water Test
1. 2 mL of extract is taken in a test tube.
2. Few drops of lime water are added to it.
3. Formation of white precipitate is observed.
4. Few drops of acetic acid and ammonia solution are added to it, which remains insoluble in white precipitate.
5. Few drops of dilute hydrochloric acid or nitric acid are added to it.
6. White precipitate is soluble, showing the presence of oxalic acid.

Calcium Chloride Test
1. 2 mL of extract is taken in a test tube.
2. 1 mL of ammonia solution is added to neutralize the solution.
3. Few drops of calcium chloride solution are added to it.
4. White precipitate is formed, showing the presence of oxalic acid.

Potassium Permanganate Test
1. 2 mL of extract is taken in a test tube.
2. Few drops of 0.1% (w/v) potassium permanganate solution are added to it.
3. Few drops of dilute sulfuric acid are added to acidify the solution and warmed.
4. The pink color of the solution is discharged, showing the presence of oxalic acid.

Silver Nitrate Test
1. 2 mL of extract is taken in a test tube.
2. Few drops of silver nitrate solution are added to it.
3. White precipitate is formed, which is soluble in ammonia, indicating the presence of oxalic acid.

Nitrous Acid (HNO_2)
Starch-iodide Test
1. One drop of extract is taken on a starch iodide paper.
2. Blue color is observed, showing the presence of nitrous acid.

Sulfanilic Acid Test
1. 2 mL of extract is mixed with few drops of sulfanilic acid.
2. Solution is warmed on water bath.
3. 1 mL of the 1% naphthylamine solution is added to it.
4. Red color is formed, showing the presence of nitrous acid.

Alkalies
Litmus Paper Test
1. One drop of extract is taken on a red litmus paper.
2. Red litmus turns blue, indicating the presence of alkalis.

Chloroplatinic Acid Test
1. 2 mL of extract is taken in a test tube.
2. Few drops of hydrochloric acid are added to neutralize the solution.
3. Few drops of chloroplatinic acid are added to it.
4. Yellow crystalline precipitate is formed, which is soluble in alcohol, indicating the presence of alkalis.

Test for Some Individual Alkalies
Sodium Hydroxide (NaOH)
Flame Test
1. Small amount of extract is applied on a glass rod.
2. The glass rod is brought on the flame.
3. Golden-yellow flame is observed showing the presence of sodium.

Potassium Antimonate Test
1. 2 mL of extract is taken in a test tube.
2. Few drops of potassium antimonate solution are added to it.
3. White crystalline precipitate is formed, which is soluble in ammonia showing the presence of sodium hydroxide.

Potassium Hydroxide (KOH)
Flame Test
1. Small amount of extract is applied on a glass rod.
2. The glass rod is brought on a flame.
3. Violet colored flame is observed, showing the presence of potassium hydroxide.

Perchloric Acid Test
1. 2 mL of extract is taken in a test tube.
2. Few drops of hydrochloric acid are added to neutralize the solution.
3. Few drops of perchloric acid are added to it.
4. White crystalline precipitate is formed, which is soluble in alcohol showing the presence of potassium hydroxide.

SCREENING/SPOT/COLOR TESTS FOR DIFFERENT POISONS

Zinc Uranyl Acetate Test
1. Two drops of extract are taken in a test tube.
2. Three to four drops of zinc uranyl acetate are added to it.
3. Yellow precipitate is observed showing the presence of potassium hydroxide.

Sodium Hydrogen Tartrate Test
1. 2 mL of extract is taken in a test tube.
2. Few drops of sodium hydrogen tartrate solution are added to it.
3. White crystalline precipitate is formed, which is soluble in ammonia showing the presence of potassium hydroxide.

Barium Hydroxide [Ba(OH)$_2$]
Flame test
1. Apply a small amount of extract on a glass rod.
2. Bring the glass rod on flame.
3. Green-colored flame is observed, showing the presence of barium hydroxide.

Ammonia or Ammonium Hydroxide (NH$_3$ or NH$_4$OH)
Nessler's Reagent Test
1. 2 mL of extract is taken in a test tube.
2. 1 mL of Nessler's reagent is added to it.
3. Yellow to brown color is observed, showing the presence of ammonia.

Mercurous Nitrate Test
1. 2 mL of extract is taken in a test tube.
2. 1 mL of mercurous nitrate reagent is added to it.
3. Black precipitate is observed, showing the presence of ammonia.

Calcium Hydroxide [Ca(OH)$_2$]
Flame Test
1. Apply a small amount of extract on a glass rod.
2. Bring the glass rod on flame.
3. Orange-red colored flame is observed, showing the presence of calcium hydroxide.

Sodium Hydroxide Test
1. 2 mL of extract is taken in a test tube.
2. 1 mL of sodium hydroxide is added to it.
3. White precipitate is observed, showing the presence of calcium hydroxide.

Ammonium Oxalate Test
1. 2 mL of extract is taken in a test tube.
2. 1 mL of ammonium oxalate is added to it.

3. White precipitate is observed, showing the presence of calcium hydroxide.

■ SCREENING/SPOT/COLOR TESTS FOR TOXIC ANIONS

The toxic anions such as nitrite, chlorate, borate, bromide, iodide, fluoride, bromate, iodate, hypochlorites, cyanide, cyanate, thiocyanates, hexacyanoferrate (II), hexacyanoferrate (III), sulfites, thiosulfate, sulfide, sulfate, nitrate, phosphate, oxalate and dichromate, etc., are isolated/extracted from tissues by dialysis. In this method, the tissue is cut into small pieces and placed in a cellophane membrane made into shape of a bag. The bag is then slowly rotated in a beaker containing 100 mL of distilled water by means of an electrical motor or mechanical device. Dialysis occurs rapidly. After 1 hour, the water in the beaker is replaced by fresh water and the bag is rotated further for half an hour. The water is then taken out, mixed with previous fraction and evaporated to a small volume in a water bath, which is used for analysis of toxic anions.

Nitrite (NO_2^-)
Starch Iodide Test
1. A filter paper is soaked in potassium iodide solution, followed by starch solution.
2. One drop of test solution is added on the soaked and dried filter paper.
3. Blue color spot is obtained, which confirms the presence of nitrite.

Diazotization Test
1. Test solution is acidified with acetic acid.
2. One drop of acidified test solution is mixed on the spot plate with a drop of 1% sulfanilic acid (in 30% acetic acid), and a drop of 0.3% α-naphthylamine (in 30% acetic acid).
3. A red spot is obtained, which confirms the presence of nitrite.

Pyrimidone Test
1. Three drops of 5% pyrimidone solution and two drops of diluted (10%) acetic acid are added to about 1 mL of test solution.
2. Solution is warmed in a water bath.
3. A violet coloration appears immediately, which confirms the presence of nitrite.

Resorcinol Test
1. Resorcinol (5 g) and ferrous ammonium sulfate (5 g) are dissolved in separate 5 mL portions of glacial acetic acid and each solution is diluted to 100 mL.
2. One drop of each of the suspected solution, resorcinol solution and ferrous solutions are placed on a Whatman® No. 1 filter paper piece.
3. Green color is developed, which confirms the presence of nitrite.

Benzidine Solution Test
1. Add a drop of suspected solution on a piece of filter paper.
2. One drop of benzidine solution is added to it.
3. Yellowish-red color is obtained, which confirms the presence of nitrite.

Indole Test
1. A few drops of the extract are placed in a semi-micro test tube.
2. A few drops of indole reagent and five drops of 0.8 M sulfuric acid are added to it.
3. A purplish coloration observed, which shows the presence of nitrite.

Sulfanilic Acid-α-Naphthylamine Test
1. A few drops of neutral or acidic solution of the extract are taken on a spot plate.
2. One drop of sulfanilic acid followed by one drop of α-naphthylamine is added to it.
3. Formation of red color is observed, which shows the presence of nitrite.

Chlorate (ClO_3^-)

Starch Solution Test
1. To a portion of the filtered liquid or dialysate, a few drops of starch solution and 1 mL of 10% potassium iodide solution are added.
2. The solution is acidified with concentrated hydrochloric acid.
3. Blue colored precipitate is obtained, which confirms the presence of chlorate.

Indigo Test
1. To 1 mL of the extract, a dilute solution of indigo in concentrated sulfuric acid is added, until the later acquires a pale blue color.
2. Dilute sulfurous or sodium sulfite solution is added to it dropwise.
3. The blue color disappears, which shows the presence of chlorate.

Manganous Sulfate—Phosphoric Acid Test
1. Two drops of the extract are taken in a micro crucible.
2. Two drops of manganous sulfate—phosphoric acid reagent are added to it.
3. Warmed rapidly over a burner and allowed to cool.
4. Violet color appears.
5. Very pale coloration may be intensified by adding a drop of 1% alcoholic diphenylcarbazide solution.
6. Deep violet color is obtained, which confirms the presence of chlorate.

Borate (BO_3^{3-})

Turmeric Paper Test
1. Acidify a portion of the sample with dilute hydrochloric acid and apply the solution to turmeric paper.
2. A brown-red color is observed, which intensifies when the paper is dried indicating the presence of borate.
3. Moisten the paper with dilute ammonia solution.
4. Green-black color is observed, which confirms the presence of borate.

Silver Nitrate Test
1. 2 mL of the extract is taken in a test tube.
2. 2 mL of silver nitrate solution is added to it.
3. A yellow precipitate appears, which is insoluble in 30% (v/v) solution of nitric acid, and slightly soluble in dilute ammonia solution.

Sulfuric Acid Test
1. Transfer a portion of the extract to an evaporating basin.
2. 1 mL of sulfuric acid and 3 mL of ethanol is added to it.
3. Solution is heated in a water bath for few minutes.
4. A green border around the flame, indicates the presence of borate.

Bromide (Br^-)

Silver Nitrate Test
1. To a portion of extract, add an equal volume of silver nitrate solution.
2. Yellow precipitate is observed.
3. The precipitate is insoluble in 30% (v/v) solution of nitric acid and slightly soluble in dilute ammonia solution, indicating the presence of bromide.

Chlorine Water Test
1. 5 mL of extract is taken in a test tube.
2. 5 mL of chlorine water and 3 mL of chloroform is added to it.
3. A yellow color, which is extracted into the chloroform layer, indicates the presence of bromide.

Chloride (Cl^-)

Silver Nitrate Test
1. 5 mL of extract is taken in a test tube.
2. 5 mL of silver nitrate solution is added to it.
3. A white crystalline precipitate is formed, which is insoluble in dilute nitric acid, but soluble in dilute ammonia or potassium cyanide or sodium thiosulfate solution, indicating the presence of chloride.

Diphenyl Carbazide Test

1. To a portion of the extract, add a small quantity of solid potassium dichromate and 1 mL of concentrated sulfuric acid.
2. The mixture is then heated gently.
3. A red color vapor (of chromyl chloride) evolves, which turns diphenyl carbazide spot on filter paper violet.

Iodide (I^-)

Lead Acetate Test

1. 1 mL of extract is taken in a test tube.
2. A few drops of lead acetate solution are added to it.
3. A yellow precipitate is obtained, which is soluble in hot water, forming a colorless solution.
4. On cooling, golden-yellow plates appear, showing the presence of iodide.

Chlorine Water Test

1. Chlorine water is added to a portion of extract dropwise.
2. 1–2 mL of carbon tetrachloride is added to it with constant shaking.
3. Free iodine may also be identified by blue color formed by starch solution.
4. If excess chlorine water is used, the solution becomes colorless (due to oxidation to colorless iodic acid).

Copper Sulfate Test

1. 2 mL of extract is taken in a test tube.
2. Few drops of copper sulfate solution are added to it.
3. Brown color precipitate is obtained, showing the presence of iodide.

Fluoride (F^-)

Calcium Chloride Test

1. 2 mL of extract is taken in a test tube.
2. 2 mL of 0.25% calcium chloride solution is added to it.
3. A white gelatinous precipitate is obtained, which is insoluble in 30% (v/v) solution of acetic acid, but slightly soluble in hydrochloric acid, showing the presence of fluoride.

Zirconium–Alizarin Test

1. Two drops of alizarin S are taken on a spot plate
2. Two drops of zirconyl chloride solution are added to it.
3. Two drops of extract are added to the mixture.
4. Appearance of yellow color indicates the presence of fluoride.

Bromate (BrO$_3^-$)
Silver Nitrate Test
1. 5 mL of the extract is taken in a test tube.
2. 2 mL of silver nitrate solution is added to it.
3. A white crystalline precipitate is obtained.
4. The precipitate obtained is soluble in hot water, rapidly soluble in dilute ammonia solution (forming a complex) and sparingly soluble in dilute nitric acid, indicating the presence of bromate.

Manganous Sulfate Test
1. Few drops of extract are taken in a semi-micro test tube.
2. Two drops of 0.25 M manganous sulfate solution are added to it.
3. Acidify the solution with dilute sulfuric acid.
4. Boiled the solution for 2–3 minutes on a water bath, and cooled.
5. Few drops of benzidine reagent and few small crystals of sodium acetate are added.
6. A blue coloration is observed, showing the presence of bromate.

Iodate (IO$_3^-$)
Silver Nitrate Test
1. 5 mL of extract is taken in a test tube.
2. 2 mL of silver nitrate solution is added to it.
3. A white curdy precipitate is obtained, which is readily soluble in dilute ammonia solution, but sparingly soluble in dilute nitric acid.
4. If the ammoniacal solution of the precipitate is treated dropwise with sulfurous acid solution, light yellow precipitate (of silver-iodide) is obtained, showing the presence of iodate.

Barium Chloride Test
1. 5 mL of extract is taken in a test tube.
2. 2 mL of barium chloride solution is added to it.
3. A white precipitate is obtained, which is soluble in hot water and dilute nitric acid, but insoluble in alcohol.
4. If the precipitate is well washed and treated with a little sulfurous acid solution and 1–2 mL of carbon tetrachloride, the organic layer is colored violet, and a white precipitate (of barium sulfate) is obtained, which shows the presence of iodate.

Starch Paper Test
1. A piece of starch paper is treated successively with a drop of 0.1 M potassium thiocyanate solution.
2. A drop of acidic solution of the sample is added to it.
3. A blue spot is obtained, which shows the presence of iodate.

Hypochlorites

Potassium Iodide-starch Paper Test
1. A drop of concentrated extract (neutral or weakly alkaline) is placed on potassium iodide-starch paper.
2. A bluish-black color is obtained, which shows the presence of hypochlorites.

Lead Nitrate Test
1. 2 mL of extract is taken in a test tube.
2. 1-2 mL of lead nitrate solution is added to it.
3. Boil the solution for few minutes.
4. A brown solid is found to separate, which shows the presence of hypochlorites.

Cobalt Nitrate Test
1. 2 mL of extract is taken in a test tube.
2. A few drops of cobalt nitrate solution are added to it.
3. A black precipitate is obtained, which shows the presence of hypochlorites.

Cyanide (CN$^-$)

Prussian Blue Test
1. 2 mL of extract is taken in a test tube.
2. 5 mL of a freshly prepared 10% solution of ferrous sulfate in freshly boiled and cooled water is added to it.
3. A greenish precipitate is formed.
4. Hydrochloric acid is added dropwise to dissolve the precipitate.
5. A blue coloration or precipitate (sometimes precipitate is formed on keeping), indicates the presence of cyanide.

Ferric Thiocyanate Test
1. 5 mL of the extract is taken in a test tube.
2. 1 mL of ammonium polysulfide is added to it.
3. The mixture is evaporated to dryness.
4. 1-2 drops of dilute hydrochloric acid are added to it and allowed to cool.
5. After cooling 1 to 2 drops of 3% ferric chloride solution is added to it.
6. A red coloration is obtained, which shows the presence of cyanide.

Cyanate (OCN)$^-$

Copper Sulfate-Pyridine Test
1. 1 mL of the extract is taken in a test tube.
2. Add dilute solution of copper sulfate to which a few drops of pyridine have been previously added.

3. A blue precipitate is formed, which is soluble in chloroform with the production of a sapphire-blue solution, showing the presence of cyanate.

Chloroform–Pyridine Test
1. A few drops of pyridine are added to 2–3 drops of a 0.25 M solution of copper sulfate.
2. 2 mL of chloroform, followed by a few drops of extract of sample is added to it.
3. The mixture is shaken briskly.
4. The chloroform layer acquires a blue color, which shows the presence of cyanate.

Cobalt Acetate Test
1. 2 mL of concentrated extract is taken in a test tube.
2. 1 mL of cobalt acetate solution is added to it.
3. Blue coloration is produced, which shows the presence of cyanate.

Thiocyanates (SCN)$^-$
Ferric Chloride Test
1. A few drops of extract are placed on a spot plate.
2. Two drops of cobalt nitrate solution are added to it.
3. A red precipitate is produced, which shows the presence of thiocyanates.

Cobalt Nitrate Test
1. One drop of the extract is mixed with one drop of 0.5 M solution of cobalt nitrate in a microcrucible.
2. Mixture is evaporated to dryness.
3. The residue becomes violet in color, which gradually fades.
4. A few drops of acetone are added to it.
5. A blue or green coloration is obtained, which shows the presence of thiocyanates.

Hexacyanoferrate (II) $[Fe(CN)_6]_4^-$
Ferrous Sulfate Test
1. 2 mL of extract is taken in a test tube.
2. A few drops of ferrous sulfate solution are added to it.
3. A white precipitate is formed, which shows the presence of hexacyanoferrate (II).

Copper Sulfate Test
1. 2 mL of extract is taken in a test tube.
2. A few drops of copper sulfate solution are added to it.
3. A brown precipitate is formed, which shows the presence of hexacyanoferrate (II).

Hexacyanoferrate [Fe(CN)$_6$]$_3^-$
Silver Nitrate Test
1. 2 mL of extract is taken in a test tube.
2. 2 mL of silver nitrate solution is added to it.
3. An orange-red precipitate is formed, which shows the presence of hexacyanoferrate (III).

Ferrous Sulfate Test
1. 2 mL of extract is taken in a test tube.
2. A few drops of ferrous sulfate solution are added to it.
3. A dark-blue precipitate (Prussian blue) is formed, which shows the presence of hexacyanoferrate (III).

Ferric Chloride Test
1. 2 mL of extract is taken in a test tube.
2. A few drops of ferrous chloride solution are added to it.
3. A brown precipitate is formed, which shows the presence of hexacyanoferrate (III).

Sulfites (SO$_3^{2-}$)
Fuchsin Test
1. A drop of fuchsin reagent is placed on a spot plate.
2. Add a drop of the neutral solution of extract.
3. The magenta color of the reagent is discharged, which shows the presence of sulfites.

Lead Nitrate Test
1. 2 mL of extract is taken in a test tube.
2. A few drops of lead nitrate solution are added to it.
3. A white precipitate is obtained, which is soluble in dilute nitric acid.

Thiosulfate
Potassium Cyanide Test
1. 2 mL of extract is taken in a test tube.
2. Solution is made alkaline by adding sodium hydroxide.
3. A few drops of potassium cyanide are added, and boiled for some time and acidified thereafter with hydrochloric acid.
4. A few drops of ferric chloride solution are added to it. A red coloration is observed, which shows the presence of thiosulfate.

Ferric Chloride Test
1. 2 mL of the extract is taken in a test tube.
2. A few drops of ferric chloride solution are added to it.
3. A dark-violet coloration appears and on standing disappears rapidly, which shows the presence of thiosulfate.

Ethylene Diamine Nickel Test
1. 2 mL of a neutral or slightly alkaline solution of the extract is taken in a test tube.
2. Few drops of ethylene diamine nickel reagent are added to it.
3. A crystalline-violet precipitate is formed, which shows the presence of thiosulfate.

Sulfide (S_2^-)
Sodium Nitroprusside Test
1. One drop of the alkaline extract is taken on a spot plate.
2. One drop of a 1% solution of sodium nitroprusside is added to it.
3. A violet coloration appears, which shows the presence of sulfide.

Methylene Blue Test
1. One drop of the extract is placed on a spot plate.
2. A drop of concentrated hydrochloric acid is added and mixed in it.
3. To this, a few grains of p-aminodimethyl aniline is added, followed by a drop of 0.5 M ferric chloride solution.
4. A clear blue coloration appears within 2–3 minutes, showing the presence of sulfide.

Sulfate (SO_4^{2-})
Sodium Rhodizonate Test
1. A drop of barium chloride solution is placed on filter paper or drop reaction paper, followed by a drop of freshly prepared 0.5% aqueous solution of sodium rhodizonate.
2. The reddish-brown spot appears on the paper, which is treated with a drop of the acid or alkaline solution of the extract.
3. The colored spot disappears, which shows the presence of sulfate.

Barium Chloride
1. 2 mL of extract is taken in a test tube.
2. A few drops of dilute hydrochloric acid are added to it.
3. 2 mL of barium chloride solution is added to it.
4. A white precipitate is obtained.
5. The precipitate is insoluble in warm dilute hydrochloric acid and in dilute nitric acid, but moderately soluble in boiling concentrated hydrochloric acid.

Potassium Permanganate–Barium Sulfate Test
1. Three drops of extract are taken in a semi-micro centrifuge tube.
2. Two drops of 0.02 M potassium permanganate solution and one drop of barium chloride are added to it.
3. A pink precipitate is obtained in which few drops of 3% hydrogen peroxide solution are added, shaken, and centrifuged.
4. A colored precipitate is formed, showing the presence of sulfate.

SCREENING/SPOT/COLOR TESTS FOR DIFFERENT POISONS

Nitrate (NO_3^-)

Brucine Test
1. A few drops of test solution are placed on a spot plate.
2. A drop of concentrated sulfuric acid and a small crystal of brucine is added and the mixture is stirred with a glass rod.
3. A blood-red color is produced, which shows the presence of nitrate.

Sulfanilic Acid-α-Naphthylamine Test
1. A few drops of neutral or acetic acid solution of the sample is mixed with one drop of sulfanilic acid and one drop of α-naphthylamine.
2. A few milligram of zinc dust is added to the above solution.
3. Red coloration indicates the presence of nitrate.

Phosphate (PO_4^{3-})

Ammonium Molybdate Test
1. 2 mL of the extract is taken in a test tube.
2. 2 mL of ammonium molybdate solution is added to it.
3. A few drops of concentrated nitric acid are added and warmed.
4. The appearance of a canary yellow precipitate is observed, which shows the presence of phosphate.

Ammonium Molybdate–Quinine Sulfate Test
1. 1 mL of extract is placed in a semi-micro test tube.
2. 1 mL of ammonium molybdate-quinine sulfate reagent is added.
3. It is warmed gently in a water bath.
4. A yellow precipitate is produced within a few minutes, showing the presence of phosphate.

Oxalate ($C_2O_4^{2-}$)

Permanganate Test
1. 1 mL of extract is taken in a test tube.
2. Two drops of dilute sulfuric acid and three drops of 1% solution of potassium permanganate are added to it.
3. The violet color disappears, which shows the presence of oxalate.

Calcium Chloride Test
1. 1 mL of the extract is taken in a test tube.
2. 1 mL of 25% solution of calcium chloride is added to it.
3. A white colored precipitate is formed instantaneously.
4. The precipitate is soluble in 30% (v/v) solution of acetic acid, but insoluble in dilute hydrochloric acid, which shows the presence of oxalate.

Chromate (CrO_4^{2-})

Barium Chloride Test
1. 2 mL of the extract is taken in a test tube.
2. 1 mL of barium chloride solution is added to it.
3. A pale yellow precipitate is obtained, which is insoluble in water and acetic acid, but soluble in dilute mineral acids, showing the presence of chromate.

Silver Nitrate Test
1. Take 2 mL of the extract in a test tube.
2. 2 mL of silver nitrate solution is added to it.
3. A brownish-red precipitate is obtained, which is soluble in dilute nitric acid and ammonia solution, but insoluble in acetic acid, showing the presence of chromate.

Lead Acetate Test
1. 2 mL of the extract is taken in a test tube.
2. A few drops of lead acetate solution are added to it.
3. A yellow precipitate is obtained, which is insoluble in acetic acid but soluble in dilute nitric acid, showing the presence of chromate.

Hydrogen Peroxide Test
1. 2 mL of acidic solution of the extract is taken in a test tube.
2. A few drops of hydrogen peroxide are added to it.
3. A deep-blue solution is obtained, which shows the presence of chromate.

Dichromate ($Cr_2O_7^{2-}$)

Barium Chloride Test
1. 2 mL of the extract is taken in a test tube.
2. 1 mL of barium chloride solution is added to it.
3. A pale yellow precipitate is formed, which shows the presence of dichromate.
4. The precipitate formation becomes quantitative if sodium hydroxide or sodium acetate solution is added.

Silver Nitrate Test
1. 2 mL of the extract is taken in a test tube.
2. 2 mL of silver nitrate solution is added to it.
3. A reddish-brown precipitate is formed, which shows the presence of dichromate.

■ SCREENING/SPOT/COLOR TESTS FOR PLANT POISONS

It has been recognized since remote antiquity that plants can contain substances that are harmful or poisonous to the human race. This is reflected in the common names of such dangerous plants. A striking feature of most of the plants which are poisonous to human beings is that these plants are also known for their curative properties. Thus, they often have a long history of use as herbal medicines. This is hardly surprising, since the active principle of such herb may provide the cure of a particular disease at one dose, and can equally cause death of the individual at another, e.g., Digitoxin. The plant poisons such as Calotropiss gigantea/Calotropis procera, Croton tiglium, Abrus precatorius, Digitalis purpurea, Nicotiana tabacum, Aconitum napellus, Datura fastuosa, Strychnine (strychnos nux-vomica), Brucine, Cannabis sativa, Opium alkaloids, Argemone mexicana, Ergot, Oleander (kaner), etc., are isolated from biological materials by solvent extraction method.

Therefore, in present section of the chapter, an attempt has been made to set out standard procedure for screening/spot/color test for plant poisons in a stepwise manner, which can be of handy reference for student/analyst/scientist/forensic toxicologist.

Calatropis gigantea/Calatropis procera
Concentrated Hydrochloric Acid Test
1. A small portion of residue of the extract is taken in a test tube.
2. Few drops of concentrated hydrochloric acid are added to it and warmed slightly.
3. A greenish-blue color is formed, which confirms the presence of Calatropis gigantea.

Concentrated Sulfuric Acid Test
1. A small portion of residue of the extract is taken a test tube.
2. Few drops of concentrated sulfuric acid are added to it.
3. A pink to purple color develops after few minutes, which confirms the presence of Calatropis gigantea.

Froehde's Test
1. A small portion of residue of the extract is taken in a test tube.
2. Two drops of Froehde's reagent are added to it.
3. A deep-green color develops, changing to blue, and finally to green color, which indicates the presence of Calatropis gigantea.

Ester Test
1. A small amount of the extracted portion is taken in the conical flask.
2. 5 mL of concentrated sulfuric acid is added to it.
3. Extract is then refluxed for 1 hour and cooled.

4. Equal amount of water is added to the extract, and then refrigerated for 1 hour.
5. A characteristic fruity odor is noticed, which indicates the presence of Calatropis gigantea.

Croton tiglium
Sodium Hydroxide Test
1. 2 mL of concentrated extract of the residue in ethanol is taken in a test tube.
2. Equal volume of 40% sodium hydroxide solution is added to the above test tube.
3. A brownish-red or reddish-violet ring develops at the junction of the two liquids.
4. This development of ring at the junction of two liquids, confirms the presence of Croton tiglium.

Bam Ford's Test
1. 2 mL of concentrated ether extract of residue is taken in a porcelain basin.
2. The solvent is evaporated off.
3. To the residue, 1% alcoholic solution of p-dimethyl amino benzaldehyde acidified with 1 mL of concentrated sulfuric acid is added dropwise.
4. A transient red color is observed.
5. On evaporating to dryness in hot water bath, the residue becomes brownish-red to purple, which changes to pale blue on adding an excess of reagent.
6. This change in color on adding excess of reagent, confirms the presence of Croton tiglium.

Abrus Precatorius
Fast Blue B-Potassium Hydroxide Test
1. The dried residue of the extract is taken in a porcelain basin.
2. Few drops of 5% ethanolic solution of fast blue B salt are added, followed by two drops of aqueous KOH solution.
3. A red to orange color is observed, which indicates the presence of Abrus precatorius.

Marquis Test
1. Dried residue of extract is taken in a porcelain basin.
2. Two drops of Marquis reagent are added to the porcelain basin.
3. Pink color is formed, which confirms the presence of Abrus precatorius.

Van-UrK Test
1. Dried residue of the extract is taken in a porcelain basin.
2. One drop of Van-Urk reagent is added to the porcelain basin.

3. A green color changing to blue is observed.
4. This green color confirms the presence of Abrus precatorius.

Special Test (Agglutination Test)
1. Two drops of the aqueous solution of residue of the extract are taken in a small test tube.
2. 2 mL of defibrinated blood (undiluted) is added to the test tube.
3. The red blood corpuscles are agglutinated into a mass, like that of sealing wax.
4. This confirms the presence of Abrus precatorius.

Nessler's Reagent Test
1. 1 mL of test solution is taken in a small test tube.
2. 2–3 drops of Nessler's reagent are added to it.
3. Orange color is formed, which confirms the presence of Abrus precatorius.

Ferric Chloride Test
1. One drop of test solution is taken on the plate.
2. One drop of $FeCl_3$ solution is added to it, and then it is heated at 110°C for 5 minutes.
3. Violet-blue solution is formed, which confirms the presence of Abrus precatorius.

Digitalis Purpurea
Antimony Pentachloride Test
1. The dried residue of the extract is taken in a small porcelain basin.
2. Five drops of mixture of ethanol and chloroform (1:1) are added and stirred with the help of glass rod.
3. The organic solvent extract is spotted on filter paper in varying amounts and sprayed with a 10% solution of antimony pentachloride in chloroform.
4. The development of yellow color changing to purple is observed.
5. On warming the spotted paper in hot air for 5 minutes, the color of spot changes to black, which indicates Digitalis purpurea.

Digitoxin Test
1. Small amount of test solution is taken in a small test tube.
2. Few drops of concentrated sulfuric acid are added to it.
3. Green color appears, which is not affected by adding bromine water, indicating the presence of Digitalis purpurea.

Digitalin Test
1. Small amount of test solution is taken in a test tube.
2. To the test solution, few drops of concentrated sulfuric acid are added.

3. A yellow color appears, which rapidly changes to blood-red color.
4. The addition of bromine water changes its color to violet-red.
5. This change in color confirms the presence of Digitalis purpurea.

Ferric Chloride Test
1. The extracted residue is taken in a test tube.
2. Few drops of a mixture of concentrated sulfuric acid and alcohol (1:1) are added in the above test tube.
3. A yellow-brown color appears.
4. When one drop of dilute solution of ferric chloride is added, the solution turns bluish-green.
5. This bluish-green color confirms the presence of Digitalis purpurea.

Nicotiana Tabacum
Mayer's Reagent Test
1. The dried residue of the extract is acidified with acetic acid, followed by addition of two drops of reagent.
2. A white or yellowish precipitate is obtained, which confirms the presence of Nicotiana tabacum.

Phosphomolybdic Acid Test
1. Dried residue of the extract is taken in a small test tube.
2. A few drops of phosphomolybdic acid are added to it and warmed.
3. A yellowish-white precipitate is obtained, which confirms the presence of Nicotiana tabacum.

Silicotungstic Acid Test
1. Dried residue of the extract is taken in a small test tube.
2. A few drops of silicotungstic acid are added.
3. A white precipitate is obtained, which indicates the presence of Nicotiana tabacum.

Dragendorff's Reagent Test
1. Dried residue of the extract is taken in a small test tube.
2. A few drops of Dragendorff's reagent are added to it.
3. An orange color solution or precipitate is obtained, which confirms the presence of Nicotiana tabacum.

Schindel Misser's Test
1. A portion of the extracted residue is taken in a test tube.
2. One drop of formalin is added, followed by a single drop of concentrated sulfuric acid.
3. A rose-red color is obtained (in excess of formalin, a green color is obtained).
4. This rose-red color indicates the presence of Nicotiana tabacum.

Roussin's Test
1. A small portion of the extracted residue is taken in a small test tube.
2. Few drops of ether are added to it and transferred to a cavity slide.
3. To it is added a drop of ethereal solution of iodine.
4. Brownish-red precipitate is formed, which after keeping for four hours changes to ruby-red needle shaped crystals (Roussin's crystals).
5. These ruby-red needle-shaped crystals indicate the presence of Nicotiana tabacum.

P-Dimethylaminobenzaldehyde Test (PDMAB Test)
1. A drop of the PDMAB reagent is taken on a watch glass.
2. A drop of concentrated aqueous solution of residue containing Nicotiana tabacum is added from the side of the watch glass.
3. Immediately, a rose-red color is developed at the junction of two drops.
4. After shaking the above solution, a violet-red color is obtained, which confirms the presence of Nicotiana tabacum.

Aconitum Napellus
Palet's Reaction Test
1. Purified extract of the residue is taken in a test tube.
2. A few drops of the mixture consisting of 2.5 g syrupy phosphoric acid and 0.1 g of sodium molybdate is added and heated over the small flame until vapor appears.
3. A violet color develops, which confirms the presence of Aconitum napellus.

Alvarez Reaction Test
1. Purified residue is taken in a porcelain dish.
2. 5–10 drops of pure bromine is added to the residue in porcelain basin and evaporated to dryness in a water bath.
3. 1–2 mL of concentrated nitric acid is added and evaporated to dryness (if nitric acid loses its color, few drops of bromine are to be added).
4. To the yellow oxidation product, 1 mL of saturated alcoholic solution of sodium hydroxide is added and again evaporated to dryness.
5. A red or brown residue is obtained.
6. It is then allowed to cool. After cooling, 5–6 drops of 10% copper sulfate solution are added to it.
7. A green color develops, which indicates the presence of Aconitum napellus.

Gold Chloride Test
1. Two drops of acetic acid solution are taken into a glass basin, and evaporated to dryness.
2. The residue is dissolved in two drops of 0.01 N hydrochloric acid.

SCREENING/SPOT/COLOR TESTS FOR DIFFERENT POISONS

3. Few drops of 5% gold chloride solution are added to it.
4. An amorphous precipitate is formed, which when crystallized shows golden-yellow needles or rectangular prisms.
5. Formation of this golden-yellow needles or rectangular prisms, confirms the presence of Aconitum napellus.

Crystal Test
1. After undertaking preparative TLC, the scrapped material around spot is taken up in acetone and the extract is evaporated to dryness.
2. One drop of 0.01 N HCl is added followed by two drops of 5% sodium carbonate solution.
3. Crystals having shape of rosettes are observed, which confirms the presence of Aconitum napellus.

Datura Fastuosa
Vitali's Test
1. The extracted residue is dissolved in 2 mL of 0.5% acetic acid
2. Two drops of acetic acid solution are taken into a porcelain basin and evaporated to dryness.
3. To the above dry residue, one drop of fuming nitric acid is added.
4. It is again evaporated to dryness in a hot water bath.
5. After cooling, a drop of alcoholic KOH is added to it.
6. Violet color is produced, which immediately changes to red and then disappears.
7. On adding a few drops of alcoholic KOH, the color reappears again. This shows the presence of Datura fastuosa.

Microscopic Test
1. Dried residue of extract of vomit or stomach contents or viscera is taken on a microscopic slide with one drop of glycerin.
2. A characteristic structure similar to eyelids, confirms the presence of Datura fastuosa.

Strychnine (Strychnos nux-vomica)
Discussed in Screening/Spot/Color test for alkaloids.

Brucine
Discussed in Screening/Spot/Color test for alkaloids.

Cannabis Sativa
Fast Blue B Test
1. A small amount of residue of the extract is placed in the test tube.
2. A very small amount of solid fast blue B reagent is added to it, along with 1 mL of chloroform and shaken.

SCREENING/SPOT/COLOR TESTS FOR DIFFERENT POISONS

3. It is then kept for 2 minutes.
4. The chloroform layer becomes purple-red in color, which confirms Cannabis sativa.

Duquenois-Levine Test
1. A small amount of the residue of the extract is placed in a test tube.
2. It is shaken with 2 mL of acetaldehyde and vanillin reagent for 1 minute.
3. 2 mL of concentrated hydrochloric acid is added to it, shaken and allowed to stand for 10 minutes.
4. If color develops, 2 mL of chloroform is added.
5. The lower (chloroform) layer becomes violet, which indicates the presence of Cannabis sativa.

Test for Differentiation between Bhang, Ganja and Charas
1. Suspected material of Cannabis is extracted in ethanol.
2. A drop of extract is taken in the cavity of a spot tile/micro-tube and two drops of chromogenic reagent 1 (p-aminophenol, 1 mg in 10 mL ethanol) is added to it.
3. It is then thoroughly mixed, followed by addition of two drops of reagent 2 (i.e., 1 g of caustic potash in 10 mL of distilled water).
   - If blue color appears → it confirms *ganja*.
   - If green color appears → it confirms *bhang*.
   - If violet color appears → it confirms *charas*.

Opium Alkaloids
Froehde's Test
1. Dried residue of the extract is taken in the small test tube.
2. Few drops of Froehde's reagent are added to the test tube.
3. A violet color changing to green, and finally blue is observed.
4. This series of change in color indicates the presence of Opium.

Marquis Test
1. Dried residue of extract is taken in a porcelain basin.
2. One drop of Marquis reagent is added to it.
3. A purple-red color is produced, which changes to violet, and finally to blue, which confirms the presence of Opium.

Husemann's Test
1. A little dried extract is taken in a porcelain basin.
2. 2–3 drops of concentrated sulfuric acid are added and heated in a water bath for 30 minutes until white fumes appear.
3. A reddish or reddish-brown or black color appears.
4. It is cooled and one drop of conc. nitric acid, and a crystal of potassium nitrate is added to it.

5. A reddish-violet color appears, which immediately changes to blood red, and then to reddish-yellow, and finally fades away, which confirms the presence of Opium alkaloid.

Urotropine Test

1. Little amount of dried extract of the residue is taken in a porcelain basin.
2. Few drops of aqueous solution of urotropine are added and warmed slightly.
3. A purple color changing to blue, and then green is observed, which confirms the presence of Opium alkaloid.

Denigès-Oliver's Test

1. Two drops of acetic acid solution are taken into a porcelain basin.
2. One drop of ammonium hydroxide, followed by two drops hydrogen peroxide (20% volume) are added.
3. The solution is then rubbed gently with a clean small clean foil of copper.
4. When the resulting effervescence ceases, a pink or wine-red color is observed, which confirms the presence of Opium alkaloid.

Acetic Acid–Hydrochloric Acid Test

1. Two drops of acetic acid solution of the extracted residue are taken into a porcelain basin.
2. The residue is then mixed with few drops of dilute hydrochloric acid, and warmed over a low flame.
3. A pink or rose-red color is obtained, which indicates the presence of Opium alkaloid.

Ferric Salt Test (for Meconic Acid)

1. Small amount of suspected material is taken on a spot plate.
2. Two drops of water are added to it.
3. The sample is then titrated until the water becomes brown.
4. One drop of this brown liquid is taken to another spot plate, and one drop of ferric salt reagent is added to it.
5. A brown-purple color appears, which confirms the presence of Opium alkaloid.
6. The meconic acid is helpful in raw and prepared Opium, but it will not be detected in crude morphine.

Argemone Mexicana

Nitric Acid Test

1. Few drops of sample are taken in a test tube.
2. Equal volume of concentrated nitric acid is added to it.
3. A crimson-orange color appears, which indicates the presence of Argemone mexicana.

Cupric Acetate Test
1. 1 mL of glacial acetic acid and 2 mL of cupric acetate solution is added to 5 mL of oil sample in the test tube.
2. It is boiled in water bath for 15 minutes.
3. Greenish discoloration occurs, which confirms the presence of Argemone mexicana.

Ferric Chloride Test
1. 2 mL of concentrated hydrochloric acid is added to 4 mL of oil.
2. It is thoroughly mixed and warmed in a boiling water bath for 4–5 minutes.
3. 1 mL of ferric chloride solution is added; and again heated in a water bath for 10 minutes.
4. A precipitate of reddish-brown color appears. The precipitate is acicular or needle-shaped when observed under a microscope, which confirms the presence of Argemone mexicana.

Ergot
Marquis Reagent Test
1. A portion of dried residue of the extract is taken in a test tube.
2. One drop of Marquis reagent is added to the test tube.
3. A brown color develops, which confirms the presence of ergot.

Vitali's Test
1. The extracted residue is dissolved in 2 mL of 0.5% acetic acid.
2. Two drops of acetic acid solution are taken into a porcelain basin and evaporated to dryness.
3. To the above dried residue, one drop of fuming nitric acid is added.
4. It is then evaporated to dryness in a hot water bath.
5. After cooling, a drop of alcoholic KOH is added to it.
6. Violet color is produced, which immediately changes to red, and then disappears.
7. On adding a few drops of alcoholic KOH, the color reappears.
8. A play of colors from dull orange to yellow and then purple is observed with the residue of the extract, which confirms the presence of ergot.

Mandelin's Reagent Test
1. A portion of the dried residue of the extract is taken in a test tube.
2. One drop of Mandelin's reagent is added to it.
3. A purple-brown color develops, which confirms the presence of ergot.

Froehde's Reagent Test
1. A portion of dried residue of the extract is taken in a test tube.
2. 1 mL of Froehde's reagent is added to the test tube.

3. Change in color from deep-green to red, gray and finally blue is observed.
4. This change in color from deep-green to red, gray and finally blue indicates the presence of ergot.

Fluorescence Test
Blue fluorescence of ethanolic solution of residue of extract is observed under UV light in case of ergot.

Sulfuric Acid Test
1. Some portion of the extract is taken in a porcelain basin and evaporated to dryness.
2. 4–5 drops of concentrated sulfuric acid are added to the dried residue, followed by a micro drop of ferric chloride solution.
3. An orange-red color is developed, which changes to deep-red which indicates the presence of ergot.

Glacial Acetic Acid–Ferric Chloride Acid Test
1. A portion of the extracted residue is taken in the 10 mL of glacial acetic acid in the test tube.
2. One drop of ferric chloride solution is added to it.
3. The above mixture is then poured cautiously into another test tube containing 2 mL of concentrated sulfuric acid.
4. A bluish–violet color is developed at the junction of two liquids which indicates the presence of ergot.

Potassium Hydroxide Test
1. Small portion of the extract is taken in a test tube.
2. 1 mL of 10% potassium hydroxide is added to it and heated gently.
3. A faint-red color is obtained, and a fishy odor is noticed which confirm the presence of ergot.

Oleander (*Kaner*)
Nerin and thevetin are two active constituents of Oleander.

Keller's Test
1. Small amount of residue of the extract is taken in a test tube.
2. The residue is dissolved in 1 mL of glacial acetic acid containing 5% ferric sulfate and the solution is layered over concentrated sulfuric acid containing 0.05% ferric sulfate.
3. An immediate crimson color in the sulfuric acid layer, and a green color in the acetic acid layer confirm the presence of nerin.
4. An immediate blue color in the acetic acid layer, and a mauve color in the H_2SO_4 layer, confirms the presence of thevetin.

Sulfuric Acid/Phosphoric Acid Test

1. The purified acid ether extract of the sample is taken in a porcelain crucible.
2. One drop of concentrated sulfuric or phosphoric acid is added and warmed in the water bath.
3. If an immediate pink color appears, it confirms the presence of nerin.
4. If yellowish-brown color slowly changing to pink is obtained which confirms the presence of thevetin.

Hydrochloric Acid Test

1. Small amount of the extract is taken in a porcelain basin.
2. 2 mL of concentrated hydrochloric acid is added, and heated for few minutes.
3. A blue/bluish-green color appears, which confirms the presence of Oleander.

Vanilline–Sulfuric Acid Test

1. Small amount of extract is taken in a porcelain basin, and heated to form a residue.
2. One drop of vanillin-sulfuric acid reagent is added to it.
3. A pink or purple color is seen, which confirms the presence of Oleander.

Furfural–Sulfuric Acid Test

1. Small amount of extract is taken in a porcelain basin, and heated to form a residue.
2. One drop of furfural–sulfuric acid reagent is added to it.
3. Violet color is seen, which confirms the presence of Oleander.

■ CONCLUSION

All the above discussed screening/spot tests can be used for qualitative assessment of different pesticides/insecticides, volatile poisons, tranquilizers, alkaloids, metallic poisons, antibiotics, drug of abuse, acids and bases, toxic anions and plant poisons, etc., after extraction/isolation from biological materials, such as viscera, blood, urine, etc.

■ FURTHER READINGS

1. Brown GP, Yang K, King MA, Rossi GC, Leventhal L, Chang A, et al. 3-Methoxynaltrexone, a selective heroin/ morphine-6-beta-glucuronide antagonist. FEBS Lett. 1997;412(1):35-8.
2. Clarke EC. Isolation and Identification of drugs, 2nd edition. London: The Pharmaceutical Press; 1986.
3. Curry AS. Analytical Methods in Human Toxicology, 1st edition. London: Macmillan Press Ltd.; 1985. pp. 249-50, 161-9.

SCREENING/SPOT/COLOR TESTS FOR DIFFERENT POISONS

4. Directorate of Forensic Science. DFS Manual of Toxicology, 1st edition. New Delhi: Selective and Scientific Publisher; 2005.
5. Feigl F. Spot tests, 2nd edition. New York: Elsevier; 1939.
6. Jaiswal AK, Kashap SK, Gupta M, Mewar SK, Rana SV. Analysis of dimethoate in viscera sample using HPTLC plates. Amity J Behav Forens Sci. 2006;2(2):85-90.
7. Jaiswal AK, Millo T, Murthy OP. Toxicology Manual Series: Article–VI Screening/spot test for volatile poisons. Intl J Med Tox Leg Med. 2009;11(3):20-7.
8. Jaiswal AK, Millo T, Murthy OP. Toxicology Manual Series: Article–VII Screening/spot test for Metallic Poisons. Intl J Med Tox Leg Med. 2009;11(4):28-37.
9. Jaiswal AK, Millo T, Murthy OP. Toxicology Manual Series: Article–VIII Screening/spot test for Toxic Anions. Intl J Med Tox Leg Med. 2009;12(1):23-32.
10. Jaiswal AK, Millo T, Murthy OP. Toxicology Manual Series: Article–IX Screening/spot test for Plant Poisons. Intl J Med Tox Leg Med. 2009;12(2):39-40.
11. Jaiswal AK, Millo T, Murthy OP. Toxicology Manual Series: Article–X Screening/spot test for Pesticides/Insecticides. Intl J Med Tox Leg Med. 2010;12(3):54-62.
12. Jaiswal AK, Millo T, Murthy OP. Toxicology Manual Series: Article–XI Screening/spot test for Drugs of Abuse. Intl J Med Tox Leg Med. 2010;12(4):50-9.
13. Jaiswal AK, Millo T, Murthy OP. Toxicology Manual Series: Article–XII Screening/spot test for Acids and Alkalis (Bases). Intl J Med Tox Leg Med. 2010;13(1):50-7.
14. Jaiswal AK, Millo T, Murthy OP. Toxicology Manual Series: Article–XIII Screening/spot test for Antibiotics. Intl J Med Tox Leg Med. 2010;13(2):77-83.
15. Jeffcoat AR, Perez-Reyes M, Hill JM, Sadler BM, Cook CE. Cocaine disposition in humans after intravenous injection, nasal insufflation (snorting), or smoking. Drug Metab Dispos. 1989;17(2):153-9.
16. Jungreis E. Spot Test Analysis. New York: John Wiley and Sons; 1984.
17. Mathiharan K, Patnaik AK. Modi's Medical Jurisprudence and Toxicology, 23rd edition. New Delhi: Lexis Nexis; 2005.
18. Parikh CK. Parikh's Textbook of Medical Jurisprudence and Toxicology, 6th edition. New Delhi: CBS Publishers and Distributors; 2005.
19. Pillay VV. Modern Medical Toxicology, 3rd edition. New Delhi: Jaypee Brothers Medical Publishers (P) Ltd.; 2005.
20. Proceedings of National Workshop on Practical and Emergency Medical Toxicology. New Delhi: AIIMS; 1998.
21. Reddy KS. The Essentials of Forensic Medicine and Toxicology, 16th edition. New Delhi: Jaypee Brothers Medical Publishers (P) Ltd.; 1997.
22. Sawynok J. The therapeutic use of heroin: a review of the pharmacological literature. Can J Physiol Pharmacol. 1986;64(1):1-6.
23. Tiwari SN. Manual of Toxicology, 1st edition. Agra: Forensic Science Laboratory; 1976.
24. Vogel AI. A Text Book of Macro and Semi Micro Qualitative Inorganic Analysis, 4th edition. London: Longman & Co.; 1964.
25. Vogel AI. A Textbook of Quantitative Inorganic Analysis, 3rd edition. London: The ELBS and Longman Publishing Co.; 1975.
26. Vogel AI. Text Book of Macro and Semi Micro Qualitative Inorganic Analysis, 5th, 3edition. London: Longman & Co.; 1982.

Chapter 5

Thin Layer Chromatography and its Applications

■ INTRODUCTION

Chromatography is the most modern and versatile method used for the separation and purification of organic compounds. The method was first discovered by Mikhail Tswett, a Russian botanist, in 1906, for the separation of colored substances into individual components. In chromatography, separation is achieved by the differential movement of individual components through a stationary phase under the influence of a mobile phase. Adsorption chromatography is based on the facts that different compounds are adsorbed on adsorbent to different degrees. Commonly used adsorbents are silica gel and alumina. When a mobile phase is allowed to move over a stationary phase (adsorbent), the components of the mixture move by varying distances over the stationary phase. There are two main types of chromatographic techniques based on the principle of different adsorption: (1) column chromatography and (2) thin layer chromatography.

Column chromatography (**Fig. 5.1**) involves separation of a mixture in a long glass tube, called column, packed with an adsorbent, the column is fitted with a stopcock at its lower end, the mixture is dissolved in a

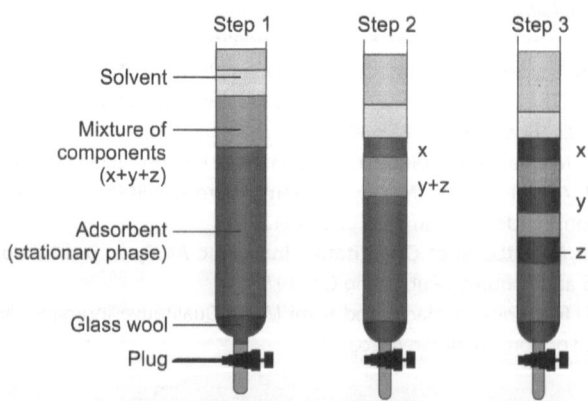

Fig. 5.1: Column chromatography.

minimum amount of solvent and transferred on the top of the adsorbent in the column. An appropriate solvent or a mixture of solvents is allowed to flow-down the column slowly. Depending upon the degree to which the compounds are adsorbed, partial or complete separation takes place. The most readily adsorbed substance is retained near the top and others come down to various distances in the column.

Thin layer chromatography (TLC) is another type of adsorption chromatography. This involves separation of the components of a mixture over a thin layer of an adsorbent. A thin layer of an adsorbent is spread over a glass plate of suitable size. The plate is called as thin layer chromatography plate. The solution of a mixture to be separated is applied as a small spot about 10-20 mm above one end of the TLC plate. The glass plate is then placed in a closed jar containing the solvent. As the solvent jar moves up the plate, the components of the mixture move up along the plate to different distances, depending on their degree of adsorption, and separation takes place.

Thin layer chromatography has found wide recognition in many fields and its sensitivity of detection offers particular advantage to the toxicologist/chemist which has increased, 10-100 times as compared to the chemical methods. It has become an important analytical tool since it can separate complex mixture in a relatively short time. It is also possible to achieve reproducibility of a very high degree by means of controlling the coating. In TLC, the individual spots are more discrete and are not diffused as in paper chromatography. In addition to the usual visualization employed with paper chromatography, reagents of corrosive nature, such as sulfuric acid, nitric acid, perchloric acid and the possible use of high temperatures with carbonization offer a much wider range of detection in this technique. The background substances which cause inherent fluorescence in paper chromatography are not encountered in the inorganic chromatographic substances used in TLC.

Basic principle of TLC: Thin layer chromatography is an adsorption chromatography which involves separation of the substances of a mixture over a thin layer of adsorbent which is supported on a glass plate or other supporting medium under the influence of mobile phase.

■ BASIC REQUIREMENT OF THIN LAYER CHROMATOGRAPHY

There are several materials/items which are necessary to perform TLC experiment without which we cannot proceed. The following items should be available in the laboratory while performing TLC experiment:
- An adsorbent
- Glass plates or other supporting medium of different size
- TLC plate holder
- TLC chamber

- Oven
- TLC plate heater
- Fume hood
- UV viewing cabinet
- TLC spray cabinet
- Digital camera
- Glass capillaries
- TLC sprayer
- Refrigerators

Adsorbents Used in Thin Layer Chromatography

Usually, the adsorbents used are highly polar in nature, and the solvents are highly nonpolar. Several compounds are being used as adsorbents in TLC. A few examples of adsorbent used for TLC are silica gel, alumina, aluminum silicate, bauxite, calcium carbonate, calcium hydroxide, calcium oxalate, calcium silicate, calcium sulfate, dicalcium phosphate, Fuller's earth, hydroxylapatite, magnesia, magnesium silicate, tricalcium phosphate, water soluble salts, zinc carbonate, cellulose, charcoal and activated carbon, dextran gels, polyamide powder, activated bentonite, sucrose, polyethylene powder, diatomaceous earth, activated perlite and baby powder, etc. Pictorial view of silica gel, which is the most commonly used adsorbent from Merck is given in **Figure 5.2**.

Glass Plates or Other Supporting Medium of Different Size

In TLC, the adsorbent is thinly coated onto a suitable support, e.g., glass plate, polyester or aluminum sheet. Glass is the most commonly used plate, because it is rigid, transparent and chemically resistant to mobile phases and easy to visualize chemicals. Glass plates are also reusable; an important consideration for analysts who make their own plates. For

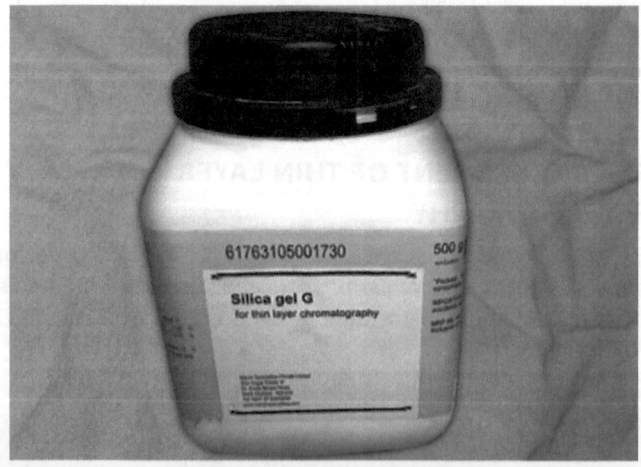

Fig. 5.2: Silica gel from Merck.

THIN LAYER CHROMATOGRAPHY AND ITS APPLICATIONS

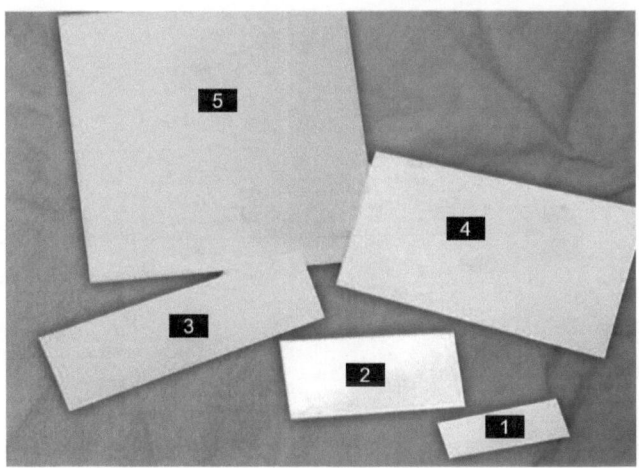

Fig. 5.3: Thin layer chromatography glass plates of different size coated with silica gel (adsorbent) (1—2.5 × 7.5 cm; 2—05 × 10 cm; 3—05 × 20 cm; 4—10 × 20 cm; 5—20 × 20 cm).

in situ densitometry quantification, the use of uniform precoated layers on glass is virtually mandatory for reproducibility and accuracy. For thin layer and preparative layer chromatography, ready-to-use glass plates of layer thickness 0.25 mm, allow safe spotting without layer damage and plates have a uniform, abrasion-resistant coating and an inert, hard-layer binder that is abrasion-resistant. Glass plates of following sizes are required for conducting the experiment. Glass plates of different sizes coated with adsorbent (silica gel) are shown in **Figure 5.3**.

Means of Holding the Plates during Coating (TLC Plate Holder)

One TLC plate holder for holding different sizes of TLC plates, such as 2.5 × 7.5 cm, 5 × 10 cm, 5 × 20 cm, 10 × 20 cm and 20 × 20 cm are also essential for TLC experiment. TLC plate holder which can hold 20 × 20 size plate easily is given in **Figure 5.4**.

Thin Layer Chromatography Chamber

Different types of TLC chambers are required for running different types of TLC plates. On top of it, the substance mixture separates by elution with a suitable solvent. The usual technique involves a single TLC run in a glass chamber. However, better separation results can be obtained through multiple runs with or without modifications in mobile phase. TLC chamber of different sizes with lid are given in **Figure 5.5**.

Oven

An oven is also essential for TLC experiment. It is used for activating the layers after coating. The silica gel on the plates becomes activated when

THIN LAYER CHROMATOGRAPHY AND ITS APPLICATIONS

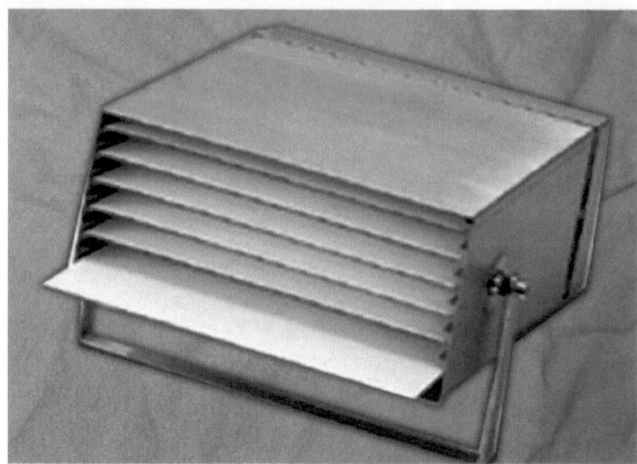

Fig. 5.4: Thin layer chromatography plate holder.

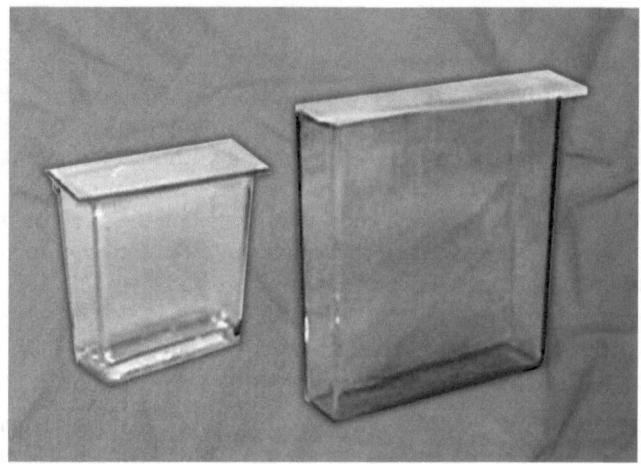

Fig. 5.5: Thin layer chromatography chambers of different size with lid.

all the water has been removed by drying in an oven. This allows for more interaction between the compound being eluted on the plate and the silica gel, which results in lower retention factor (R_f). The picture of oven is given in **Figure 5.6**.

TLC Plate Heater

Thin layer chromatography plate after spraying should not be exposed to direct sunlight. At least one TLC plate heater should be available in the laboratory for drying of the TLC plate after spraying with visualization reagent. The TLC plate heater is designed for heating TLC plates to a given temperature, while insuring homogenous heating across the plate. Pictorial view of TLC plate heater is shown in the **Figure 5.7**. The 200 × 200 mm

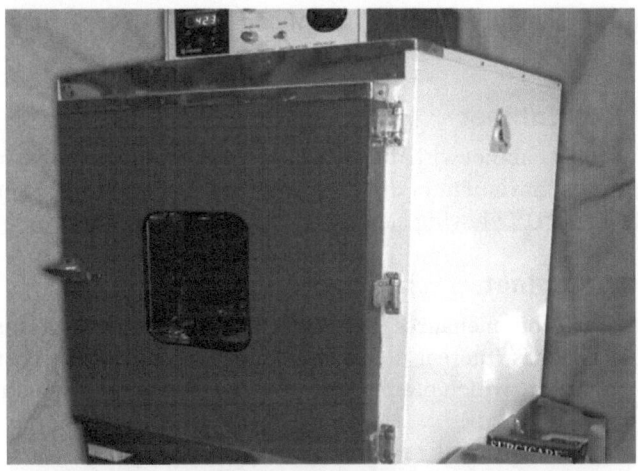

Fig. 5.6: Oven for activating thin layer chromatography plates.

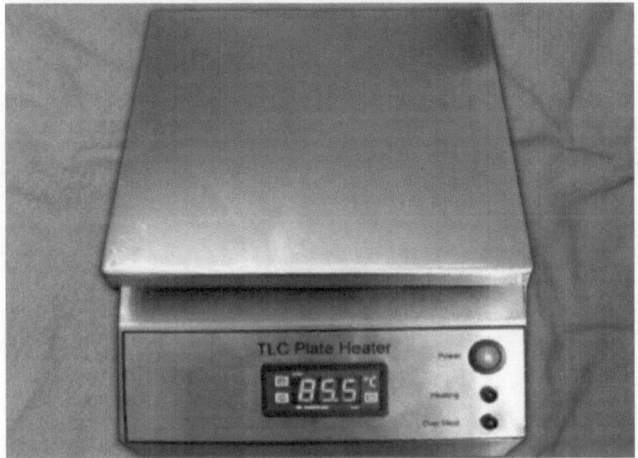

Fig. 5.7: Thin layer chromatography plate heater from TABA TEB Company.

heating surface has a grid to facilitate correct positioning of the TLC plate. The other advantages of the TLC plate heater are:
- Actual temperature is displayed digitally
- Temperature is selectable between 25°C and 200°C
- Plate heater is protected from overheating

Fume Hood

Fume hood is very essential for TLC. While preparing the samples for TLC (toxin, pesticide, poisons, etc.) there is a danger of it being absorbed by the skin or of it being inhaled, which can cause allergies or even other serious side effects. Hence, this work must always be carried out in fume hoods. All the solvents should be opened and measured in fume hood. Even the

THIN LAYER CHROMATOGRAPHY AND ITS APPLICATIONS

TLC chamber should be kept in fume hood during development. Simple type of fume hood for TLC is given in **Figure 5.8**.

UV Viewing Cabinet

One UV viewing cabinet with dual wavelength 254/366 nm is also required for viewing the movement of different spots during TLC experimentation. Pictorial view of UV viewing cabinet is given in **Figure 5.9**.

TLC Spray Cabinet

The TLC spray cabinet ensures the complete removal of reagent mist while spraying TLC plates. There is no deflection of the spray jet before it reaches the chromatogram, which often occurs in a normal laboratory fume hood.

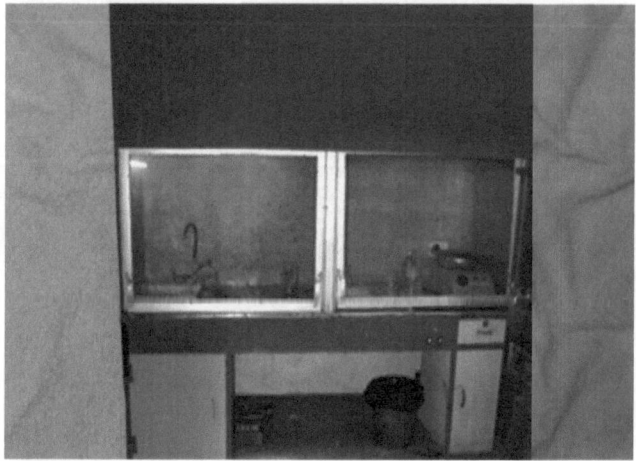

Fig. 5.8: Fume hood.

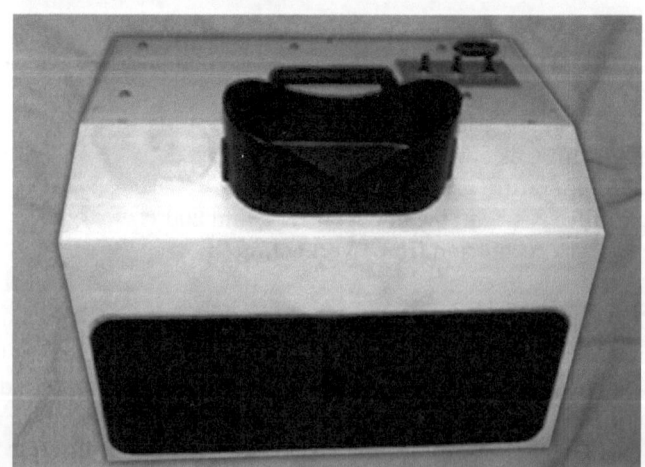

Fig. 5.9: UV viewing cabinet from JSGW.

THIN LAYER CHROMATOGRAPHY AND ITS APPLICATIONS

The TLC spray cabinet is made of polyvinyl chloride (PVC). The blower which has a radial fan driven by a motor outside of the fume duct produces airflow. Pictorial view of TLC spray cabinets is given in **Figure 5.10**.

Digital Camera

One good quality digital camera, which will take the photograph of the chromatograms in the day light at a distance 30–50 cm, should be available. A pictorial view of digital camera is given in **Figure 5.11**.

Glass Capillaries

Graduated/nongraduated glass capillaries are also required for spotting sample as well as standard during experiment. It is available in packets of 50 pieces and 100 pieces. The pictorial view of capillaries is given in **Figure 5.12**.

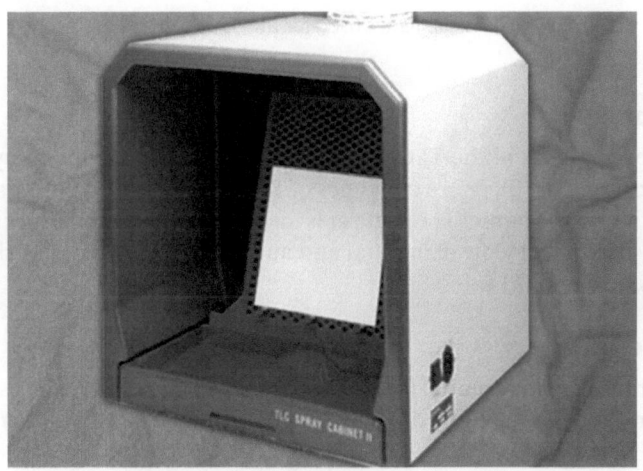

Fig. 5.10: TLC spray cabinet from CAMAG®.

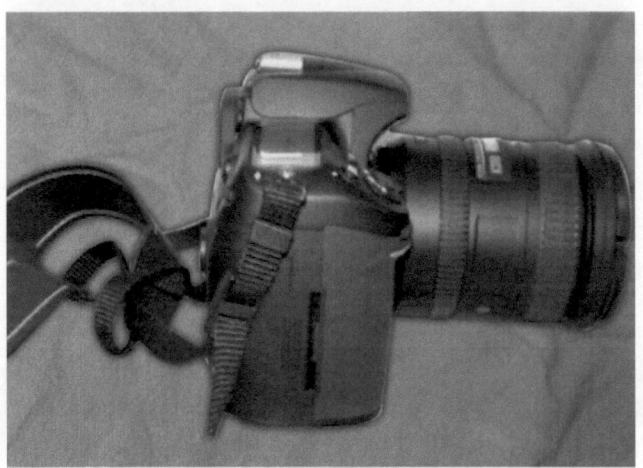

Fig. 5.11: Digital camera from Nikon.

THIN LAYER CHROMATOGRAPHY AND ITS APPLICATIONS

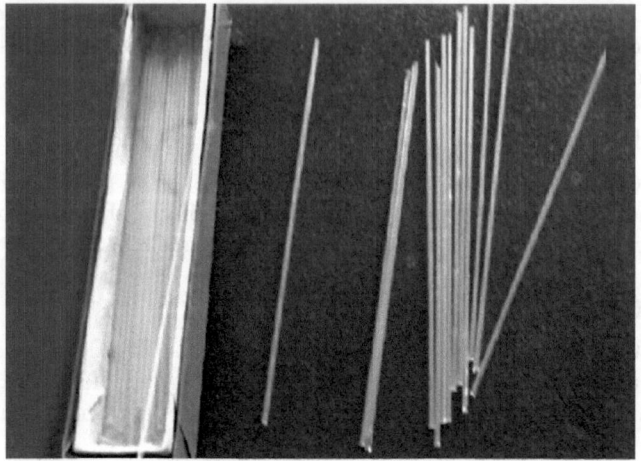

Fig. 5.12: Glass capillaries used for thin layer chromatography.

TLC Sprayer

After development of the TLC plate, we need TLC sprayer for spraying the visualizing agent. There are two types of TLC sprayer, one is automatic, and other is manual. Manual TLC sprayer is made up of the glass connected with the valve. Pictorial view of manual and automatic TLC sprayer is shown in **Figures 5.13** and **5.14**.

Refrigerator

Refrigerator is also essential for TLC for storage of standard and its solution. Refrigerator of either 100 L or 150 L is sufficient for TLC experiment.

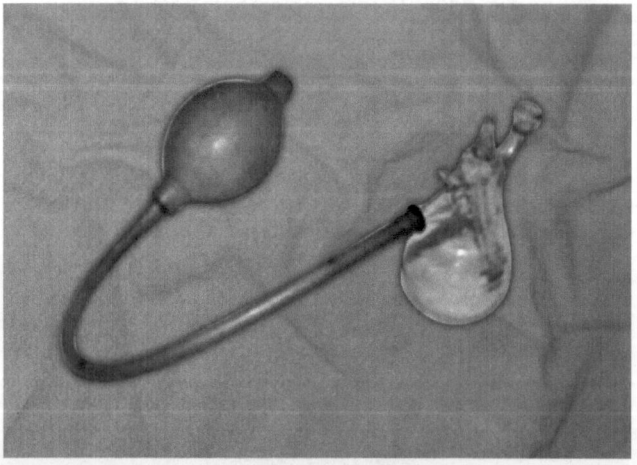

Fig. 5.13: Glass TLC sprayer.

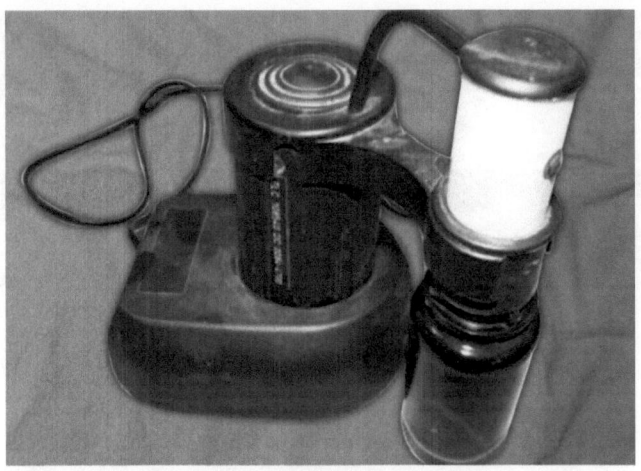

Fig. 5.14: Automatic TLC sprayer (Merck).

■ TYPES OF THIN LAYER CHROMATOGRAPHY PLATES

There are two types of the TLC plates, one is handmade plate, and other is precoated plate.

Handmade Plates

Thin layer chromatography plates manually made in laboratory are called handmade TLC plates. For this, a tablespoon of silica gel is mixed with one tablespoon of water. It is mixed to get uniform suspension. Small amount of suspension is poured on the plate very carefully. Make sure, you are not holding plate by the sides—that will cause suspension to spill over the edge of the plate as soon as it touches your fingers.

Tilt plate carefully from side to side until suspension covers all plate as a thin liquid layer. The plate is kept in a safe place on horizontal surface to dry. Different steps involved in handmade TLC plates are shown in **Figure 5.15**.

Precoated Plates

Precoated plates are used for analytical TLC, high performance analytical TLC, or preparative TLC. The solvent used on these plates are carefully standardized and controlled. Each TLC plate is characterized by narrow particle size, pore volume distribution, standardized surface area activity, and high resolution capacity. Precoated products are stable and economical with uniform feature, hard and abrasion-resistant coating. F_{254} is a fluorescent indicator with a 254 nm excitation wavelength. F (254 + 366) is a fluorescent indicator with 254 nm and 366 nm excitation wavelengths.

F_{254} is an acid-stable fluorescent indicator with a 254 nm excitation wavelength. Vacuum-sealed plates exclude moisture and have a convenient hard surface for writing. Pictorial view of precoated TLC plates is shown in **Figure 5.16**.

THIN LAYER CHROMATOGRAPHY AND ITS APPLICATIONS

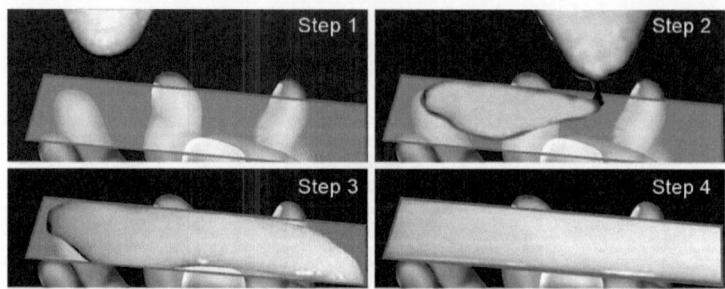

Fig. 5.15: Handmade TLC plates.

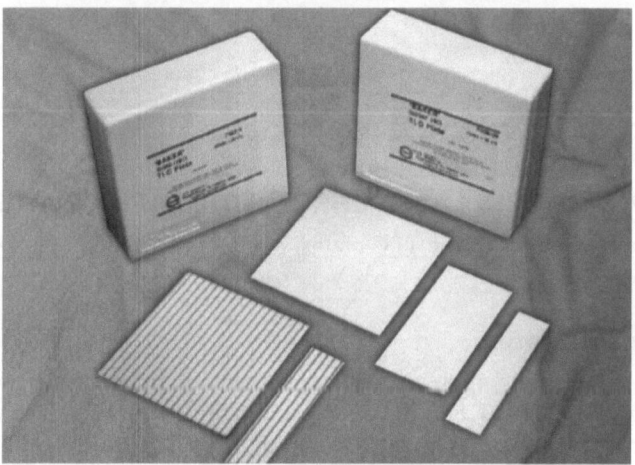

Fig. 5.16: Precoated TLC plates from Merck.

Important Points about Handmade Plates and Precoated Plates

1. Generally, results on handmade plates are less reproducible than precoated plates.
2. The quality of handmade TLC plates should be carefully monitored. Activation, i.e., heating at 100°C for 30 minutes before use may be helpful in maintaining performance.
3. Preparing TLC plates by dipping glass plates into slurry of silica with subsequent drying gives very variable results and is not to be recommended.
4. It is advised to use an applicator to apply the stationary phase, on the plate so as to get a uniform and thin layer on the plate.
5. Lack of uniformity and thinness can badly affect the success of the experiment.
6. Experience suggests that it is best to standardize on a particular brand of commercially available plates, such as Silica gel GF_{254}. However, even with commercially available precoated plates, batch-to-batch variations in retention time, and also in sensitivity may be encountered.

PREPARATION OF THIN LAYER CHROMATOGRAPHY PLATES

Setting-out the Glass Plates and Preparing the Spreader

The plates must be carefully cleaned and completely free of grease. The plates are thoroughly washed with a vim powder or left for some hours in chromic acid solution. They are then thoroughly brushed under running tap water, rinsed with distilled water and dried at room temperature. They may also be rubbed dry with liquid free absorbent paper. It is not advisable to rinse them with usual organic solvents. The aligning tray, approximately 110 cm long, is placed on the bench with its short run of the right five 20 × 20 cm glass plates of equal thickness placed on the tray. To prevent them from sliding about on the baseboard, they can be stitch down with a little water. The left and right hand of the row of plates are completed with two 5 × 20 cm plates. The top of the spreader is opened and it is then placed on the left hand and plate with the lever of the tipping mechanism pointing to the right.

Preparation of Suspensions

For silica gel or silica gel G plates: 25 g of silica gel (silica gel G) in 200 mesh is shaken thoroughly with 50 mL distill water in 250 mL flask-fitted with stopper for 30 seconds to get homogeneous slurry.

For alumina plates: 25 g of aluminum oxide G is shaken with 55 mL distilled water in a 250 mL flask-fitted with stopper for 30 seconds to get homogeneous slurry.

For cellulose plates: 15 g of fibrous cellulose is shaken with 100 mL distilled water in a 250 mL flask-fitted with stopper for 30 seconds to get homogeneous slurry.

For silica gel with starch: 30 g of silica gel with starch is mixed with 90 mL of boiling water in a 250 mL flask and shaken to get homogeneous slurry.

For acetylated cellulose and $CaSO_4 \cdot \frac{1}{2} H_2O$ plates: Suspend 30 g of acetylated cellulose and 4.5 g of $CaSO_4$ in a mixture containing 60 mL of water and 10 mL of methanol. Stir it in an electric stirrer for 30 seconds to get homogeneous slurry. Sometime, air bubbles get trapped, which can be removed by pouring 2–3 mL of methanol over slurry, followed by shaking. Use the slurry prepared within 10 minutes for coating the plates.

For basic silica gel plates: Mix silica gel with 0.1 N NaOH, Sorensen buffer (pH 6.8) or 0.15M sodium acetate solution in place of water.

For acidic silica gel plates: Prepared by using 0.2M oxalic acid or 2.5% (v/v) sulfuric acid solution in place of water.

For fluorescent plates: Prepared by using a 0.04% solution of fluorescein in place of water to prepare the slurry.

Coating of Plates

When suspension is ready, the same should be sprayed on the TLC plate either manually, or by using TLC spreader on suitable size of TLC plate to get homogeneous layer. During use of spreader, the suspension is poured into the spreader and the lever twisted through 180°. When slurry can be seen coming out, the process of coating has begun. The lever is again turned opposite 180° to prevent any liquid still remaining in the spreader from running out.

Treatment of the Plates after Coating

After coating, plate should be treated with several processes such as drying, activation, storage, etc.

Drying: The plates are left in position until their surface has become completely dry (about 10–20 min). It is then best to leave them to dry in air overnight, when layers, that adhere particularly well, are obtained. These dried layers are adequate for many separations.

Activation: The plates are placed in a drying cabinet, i.e., oven, but not before they have set, i.e., when the surface is wet. Time and temperature of heating are determined by the required activity of thin layers. Heating at 105°C for 30 minutes gives an activity about equal to that of standardized neutral alumina "Merck" (Grade II/III). Layers with greater adsorption activity are obtained by heating for longer time at higher temperature.

Storage: Since active plates become deactivated in moist air, they are stored over a desiccant (silica gel, activated alumina, calcium chloride, etc.) in a desiccator of 30 cm internal diameter, or in a plate cabinet. If hot plates are placed in the desiccator, the tap must be left open, so this is provided with a short drying tube filled with silica gel.

Testing of silica gel G plates: The layers should be uniform in appearance by both transmitted and reflected lights. The surface must be smooth with no coarse grains visible. They must adhere sufficiently well, so that they are markedly damaged if rubbed lightly with the finger.

■ SOLVENTS/MOBILE PHASE USED FOR THIN LAYER CHROMATOGRAPHY

In order to obtain reproducible results, only pure solvents must be used in chromatography. Solvents that undergo chemical changes should preferably be freshly prepared. If the substances remain near the base line when chromatographed, either a more strongly elutive solvent is chosen, or a more strongly elutive component is added to the solvent being used, and if the substances migrate rapidly, a more weakly elutive solvent is used. Mixture of two or three solvents of different polarity gives better separation than chemically homogeneous solvents. Solvent systems for analysis of different samples, such as pesticides, barbiturates, narcotics, tranquilizers are given in **Table 5.1**.

Table 5.1: Developing solvent system/mobile phase for different compounds.

S. No.	Solvent system	Solvent ratio
\multicolumn{3}{c}{Organophosphorous}		
1.	Hexane: Acetone	8: 2
2.	Chloroform: Acetone	7: 3
3.	Hexane: Benzene: Methanol: Acetone	5: 3: 1.9: 0.1
4.	Benzene: Chloroform: Methanol: Acetic acid	7: 2: 1: 0.1
5.	Hexane: Benzene: Chloroform	7: 2: 1
6.	Hexane: Benzene: Ethyl acetate: Acetic acid	6: 2.5: 1.5: 0.1
7.	Benzene: Chloroform: Acetone	6: 3: 1
8.	Cyclohexane: Chloroform	7: 3
9.	Petroleum ether: Acetone	7: 3
10.	Benzene: Methanol	6: 4
11.	Chloroform: Liquid Paraffin	9: 1
12.	Hexane: Dioxane: Acetic acid	7.9: 2: 0.1
13.	Hexane: Dioxane	8: 2
14.	Chloroform: Ether	8: 2
15.	Hexane: Chloroform	8: 2
16.	Hexane: Acetone: Methanol: Acetic acid	6.3: 3: 1: 0.2
17.	Hexane: Benzene: Ethyl acetate: Acetic acid	6: 2.5: 1.5: 0.5
18.	Hexane: Benzene: Methanol: Acetic Acid	5: 3: 1.9: 1
19.	Benzene: Chloroform: Methanol: Acetone	5: 3: 1.5: 0.5
20.	Benzene: Chloroform: Acetic acid	6: 4: 0.5
21.	Gardona: Chloroform: Acetone	5: 5: 0.5
22.	Petroleum ether: Benzene: Ethyl acetate	6.5: 3: 0.5
23.	Hexane: Xylene: Ethyl acetate: acetone	6: 1.5: 0.5: 1.5
24.	Hexane: Ether	1: 1
\multicolumn{3}{c}{Carbamates}		
1.	Cyclohexane: Acetone	8: 2
2.	Benzene	10
3.	Hexane: Acetone	8: 2
4.	Hexane: Benzene: Methanol: Acetone	5: 3: 1.9: 0.1
5.	Benzene: Chloroform: Methanol: Acetic acid	7: 2: 1: 0.1
6.	Benzene: Hexane: Chloroform: Methanol: Acetic acid	5: 3: 1.5: 0.5: 0.1
7.	Hexane: Benzene	6: 4
8.	Hexane: Benzene: Petroleum ether	6: 3: 1
9.	Hexane: Ethyl acetate: Chloroform: Acetone	5: 3: 1: 1

Continued

THIN LAYER CHROMATOGRAPHY AND ITS APPLICATIONS

Continued

S. No.	Solvent system	Solvent ratio
10.	Benzene: Chloroform: Acetone	6: 3: 1
11.	Hexane: Benzene: Chloroform: Acetic acid	6: 2: 2: 0.1
12.	Toluene: Ethyl acetate	8: 2
13.	Ethanol: Water: Acetic acid	6.5: 2.5: 1
14.	Benzene: Ethyl acetate	5: 1
15.	Toluene: Ether: Ethyl acetate	6: 3: 1
16.	Chloroform: Acetonitrile: Acetone	4: 1: 1
17.	Ether: Hexane	4: 1
18.	Toluene: Ethyl acetate	8: 2
Organochloro compound		
1.	Hexane: Acetone	9: 1
2.	Hexane: Benzene: Methanol: Acetic acid	5: 3: 1.9: 0.1
3.	Benzene: Chloroform: Methanol: Acetic acid	5: 3: 1.9: 0.1
4.	Benzene: Hexane: Chloroform: Methanol: Acetic acid	5: 3: 1.5: 0.5: 0.1
5.	Hexane: Benzene: Chloroform	7: 2: 1
6.	Hexane: Benzene: Ethyl acetate: Acetic acid	6: 2.5: 1.5: 5
7.	Hexane: Chloroform: Benzene: Acetic acid	6: 3: 1: 0.5
8.	Hexane: Ethyl acetate: Chloroform: Acetone	5: 3: 1: 1
9.	Benzene: Chloroform: Acetone	6: 3: 1
10.	Hexane: Benzene: Chloroform: Acetic acid	6: 2: 2: 0.5
11.	Hexane: Ethyl acetate	9: 1
12.	Hexane: Benzene: Ethyl acetate	6: 4: 1
13.	Hexane: Ether	8.5: 1.5
14.	Petroleum ether: Liquid paraffin	9: 1
15.	Cyclohexane: Liquid paraffin	8.5: 1.5
16.	Cyclohexane: Methylene dichloride	9: 1
17.	Petroleum	10
Pyrethroid		
1.	Benzene: Hexane: Chloroform	4.5: 4.5: 1
2.	Benzene	100
3.	Cyclohexane: Toluene	7: 3
4.	Petroleum ether: Diethyl ether	9: 1
5.	Cyclohexane: Toluene	6: 4
6.	Hexane: Acetone: Acetic acid	5: 5: 0.1
7.	Toluene: Diethyl ether: Acetic acid	7.5: 2.5: 0.1
8.	Hexane: Chloroform: Acetic acid	9: 5: 0.5

Continued

Continued

S. No.	Solvent system	Solvent ratio
9.	Hexane: Benzene	4.5: 5.5
10.	Hexane: Chloroform: Benzene	4.5: 0.5: 5
11.	Hexane: Chloroform	7: 3
12.	Benzene: Carbon tetrachloride	6: 4
13.	Hexane: Benzene: Acetone	4.5: 4.5: 1
14.	Hexane: Ether	4: 1
15.	Chloroform: Acetic acid	9.9: 0.1
16.	Toluene: Hexane	5: 5
17.	Hexane: Ether	20: 1
18.	Toluene: Ether: Acetic acid	7.5: 2.5: 0.1
19.	Butanol: Acetic acid: Water	6: 1: 1
20.	Hexane: Toluene: Acetic acid	3: 15: 2
21.	Methanol: Water	8: 2
22.	Hexane: Chloroform	6: 4
23.	Benzene saturated with formic acid: Ether	8.9: 1.1
24.	Hexane: Benzene: Acetone	7: 3: 0.1
25.	Toluene: Ether: Acetic acid	7.5: 2.5: 0.2
Barbiturates		
1.	Ethyl acetate: Methanol: Ammonia	8.5: 1: 0.5
2.	Chloroform: Acetone	8: 2
3.	Benzene: Acetic acid	9: 1
4.	Dioxane: Benzene: Ammonium hydroxide	2: 7.5: 0.5
5.	Chloroform: Acetone	9: 1
Tranquilizers		
1.	Chloroform: Acetone	8: 2
2.	Chloroform: Methanol	9: 1
3.	Cyclohexane: Toluene: Diethylamine	7.5: 1.5: 1
Narcotics		
1.	Cyclohexane: Toluene: Diethylamine	7.5: 1.5: 1
2.	Methanol: Concentrated ammonia	9: 1
3.	Chloroform: Methanol	9: 1

■ APPLYING THE SUBSTANCE ON THIN LAYER CHROMATO-GRAPHY PLATE/LOADING OF SAMPLE AND STANDARD

The mixtures to be separated are applied to the starting line of the chromatogram as in paper chromatography. This line is usually about 1.5–2.0 cm from the edge of the plate. Suitable pipettes or capillary tube

THIN LAYER CHROMATOGRAPHY AND ITS APPLICATIONS

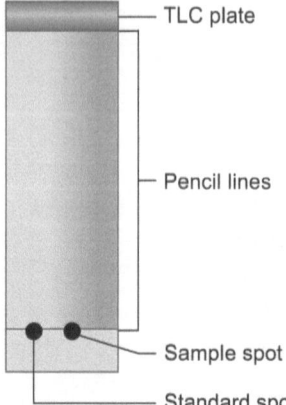

Fig. 5.17: Loading of sample and standard on thin layer chromatography (TLC) plate.

are used for applying the substances. Sharp micropipettes with a volume of 10 μL are very convenient. Blood sampling pipettes, used in blood counts are also suitable. The diameter of starting spots should be kept as small as possible. Less concentrated solutions are applied several times in succession, allowing them to dry out for a short time between each application. Lyophilic substances should preferably be applied in a nonpolar solvent. The simplest method is to number the spots from left to right, and record in a note-book the substances that have been applied. This information can also be written on the plate. **Figure 5.17** shows the loading of sample and standard on TLC plate.

■ OPERATION/DEVELOPMENT OF CHROMATOGRAM

The tank is filled to a depth of about 10 mm with the solvent and covered with glass plate. The coated plate with the substances to be separated is placed layer side down on the frame of the separation chamber, and is fastened to the latter with two chips. Where the plate rests on the support edges of the frame, the layer has previously been wiped off with a finger. The chamber is now so positioned in the cylindrical tank containing the solvent that the liquid can enter the openings into the chamber and rinse the layer. **Figure 5.18** shows the development of chromatogram.

■ DETECTION REAGENTS/SPRAYING REAGENTS FOR VISUALIZING THE CHROMATOGRAM

Compounds not characterized by the possession of color, strong absorption to UV or fluorescence have to be rendered visible by special detection reagents applied to the layer by means of a spray. Different spraying reagent with their preparation, spraying procedure and application are given in **Table 5.2**.

THIN LAYER CHROMATOGRAPHY AND ITS APPLICATIONS

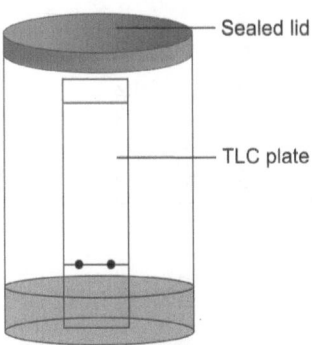

Fig. 5.18: Development of chromatogram.

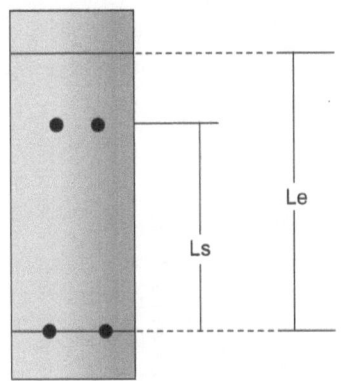

Fig. 5.19: Calculation of R_f value by measuring Ls and Le.

RETENTION FACTOR

Retention factor (R_f) is defined as the ratio of distance traveled (**Fig. 5.19**) by analyte to the distance traveled by solvent. It is also known as retardation factor. It is represented by R_f. If the retention factor of the compound and the sample are same, then we can say that the sample contains the compound as in the standard. R_f can be calculated by using following formula:

$$R_f = \frac{\text{Distance traveled by analyte (Ls)}}{\text{Distance traveled by solvent font (Le)}}$$

Factors Affecting R_f Values

The reproducibility of R_f value depends upon various factors as mentioned here.

1. *Quality of the layer material:* It is best to use, only material from a single delivery during a series of experiments, as it can vary sometimes from batch to batch.
2. *Activation grade of the layer, humidity*: Activity is determined by time and temperature of heating. Therefore, plates must receive always identical pretreatment, because relative humidity at the time of application of the samples and during development in the chromatography tank is also of great importance.
3. *Layer thickness, preparation of the layer:* The effect of the layer thickness from 0.2–0.3 mm can be ignored.
4. *Quality of the solvent:* Only very pure solvents must be used.
5. *Tank saturation:* R_f values are strongly influenced by saturation of the atmosphere in the chromatography tank with vapor.
6. *Technique:* Ascending to horizontal or descending methods.
7. Development distance and distance of the starting point from the surface of the solvent.
    - Surface of the solvent – starting point.
    - Surface of the solvent – solvent front.

THIN LAYER CHROMATOGRAPHY AND ITS APPLICATIONS

Table 5.2: Different spraying reagents with their preparation, spraying procedure and application.

S. No.	Spraying reagent	Preparation	Spraying procedure	Application
1.	Aluminum chloride	1 g of aluminum chloride is dissolved in 100 mL of ethanol	Solution sprayed on developed plate and dried	Flavonoids
2.	Ammonium molybdate	Solution I: 1M perchloric acid is dissolved in water/acetone (1:1) Solution II: (Ammonium molybdate Soln): 5g $(NH_4)_6Mo_7O_{24} \cdot 4H_2O$ is dissolved in 35 mL semi-conc. nitric acid and 65 mL water. Solution III (Tin (II) chloride Soln): 0.5 g $SnCl_2 \cdot H_2O$ is dissolved in 100 mL 0.5M hydrochloric acid.	Sprayed with solution I and II and finally with solution III and heated to 60°C	Phosphoric acid derivatives
3.	p-Anisaldehyde-acetic acid	0.5 mL p-anisaldehyde is dissolved in 50 ml glacial acetic acid and 1 mL 97% sulfuric acid.	Solution sprayed on plate and heated to 105°C	Phenols, sugars, steroids, and terpenes
4.	p-Anisaldehyde – ethanol	1 mL p-Anisaldehyde, 1 mL 97% sulfuric acid is dissolved in 18 mL ethanol	Solution sprayed on plate and heated to 110°C	Sugars
5.	p-Anisidine Hydrochloride	3% p-anisidine hydrochloride in n-butanol	Solution sprayed on plate and heated to 100°C for 2–10 min	Carbohydrates and sugars
6.	Anisidine phthalate	1.23 g p-anisidine and 1.66 g phthalic acid is dissolved in 100 mL of 95% ethanol	Solution sprayed on plate	Carbohydrates and reducing sugars
7.	Antimony (III) chloride	25 g antimony (III) chloride is dissolved in 75 mL chloroform/a saturated solution of antimony (III) chloride in chloroform or carbon tetrachloride	Solution sprayed on plate and heated to 100°C for 10 min	Vitamins A and D, steroids and terpenes
8.	Alkaline fast blue B Salt	0.1 g of fast blue B salt is dissolved in 100 mL of 10% aqueous sodium hydroxide solution	Freshly prepared solution sprayed on plate	Insecticides
9.	Bromocresol green	0.1 g bromocresol green is dissolved in 500 mL ethanol and 5 mL 0.1M NaOH	Solution sprayed on plate	Organic acids

Continued

Continued

S. No.	Spraying reagent	Preparation	Spraying procedure	Application
10.	Bromothymol blue	0.1% bromothymol blue in 10% aqueous ethanol and made alkaline with NH_4OH.	Solution sprayed on plate	Lipids and phospholipids
11.	Bromine/carbon tetrachloride	10% bromine in carbon tetrachloride.	Chromatogram is placed in a chamber with the solution without contact with the liquid	Organophosphorus Pesticides
12.	Bromophenol blue	Solution I: 0.5 g of bromophenol blue is dissolved in 10 Ml of acetone. Solution II: 1 g of silver nitrate is dissolved in 100 mL of distilled water, and then 30 mL is removed from Soln II, and made up to 100 mL with acetone. 90 mL of solution II is mixed with 10 mL of Solution I, which is called bromophenol blue.	Solution is sprayed on plate followed by acetic acid	Organophosphorus Insecticides
13.	Cobalt acetate-o-toluidine reagent	Solution I (Cobalt acetate solution): 5 g of cobalt acetate is dissolved in 100 mL of distilled water Solution II: (o-toluidine reagent): 1 g of o-toluidine is dissolved in 100 mL of 10% (v/v) acetic acid.	Sprayed with solution I and then with solution II	Organophosphorus Insecticide
14.	Ceric ammonium nitrate reagent	Solution I (1% ceric ammonium nitrate): 1 g of ceric ammonium nitrate is dissolved in 100 mL of 20% (v/v) HCl acid. Solution II: (1% sodium nitrite solution): 1 g sodium nitrite is dissolved in 100 mL of distilled water. Solution III: (10% sodium hydroxide solution): 10 g of sodium hydroxide is dissolved in 100 mL of distilled water.	Sprayed with solution I and II and finally with solution III	Carbaryl
15.	Cobalt thiocyanate	Solution I (2.5% cobalt thiocyanate): 2.5 g of cobalt thiocyanate is dissolved in 100 mL of water. Solution II (16% HCl): 16 mL HCl is dissolved in 100 mL of water.	Sprayed with solution I and then with solution II	Cocaine and heroin

Continued

THIN LAYER CHROMATOGRAPHY AND ITS APPLICATIONS

Continued

S. No.	Spraying reagent	Preparation	Spraying procedure	Application
16.	Chloranil reagent	1% tetrachloro-p-benzoquinone in toluene.	Solution sprayed on plate	Phenol
17.	Copper sulfate/phosphoric acid	10% copper (II) sulfate in 10% phosphoric acid.	Solution sprayed on plate and heated to 110°C for 5–30 minutes	Polymer bound TLC plates
18.	DDQ reagent	2% 2,3-dichloro5,6-dicyano-1,4-benzoquinone in toluene.	Solution sprayed on plate	Phenols
19.	Dichlorofluorescein	0.2% dichlorofluorescein in 96% ethanol.	Solution sprayed on plate	Sweeteners saccharine and cyclamate
20.	Dichlorofluorescein/fluorescein sodium salt	0.1% of dichlorofluorescein in ethanol solution.	Solution sprayed on plate	N-substituted barbiturates
21.	2,6-Dichloroquinone-4-chloroimide	0.5–2% solution of 2,6-dichloroquinone-4-ch oroimide in ethanol.	Solution sprayed on plate	Antioxidants, phenols, amines, phenoxyacetic acid herbicides, etc.
22.	p-Dimethylaminobenzaldehyde	1% p-dimethyl aminobenzaldehyde in 5% hydrochloric acid and 5% ethanol.	Solution sprayed on plate	Sulfonamides
23.	2,4-Dinitrophenylhydrazine (DNPH)	0.4 g 2,4-DNPH is dissolved in 100 mL 2N hydrochloric acid and 1 mL of ethanol is added to it	Solution sprayed on plate	Aldehydes and ketones
24.	Diphenylamine	10 mL of 10% diphenylamine in ethanol, 10C mL HCl and 80 mL glacial acetic acid are mixed.	Solution sprayed on plate	Glycosides, glycolipids
25.	Dragendorff's reagent	1 g of bismuth sub nitrate is dissolved in 3 mL of 10 M of hydrochloric acid. It is diluted to 20 mL. 1 g of potassium iodide is dissolved to it. If black precipitate of bismuth tri-iodide appears, it is dissolved in 2 M HCl.	Solution sprayed on plate	Alkaloid
26.	Diphenylcarbazone	0.1% s-diphenylcarbazone in 95% ethanol.	Solution sprayed on plate	Barbiturates

Continued

THIN LAYER CHROMATOGRAPHY AND ITS APPLICATIONS

Continued

S. No.	Spraying reagent	Preparation	Spraying procedure	Application
27.	2, 2′-Diphenylpicryl-hydrazyl (DPPH)	15 mg of 2, 2′-DPPH is dissolved in 25 mL chloroform	Solution sprayed on plate	Aldehydes and ketones
28.	Dithizone	20 mg dithizone is dissolved in 100 mL acetone and stored in a brown bottle in refrigerator.	Sprayed with dithizone solution, followed by 25% ammonia solution	Heavy metal ions
29.	Emerson reagent	Solution I [0.5 % mercuric (II) Nitrate solution]: 0.5 g of mercuric (II) nitrate is dissolved in 100 ml of distilled water. Solution II (1% Potassium hexacyanoferrate): 1 g of potassium hexacyanoferrate is dissolved in 100 mL of distilled water.	Sprayed with solution I and then with solution II	Insecticide
30.	Ferric chloride/sulfuric acid	2 g $FeCl_3$ is dissolved in 83 mL n-butanol and 15 mL conc. sulfuric acid.	Solution sprayed on plate	Polymer bound TLC plates
31.	Flavone reagent	1% solution of ethanolamine diphenyl borate in methanol.	Solution sprayed on plate	Flavonoids
32.	FPN reagent	5 mL of a 5% (w/v) solution of ferric chloride in water, 45 mL of 20% (w/w) perchloric acid and 50 mL of 50% (w/w) nitric acid are mixed together.	Solution sprayed on plate	Basic drug
33.	Formaldehyde/phosphoric acid	0.03 g formaldehyde is dissolved in 100 mL of 85% phosphoric acid with stirring at room temperature. The reagent is stable for several weeks.	Sprayed with the prepared solution	Steroid, alkaloids, steroid, sapogenins and phenothiazine derivatives
34.	Furfural/sulfuric acid	Solution I: 1% solution of furfural in acetone. Solution II: 10% solution of sulfuric acid in acetone.	Sprayed plate with I, then II	Carbamate esters
35.	Formaldehyde-sulfuric acid	4 parts of sulfuric acid is mixed with 6 parts of formalin.	Solution sprayed on plate	Benzodiazepines/Phenothiazine

Continued

Chapter 5

207

THIN LAYER CHROMATOGRAPHY AND ITS APPLICATIONS

Continued

S. No.	Spraying reagent	Preparation	Spraying procedure	Application
36.	Forrest reagent	Equal volumes of a 0.2% solution of potassium dichromate, 30% (v/v) solution of sulfuric acid, 20% (v/v) solution of perchloric acid and 50% solution of nitric acid are mixed together.	Solution sprayed on plate	Phenothiazines
37.	Gentian violet–bromine	0.1% gentian violet (crystal violet) in methanol.	Sprayed and then placed in a tank containing bromine vapor	Lipids
38.	Gibb's reagent	3% 2,6-dibromo-N-chloro-p-benzoquinone imine in toluene or methanol.	Solution sprayed on plate	Phenols
39.	Griess reagent	Solution I (5% of sodium nitrite solution): 5 g sodium nitrite is dissolved in 100 mL 10% (v/v) acetic acid solution. Solution II (0.1% 1-Napthyl amine solution): C 1 g of 1-napthyl amine is dissolved in 10 mL of glacial acetic acid and to 100 mL of distilled water. Solution III (0.5% stannous chloride solution): 5% stannous chloride in 100 mL of 50% HCl solution (v/v).	Sprayed with solution I and II and finally with solution III	Organophosphorus compound
40.	Hydroxylamine/iron (III) chloride	Solution I: Equal volume of 7% hydroxyl ammonium chloride in methanol is mixed with 7.2% KOH in methanol and filtered. Solution II: 2% solution of iron (III) chloride in 1% aqueous HCl.	Sprayed with solution I and then with solution II	Amides, lactones, carboxylic acid esters and anhydrides
41.	Iodine vapor	Chamber is charged with some crystals of iodine.	Developed and dried chromatogram is placed in iodine vapor	Many organic compounds

Continued

THIN LAYER CHROMATOGRAPHY AND ITS APPLICATIONS

Continued

S. No.	Spraying reagent	Preparation	Spraying procedure	Application
42.	Iron (III) chloride/potassium hexacyanoferrate/sodium arsenate (Patterson and Clements)	Solution I: 2.7% iron (III) chloride hexahydrate in 2N HCl Solution II: 3.5% potassium hexacyanoferrate in water Solution III: 3.8 g arsenic trioxide is dissolved in 25 mL 2N NaOH solution, heated slightly, cooled and mixed with 50 ml 2N sulfuric acid and made upto 200 ml with water. 5 ml solution I, 5 mL solution II and 1 mL solution III is mixed immediately before use.	Solution sprayed on plate	Iodine compounds
43.	Iodoplatinate solution	2 mL of 5% solution of platinic chloride in 2 N HCl and 5 g of potassium iodide are mixed in 98 mL of water with stirring.	Solution sprayed on plate	Alkaloids
44.	Koppanyi-Zwikker reagent	1% solution of cobalt nitrate in ethanol and then 0.1 mL of pyrolidine is added.	Solution sprayed on plate	Sulfonamides
45.	Lead tetraacetate/2,7-dichlorofluorescein	Solution I: 2% (w/v) lead tetra-acetate in glacial acetic acid. Solution II: 1% (w/v) 2,7-dichlorofluorescein in ethanol 5 mL of each Solution I and II are mixed, filled to 200 mL with dry toluene. This solution is stable for only about 2 hours.	Solution sprayed on plate	Vicinal diols, and phenols
46.	Mandelin's reagent	1% solution of vanillin in conc. sulfuric acid or 0.5 g vanillin is dissolved in 100 mL sulfuric acid/ethanol (40:10) Note: This reagent can only be used with G (gypsum) binder plates, since it will char the polymer binders in the harder layer plates.	The prepared solution is sprayed at 120°C until maximum color formation	Steroids
47.	Mercury (II) chloride/diphenylcarbazone	Solution I: 2% ethanolic mercury (II) chloride Solution II: 0.2% ethanolic diphenylcarbazone. Mixed in equal parts of solution I and II freshly before use.	Solution sprayed on plate	Barbiturates
48.	Mercury (II) chloride/dithizone	1:1 mixture of 1–2% mercury (II) chloride in ethanol and 0.1–0.2% dithizone in ethanol (prepared freshly)	—do—	Barbiturates

Continued

THIN LAYER CHROMATOGRAPHY AND ITS APPLICATIONS

Continued

S. No.	Spraying reagent	Preparation	Spraying procedure	Application
49.	4-Methoxybenzaldehyde/sulfuric acid/ethanol	4-methoxybenzaldehyde/sulfuric acid/ethanol (1:1:9)	—do—	Erythromycin
50.	Methyl yellow	0.1 g methyl yellow (N, N-dimethyl-4-phenylazoaniline) is dissolved in 75 mL ethanol and 25 mL water	—do—	Chlorinated insecticides
51.	Molybdatophosphoric acid	250 mg molybdatophosphoric acid is dissolved in 50 mL ethanol. The reagent solution is stable for only 10 days even in the dark.	Solution sprayed on plate and heated to 120°C.	Alcohols, lipids, fatty acids and steroids
52.	Mercuric nitrate-potassium Hexacyanoferrate reagent	Solution I (0.5% mercuric (II) Nitrate solution): 0.5 g of mercuric (II) nitrate is dissolved in 100 mL of distilled water. Solution II (1% Potassium hexacyanoferrate): 1 g of potassium dissolved in 100 mL of distilled water.	Sprayed with solution I and then with solution II	Insecticide
53.	Mercurous nitrate reagent	1 g of mercurous nitrate is dissolved in 100 mL of water followed by addition of a few drops of concentrated nitric acid	Solution sprayed on plate	OP insecticides, barbiturates
54.	Marquis reagent	One volume of formalin is mixed with nine volume of concentrated sulfuric acid.	Solution sprayed on plate	Benzodiazepines alkaloids
55.	Mercuric chloride-diphenyl carbazone Reagent	Solution I: (Diphenyl carbazone solution): 0.1 g of diphenyl carbazone is dissolved in 50 mL of ethanol. Solution II: (Mercuric chloride solution): 0.1 g of mercuric chloride is dissolved in 50 mL of ethanol.	Sprayed with solution I and then with solution II	Barbiturates
56.	Nickel amine reagent	Solution I (Nickel amine reagent): Equal volumes of 5% (w/v) aqueous nickel chloride solution and 30% ammonia are mixed. Solution II: (20% Sodium hydroxide solution): 20 g of sodium hydroxide is dissolved in 100 mL of distilled water.	Sprayed with solution I and then with solution II	Endosulfan

Continued

THIN LAYER CHROMATOGRAPHY AND ITS APPLICATIONS

Continued

S. No.	Spraying reagent	Preparation	Spraying procedure	Application
57.	Ninhydrin	0.2 g ninhydrin is dissolved in 100 mL ethanol.	Solution sprayed on plate and heated to 110°C	Amino acids, amines, amino sugars
58.	Ninhydrin/cadmium acetate	1 g ninhydrin and 2.5g cadmium acetate is dissolved in 10 mL glacial acetic acid and made upto 500 mL with ethanol.	Solution sprayed on plate and heated to 120oC for 20 min	Amino acids and heterocyclic amines
59.	Ninhydrin/pyridine/glacial acetic acid	1% ninhydrin in pyridine/glacial acetic acid (5:1, v/v).	Solution sprayed on plate and heated to 100°C for 5 min	Peptides
60.	Nitric acid/ethanol	50 drops of 65% nitric acid in 100 mL ethanol.	Solution sprayed on plate and heated to 120°C for sometime	Amines and alkaloids
61.	Orcinol (Bial's reagent)	0.1 g orcinol is dissolved in 40.7 mL conc. HCl, 1 mL of 1% ferric (III) chloride is added to it and diluted to 100 mL with water.	Sprayed and heated at 80°C for 90 minutes	Glycosides, glycolipids
62.	Potassium iodate starch reagent	Solution I (Potassium Iodate): 5 g of potassium iodate is dissolved in 100 mL of distilled water. Solution II (Starch solution): 1 g of soluble starch is dissolved in 100 mL of boiled water. The solution is cooled thereafter, for preservation. 25 mL of solution I is mixed with 2 mL of solution II immediately before use.	Solution sprayed on plate	Organophosphorus Insecticides
63.	Palladium chloride solution	0.5 g of palladium chloride is dissolved in 100 mL 2 N HCl acid.	Solution sprayed on plate	Insecticides
64.	Phenyl hydrazine hydrochloric reagent	Equal volume of 1 % (w/v) aqueous solution Phenyl hydrazine hydrochloride in 10 % (w/v) aqueous solution of sodium hydroxide.	Solution sprayed on plate	Carbaryl
65.	Paraffin oil	1% paraffin oil in hexane	Solution sprayed on plate	Enhancement of fluorescence spots–more stable and greater intensity

Continued

Chapter 5 — THIN LAYER CHROMATOGRAPHY AND ITS APPLICATIONS

Continued

S. No.	Spraying reagent	Preparation	Spraying procedure	Application
66.	m-Phenylenediamine	3.6 g m-phenylenediamine dihydrochloride is dissolved in 100 mL 70% ethanol.	Sprayed and heated at 105°C	Reducing sugars
67.	o-Phenylenediamine – trichloroacetic acid	0.05 g 1,2-phenylenediamine is dissolved in 100 mL 10% aqueous trichloroacetic acid.	Solution sprayed on plate and heated to 100°C for not more than 2 minute	Alpha-keto acids
68.	p-Phenylenediamine – phthalic acid	0.9 p-phenylenediamine and 1.6g phthalic acid are dissolved in 100 mL of 1-butanol saturated with water.	Sprayed and heated at 100–110°C	Conjugated 3-ketosteroids
69.	Phenylhydrazine sulfonate	Solution I: 3.5g phenylhydrazine 4-sulfonic acid hemihydrate is dissolved in 10 mL water and 20 mL 1N NaOH solution. Solution II: 30 mL 1N sodium hydroxide solution is mixed with 40 mL acetone.	Sprayed with Solution I, dried and then sprayed with Solution II	Some antimicrobial compounds
70.	Phosphoric acid	85% phosphoric acid in water (1:1, v/v).	Solution sprayed on plate and heated to 120°C for 10–15 minutes	Sterols, steroids, and bile acids
71.	Phosphoric acid – bromine	Solution I: 10% aqueous phosphoric acid solution Solution II: 2 mL saturated aqueous potassium bromide, 2 mL saturated solution of aqueous potassium bromate, and 2 mL 25% hydrochloric acid are mixed.	Sprayed with solution I and heated 12 minutes at 120°C and sprayed lightly with solution II	Digitalis glycosides
72.	Phosphomolybdic acid	250 mg molybdatophosphoric acid is dissolved in 50 mL ethanol. The reagent solution is stable for only 10 days even in the dark.	Solution sprayed on plate and heated to 120°C	Alcohols, bile acids, lipids, fatty acids, steroids
73.	Phosphotungstic acid	20% phosphotungstic acid in ethanol	Sprayed and heated at 110°C for 5–15 minutes	Cholesterol, lipids and steroids
74.	Pinacryptol yellow	100 mg pinacryptol yellow is dissolved in 100 mL hot water or ethanol.	Solution sprayed on plate	Sweeteners

Continued

Continued

S. No.	Spraying reagent	Preparation	Spraying procedure	Application
75.	Potassium dichromate/sulfuric acid (chromosulfuric acid)	5 g potassium dichromate is dissolved in 100 mL conc. Sulfuric acid.	Solution sprayed on plate	Organic compounds
76.	Potassium permanganate/sulfuric acid	1.6% potassium permanganate in conc. sulfuric acid	Sprayed with prepared solution	Organic compounds
77.	Rhodamine 6 G	1 mg Rhodamine 6 G is dissolved in 100 mL acetone.	Solution sprayed on plate	Lipids
78.	Rhodamine B solution	0.5 g of Rhodamine B is dissolved in 100 mL of ethanol.	Solution sprayed on plate	Insecticides
79.	Stannic chloride	10 mL tin (IV) chloride is dissolved in 160 mL equal volumes of chloroform and glacial acetic acid.	Solution sprayed on plate and heated to 100°C for 5–10 min	Triterpenes, steroids, phenols
80.	Silver nitrate/hydrogen peroxide	0.1 g silver nitrate is dissolved in 1 mL water, 10 mL 2-phenoxyethanol is added to it, made up to 200 mL with acetone and one drop hydrogen peroxide (30% solution) is added to it.	Solution sprayed on plate	Halogenated hydrocarbons
81.	Sodium azide	Solution I: 0.5% solution of soluble starch Solution II: 3.5% sodium azide in 0.1 N iodine solution	Sprayed with solution I, dried and sprayed with solution II	Antibiotics
82.	Sodium 1,2-naptha-quinone-4-sulfonate (NZS reagent)	Solution I: 0.1 N NaOH is prepared. Solution II: Saturated solution of reagent in 1:1 ethanol: water.	Sprayed with solution I and then with solution II	Thiazide drugs, basic drugs with primary amino groups
83.	Sodium nitrite/hydrochloric acid	1 g sodium nitrite is dissolved in 100 mL hydrochloric acid.	Solution sprayed on plate and heated to 100°C	Indoles and thiazoles
84.	Sodium nitroprusside/hydrogen peroxide	2 mL 5% aqueous sodium nitroprusside, 1 mL 10% aqueous sodium hydroxide and 5 mL 3% aqueous hydrogen peroxide is mixed and diluted with 15 mL water. This solution can be stored for several days in the refrigerator.	Solution sprayed on plate	Guanidine, urea, thiourea and derivatives, creatine and creatinine

Continued

Continued

S. No.	Spraying reagent	Preparation	Spraying procedure	Application
85.	Sodium nitroprussate/potassium hexacyanoferrate (III)	1 volume part each of 10% aqueous sodium hydroxide, 10% sodium nitroprussate, and 10% potassium hexacyanoferrate (III) in 3 volume parts water are mixed and allowed to stand for at least 20 min at ambient temperature before use. Stored in the refrigerator, it is stable for several weeks.	The reagent solution is mixed with an equal part of acetone and sprayed	Aliphatic nitrogen compounds, cyanamide, guanidine, urea, thiourea and derivatives, creatine, and creatinine
86.	Tetracyanoethylene-toluene reagent	0.5–1.0 g tetracyanoethylene is dissolved in dichloromethane or toluene.	Solution sprayed on plate	Aromatic hydrocarbons and heterocyclics, aromatic amines, and phenols
87.	Tetranitrodiphenyl	Solution I: Saturated solution of 2,3′,4,4′-tetranitro-diphenyl in toluene. Solution II: 10% potassium hydroxide solution in 50% aqueous methanol.	Sprayed with solution I, dried at room temperature and then sprayed with solution II	Cardiac glycosides
88.	Tollen's Reagent	10 g of silver nitrate is dissolved in 100 mL of water followed by addition of a few drops of nitric acid. After sometime NH_3 solution is added drop-wise when a precipitate appears, which gets dissolved on adding excess of ammonia.	Solution sprayed on plate	Organophosphorus insecticide
89.	Tetrazolium blue	1:1 mix of 0.5% methanolic tetrazolium blue solution and 6M NaOH in water omethanol (freshly prepared).	Sprayed with the prepared solution	Corticosteroids
90.	Thymol/sulfuric acid	0.5 g thymol is dissolved in 95 mL ethanol, and added 5 mL 97% sulfuric acid with caution.	Sprayed and heated for 15–20 minutes at 120°C	Sugars
91.	Tin (IV) chloride	10 mL tin (IV) chloride is dissolved in 160 mL equal volumes of chloroform and glacial acetic acid	Solution sprayed on plate and heated to 100°C for 5–10 minutes	Triterpenes, sterols, steroids, phenols.

Continued

Continued

S. No.	Spraying reagent	Preparation	Spraying procedure	Application
92.	o-toluidine, diazotized	Solution I (toluidine solution): 5g o-toluidine and 14 mL conc. hydrochloric acid are mixed in 100 mL water. Solution II (Nitrate solution): 10% aqueous sodium nitrate solution is prepared fresh. 20 mL solution I and 20 mL Solution II is mixed at 0°C with constant stirring. The spray solution is stable for about 2–3 hours.	After spraying, it takes several hours to form colored spots	Phenols
93.	p-Toluenesulfonic acid	20% p-toluenesulfonic acid in chloroform.	Solution sprayed on plate and heated to 100°C for few minutes	Steroids, flavonoids and catechins
94.	Tungstophosphoric acid	20% phosphotungstic acid in ethanol.	Sprayed with prepared solution and heated at 110°C for 5–15 minutes or until maximum visualization of the spots occurred	Cholesterol and steroids
95.	Urea/hydrochloric acid	5 g urea is dissolved in 20 mL 2M HCl, made up to with 100 mL ethanol.	Solution sprayed on plate heated to 100°C	Sugars
96.	Vanillin/potassium hydroxide	1 g vanillin is dissolved in 50 mL 2-propanol.	Sprayed with 1 mL 1M KOH solution filled up to 100 mL with ethanol and dried for 10 min at 110°C.	Amines and amino acids
97.	Vanillin/phosphoric acid	1 g vanillin is dissolved in 100 mL 50% aqueous H_3PO_4	Solution sprayed on plate and heated to 110°C for 5–30 minutes	Polymer bound TLC plates
98.	Zwikker's reagent	40 mL of 10% solution of copper sulfate in 10 mL of pyridine and made up to 100 mL with water.	Solution sprayed on plate.	Barbiturates
99.	Zinc-chloride diphenylamine reagent	0.5 g of diphenylamine and 0.5 g of zinc chloride are dissolved in 100 mL of acetone	Solution sprayed on plate.	Organochloro Insecticide

(Conc.: concentrated; Soln: solution)

THIN LAYER CHROMATOGRAPHY AND ITS APPLICATIONS

8. *Amount of substance*: R_f depends upon the amount of the substance applied. Differences are noticeable at very low and especially, at very high concentrations.
9. *Impurities*: Effected by the presence of impurities.
10. *Temperature*: A constant temperature is not so important for TLC as in paper chromatography.

Advantages of Thin Layer Chromatography

1. TLC is a simple procedure for chromatographing.
2. TLC can be performed on an analytical and preparative scale.
3. It may be applied to almost the entire spectrum of compounds.
4. Due to its rapid speed, it can be employed for checking the course of chemical reactions in laboratory.
5. TLC can be used for detecting adulteration of foods as well as decomposition of foods.
6. Compounds which are encountered in trace amounts can be easily detected by TLC.
7. TLC is of great help in chemical toxicology.
8. In chemical laboratory, morphological appearance of tissues can be associated with their chemical composition, which can be detected by TLC.
9. The great advantages of TLC are often most profitably exploited when TLC is employed in conjugation with other methods of analysis.
10. TLC is a rapid investigative tool by which, results can be available in minimum time.

Superiority of Thin Layer Chromatography over Paper and Column Chromatography

1. It requires less amount of substance than both the techniques.
2. It is less time consuming.
3. The separation is very great in TLC as compared to column and paper chromatography.
4. Even strong acid can be safely sprayed on chromatoplates.
5. For many purposes, TLC plates may be heated in an oven for several hours without causing any damage to it.
6. Capacity of thin layers of an adsorbent in TLC is higher than that of paper chromatography.
7. Due to thin layers, it has physical strength, therefore ascending techniques are preferred for this type of chromatography. Because of lack of physical strength in paper, descending techniques are usually used in paper chromatography.
8. In TLC even corrosive reagents may be coated on glass plates. These reagents will, however, destroy paper chromatogram.
9. TLC method does not demand laboratory requirement.
10. It can be handled with minimal operator training and cost for toxicological applications.

STANDARD OPERATING PROCEDURE FOR THIN LAYER CHROMATOGRAPHY (SOP FOR TLC)

Step 1: Preparation of Thin-layer Plates

1. Select the type of plate. Plate can be of metal (aluminum) or of plastic, though the usual practice is of using the glass plates.
2. Select the size of TLC plate. The usual size of the plate is 20 × 20 × 0.5 cm, although smaller sizes may be used.
3. The plate must be cleared with a detergent in order to make it clear and completely free of any grease. The plate can then be dried in a hot air oven.
4. Select suitable adsorbent, such as silica gel, alumina, etc.
5. The adsorbent silica gel is prepared by taking silica gel and water in the ratio of 1:2 (one part of silica gel, two parts of water), it is continuously stirred in order to prevent the formation of lumps.
6. Once thick slurry is formed, it is immediately poured on TLC plate and spread uniformly by tilting the plate or by using TLC applicator. Precaution should be taken that the silica gel is spread uniformly over the plate as a thin film (0.1-0.2 mm). Lack of uniformity can affect retention capacity of the adsorbent.
7. The TLC plate is then air dried for 20 minutes.
8. The TLC plate is then placed in the oven at 100°C for 30 minutes in order to activate it.
9. After the plate is prepared, it should be kept dry and free of moisture, as silica gel is hygroscopic and tends to absorb water. Prepared TLC is given in **Figure 5.20**.

Step 2: Sample Application

1. The plate should be prepared by marking the origin by drawing a light pencil line at least 1-2 cm from the bottom of the plate, care should be taken not to disturb the silica surface in any way.
2. A line should then be drawn on the plate 10 cm above the origin to indicate the optimum position of the solvent front, other distances may be used if required.

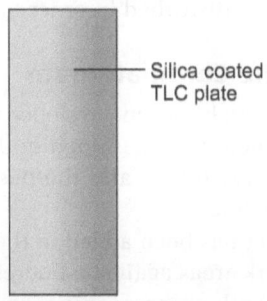

Fig. 5.20: Prepared thin layer chromatography (TLC) plate.

THIN LAYER CHROMATOGRAPHY AND ITS APPLICATIONS

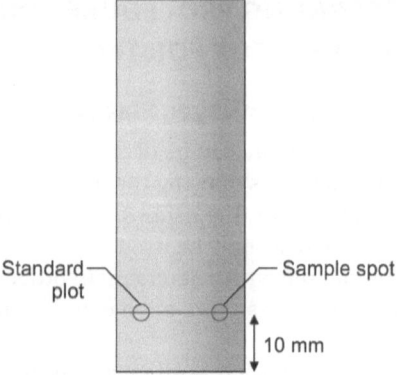

Fig. 5.21: Spotting of sample and standard on thin layer chromatography plates.

3. The samples and standards should be applied at the line with sufficient distance. Sample loading should be performed carefully using a micropipette or syringe or capillary, so as to form "spots" of not more than 5 mm in diameter.
4. If larger spots are produced, then resolution will be impaired when the chromatogram is developed.
5. The volume of solvent applied should be kept to minimum, as 5–10 µL of solution containing about 10 µg of analyte is suitable.
6. .Spotting of sample as well as standard is shown in **Figure 5.21**.

Step 3: Developing the Chromatogram
1. Add suitable amount of solvent in chromatography chamber.
2. The solvent should be added at least 30 minutes before the chromatogram is to be developed to saturate the atmosphere with solvent vapors.
3. The chromatogram is developed by placing the loaded plate in the equilibrated tank, ensuring that the level of the solvent is above the bottom edge of the silica layer on the plate, but below the level of the spots applied to the plate (**Figs. 5.22** and **5.23**).
4. The plate should be observed to insure that the solvent front is being drawn up uniformly. The mobile phase movement is primarily due to capillary forces and, as the stationary phase is dry.
5. This set-up must not be disturbed in order to obtain effective result.

Step 4: Visualizing the Chromatogram
1. When the chromatogram has been developed then the plate is air dried.
2. The chromatogram should be examined under UV light (254 and 366 nm) in a suitable enclosed box, and the positions of any fluorescent compounds ("spots") noted.
3. If a fluorescent marker has been added to the silica, many substances present appear as dark areas against a fluorescent background.
4. The plate is sprayed with chromogenic reagent by using TLC sprayer (**Fig. 5.24**).

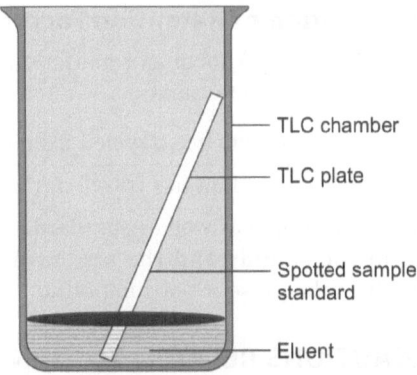

Fig. 5.22: Thin layer chromatography (TLC) plate placed in a beaker.

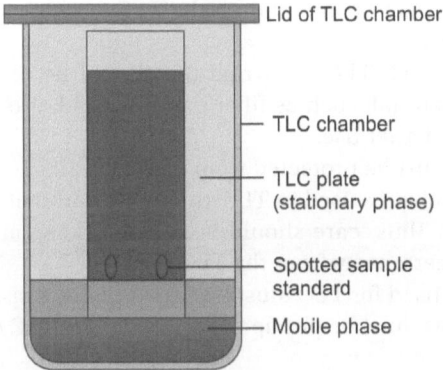

Fig. 5.23: Position of mobile phase and spots on the plate.

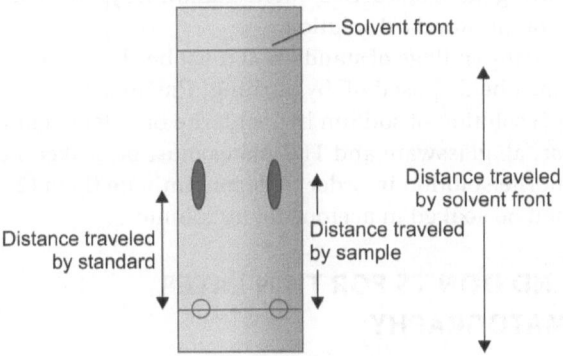

Fig. 5.24: Visualization of thin layer chromatography plate.

5. In clinical toxicology, the use of chromogenic chemical detection reagents generally gives more useful information. Plates can be dipped in reagent, but unless special precautions are taken, the structure of the silica tends to be lost and the chromatogram destroyed.

THIN LAYER CHROMATOGRAPHY AND ITS APPLICATIONS

Step 5: Result/Calculation of Retention Factor

1. Retention factor (R_f) is also known as retardation factor and can be calculated by using following formula:

$$R_f = \frac{\text{Distance the analyte has traveled from the origin}}{\text{Distance the solvent font has traveled from the origin}}$$

2. Calculate R_f value for sample as well as standard.
3. If the R_f value of the sample and the standard is same, then we qualitatively confirm the presence of compound.

■ SAFETY PRECAUTIONS RELATED TO THIN LAYER CHROMATOGRAPHY

1. For carrying out TLC of toxin, an area in the laboratory should be reserved for this purpose and all the TLC work must be restricted to that area only.
2. Surface on which TLC is carried out should be a non-absorbent. If absorbent material, such as filter paper is used, it must be discarded and destroyed after use.
3. This region must be protected from direct sunlight.
4. Most of the solvents used in TLC are highly flammable and are highly combustible. Thus, care should be taken to keep apparatus such as heaters, burners, away from the TLC area.
5. The solvents used for TLC must be stored in fire resistant cabinets.
6. Warning signs must be put up in regions where TLC of toxins is being carried out.
7. The toxins (solute) used for TLC should be of least strength and stored carefully in small containers.
8. TLC spotting must be carried out in shallow trays that can contain the spillage of the standard solution.
9. In case of any spillage of standard, it must be cleared with filter paper, and it must be disposed off by burning. The area can then be sprayed with a 4% solution of sodium hypochlorite or a detergent to clear it.
10. After use, all glassware and TLC plates must be soaked in 1% sodium hypochlorite solution in order to decontaminate them (2 hours). They must then be soaked in acetone for 30 minutes.

■ DO'S AND DON'TS FOR THIN LAYER CHROMATOGRAPHY

Do's

1. While preparing the samples for TLC (toxin, pesticide, poisons, etc.), there is a danger of it being absorbed by the skin or of it being inhaled, which can cause allergies or even other serious side effects. Hence, this work must always be carried out in fume hoods.

2. Most of the solvents used are highly toxic and carcinogenic (benzene, petroleum ether, etc.) they are also volatile, hence gloves and surgical masks which covers mouth and nose must be used.
3. Safety spectacles must be used at work throughout the entire process.
4. A laboratory coat must be worn, as several dyes and spraying reagents are used which can stain clothes.
5. Spraying of TLC plates must be carried out in fume hoods or spray cabinets.
6. When viewing the plates under UV, the eyes should be protected by wearing spectacles or should be viewed through UV filters.

Don'ts

1. Do not eat, drink or smoke around areas where TLC is being carried out.
2. The used organic solvents must never be dumped in the sink. It must be disposed off into an appropriate waste bottle. (Chloroform can produce fumes which are toxic).
3. Do not force dry the spot with drier on the plates.
4. Do not keep plates in open air, in order to protect them from moisture.
5. Do not disturb the TLC set up, once the solvent starts to run the plate.
6. Do not mix all organic solvents in a waste bottle, as they can form an explosive mixture.
7. Do not force dry the spots by blowing air.

■ FORENSIC APPLICATIONS OF TLC

Analysis of Basic Drugs

Thin layer chromatography technique is very useful for the detection of basic drugs. TLC condition and data for screening of some common basic drugs is as follow:
- Solvent system: Methanol: Ammonia (100:1.5) (v/v)
- Plate: Silica gel G (0.2 mm thickness)
- Development: Ascending technique
- Spray reagent:
    - Iodoplatinate solution: Violet/blue violet/brown violet/(for alkaloids), gray violet spots
    - Dragendorff's reagent: Orange spots (alkaloids and benzodiazepines).

Analysis of Barbiturates

Barbiturates such as barbital, phenobarbital, and secobarbital can be easily analyzed by TLC. The TLC condition such as stationary phase, solvent system, spray reagent and visualization methods are given in **Table 5.3**.

Analysis of Tranquilizers

Thin layer chromatography is very useful for the analysis of tranquilizers such as diazepam, chlorpromazine, etc. The different solvent system,

THIN LAYER CHROMATOGRAPHY AND ITS APPLICATIONS

■ **Table 5.3:** Thin layer chromatography parameters for the analysis of barbiturates.

Stationary phase	Solvent system	Spray reagent	Visualization method
Silica gel G	1. Ethylacetate: Methanol: Ammonia (85:10:5) 2. Chloroform: Acetone (80:20) 3. Benzene: Acetic acid (90:10) 4. Dioxane: Benzene: Ammonium hydroxide (20:75:5) 5. Chloroform: Acetone (90:10)	1. Mercuric chloride – diphenyl carbazone reagent 2. 0.2% aqueous potassium permanganate solution spray 3. Saturated mercurous nitrate spray.	The plates must be dried prior to visualization. This can be done at 120°C for 5 minutes in an oven.

■ **Table 5.4:** Thin layer chromatography parameters for the analysis of tranquilizer.

Stationary phase	Solvent system	Spray reagent	Visualization method
Silica gel G	1. Chloroform: Acetone (80:20) 2. Chloroform: Methanol (90:10) 3. Cyclohexane: Toluene: Diethylamine (75:15:10)	1. FPN spray- (brown-red spot) 2. Acidified potassium iodoplatinate reagent. (yellow spot)	The plates must be dried prior to visualization This can be done at 120°C for 5 minutes in an oven, to remove all traces of diethylamine

■ **Table 5.5:** Thin layer chromatography (TLC) parameters for analysis of narcotics.

Stationary phase	Solvent system	Spray reagent	Visualization method
Silica gel G	1. Cyclohexane: Toluene: Diethylamine (75:15:10) 2. Methanol: Concentrated Ammonia (100:1.5) 3. Chloroform: Methanol (90:10)	1. Acidified potassium iodoplatinate reagent (yellow spot) 2. Dragendorff's Reagent (orange color spot)	UV light 224 nm, plate should be dried well

spray reagent and visualization methods for screening of some common tranquilizers are given in **Table 5.4**.

Analysis of Narcotics

Thin layer chromatography is used to analyze various narcotic drugs, such as morphine, cocaine, heroin, etc. TLC condition and data for screening of narcotic drugs is given in **Table 5.5**.

Analysis of Pesticides

Pesticides such as organophosphorus, organochloro compounds, carbamates, pyrethroids, etc., can be easily analyzed by TLC. The TLC conditions such as stationary phase, solvent system, spray reagent, and visualization methods are given in **Table 5.6**.

Table 5.6: Thin layer chromatography (TLC) parameters for analysis of pesticides.

Pesticides	Developing reagent	Spraying Reagent	Color of the spot
Organophosphorus	Hexane: Acetone (8:2) Chloroform: Acetone (7:3)	1. Mercurous nitrate reagent 2. Mercuric nitrate potassium hexacyanoferrate reagent 3. Potassium iodate starch reagent 4. Cobalt acetate-o-toluidine reagent 5. Griess reagent 6. Phenyl hydrazine hydrochloride and hydrochloric acid solution	1. Black 2. Bluish-green 3. Violet 4. Blue 5. Pink-orange 6. Yellowish-red turns red
Organochloro compounds	Hexane: Acetone (9:1) Cyclohexane: Acetone (8:2)	1. Zinc chloride diphenylamine reagent 2. o-toluidine reagent 3. Ethanolic silver nitrate and concentrated ammonium hydroxide 4. Diphenylamine in alcohol 5. Nickel amine reagent (sodium hydroxide sprayed earlier)	1. Bluish green 2. Bluish green 3. Black (UV-366 nm) 4. Green gray spots 5. Grayish-black
Carbamate	Hexane: Acetone (8:2) Chloroform: Acetone (7:3)	1. Diazotized sulfanilamide/sulfanilic acid reagent (sodium hydroxide sprayed earlier) 2. Chloranil reagent 3. Palladium (II) chloride 4. Congo red 5. Bromine fluorescence 6. Silver nitrate 7. Tollen's reagent 8. Alkaline fast blue salt 9. Phenyl hydrazine hydrochloride reagent 10. Ceric ammonium nitrate reagent (sodium hydroxide sprayed earlier)	1. Orange or violet 2. Red 3. Yellow 4. Red 5. Yellow 6. Black 7. Black 8. Red/Violet 9. Red 10. Violet

Continued

Continued

Pesticides	Developing reagent	Spraying Reagent	Color of the spot
Pyrethroid	1. Petroleum ether: Diethyl ether (9:1) 2. Cyclohexane: Toluene (7:3) 3. Hexane: Acetone: Acetic Acid (25:25:1) 4. Hexane: Chloroform: Acetic acid (9:5:0.5)	1. Sodium hydroxide followed by phosphomolybdic acid 2. Bromine followed by o-toluidine 3. Silver nitrate	1. Black 2. Black 3. Black

■ MEDICOLEGAL ASPECTS

Thin layer chromatography is commonly used as screening test for various drugs. It is a reliable qualitative test. TLC test results are admissible as forensic evidence, in the court of law. However, it has to be confirmed by more specific instrumental techniques. It can give an idea about the presence and absence of the drug and be used as corroborative evidence.

■ CONCLUSION

Thin layer chromatography has been used as a broad-spectrum screening test for detection of various drugs of abuse. The method is most inexpensive and does not require any sophisticated instrumentations. TLC results are qualitative and cannot be quantified. Therefore, it gives positive or negative results. The major drawbacks of TLC are its low sensitivity (1,000–2,000 ng/mL) and specificity as compared to other instruments. Thus, negative TLC results are not always negative by other analytical methods. TLC relies on a reproducible migration pattern by the drugs on a thin layer absorbent, such as silica gel coated on glass plates. Characterization of particular drug is achieved by color reactions produced by spraying the plate with color complexing reagents. It is very good test for an emergency case where drugs taken are not known, but presence or absence of a drug is necessary to start the specific treatment. In TLC, it should be understood that whether a sample is positive or negative, it often depends upon the concentration of the drug in a sample or the sensitivity of cutoff value of the assay. For most drugs of abuse, the cutoff value by TLC is 1,000–2,000 ng/mL. A urine sample may be negative by TLC, but the sample can be positive by other methods. Therefore, cutoff value is very critical in determining if the sample is positive or negative for a particular drug. Often, the cutoff value of assay is set high to avoid false positive especially for legal purpose. False positive results are quite unusual by TLC, but they can be confirmed with a more specific test. Thus, very low level substance is not easily determined by TLC.

■ FURTHER READINGS

1. Adloff RO, List GR. Synthesis and analysis of Symmetrical and nonsymmetrical disaturated/monounsaturated triaciglyserols. J Agric Food Chem. 2003;51:2096-9.
2. Berezkin VG, Mardanov RG, Maliovska I, Rozylo JK. Thin layer chromatography with an isolated support and forced flow of the mobile phase. J Planar Chromatography. 2002;15:377-9.
3. Bicchi C. Simultaneous determination of six triozolic pesticides in Apple and Pear Pulps by liquid chromatography with Ultraviolet Diode Array detector. AOAC. 2001;85(5):1543-50.
4. Campbell A, Chejlana MJ, Sharma J. Use of a modified flatbed scanner for documentation and quantification of thin layer chromatography detected by fluorescence quenching. J Planar Chromatography. 2003;16:244-6.
5. Carpinella MC, Giorda LM, Ferrayoli CG, Palicos SM. Antifungal effects of different organic extracts from Melia azedarach L. on phytopathogenic fungi and their isolated active components. J Agric Food Chromatography. 2003;51:2506-11.
6. Chun OK, Kang HG, Kim MH. Multiresidue method for determination of Pesticides in Korean Domestic Crops by Gas Chromatography/mass Selective Detection. AOAC. 2003;86(4):823-31.
7. Flieger J, Szmilo H, Gielzak-Koewien K, Matosicuk D. Effect of impregnation condition on structure and chromatographic behavior of TLC adsorbents modified with Cu(II) and Ni(II) salts. J Planar Chromatography. 2002;15:354-60.
8. Getz ME, Wheel HG. Thin layer chromatography of organophosphorus insecticides with several adsorbent and ternary solvent systems. J Assoc off Analytical Chemistry. 1968;51:1101-7.
9. Gorsel TA, Bricker JD. Principles of clinical Toxicology. New York: Raven Publishers; 1994.
10. Hack MH, Helmy FM, Mueller TE, Ajuracka M. Further TLC evidence of the preferential deacylation of a cardiolipin and N-acyl phosphatidyl ethanolamine product in mammalian myocardia, fetal and adult. An *in vitro* study. J Planar Chromatography. 2002;15:396-403.
11. Janoszka B, Warzecha L, Dobosz C, Bodzek D. Determination of 7-Ketocholesterol and 7-hydroxycholesterol in meat samples by TLC with densitometric detection. J Planar Chromatography. 2003;16:186-91.
12. Karthrin A, Reich E, Blatter A, Markus V. Validation of standardized high performance thin layer chromatography method for quality control and stability testing of herbals. J AOAC. 2003;86(5):909-15.
13. Laboratory procedure manual: Forensic Toxicology. New Delhi: Selective and Scientific Books Publisher and Distributors; 2005.
14. Malinowska I, Rogglo JK, Rason AK. The effect of electric fields on solute migration and mixture separation in TLC. J Planar Chromatography. 2002;15:418-24.
15. Marutoiu C, Filip M, Tigae C, Coman V, Gresu R, Marcu G. Synthesis and characterization of alumina R chemically modified with n-octyl for use as a stationary phase in TLC. J Planar Chromatography. 2003;16:183-5.
16. Meaga G, Dayan FE, Wedge DE. Activity of quinines on colletotrichum species. J Agric Food Chem. 2003;51:3824-8.
17. Meireles LA, Guedes AC, Malcata FX. Lipid class composition of the microlaga Pavlova lutheri: Eicosapentaenoic and docosahexaenoic acid. J Agric Food Chem. 2003;51: 2237-41.

18. Mohammad A, Agarwal A, Kumar S. Use of water–in-oil microemulsion as mobile phase in complexation TLC of amino acids an silica layers impregnated with metal cations. J Planar Chromatography. 2003;16:220-6.
19. Nyiredy S. Fully on line TLC/HPLC with diode assay detection and continuous development. Part 1: Description of the method and basic possibilities. J Planar Chromatography. 2002;15:454-7.
20. Orinak A, Artinghaus HF, Vering G, Justinova M, Orinakova R, Turcaniova L, et al. New interfaces for coupling TLC with TOF SIMS. J Planar Chromatography. 2003;16:23-7.
21. Poole IC, Poole SK. Modern Thin Layer Chromatography. Analytic Chem. 1989;61:257a-1269a.
22. Poole IC, Poole SK. Recent advances in Chromatography. Analytic Chem Acta. 1989;216:109-45.
23. Prus W, Sazewicz M, Kowalska T. Thermal aromatization of selected TLC type aliphatic chemically bonded stationary phases as monitored by use of HPLC-DAD. J Planar Chromatography. 2002;15:324-33.
24. Pyka A, Niestroj A, Szarkovicz A, Sliwiok J. Use of TLC and RPTLC for separation of nicotinic acid derivatives. J Planar Chromatography. 2002;15:410-13.
25. Pyka M, Dolowy M. Separation of selected bile acids by TLC (I). J Liq Chromatogr Rel Technol. 2003;26:1095-108.
26. Rack KD, Coats JR. Comparative degradation of organophosphorus insecticide in soil: specificity of enhanced microbial degradation. J Food Chem. 1990;36:193-9.
27. Rack KD, Coats JR. Enhanced Biodegradation of Pesticides in the environment. ACS Symposium series 426. Washington DC: American Chemical Society; 1990.
28. Reich E, Schibli A. High performance Thin Layer Chromatography for the analysis of medicinal plants. New York: Thieme Medical Publishers, Inc.; 2006.
29. Reiffova K, Vicova VP, Orinak A, Florida K, Gondova T. Preliminary TLC analysis of fructoligo saccharides as feed additives. J Planar Chromatography. 2003;16:52-7.
30. Salwa MD. Monitoring of Pesticide residues in Egyptian fruit and vegetables during 1996, 2001. AOAC. 2001;84(2):519-31.
31. Sanganalmath PU, Yogaraje CV, Gowtham MD, Nayak VG, Mohan BM. Quantitative Densitometric determination of Quinolphos in Postmortem Blood by HPTLC. Int J Med Toxicol Legal Med. 2007;9(2):30-3.
32. Sethi PD. High Performance Thin Layer Chromatography: Quantitative analysis of pharmaceutical formulation. New Delhi: CBS Publishers and Distributors; 2012.
33. Sharma BK. Instrumental Methods of Chemical Analysis, 16th edition. Meerut: Krishna Prakashan Media (P) Ltd;1997.
34. Sharma VK, Jadhav RK, Rao GJ, Sarf AK, Chandra H. High performance liquid chromatographic method for the analysis of organophosphorus and carbamate pesticides. Forensic Sci Int. 1990;48(1):21-5.
35. Shukla Y, Singh A, Mehrotra NK. Evaluation of carcinogenic and carcinogenic potential quinolphos in mouse skin. Cancer Lett. 2007;148:1-7.
36. Singhe CJ, Botah N, Aoki NT, Wada S. Phenolics composition and antioxidant activity of Sweet basil ocimum basilicum L. J Agric Food Chromatography. 2003;51:4442-9.
37. Skibinski R. Determination of fluoxetine and paroxetine in pharmaceutical formulation by densitometric and video densitometric TLC. J Planar Chromatography. 2003;16: 19-22.

38. Tomlin C. A world compendium: the pesticide manual. London: Crop Protection Publication; 1995.
39. Valverde A. Chromatography pesticides residue analysis: introduction AOAC. 2000;83(3):679.
40. Vovk B, Simonovska S, Andrensek T, Yrjonen P, Vuorela H. Rotation planar extraction and medium pressure solid-liquid extraction of onion (Allium cepa). J Planar Chromatography. 2003;16:16-70.
41. Willard HH. Instrumental Methods of Analysis. 6th edition, CBS Publishers and Distributors, Delhi; 1986.
42. Yagüe C, Bayarri S, Lázaro R, Conchello P, Ariño A, Herrera A. Multiresidue determination of organochlorine pesticides and polychlorinated biphenyls in milk by Gas Chromatography with electron capture detector after extraction by matrix solid-phase dispersion. J AOAC. 2001;84(5):1561-8.

Chapter 6

Gas Chromatography and its Applications

■ INTRODUCTION

The Russian botanist, Mikhail Tsvet (Mikhail Semyonovich Tsvet), invented the first chromatography technique in 1901 during his research on chlorophyll. He used a liquid-adsorption column containing calcium carbonate to separate plant pigments. The method was described on December 30, 1901 at the XI Congress of Naturalists and Doctors. The first printed description was in 1903 in the Proceedings of the Warsaw Society of Naturalists, Section of Biology; German graduate student Fritz Prior developed solid state gas chromatography (GC) in 1947. Archer John Porter Martin, who was awarded the Nobel Prize for his work in developing liquid–liquid (1941) and paper (1944) chromatography, laid the foundation for the development of GC and he later produced liquid-gas chromatography (1950). Erika Cremer laid the groundwork and oversaw much of Prior's work. Modern GC was invented by Martin and James in 1952 and has become one of the most important and widely applied analytical techniques in modern chemistry. The technology of chromatography advanced rapidly throughout the 20th century. Researchers found that the principles underlying Tsvet's chromatography could be applied in many different ways, giving rise to the different varieties of chromatography.

Chromatography basically involves separation due to difference in the equilibrium distribution of sample components between two different phases. One of the phase is *mobile phase* and the other is *stationary phase*. On the basis of mobile phase, chromatography is divided into two classes:
1. *Gas chromatography*: Mobile phase is gas
2. *Liquid chromatography*: Mobile phase is liquid

■ GAS CHROMATOGRAPHY

Gas chromatography is basically a separation technique, in which the compounds of a vaporized sample are separated and fractionated as a consequence of partition between a mobile gaseous phase and a stationary phase held in the column. Partition takes place between gas and liquid or

gas and solid. Thus, according to the nature of stationary phase, GC may be divided into two classes:
1. *Gas-solid chromatography (GSC)*: Fixed phase or stationary phase consists of solid material such as granular silica
2. *Gas-liquid chromatography (GLC)*: Fixed phase or stationary phase is a nonvolatile liquid held as thin layer on a solid support
   The experiment involves generally GLC for most applications.

■ TECHNIQUES OF GAS-LIQUID CHROMATOGRAPHY

Gas-liquid chromatography or simply GC is a common type of chromatography used in analytical chemistry for separating and analyzing compounds that can be vaporized without decomposition.

Block diagram of a GLC apparatus is given in **Figure 6.1**. The gas flow is held constant by suitable controls and a device can be attached to the gas outlet for measuring flow rate. The column is kept in a thermostat oven. To avoid condensation, the injector and detector must be maintained at a constant temperature higher than column temperature. Thus, these components are thermostated as well. Different GLC instruments are given in **Figures 6.2A** to **F**. The basic apparatus consists of the following main components, which will be discussed one by one.
- Carrier gas
- An injection port of sample
- Column
- Detector

Carrier Gas

The term carrier gas was introduced by A J P Martin, the inventor of gas chromatography who used it as an alternative term for the mobile phase; obviously, the term could only be used as such in GC. The term has persisted and is still used synonymously for a gaseous mobile phase. Few points about carrier gas are:
1. It should be inert
2. It should be available at low cost

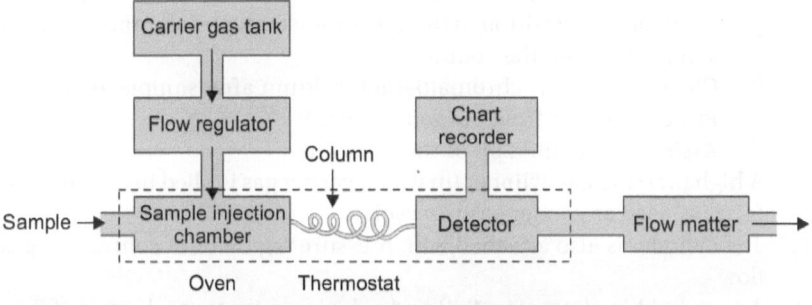

Fig. 6.1: Gas-liquid chromatography.

GAS CHROMATOGRAPHY AND ITS APPLICATIONS

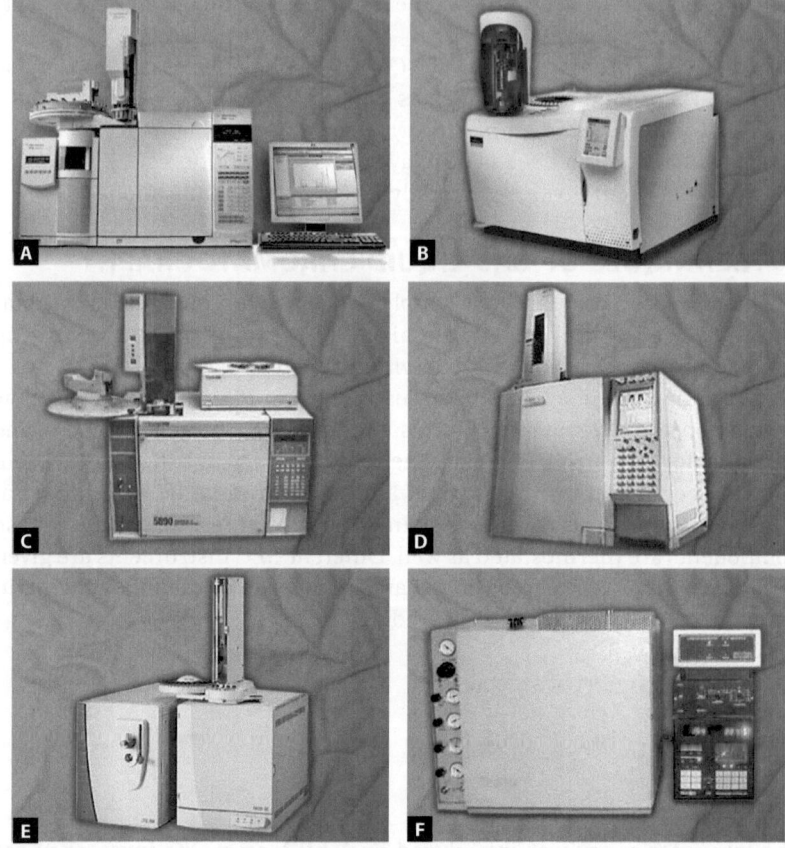

Figs. 6.2A to F: Gas chromatograph by different manufacturers. (A) Agilent; (B) Perkin Elmer; (C) HP; (D) Shimadzu; (E) Thermo Fisher; and (F) Nucon.

3. It should allow the detector to respond in an adequate manner
4. He, Ar, H_2, and N_2 fulfill all the above requirements and hence, these gases are most commonly used as carrier gas
5. N_2 is the most popular carrier gas used in GC
6. The basic purposes of carrier gas are:
    a. Push the sample through the gas chromatograph column, i.e., sweep sample through the column
    b. Clean out the gas chromatograph column after sample analysis
    c. Protect column from oxygen exposure
    d. Assists in the function of the detector
7. A high pressure gas cylinder (in which carrier gas is filled in compressed form) is used as carrier gas reservoir
8. The cylinder is also attached with pressure regulator to control the gas flow
9. A soap bubble meter (**Fig. 6.3**) and a device to measure the rate of flow of carrier gas

GAS CHROMATOGRAPHY AND ITS APPLICATIONS

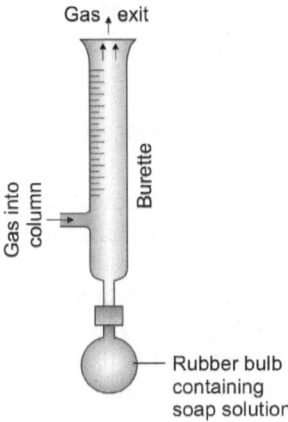

Fig. 6.3: Soap bubble meter.

The carrier gas of a gas chromatograph is very important. It varies for the gas chromatograph used, but in general, the gas must be chemically inert, dry, and free of oxygen. These conditions are required because otherwise, the carrier gas might chemically react and interfere with the surface of the gas chromatograph.

Injection Port

Injection port is very important in GLC. Schematic diagram of sample injection system is shown in **Figure 6.4**. Few important points about the injection port are:
- The injector port is heated to a temperature, which will insure rapid vaporization, but not thermal degradation of the solute molecule
- The port is made up of heavy mass that is maintained at an elevated temperature and contains a pliable septum through which samples are injected

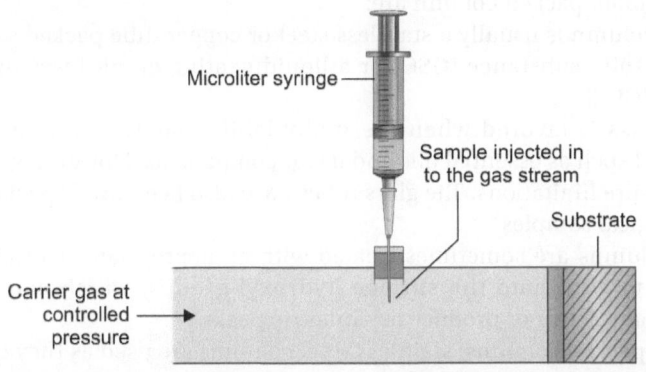

Fig. 6.4: Sample injection system.

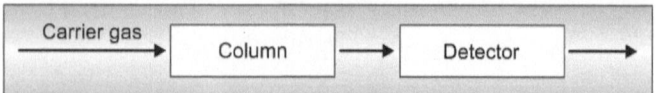

Fig. 6.5: Arrangement of carrier gas, column, and detector.

- The port is designed for instantaneous injection and vaporization of a sample, so that the sample is introduced immediately into a column
- Liquids are introduced with syringe of 0.1–100 μL capacity
- The liquid is drawn into the syringe a number of times to remove any air bubble and injected very rapidly into the gas stream
- For gases, a gas-tight syringe of 1.0–10.0 μL capacity can be used
- The solid may be dissolved in a suitable solvent and then injected as solution
- Sample, which cannot be vaporized at the operating temperature, must always be avoided

Column

The column is the heart of GLC. The different solutes in the vaporized samples are separated from each other by virtue of their different interaction with column packing. As the solute emerges individually from the end of the column, they enter the detector. The schematic diagram of carrier gas, column, and detector is given in **Figure 6.5**.

The two commonly used columns are packed column and capillary column (open tubular column). As a result of the simpler injection procedure and the more precise sampling method, the packed column tends to give greater quantitative accuracy and precision. However, despite its problems with sample injection, the open tubular column is seen as the "state of the art" column and is by far the most popular column system.

Packed Column

Packed column is very important in GLC, which is shown in **Figure 6.6**. Few points about packed column are:
- Packed column is usually a stainless steel or copper tube packed with either a solid substance (GSC) or a liquid coating on an inert solid support (GLC)
- Pyrex glass is favored when thermally labile materials are being separated such as essential oils and flavor components. However, glass has pressure limitations. The glass tubes have also been used specially for biological samples
- Glass columns are sometimes treated with an appropriate silanizing reagent to eliminate the surface hydroxyl groups, which can be catalytically active or produce asymmetric peaks
- For long packed columns, stainless steel columns are used as they can easily tolerate the necessary elevated pressures

GAS CHROMATOGRAPHY AND ITS APPLICATIONS

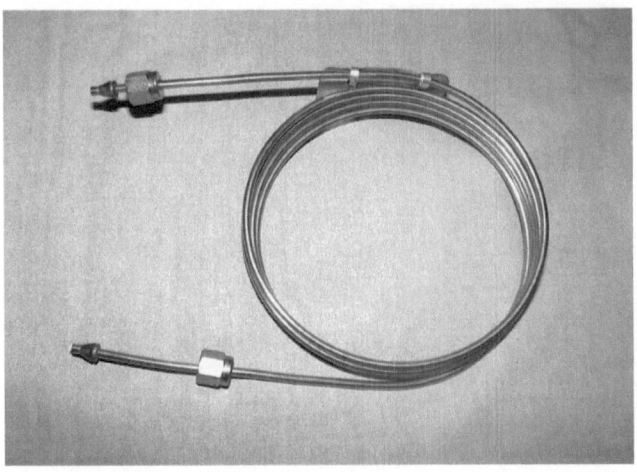

Fig. 6.6: Packed column.

- Short columns can be straight and installed vertically in the chromatograph. Longer columns can be U shaped but columns more than a meter long are usually coiled
- The columns can be constructed of any practical length and relatively easily installed. Length of tube is 5–50 feet
- Stainless steel columns are usually washed with dilute hydrochloric acid, then with water followed by methanol, acetone, methylene dichloride, and n-hexane. Washing procedure removes any corrosion products and traces of lubricating agents used in the tube drawing process
- The column is placed in an oven such that the temperature can be easily controlled. Ordinarily, the tubes are folded or coiled, so that they can be conveniently fitted into a thermostat
- The diameter of metal or glass tube is 1/4" or 0.25 inch

Capillary Column (Open Tubular Column)

Second type of column is capillary column, which is also known as open tubular column. Capillary column is shown in **Figure 6.7**. Few points about capillary column are:
- Capillary column is fabricated from capillary tubing, the bore of which is coated with very thin film of the liquid phase
- The column diameter is 1/16" or less
- These columns are available in length up to 200 m because of the fact that they have very low pressure drop
- These columns, however, have low sample capacities and these are used for partition
- Capillary columns are fabricated from stainless steel or quartz. Metal capillary columns must be carefully cleaned to remove traces of

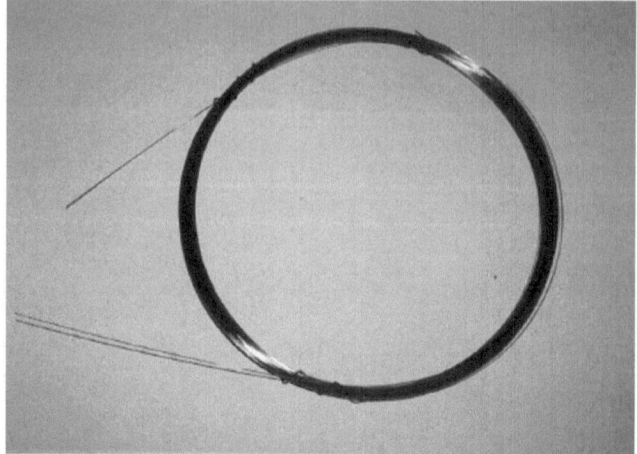

Fig. 6.7: Capillary column.

extrusion lubricants before they can be coated, usually by washing with methylene dichloride, methanol, and then water
- After removing oil and grease, the columns are washed with dilute acid to remove metal oxides or other corrosion products that may remain adhering to the walls, washed with water and then again washed with methanol and methylene dichloride
- Metal columns provide the high efficiencies expected from open tubular columns and were used for the analysis of petroleum, fuel oils, etc. Metal columns, however, have some disadvantages as they although easily coated with dispersive stationary phases (e.g., squalane, Apiezon grease, etc.) and they are not so easily coated with the more polar stationary phases such as CARBOWAX-R.
- Metal can also react directly with some materials by chelation and adsorb polar material, which results in asymmetric and tailing peaks
- Nevertheless, metal columns are rugged, easy to handle and easy to remove, and replace in the chromatograph; consequently, their use has persisted in many application areas, despite the introduction of fused silica columns.
- Open tubular columns are broadly divided into two classes:
  i. Porous layer open tubular (PLOT) columns (**Fig. 6.8A**)
  ii. Wall-coated open tubular (WCOT) columns (**Fig. 6.8B**)
- The PLOT columns are largely used for gas analysis and the separation of low molecular weight hydrocarbons
- The internal diameter of PLOT columns ranges from 320 to 530 μm with a porous layer that can be 5–50 μm thick
- The internal diameter of WCOT columns ranges from 100 to 530 μm with a porous layer that can be 0.1–8 μm thick

GAS CHROMATOGRAPHY AND ITS APPLICATIONS

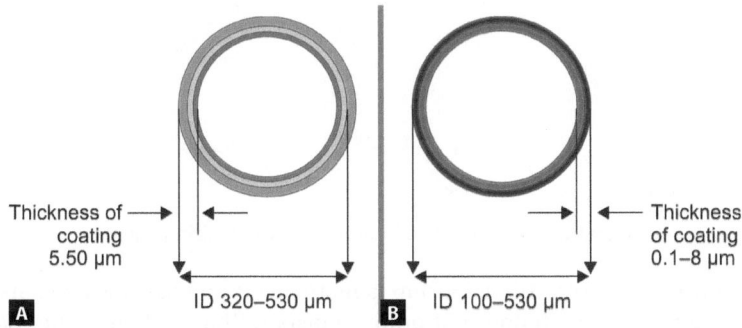

Figs. 6.8A and B: Open tubular column. (A) Porous layer open tubular (PLOT); and (B) Wall-coated open tubular (WCOT).

- The technique of coating the walls with solid particles is again largely proprietary, but stable and reproducible columns can be prepared and are commercially available
- For example using the PLOT column to separate and determine the impurities in a 2,3-butadiene sample. The PLOT column used was 50 m long, 0.32 mm ID, and coated with a 5-µm layer of aluminum oxide modified with potassium chloride
- The separation was carried out by programming the column temperature from 100 to 200°C at 6°C/min

Solid Support for Gas-liquid Chromatography

The main purpose of the solid phase or solid support is to provide support to the thin uniform film of liquid phase. The most important requirements of a solid support are:
1. It should be porous and should have a large surface area
2. It should be capable of providing good mechanical strength
3. It should consist of small, uniform, and spherical particles
4. It should be chemically inert
5. It should be readily wetted by the liquid phase to give uniform coating

Various supports have been fashioned from powdered Teflon, alumina, carborundum, and microglass beads, but the most commonly used support is diatomaceous earth or kieselguhr, which is commercially available in the form of chromosorb N, chromosorb P, fire brick, anachrom U, anachrom A, porapak Q, glass beads, celite, dicalite, sterchamol, etc.

Diatomaceous earth, being a form of hydrated silica, contains many hydroxyl groups on its surface. These can serve as sites at which solute molecules can be adsorbed. This is most undesirable because it causes tailing of peak, as it results in sluggish release of solute from the liquid film to the carrier gas. The most effective methods of reducing this effect are to treat the solid with a silanizing agent such as hexamethyldisilazane (HMDS). The support is treated with HMDS, which replaces the hydrogen of the silanol group with a trimethylsilyl radical (**Fig. 6.9**).

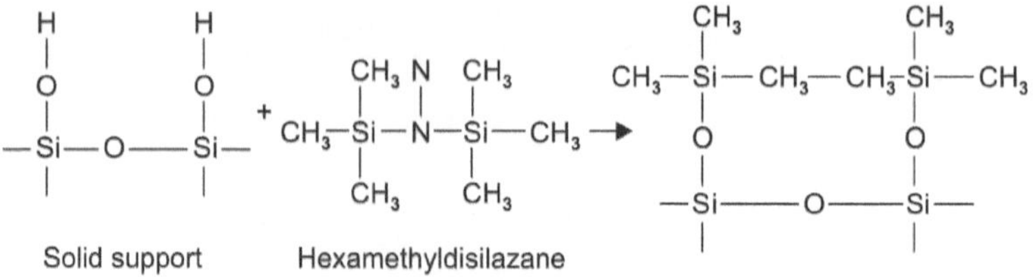

GAS CHROMATOGRAPHY AND ITS APPLICATIONS

Fig. 6.9: Treatment of solid support with silanizing agent.

In this way, polar silanol group is methylated and assumes dispersive characteristics, which does not produce peak tailing. Although the major contributors to adsorption by support are the silanol groups, radical adsorption comes from the presence of traces of heavy metals such as iron, arsenic, etc., which can be removed by acid washing prior to silanization.

Teflon was explored as a possible alternative of diatomaceous earth. Teflon powder proved to have little adsorption, but extremely difficult to pack into a column and hence, it is very rarely used in general GLC.

Glass beads have also been used as support for packed GC column, if silanized have little adsorption. Being nonporous, all the stationary phase must reside on the surface of the beads, which gives them limited loading capacity.

The macroporous polymer beads are used as support as well as adsorbents. They exhibit significant adsorption as the support itself acts as a stationary phase and makes contribution to retention. All the three types of support are commercially available. None of these supports, however, are completely devoid of adsorptive properties.

Coating the Supports

It is important to have a correct measure of the amount of stationary phase that has been placed on a support for retention time, reproducibility, and qualitative accuracy. The reproducibility of the coating procedure may have particular significance when the analytical results are to be used for forensic purposes. The material can be coated by the following three methods:

1. *Coating by direct addition method*: Coating by direct addition would appear to be the ideal quantitative method of preparing the column packings. A known amount of stationary phase is added directly to a known mass of support contained in a beaker. The material is well mixed by rotating the flask for several hours. The efficiency of the column slowly increases with use, as the stationary phase distributes itself more evenly throughout the packing. It may take several weeks of use for the column to give a constant maximum efficiency.
2. *Coating by filtration method*: The filtration method gives a packing with the stationary well distributed over the support, but the loading cannot be accurately calculated. A known weight of stationary phase is dissolved in sufficient solvent to provide excess liquid when mixed with a weighed amount of the support. The mixture is filtered and the volume of the filtrate is measured. From the volume of filtrate,

the amount of solvent remaining on the support can be calculated and hence, this stationary phase loading can be measured. The bed is then sucked dry, the solvent is evaporated, and the coated support is packed into the column. The amount of stationary phase on the support cannot be determined accurately by this method due to solvent losses by evaporation.

3. *Coating by slurry method*: In the slurry method of coating, a known amount of the support is placed in the flask of a rotary evaporator and the required mass of stationary phase is added. A measured volume of volatile solvent is then added in sufficient quantity to produce free-flowing slurry. The flask is then rotated at room temperature for 10–15 minutes to insure complete mixing. The rotating flask is then heated and the solvent is removed by evaporation. When the packing appears dry, the material is then heated to about 140–150°C in an oven to remove the final traces of solvent. This method of coating gives an extremely homogeneous surface distribution of stationary phase throughout the support and an accurate value for the stationary phase loading. The slurry method of coating is the one that is recommended.

Column Packing/Column Coating
For Packed Column
Short columns are straight and can be packed vertically.

The packing is added, approximately 0.5–0.6 mL at a time and the column is tapped until the packing has settled. Next portion of packing is then added and the process is repeated until the column is full. U-shaped columns are packed in the same manner. Columns up to 50 feet long can be packed in a series of Us and then each U column joined with a low dead volume connection. Glass columns are usually filled through an opening at the top of each U, which is terminated in a plug of wool. These long packed columns could be operated at a maximum of 200 psi and could provide efficiencies of up to approximately 5,000 theoretical plates. However, straight columns are clumsy to use and occupy a large amount of space, which are often difficult to accommodate in thermostat. The coiled column, although more difficult to pack, has been readily accepted for packing of such column and special procedure has been adopted. In this procedure, the packing is placed in a reservoir attached to a gas supply that forces the packing through the column. The column exit is connected to a vacuum pump. A wad of quartz wool is placed at the end of the column. The vacuum and gas flow are turned on simultaneously and the packing is swept rapidly through the column. This causes the material to be slightly compacted along the total length of the column (**Fig. 6.10**). The procedure is a little tedious and the success rate is about 85–90%.

For Capillary Column (Open Tubular Column)
A deactivation program for silica and soft glass columns that is suitable for most applications would first entail an acid wash. The column is filled with

GAS CHROMATOGRAPHY AND ITS APPLICATIONS

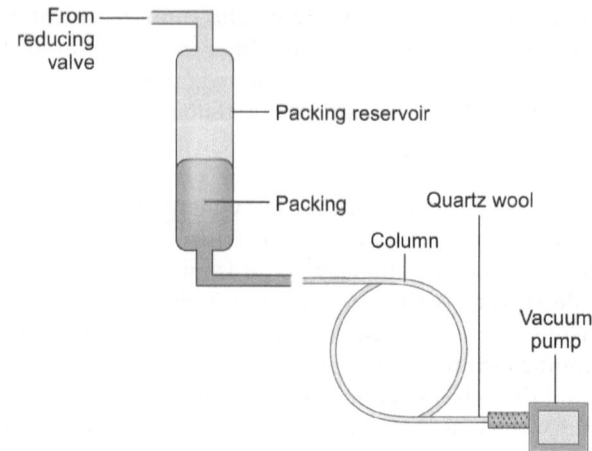

Fig. 6.10: Packing of coiled column.

10% (w/w) hydrochloric acid, the ends sealed, and the column is then heated to 100°C for 1–2 hours. It is then washed free of acid with distilled water and dried. The column is then filled with a solution of HMDS contained in a suitable solvent, sealed, and again heated to the boiling point of the solvent for 1.5 hours. This procedure blocks any hydroxyl groups that were formed on the surface during the acid wash. The column is then washed with the pure solvent, dried in a stream of pure nitrogen, and is then ready for coating.

Capillary columns can be coated internally with a liquid stationary phase or with polymeric materials that can be polymerized to form a relatively rigid, internal polymer coating. There are two methods for coating of open tubular column, one is the dynamic method and the other is static method.

1. *Dynamic coating*: A plug of solvent containing the stationary phase is placed at the beginning of the column. The strength of the solution determines the thickness of the stationary phase film. In general, the film thickness of a capillary column ranges from 0.25 mm to about 1.5 mm. A 5% w/w of stationary phase in the solvent will produce a film thickness of about 0.5 mm. However, this is only approximate, as the film thickness is also determined by the physical properties of the surface and the solvent and the stationary phase. The coating procedure is given in **Figure 6.11**. After the plug has been run into the front of the column, pressure is applied to the front of the column to

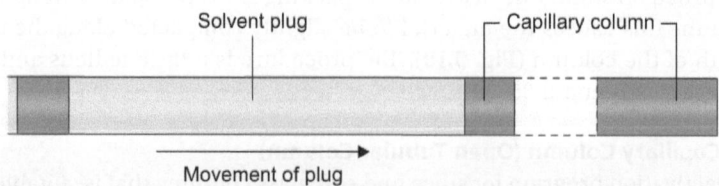

Fig. 6.11: Dynamic coating of open tubular column.

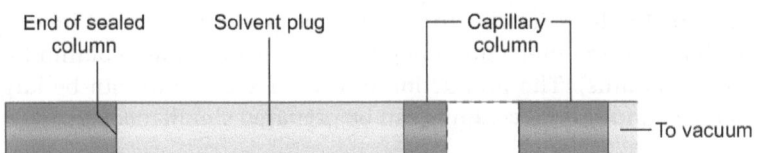

Fig. 6.12: Static coating method.

force the plug through the column at 2-5 mm/s, which will take about 5-6 hours for the plug to pass through a 60 m column. When the plug has passed through the column, the gas flow is continued for about an hour. The gas flow should not be increased too soon or the stationary phase solution on the walls of the tube is displaced forward in the form of ripples, which produces a very uneven film. After an hour, the flow rate may be increased and the column stripped of solvent. The traces of the solvent are removed by heating the column above the boiling point of the solvent. Complete solvent removal can be identified by connecting the column to a detector and observing the baseline drift.

2. *Static coating*: The whole column is filled with a solution of the stationary phase and one end is connected to a vacuum pump. When the solvent evaporates, the front retreats back down the tube leaving a coating on the walls. The static coating procedure is shown in **Figure 6.12**. The column is filled with a solution of stationary phase having a concentration appropriate for the deposition of a film of the required thickness. Again the required concentration will depend on the stationary phase, the solvent, the temperature, and the condition of the wall surface. Generally, the optimum solvent concentration is not predictable and requires some preliminary experiments to be carried out to determine the best coating conditions.

After filling, one end of the column is sealed and the other end is connected to a high vacuum pump and placed in an oven and the solvent evaporates and the front retreats leaving a film of solution on the walls. The solvent then evaporates from this film and the stationary phase remains as a thin coating on the wall. The procedure is continued till all the solvent has evaporated. The procedure needs no attention and hence, it can be carried out overnight. The static procedure is more repeatable than the dynamic method, but it produces columns having similar performance to those dynamically coated. Column stability depends on the stability of the stationary phase film, which depends on the constant nature of the surface tension forces that hold it to the column wall. These surface tension forces can be reduced with an increase in temperature. As a consequence, the film can suddenly break up. Hence, it would be highly desirable if the stationary phase was bonded to the column walls or polymerized in situ. Such coatings are known as immobilized stationary phases and cannot be removed by solvent washing.

GAS CHROMATOGRAPHY AND ITS APPLICATIONS

The difficulties involved in preparing packed columns have also contributed to the preferential popularity of the capillary column (open tubular columns). The production of capillary columns can be largely automated and several columns can be prepared simultaneously.

Liquid Phase (Stationary Phase)

The stationary phase is a polymer that is coated onto the inner wall of the fused silica tubing or adsorbed on solid support. The thickness, uniformity, and chemical nature of the stationary phase are very important. In general, the most important requirements of a liquid phase are as follows:
- It should be a good solvent for the component of the sample
- It should be thermally stable
- The solvent power of the liquid phase should be different for each component of the sample
- It should be chemically inert toward the sample
- It should be of low volatility

The most common capillary stationary phase is silicon polymer (**Fig. 6.13A**). The type and amount of substitution on the polysiloxane backbone distinguishes each phase. For example (5% phenyl), methyl phase has two phenyl groups bonded to 2.5%, by number, of the silicon atoms and 97.5% of silicon atoms have methyl groups bonded to them. Some common solvents (stationary phase) and their uses are given in **Table 6.1**.

Another widely used liquid phase is polyethylene glycol (**Fig. 6.13B**). Carbowax 20M is one of the most used polyethylene glycol as a liquid phase. The major disadvantage of polyethylene glycol is their high susceptibility to

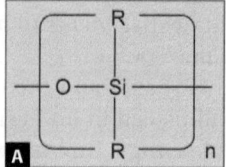 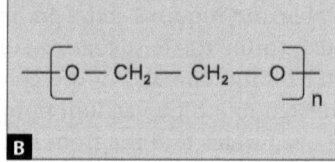

Figs. 6.13A and B: Stationary phase. (A) Silicon polymer where R may be CH_3, $-CH_2-CH_2-CH_2CN$, $-CH_2CH_2CF_2$, $-C_6H_5$; and (B) Ethylene glycol polymer.

Table 6.1: Common solvents (stationary phase).

Stationary liquid phase	Temperature (°C)	Applications
Squalane	142–150	Hydrocarbons
Apiezon L grease	250–310	Alcohols, aldehydes, ketones, fatty acids, and pesticides
Silicone oil (DC-550)	180–210	A wide variety of compound types
Silicon rubber gun (SE-30)	300–360	Drugs, alkaloids sugar, and pesticides
Carbowax 20M	200–250	Alcohol, aromatics, gases, and pesticides
Carbowax 200	150	Aldehyde and ketones

GAS CHROMATOGRAPHY AND ITS APPLICATIONS

Table 6.2: Commercially available stationary phases in GLC.

SE-30	Nonpolar
QF-1	Semipolar
OV-17	Semipolar
OV-225	Semipolar
OV-210	Semipolar
DC-200	Nonpolar
Apiezon L	Nonpolar
DC-11	Nonpolar
DEGS	Polar
Carbowax 20M	Polar
XE-60	Polar

(DEGS: diethylene glycol succinate; GLC: gas-liquid chromatography)

structure damage by oxygen at elevated temperature. Some commercially available stationary phases in GLC are given in **Table 6.2**.

A new class of capillary column contains a gas-solid adsorption type of stationary phase. For example, porous layer open tubular or PLOT column.

Detectors

General requirements of GC detectors are: High sensitivity, physically suitable, capable of operating upto a maximum column temperature of about 350°C, ease of operation, no response to undesired compounds, response to compounds for which analysis is required, an output signal which is a linear function of concentration of sample in the detector, linear response extending to high concentration, etc. Based on above physical properties, there are several types of detectors such as flame ionization detector (FID), electron capture detector (ECD), thermal conductivity detector (TCD), flame photometric detector (FPD), cross-section detection, argon ionization detector (AID), gas density balance detector (GDBD), helium ionization detector (HID), photoionization detector (PID), microdetector, piezoelectric absorption detector, microwave-excited discharge detector, flame thermocouple detector, argon triode detector, etc.

Flame Ionization Detector

Flame ionization detector is the most commonly used detector. Schematic diagram of FID is given in **Figure 6.14**. Few important points of FID are:
- The FID is used for hydrocarbons and many carbon-containing compounds with limits of detection in the picogram range
- The FID evolved from the flame thermocouple detector, in which a stream of hydrogen is burnt at a small jet, over which a thermocouple is situated

GAS CHROMATOGRAPHY AND ITS APPLICATIONS

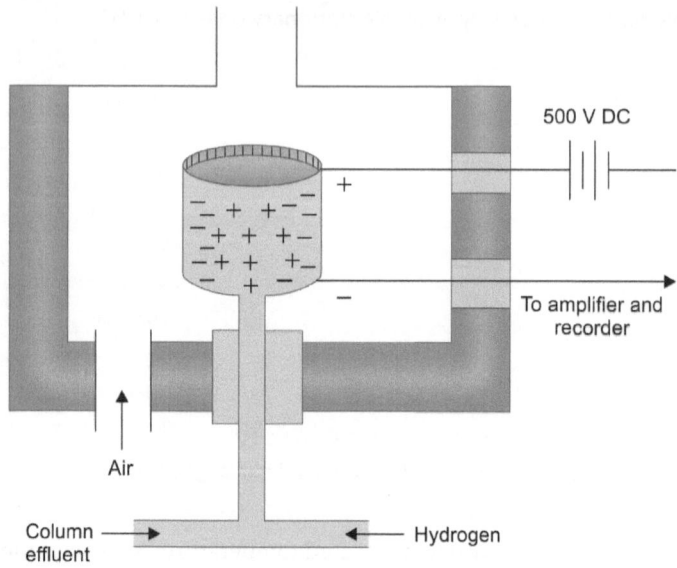

Fig. 6.14: Flame ionization detector (FID).

- The mobile phase from the GC column is fed into the hydrogen stream and when a solute is eluted, the temperature of the flame increases together with the thermocouple output. The thermocouple output is monitored by a backing off circuit and a potentiometric recorder
- In the FID, the thermocouple is replaced by an electrode situated away from the flame and a potential of a 100–200 V applied between the jet and the electrode. This potential collects any ions or electrons formed in the flame during combustion of an eluted solute, which is monitored as an increase in ion current by a high-impedance amplifier
- During the elution of a carbon-containing substance, it is thought that microscopic particles of carbon are formed that thermally emit electrons and which provide the signal current to the high-impedance amplifier
- Except for a very few organic compounds (e.g., carbon monoxide), the FID detects all carbon-containing compounds
- The gaseous eluents from the column are mixed with separately plumbed in hydrogen and air and all are burned on the jet's tip
- The detector housing is heated so that gases produced by the combustion (mainly water) do not condense in the detector before leaving the detector chimney
- To maintain the best analytical conditions, additional gas must be constantly passed through the detector. This gas makes up the additional needed gas flow and so is termed as makeup gas. Since the makeup gas needs to be inert so that its addition does not upset the fuel and oxidant balance and also it needs to be added in relatively large amounts, nitrogen is usually the gas of choice. Helium would also work but is a nonrenewable resource and more expensive

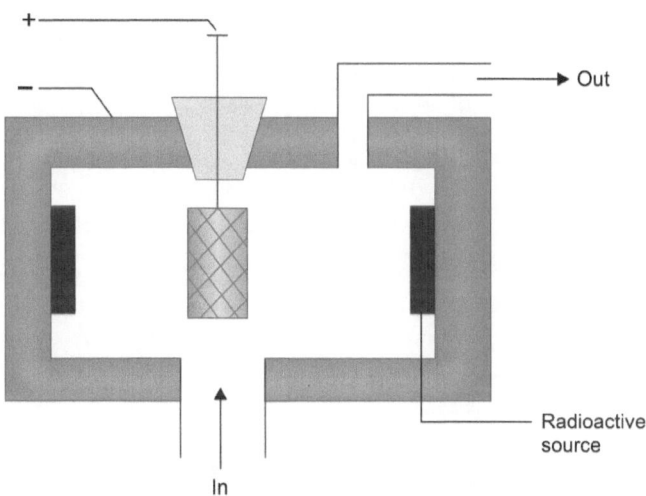

Fig. 6.15: Electron capture detector (ECD).

- Fuel and air are turned on at a predetermined flow rate, ignitor is lit, and the flame ignited. After the flame is confirmed burning, makeup gas flow is turned on. The flame stabilizes within an hour or less and then is routinely left on continuously to maintain the lowest signal background and therefore produce the lowest detection limits
- Turning off the flame involves first shutting off the fuel flow which extinguishes the flame and then the oxidant and makeup gas flow are closed.

Molecules that contained only carbon and hydrogen respond best with this detector, but the presence of heteroatoms such as nitrogen and sulfur decrease the detector's response.

Electron Capture Detector

Electron capture detector is very useful detector for halogenated compounds. Schematic diagram of ECD is given in **Figure 6.15**. Some important features are:
- Gas chromatography with an ECD is a very sensitive method and is well suited for analysis of polyhalogenated organic compounds
- In the ECD, a beta emitter, such as radioactive tritium or ^{63}Ni, is used to ionize the carrier gas
- Fast beta particles generated by the radioactive source collide with the molecules of the carrier or makeup gas. By impact ionization, free slow-moving electrons are produced, which generate a measurable and steady current
- If the GC effluent contains organic molecules with electronegative functional groups, such as halogens, phosphorus, and nitro groups, electrons will be captured and the current will be reduced

GAS CHROMATOGRAPHY AND ITS APPLICATIONS

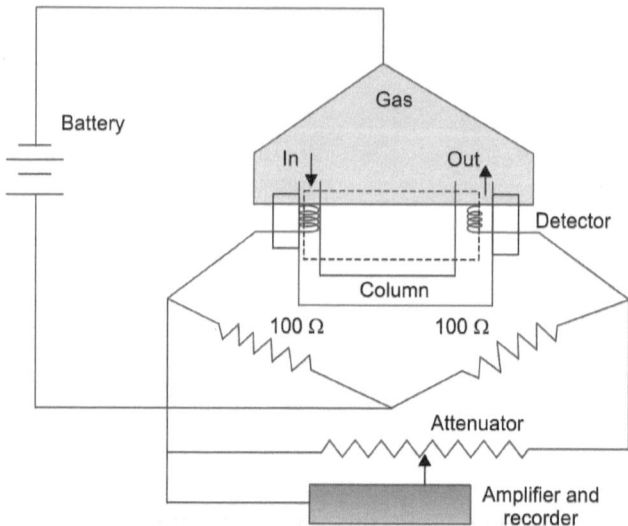

Fig. 6.16: Thermal conductivity detector (TCD).

- In comparison to a signal without sample compounds, the reduction in electron flow is proportional to the quantity of electrophile sample components
- An important facet of GC with an ECD is the carrier gas. The carrier gas transfers the sample from the injector through the column and into the ECD
- Because the ECD is sensitive to water, the carrier gas must be dry. Halocarbon-free helium or nitrogen is, therefore, recommended as carrier gas for the ECD
- To generate free slow-moving electrons, the ECD requires nitrogen or methane, where methane is used in a form of a methane/argon mixture. Both nitrogen and the methane mixture are used as detector gases as well as carrier gases.

Thermal Conductivity Detector

Schematic diagram of TCD is given in **Figure 6.16**. Few important points of TCD are:
- Thermal conductivity detectors are based upon change in the thermal conductivity of the gas stream
- The TCD is truly a universal detector and can detect air, hydrogen, carbon monoxide, nitrogen, sulfur oxide, inorganic gases, and many other compounds
- The TCD is a nonspecific and nondestructive detector. For most organic molecules, the sensitivity of the TCD is lower as compared to the FID
- The sample components in the carrier gas pass into the measuring channel. A second channel serves as a reference channel where only

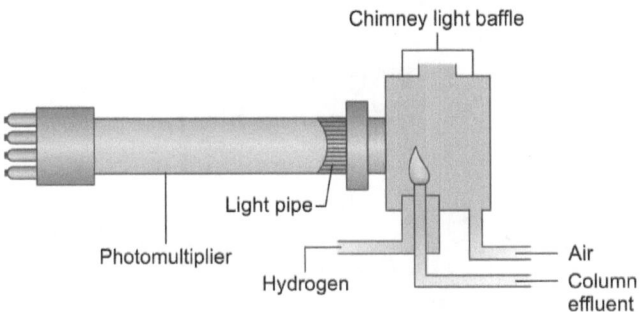

Fig. 6.17: Flame photometric detector (FPD).

pure carrier gas flows. Electrically-heated resistance wires are located in both channels
- The difference in thermal conductivity between the column effluent flow (sample components in carrier gas) and the reference flow of carrier gas alone produces a voltage signal proportional to this difference. The signal is proportional to the concentration of the sample components
- Chemically active compounds, such as acids and halogenated compounds, should be avoided when using TCD, since they can attack the filament (wires) and thereby, change the resistance and permanently reduce the detector sensitivity.
- Oxidizing substances, such as oxygen, can also damage the filament and a leak-free environment should be maintained
- In the GC-TCD, the carrier gas is both used to transfer the sample through the column and into the TCD detector and as a reference gas
- With the GC-TCD, the reference gas and the detector gas must be the same as the carrier gas
- As for any GCs, the carrier gas must be inert and may not be adsorbed by the column material. Helium is typically used as the carrier gas for the TCD because of its high thermal conductivity. However, nitrogen, argon, or hydrogen is also used as carrier gases with GC-TCD

Flame Photometric Detector

Schematic diagram of FPD is given in **Figure 6.17**. Few important points of FPD are:
- This type of detectors is based on the luminous emission from a hydrogen-rich flame in the presence of compounds containing either sulfur (394 nm) or phosphorus (526 nm). The determination of sulfur- or phosphorus-containing compounds is the job of the FPD
- The detector consists of a hydrogen air burner and a photomultiplier. The latter is so located as to see only the upper part of the flame, which does not emit appreciable in the absence of S and P
- The selection of S or P may be carried out by using interchangeable optical filters. Optical filters are used to select the wavelength range of the emission, which is characteristic of specific atoms

GAS CHROMATOGRAPHY AND ITS APPLICATIONS

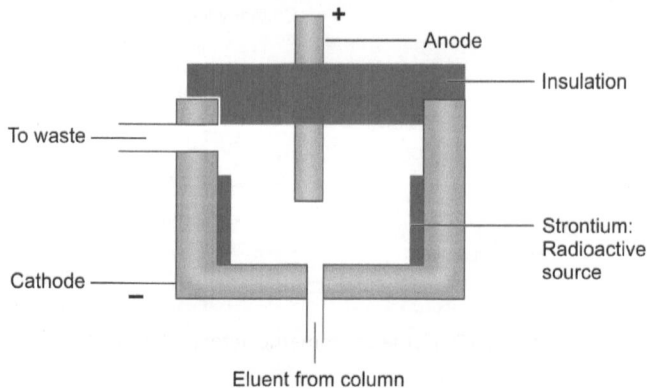

Fig. 6.18: Argon ionization detector (AID).

- The detector is very specific, depending on the choice of optical filters. It can detect the S- and P-containing compounds down to 10–30 ppmv, but the detector is nonlinear. The reason to use more than one kind of detector for GC is to achieve selective and/or highly sensitive detection of specific compounds encountered in particular chromatographic analysis
- A serious problem that can occur in the FPD is the quenching or reabsorption of the light emitted by the selected species. Hydrocarbon quenching can occur when the peak containing sulfur is coeluted with another hydrocarbon in relatively high concentration
- The drawback here being that the filter must be exchanged between chromatographic runs, if the other family of compounds is to be detected.

Argon Ionization Detector

Schematic diagram of AID is given in **Figure 6.18**. Few points are:
- The very first argon detector sensors used is an automobile sparking plug as the electrode, the ceramic seal being a very efficient insulator at very high temperatures
- Inside the main cavity of the sensor, there is a (90 Sr) source contained in silver foil.
- This tenuous layer protecting the radioactive material is rather vulnerable to mechanical abrasion, which could result in radioactive contamination
- The decay of 90 Sr occurs in two stages, each stage emitting a β-particle producing the stable atom of 90 Sr
- The electrons produced by the radioactive source are accelerated under a potential that ranged from 500 to 2,000 V, depending on the dimensions of the sensor and the geometry of the electrode

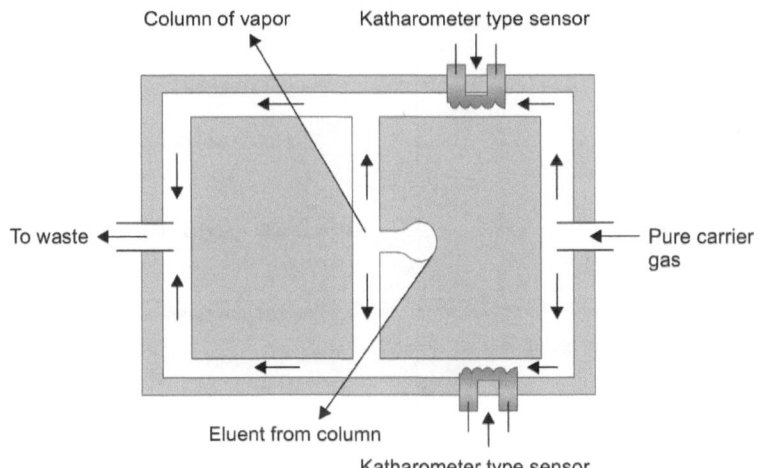

Fig. 6.19: Gas density balance detector (GDBD).

Gas Density Balance Detector

Schematic diagram of GDBD is given in **Figure 6.19**. Some important points are given below:
- The GDBD was originally described in the early 1950s and was the first in-line GC detector to be invented. In its original form, it consisted of a Wheatstone network of tubes drilled out of a high conductivity copper block
- The two tubes were connected at the center through a cylindrical convection chamber about 2 cm in diameter and 3–4 mm wide
- A looped heater situated in the chamber and twin thermocouples consisting of two copper wires 0.001 in OD with 2 mm of constantan wire of the same diameter arc welded between them are placed above the heater wires
- It was arranged that the thermocouple junctions are situated about 2 mm from the heater wires and thus, with no solute present is heated by convection to the same temperature. When a solute is present in one tube, due to the increase in vapor density of the tube contents, a pressure difference develops across the joining tube
- Because the detector responds to the vapor density of the solute, the device could also be used to determine the molecular weight of a solute
- The sensitivity of the detector is about 5×10^{-7} g/mL. The detector did not become very popular because it is difficult to make

Helium Ionization Detector

Schematic diagram of HID is given in **Figure 6.20**. Few important points of HID are:
- The HID is a universal detector, responding to all molecules except neon

GAS CHROMATOGRAPHY AND ITS APPLICATIONS

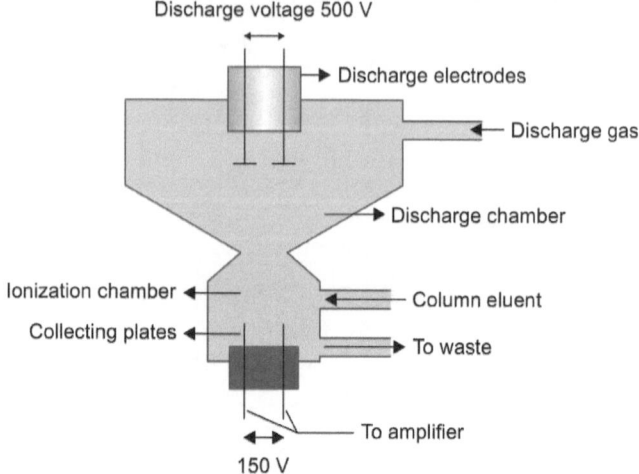

Fig. 6.20: Helium ionization detector (HID).

- It requires only helium carrier and makeup gas and is sensitive to the low ppm range and particularly useful for volatile inorganics to which the FID and other selective detectors will not respond such as NO_2, CO, CO_2, O_2, N_2, H_2S, and H_2
- It is a robust detector that, unlike TCD, it has no filaments to burn out. The helium detector works exactly on the same principle as the argon detector, but metastable helium atoms are produced by the accelerated electrons instead of metastable argon atoms
- Metastable helium atoms, however, have an energy of 19.8 and 20.6 eV and thus, can ionize, and consequently detect the permanent gases and, in fact, the molecules of all other volatile substances
- As a consequence, contaminants in the helium can be extremely deleterious and the helium must be extremely pure or the production of the metastable helium atom production will be quenched by traces of any other permanent gases that may be present
- When first developed, very complicated helium purifying chain was necessary to insure its optimum operation. However, with high purity helium becoming generally available, the detector can now be used to detect concentrations of organic vapors at 10-13 g/mL or less

Photoionization Detector

Schematic diagram of PID is given in **Figure 6.21**. Some features are:
- In PID, compounds eluting into a cell are bombarded with high-energy photons emitted from a lamp. Compounds with ionization potential below the photon energy are ionized. The resulting ions are attracted to an electrode, measured, and a signal is generated
- A potential difference is applied and the resulting ionization current is detected

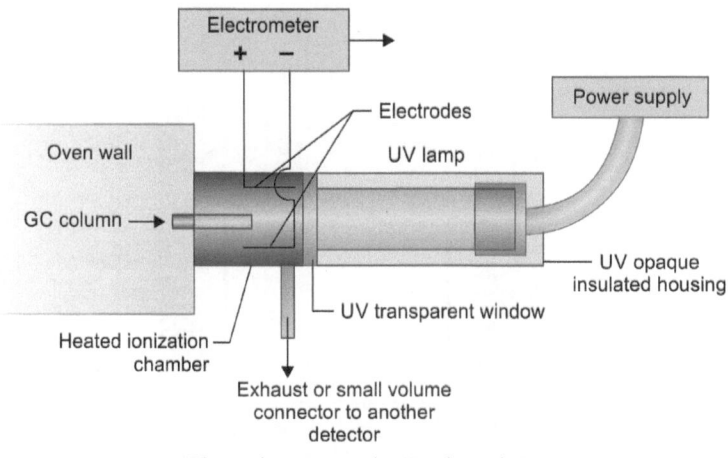

(GC: gas chromatography; UV: ultraviolet)

Fig. 6.21: Photoionization detector (PID).

- The detector is only useful for substances with ionization potentials below 11 eV. This makes it quite useful for detecting one component of a combined eluent when the other component, for instance nitrogen, has a high ionization potential
- The detector has a small linear dynamic range and is capable of detecting substances below 1 ppmv. Usually, it is used for aromatics and olefins
- The PID is nondestructive, so the sample can be routed through the PID and onto other detectors

Microdetector or Microargon Detector

Schematic diagram of microargon detector (MAD) is given in **Figure 6.22**. Some important features are:

- The microdetector is designed to have a very small effective sensing volume to facilitate its use with capillary columns, where the flow rate may be as low as 0.1 mL/min or less
- In the MAD sensor, the anode is withdrawn into a small cavity, about 2.5 mm in diameter
- This insures that the electrons can only reach the anode along a restricted path and the electric field around the electrode resides within a few diameters of the anode tip
- The anode is tubular in form and the capillary column can slide-up inside the anode, until it is within a millimeter or so of the electric field
- Metastable argon atoms are formed as a cloud around the anode tip and any solute molecules eluted from the column immediately pass through this cloud and are ionized
- At the other end of the sensor, there is another inlet that provides a scavenger flow of argon that rapidly removes the solute from the cell through two holes at the bottom of the anode cavity. This procedure reduces the effective sensor volume to less than a microliter and thus, allows the efficient use of a capillary column

GAS CHROMATOGRAPHY AND ITS APPLICATIONS

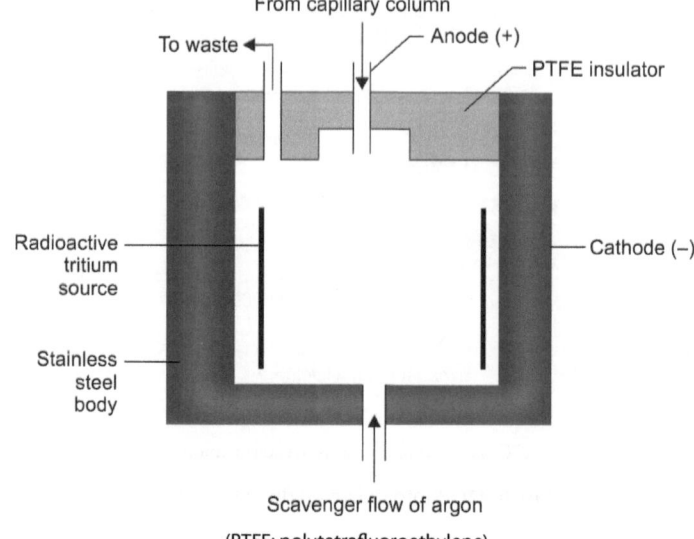

(PTFE: polytetrafluoroethylene)

Fig. 6.22: Microdetector.

Mass Detector

Few points are discussed below:
- The first mass detector was developed by Bevan and Thorburn during the 1960s for GC. The mass detectors, developed to date, can only function with packed columns, as adequate sample must be placed on the column for the mass measuring device to respond
- The mass detector actually weighs the mass of solute eluted from the chromatographic column continuously over a predetermined period of time
- Bevan and Thorburn utilized a recording microbalance on which it was placed a small, light adsorption tube. The tube had to have sufficiently low flow impedance to insure that the balance was not disturbed by the flow of carrier gas. However, at the same time, the system needed high absorption efficiency, so that it would be able to quantitatively adsorb all the eluted solutes
- The tube was about 10 mm in diameter and about 50 mm in length and the eluent from the GC column entered the center of the tube from a glass jet that protruded into one end of the tube and was arranged so that it did not touch the sides of the adsorption tube
- The adsorbent was coated on the inside wall of the tube. The detector obviously gave an integrated response, which resulted in a stepped curve, the height of each step representing the mass of each eluted solute
- Lawrence and Scott developed a mass detector, working on the same principle for use in liquid chromatography
- A flash heating tube was hung from the arm of a microbalance which was situated in an oven held at a sufficiently high temperature to flash

evaporate the mobile phase as it fell into the tube. The momentum of the solvent falling into the flash heater produced a constant offset on the balance, but as each solute was eluted, a step equivalent to its mass was produced on the recording balance chart
- The sensitivity of the mass detector was limited to the mass sensitivity of the balance
- Other type of detectors have, from time to time, been called mass detectors, but they have not actually measured the eluted mass directly, but gave an output that was related to the mass and as a consequence, were not, truly mass detectors

■ TERMS USED IN GAS-LIQUID CHROMATOGRAPHY

Chromatogram

A graphical presentation of detector response, concentration of analyte in the effluent, or other quantity used as a measure of effluent concentration versus effluent volume or time is called chromatogram (**Fig. 6.23**).

Retention Time

The maximum time required for the solute peak to reach the detector in GLC is called retention time. It is represented by T_R. In **Figure 6.24**, the retention time of A, B, and C are approximately 2.5, 6.0, and 9.0 minutes, respectively.

Retention Volume

Retention volume of a component is the volume of gas required to carry a component maximum through the column.

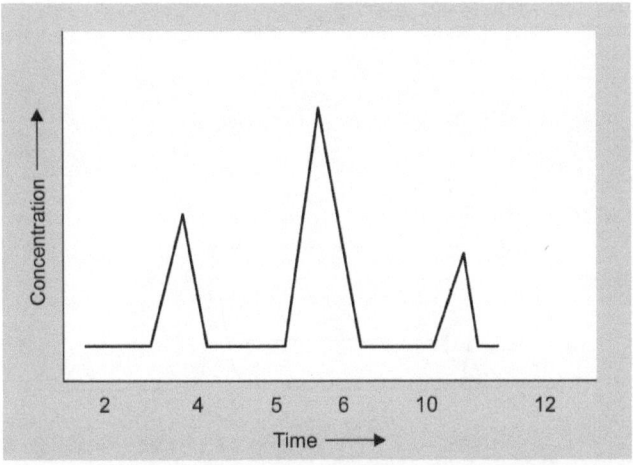

Fig. 6.23: Chromatogram of different analytes.

GAS CHROMATOGRAPHY AND ITS APPLICATIONS

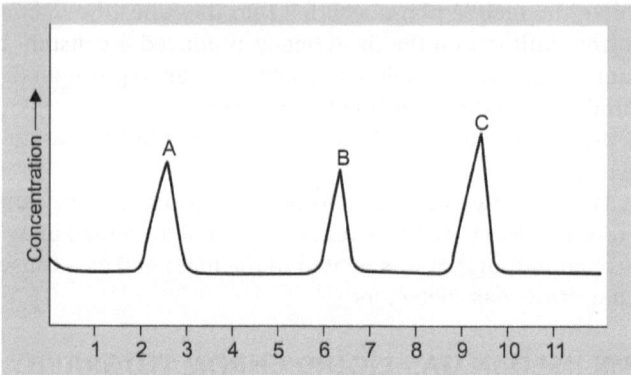

Fig. 6.24: Chromatogram showing separation of A, B, and C and the retention time for A = 2.5 minutes, B = 6 minutes, and C = 9 minutes.

Corrected Retention Time

The corrected retention time of a solute is the retention time minus the retention time of a completely unretained solute. For GC, an air peak is often used as a nonretained peak. If the mobile phase is compressible, i.e., the mobile phase is a gas, a pressure correction must be applied, which is a function of the column inlet-outlet pressure ratio.

Adjusted Retention Time (T_R')

An analyte retention time (T_R) minus the elution time of an unretained peak (T_m) is called adjusted retention time (T_R'). T_R' is also equivalent to the time the analyte spends in the stationary phase. T_R', T_R, and T_m are given in **Figure 6.25**.

$$T_R' = T_R - T_m$$

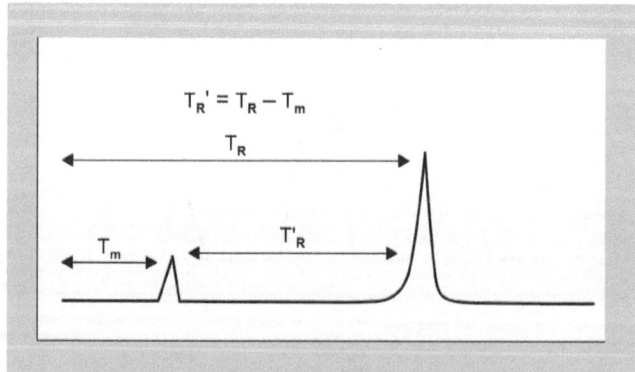

Fig. 6.25: Chromatogram showing T_R', T_R, and T_m.

Capacity Factor (k)

Expression that measures the degree of retention of an analyte relative to an unretained peak, where T_R is the retention time for the sample peak and T_m is the retention time for an unretained peak. A measurement of capacity will help determine whether retention shifts are due to the column (capacity factor is changing with change in retention time) or the system (capacity factor remains constant with change in retention time). Thus, the higher the capacity factor, the longer the retention time.

$$k = \frac{T_R - T_M}{T_M}$$

Flow Rate

The volumetric flow of the carrier gas in mL/min is called flow rate.

Theoretical Plate

Column efficiency is expressed as the number of theoretical plates. The higher the number of theoretical plates, the higher the column efficiency and its potential to resolve two closely eluting solutes. Decreasing column diameter will increase the number of theoretical plates, thus higher column efficiency. In general, thinner film of column will have higher efficiencies than corresponding thicker film column. The number of theoretical plates per meter is the usual method for reporting efficiency. Number of theoretical plates (N) is given by formula:

$$N = \frac{5.545 - T_R}{W_h}$$

where,
N = Number of theoretical plates
T_R = Retention time
W_h = Peak width at half height (in units of time)

Effective Theoretical Plates (N_{eff})

A measure of a column performance that accounts for the effects of unretained elution time. It is represented by N_{eff} and defined as:

$$N_{eff} = \left(\frac{T'_R}{\sigma}\right)^2$$

where, T'_R is adjusted retention time and "σ" is standard deviation of the peak.

Height Equivalent to a Theoretical Plate

The height equivalent to a theoretical plate (HETP) is a measure of column efficiency which is equivalent to the ratio of column length to the number of theoretical plates. A chromatographic column can be assumed to be made up of a large number of theoretical plates, which are analogous to those in a distillation column. The greater the number of these plates in a column, the better is the separation.

$$N = \frac{5.545 - T_R}{W_h}$$

where, L is the length of the column and N is the number of theoretical plates. HETP is based on actual (T_R) rather than adjusted retention times (T'_R).

Height Equivalent to an Effective Plate (HEEP) (H_{eff})

It is the ratio of length of column to the effective theoretical plate.

$$H_{eff} = \frac{L}{N_{eff}}$$

where, L = Column length

The smaller the N_{eff}, the more efficient the column's performance.

Peak Width (W)

Peak width can be expressed in time or volume. There are a number of ways to measure peak width such as tangential width and width at half height. Tangential width measures the baseline between two tangents taken from the peak inflection points and the baseline (**Fig. 6.26**). Width at half height measures width between the peaks measured at 50% peak height.

Resolution

Resolution is a measure of the separation of two peaks, taking into account both the difference in elution time and the peak width. It is represented as R_S and defined as:

$$R_S = \frac{t_1 + t_2}{0.5 \, (W_1 + W_2)}$$

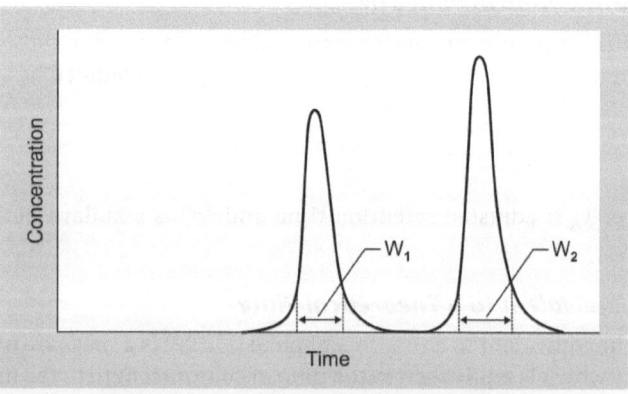

Fig. 6.26: Chromatogram showing peak width.

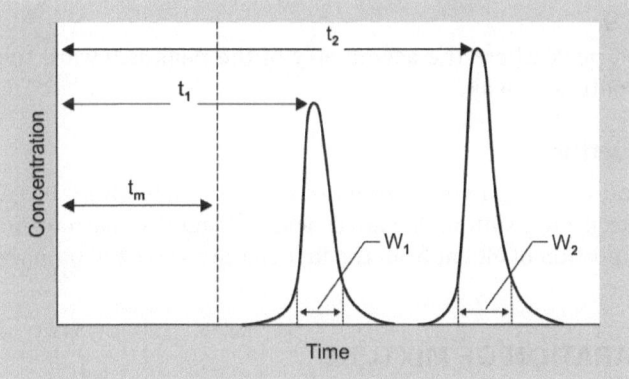

Fig. 6.27: Chromatogram showing resolution of two peaks.

where, t_1 and t_2 are the two retention times and W_1 and W_2 are peak widths (**Fig. 6.27**).

Selectivity (α)

Selectivity is the relative retention of two adjacent peaks. Selectivity can be calculated using capacity factors or retention volumes.

$$\alpha = \frac{k_2}{k_1} = \frac{(v_2 + v_1)}{(v_1 + v_0)}$$

where, α is selectivity, k_2 and k_1 are capacity factors, v_1 and v_2 are retention volumes, and v_0 is the void volume.

Coating Efficiency

Coating efficiency (CE) is a comparison between actual column efficiency and its theoretical maximum efficiency. CE is not the amount of column coated with phase or the amount of column coated as the prescribed film thickness.

Coating efficiency is defined as:

$$CE\% = \frac{H_{theoretical}}{k_{actual}} \times 100$$

Sensitivity

An estimation of the smallest analyte signal that can be detected by the method is called sensitivity. It is usually specified as a signal-to-noise ratio of 2.

Sample Capacity

The amount of sample that can be injected onto a column without overloading is called sample capacity. Often it is expressed as grams of sample per gram of packing.

Fronting
Distorted peak where the asymmetry of the peak is toward the front is called fronting of peak.

Heartcutting
A method of using two columns of different selectivity to gain more information on a sample is called heartcutting. In heartcutting, only a selected portion of eluent from the first column is passed onto the second column.

■ SEPARATION OF MIXTURE
Suppose we have to separate a mixture containing five components a, b, c, d, and e in GLC on the column. Chromatogram for separation of five components a, b, c, d, and e is given in **Figure 6.28**. It should be noted that:
- Components having negligible solubility in liquid phase move rapidly through the column
- Ideally, bell-shaped elution curves are obtained
- Component a in the above separation is least strongly dissolved, while compound e is most strongly dissolved
- If same sample is again injected into the same column, under the same circumstances of temperature and carrier gas flow rate, then an identical result is obtained
- If pure component b is injected instead of a mixture, the result is single peak in the same position as b

Efficient separation of compounds in GC is dependent on the movement of compound through column at different rates. The rate at which a compound travels through GC system depends on the following factors:
1. The number of theoretical plates increases with a decrease in particle size or increase in surface area. In general, a 60/80 mesh particle size is used in a 0.25 inch column

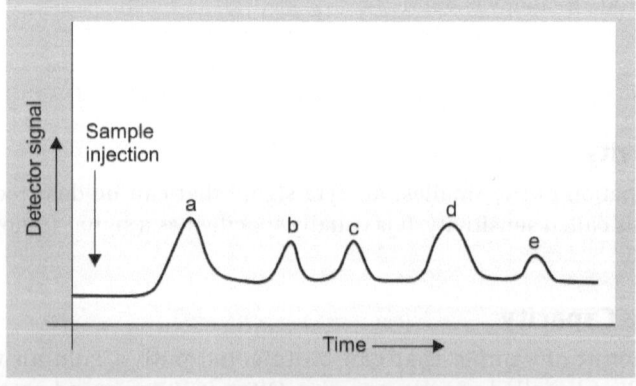

Fig. 6.28: Chromatogram of a five-component mixture.

2. The maximum efficiency can be obtained with an optimum flow rate, i.e., the rate of flow should neither be too low nor too high
3. Stationary phase is a very important factor in determining the efficiency of the column. The best separation is obtained when the liquid stationary phase is structurally similar to the compounds being separated
4. Low boiling (volatile) components will travel faster through the column than high boiling components
5. Polar compounds will move more slowly, especially if the column is polar
6. Usually, all components will move slower on polar columns, but polar compounds will show a larger effect
7. Speeding up the carrier gas flow increases the speed with which all compounds move through the column
8. The number of theoretical plates increases with an increase in the length of the column. But there is a practical limit to the length of the column because long columns may create problems relating to the gas flow. 1-10 m long columns are most common
9. The number of theoretical plates increases with a decrease in the diameter of the column. Columns having a diameter of 0.25 inch are most common
10. The temperature should be high enough to maintain the sample in the vapor state. Raising the column temperature speeds up all the compounds in a mixture

■ GAS CHROMATOGRAPHY DERIVATIZATION

Sample volatility and thermal stability are very important in GLC applications. If a sample does not possess these important properties, GLC analysis is highly unproductive. Derivatization techniques have been developed to solve these issues to insure best separations. The replacement of active hydrogen from functional groups, such as -COOH, -OH, -NH, -SH, etc., by alkyl group, acyl group, etc., is called derivatization. It can be achieved by following three ways.

1. *Silylation*: Silylation is the most widely used derivatization procedure for sample analysis by GLC. Silylation reagents are popular because they are easy to use and readily form derivatives. In silylation, active hydrogen is replaced by an alkylsilyl group such as trimethylsilyl (TMS) or *tert*-butyldimethylsilyl (*t*-BDMS), dimethylchlorosilane, tetramethyldisilazane, etc. Silyl derivatives are more volatile, less polar, and more thermally stable. As a result, GLC separation is improved and detection is enhanced. Silylation reagents are generally moisture sensitive, requiring them to be sealed under nitrogen to prevent deactivation. The derivatives of TMS reagents are also moisture sensitive. Both TMS and *t*-BDMS reagents are used in a variety of GLC applications.
2. *Acylation*: Another method of derivatization is acylation. As with silylation, acylation is used to replace an active proton, rendering a

compound less polar. Common classes of compounds subjected to acylation are alcohols, amino acid, and primary and secondary amines. Amino acids are usually esterified to the methyl or butyl ester prior to acylation. Typical reagents are acetic anhydride, a trifluoroacetic anhydride dissolved in pyridine and dimethylformamide. Acylation reagents offer the same types of advantages available from silylation reagents. In addition, acylating reagents provide the distinct advantage of introducing electron capturing groups thus, enhancing detectability during analysis. The acyl halides and acyl derivatives are highly reactive and are suitable for use where steric hindrance may be a factor.

3. *Alkylation/Esterification*: Next method of derivatization is alkylation. Alkylation reagents reduce molecular polarity by replacing active hydrogen with an alkyl group. These reagents are used to modify compounds having acidic hydrogen such as carboxylic acids and phenols. Carboxylic acid analogs, principally long-chain fatty acids, can be derivatized by using HCl in methanol or diazomethane. Amino acids can be esterified by reaction with butanol in 3 N HCl at 150°C temperature for 10 minutes. Alkylation reagents can be used alone to form esters, ethers, and amides or they can be used in conjunction with acylation or silylation reagents. Due to the availability of reagents, esterification is the most popular method of alkylation. Alkylation reagents are available in several configurations that enable the formation of a variety of esters. Alkyl esters are stable and can be formed quickly and quantitatively. In addition to the formation of simple alkylation, reagents can be used in extractive procedures where biological matrices may be present.

■ ACCESSORIES AND SPARES USED IN GAS-LIQUID CHROMATOGRAPHY

Injector Septa

It is recommended that septa (**Fig. 6.29**) should be replaced after 50 manual injections or 100 autosampler injections. Any leak in septa will allow air to enter the column, which will rapidly damage the column. Septa will have to be replaced more frequently when using large diameter needles or needles with burrs. Over tightening, the septum cap will reduce septa life. The column temperature should be reduced to 40°C or less when changing the septa. One should wear gloves while changing the septa. Reduced column lifetime will result, if air is introduced into the carrier gas (column) at elevated temperature.

Guard Columns

A guard column is a short length of deactivated fused silica tubing about 0.5–1.0 m installed between the inlet and the column. The tubing serves two functions, one as a guard column and the other as a retention gap. As

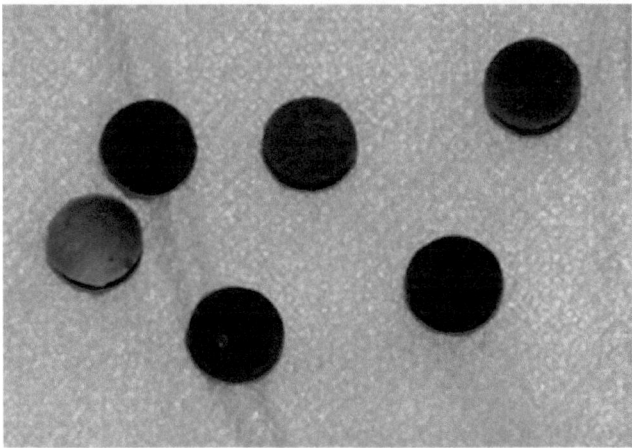

Fig. 6.29: Gas-liquid chromatography (GLC) septa.

a guard column, it catches nonvolatile residues, which prevent them from reaching the column. As a retention gap, the tubing allows larger amount of solvents with polarities unlike that of the stationary phase to be injected without adversely affecting peak shapes.

Unions

Glass or stainless steel unions may be used to join the column to the guard column. Glass press-fit unions replace stainless steel and resin methods of joining two pieces of fused silica tubing. The glass unions form a gas-tight seal by a minor compression of the polyimide coating on the column. There is no need for wrenches glue or ferrules. These unions are very lightweight and have very little thermal mass; they track oven temperature and eliminate the possibility of a cold or hot spot in the sample path. Because the glass unions have a similar expansion coefficient to fused silica tubing, they expand and contract together and can be used over a wide temperature range from −55°C to 345°C. By proper installation, they exhibit no solvent tailing or fronting.

Traps

Different traps (**Fig. 6.30**) are recommended, even if high purity carrier gases are used. Trace amounts of contaminants can cause baseline irregularities, detector noise, and possible column damage. Contaminated detector gases can lead to artificially high baseline readings and poor performance. Several types of traps are designed to remove moisture, oxygen, hydrocarbons, and other contaminants from the gas supply. Common trap systems are moisture trap, high capacity oxygen trap, and glass indicating oxygen trap. The moisture trap should be first in line because moisture will quickly deactivate the oxygen traps. The high capacity oxygen trap should be installed second followed by a glass indicating oxygen trap.

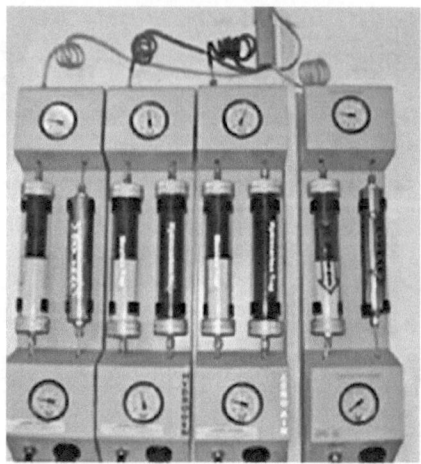

Fig. 6.30: Different traps used for different gases.

Moisture Traps

A moisture trap should be installed in the carrier and detector gas lines. It will remove trace levels of water, some nonpermanent gases, and light hydrocarbons. Two types of absorbents are available. Both contain blue indicator. Molecular sieve 4A will trap humidity. Molecular sieve 5A will trap water, some nonpermanent gases, and small hydrocarbons. Molecular sieve 13X will trap larger hydrocarbons, in addition to most of the impurities trapped by the molecular sieve 5A material.

Oxygen Traps

Trace levels of oxygen in the carrier gas can shorten the life of a column. The polyethylene glycol-based phases, such as DB-WAX, DB-FFAP, and Carbowax, are readily oxidized at elevated temperatures. Polysiloxane phases can also be irreversibly damaged via oxidation at high temperature, but much more slowly than polyethylene glycol-based phases. Oxygen has a deleterious effect on many GC detectors. Oxygen degrades the performance of electrolytic conductivity detectors, reduces filament lifetime in a thermal conductivity detector, and reduces the linearity and sensitivity of electron capture detectors. Both the column and detector benefit when oxygen is removed from the carrier gas supply.

High Capacity Oxygen Traps

The most efficient oxygen traps are 99% efficient at reducing oxygen in carrier gases, such as helium and nitrogen, at 99.999% purity. A 10- to 50-fold reduction in oxygen in the gas is often obtained. These traps will effectively remove oxygen from argon-methane mixture, which is used with ECDs without disturbing the ratios of these gases. Metal-bodied traps avoid the signal noise associated with any plastic-bodied trap. These traps will need periodic replacement. The use of an indicating oxygen trap is recommended to determine when the high capacity oxygen trap needs replacement.

Glass Indicating Oxygen Traps

A glass indicating oxygen trap should be placed downstream of the high capacity oxygen trap, as a means of indicating when to replace the high capacity nonindicating trap. This will prevent premature disposal of the high capacity oxygen trap. The indicating material undergoes a color change as it is depleted. The high capacity oxygen trap must be replaced immediately upon the first indication of color change in the indicating trap. Fully expired oxygen traps will recontaminate the gas with previously trapped materials. The indicating oxygen trap will rapidly expire, if used as the solitary oxygen trap in the system or for prolonged periods, after the high capacity oxygen trap has expired.

■ DO'S AND DON'TS FOR GAS-LIQUID CHROMATOGRAPHY

Do's

1. Routinely inspect and replace injection port septum to reduce the risk of leaks and septa particle contamination
2. Change the septum daily, especially if the instrument is in heavy use
3. Always replace the column ferrules when you install a new column or perform column maintenance. A leaking ferrule will allow oxygen into the carrier gas, shortening column life. A leak can also cause variation in retention time, baseline difference, and sample loss
4. Gas chromatography user should routinely inspect and replace the inlet liner to eliminate contaminants and active sites that will lead to poor chromatography
5. Carrier gas should be always of high purity
6. Use always double stage regulators for carrier gas as well as for hydrogen gas
7. For starting GLC, first open carrier gas then switch on the power line
8. Confirm baseline linearity by giving two or three injection of any solvent, preferably acetone before sample analysis
9. Calibrate GLC twice in a year by using solvents such as dodecane or n-octane
10. Open hydrogen gas only when the GLC attains the column temperature, injection temperature, etc.
11. After completing sample analysis, first close the hydrogen gas and then put GLC in cooling condition by passing carrier gas and then in last, close nitrogen gas and main switch
12. Before leaving the room, just insures the gases are closed properly
13. Use soap solution for testing any gas leakage at joints
14. For opening gas, first open cylinder valve and then rotate regulator valve in clockwise direction
15. For closing gas, first close cylinder valve and then rotate regulator valve in anticlockwise direction

16. Use Teflon ribbon at joints for avoiding any leakage
17. Power supply should be given through uninterruptible power supply (UPS) only
18. Clean the syringe with proper solvents
19. Check for leaks at the injector and detector using a thermal conductivity detector
20. Cool all heated zones and visually inspect oxygen and moisture traps and replace, if necessary, during column installation
21. Visually inspect injector and detector sleeves and replace, if broken or dirty
22. Cut approximately 10 cm from each column end, insert a nut, and an appropriately sized ferrule on both column ends during installation of capillary column
23. Condition the column at its maximum operating temperature
24. The injector port is heated to a temperature, which will insure rapid vaporization, but not thermal degradation of the solute
25. The liquid is drawn into the syringe a number of times to remove any air bubble and injected very rapidly into the gas stream
26. A soap bubble meter is used for measurement of flow rate
27. Sample should be dissolved in volatile solvents only
28. Inject standard sample before and after the test sample for quantification
29. Use always AR grade chemicals and reagents for the instrument
30. Instrument should be in annual maintenance contract (AMC) for its maintenance and power supply should be given through UPS only

Don'ts

1. Do not open the oven chamber during analysis
2. Do not close carrier gases before the instrument attains cooling temperature
3. Do not touch septum with naked hand, use gloves always
4. Flow of hydrogen should not be too high or too low
5. Do not switch off the GLC directly, first bring it in cooling condition, i.e., column temperature should reach up to 30°C and then put it off
6. Do not close the carrier gas until column temperature reaches up to 30°C
7. Do not use single-stage regulator
8. Do not inject any aqueous sample in GC
9. Do not allow the solution which is thermally unstable
10. Do not use soaps or liquids to check for leaks at the injector and detector
11. Column temperature should not exceed the phase's maximum operating temperature
12. Do not use GLC for inorganic substance analysis
13. There should be no air bubbles in the syringe while injecting samples in the GC
14. Do not allow the inject sample in GC until clear baseline is obtained
15. Do not open hydrogen gas until all the other parameters are achieved

■ HEADSPACE GAS CHROMATOGRAPHY

Headspace GC is a simple GC unit with a modified injection system, consisting of headspace generator. The "headspace" is the gas space in a chromatography vial above the sample. Headspace analysis is, therefore, the analysis of the components present in the gas. Headspace GC is used for the analysis of volatiles and semivolatile organics in solid, liquid, and gas samples. The volatile or nonvolatile sample to be tested is placed inside a vial (**Fig. 6.31**), which is used to perform the headspace analysis. The vial will also contain a dilution solvent and a matrix modifier. On heating, the volatile components accumulate at the headspace (the empty space above the sample). This gaseous phase from the headspace can be directly injected into the GC for separation.

There are three types of headspace autosamplers namely, syringe injection, balanced pressure, and pressurized loop.

Syringe Injection System

Syringe injection is the most commonly used method of headspace sampling (**Fig. 6.32**). Common steps involved in syringe injection system are given below:
- *Step 1*: The syringe is heated and agitated in an oven until equilibrium is reached
- *Step 2*: An aliquot of the headspace is extracted using a heated syringe
- *Step 3*: The collected headspace is injected directly into the GC

The syringe must be heated above the temperature of the oven in step 1 to avoid risk of condensation and carryover between samples. After injection, the syringe is flushed with nitrogen or any other inert gas before using it for another sample. Syringe injection system has following advantages:
- Highly reproducible results are obtainable
- Low carryover between samples, if performed properly

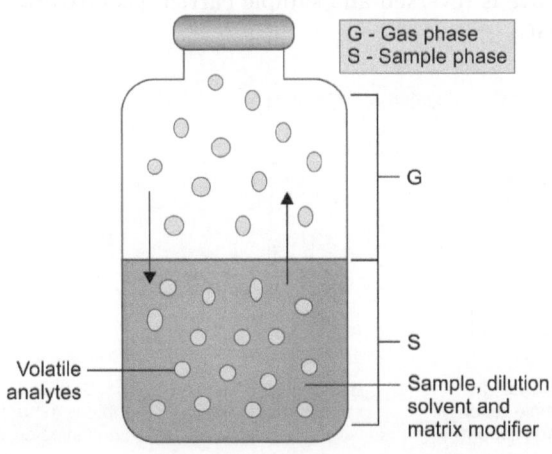

Fig. 6.31: Vial used in gas chromatography (GC) headspace technique.

GAS CHROMATOGRAPHY AND ITS APPLICATIONS

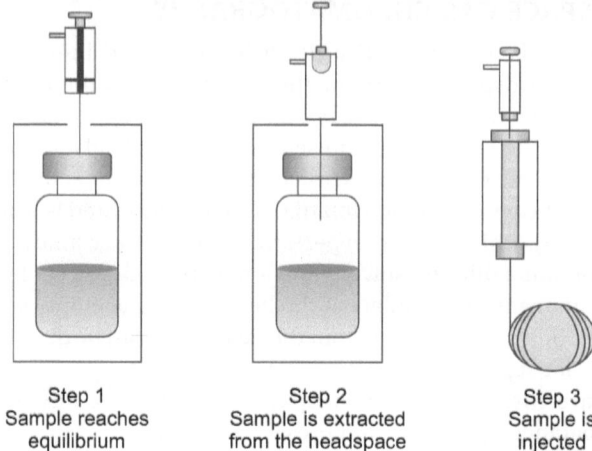

Fig. 6.32: Different steps involved in syringe injection system.

- Fast transfer of sample to GC, as extraction of sample is not necessary
- As a simple syringe is used, sample size and injection speed can be easily controlled
- As this is just an attachment to the GC, therefore sample injection through the traditional injection port is always possible when necessary

Balanced Pressure System

This system uses a seamless syringe to incorporate the sample from the headspace vial into the carrier gas stream directly (**Fig. 6.33**). Common steps involved in balanced pressurized system are given below:
- *Step 1*: A normal headspace vial is incubated in an oven till the sample reaches equilibrium
- *Step 2*: Pressurization of vial with carrier gas
- *Step 3*: Valve is reversed and sample carrier gas mixture is redirected into the GC

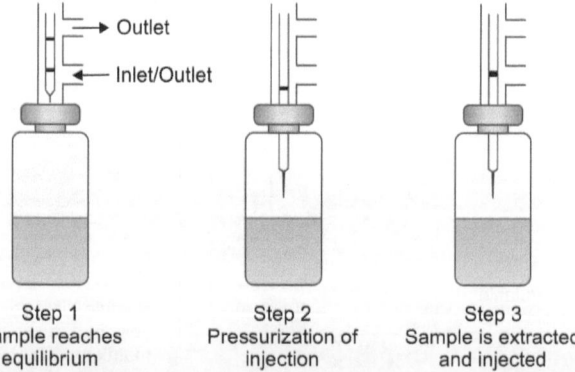

Fig. 6.33: Different steps involved in balanced pressurized system.

GAS CHROMATOGRAPHY AND ITS APPLICATIONS

The balanced pressurized system has several merits such as accuracy, manual interference is reduced as sample injection is done automatically, and fast transfer of sample to GC, as extraction of sample is not necessary.

The balanced pressurized system has also several demerits such as the absolute volume of injected sample is unknown, therefore, quantification is complex, chances of carryover are more, and the injection port is always occupied, and therefore, not available for manual use.

Pressurized Loop System

This is a balanced pressurized system modified with a complex system of valves (a loop which regulates gas flow between two ends).

Different steps of pressurized loop system (**Fig. 6.34**) are:

Step 1: Sample is pressurized in this step

Step 2: Sample is extracted into the loop from the headspace by turning the loop valve

Step 3: Once the loop is filled, the loop is turned to redirect the gas flow and resulting in the sample being flushed into the transfer line, leading to the GC.

The pressurized loop system has several merits such as this system allows high temperatures, so samples which are not highly volatile can also be analyzed.

■ TECHNICAL SPECIFICATIONS FOR GAS-LIQUID CHROMATOGRAPHY

Basic System

Basic system with EPC controls for carrier/detector zone gases. All parameters should be stored as a part of method for better analysis, reproducibility, and to meet the regulatory compliance.

Oven and Pneumatic Control System

1. Temperature up to 450°C
2. Approximately 10 programmable temperature ramps or higher

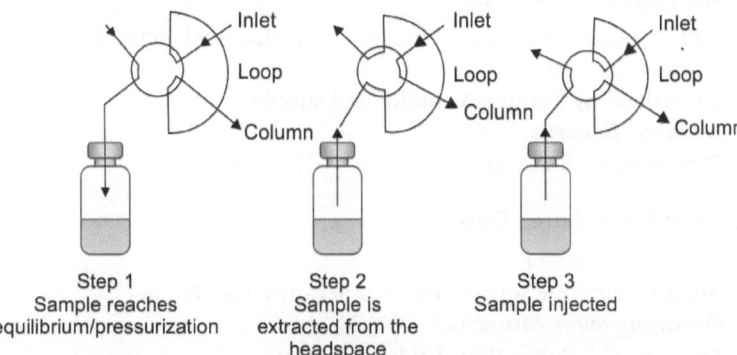

Fig. 6.34: Different steps involved in pressurized loop system.

3. Heating rate minimum 0.1°C/min up to 100°C/min or higher
4. Cooling time from 450 to 50°C in <4 minutes
5. Oven size—approximate 11 L
6. Method storage of minimum 5 methods built in basic GC
7. Programmable pneumatic control for injector and detector for flow and pressure as well. Carrier gas, inlet, oven, and detector should be computer controlled.
8. *Chromatography performance*: Retention time repeatability: Approximately <0.008

Split-splitless injector with EPC, temperature range ambient to 450°C, and packed column injector with EPC with wide-bore column adopter.

Detectors

Flame Ionization Detector

1. Autoignition of flame in FID and monitoring the same operating temperature from ambient to 450°C
2. *Detectability*: Approximately 2 pgC/s
3. Dynamic linearity better than >10^6
4. Makeup gas is not required due to zero dead volume design

Thermal Conductivity Detector

1. *Temperature range*: Up to 450°C
2. *Dynamic range*: 10^5
3. *Sensitivity*: 20,000 mV.mL/mg (decane)

Flame Photometric Detector

1. Double flame techniques for selective detection of sulfur and phosphorus compounds
2. High voltage unit for photomultiplier and supply for the ignitor
3. Sensitivity range selectable from 10^{-9} to 10^{-12} A/mV
4. *Dynamic range*: 10^7 phosphorus
5. Logarithmic program for sulfur calibration

Electron Capture Detector

1. Nickel-63 source mounted in a sealed cylindrical chamber
2. Central electrode
3. Linearized by frequency modulated supply
4. *Dynamic linearity*: 5.10^4
5. *Detectability*: Better than 4.10^{-15} g/s of lindane

Nitrogen Phosphorus Detector

1. Head adaptable on FID body
2. Alkaline ceramic source with temperature regulation
3. *Operating temperature*: 600–700°C
4. *Linearity (L)*: Better than 10^6 for nitrogen
5. *Detectability*: 10^{-13} g/s nitrogen and 5×10^{-14} g/s phosphorus

Headspace Sampler
1. Headspace sampler 10 vials capacity or more
2. The platen heater must be able to achieve and maintain constant temperature up to 300°C ± 0.1°C
3. The headspace autosampler must have electronic flow control
4. The headspace autosampler must come with software that controls the autosampler

Accessories and Spares
1. Capillary columns—for pesticides, drugs, and alcohol analysis (one each)
2. Packed columns—OV-101 and SE-30 (one each)
3. *Syringes*: 10 µL, 25 µL (five each), and 100 µL, 500 µL (one each)
4. Gas-tight syringe
5. Set of aluminum crimps vials (pk/1,000) for headspace
6. Aluminum crimper for vials
7. Necessary starter kit and control S/W to be offered

Control Unit
1. Optimized for the latest windows platform with user-friendly software. It can acquire and process/control multichromatographic instruments parameter and complete software for headspace and autosampler
2. Branded desktop with TFT screen, with latest configuration
3. Laser printer with good speed
4. Online 5 KVA UPS with inbuilt batteries and 30 minutes backup or suitable as per the system requirement
5. H_2, N_2, and zero air gas cylinders with double stage regulators
6. Gas station for all gas cylinders with purifiers
7. Complete operational training to be provided to working analyst at site
8. Clearly mention and quote any other specific accessory or preinstallation requirements for your system.

This is a general specification, which can be changed as per the laboratory requirement.

■ FORENSIC APPLICATIONS OF GAS-LIQUID CHROMATOGRAPHY

Identification and Quantification of Pesticides by Gas-liquid Chromatography

Suicide by consuming pesticide is a common cause of death. Majority of the Indian population live in rural areas who are mostly farmers. Recently, there has been series of suicides by farmers in different states of India due to tragedy of crop failure and financial burden. Most of them have died due to pesticide poisoning as it is easily available. There has also been occupational disease due to chronic exposure to pesticides by contamination of groundwater. In recent news, there was allegation of detecting pesticides in soft drinks such as coca cola. In all these cases, GLC plays a significant role in analyzing the pesticides content in the biological material.

Gas-liquid chromatography is preferably used for analysis of volatile and thermostable pesticides. In recent years, capillary columns have almost completely replaced the packed columns owing to their high resolving power, which allows the separation of a large number of pesticides with similar characteristics. The most frequently used detectors include ECD, NPD, FPD, and MSD. The ECD has been the detector mostly used in pesticide residue analysis. The parameters used for analysis of various types of pesticides are given below:

Organophosphorus Insecticides

NPD is used in pesticide residue analysis because of its selectivity for phosphorus and nitrogen-containing compounds. The FPD, in phosphorus mode, has frequently been the instrumental technique of choice for the analysis of organophosphorus pesticides. The purified extract may be subjected to GLC analysis using NPD detector under following conditions:
- *Column*: 5 m × 0.53 mm, OV-17 (50% phenyl siloxane and 50% methyl siloxane) megabore column of 2.0 μm thickness
- *Initial temperature*: 110°C
- *Final temperature*: 290°C
- *Rate*: 10°C/min
- *Final temperature hold*: 5 minute
- *Hydrogen flow*: 3.5 mL/min
- *Air flow*: 100 mL/min
- *Nitrogen flow*: 7 mL/min
- *Detector*: NPD
- *Injection volume*: 1 μL

Flame photometric detector is also used for detection of organophosphorus compound. GLC conditions for FPD are as follow:
- *Column*: 30 m × 0.53 mm, SPB-608 of film thickness 2.0 μm
- *Oven temperature*: 150°C (0.5 min) to 230°C at 6°C/min, holding at 230°C for 2 minutes, then to 245°C at 3°C/min
- *Carrier gas*: Helium
- *Flow rate*: 8 mL/min
- *Detector*: FPD
- *Injection volume*: 1 μL

Organochlorine Insecticides

Organochlorine insecticides, such as dichlorodiphenyltrichloroethane (DDT), benzene hexachloride (BHC), lindane, endosulfan, etc., are being extensively used in agriculture and also familiar in domestic applications. New varieties of these pesticides are emerging every year. Owing to the easy availability, these pesticides are frequently misused in homicidal and suicidal poisoning cases. Accidental poisoning cases are also known. GLC is also used for identification of organochlorine compound in biological and

nonbiological matrices. ECD is the most suitable detector for analysis of organochlorine insecticides. GLC conditions for organochlorine compound are given below:
- *Column*: 6 × 4 mm, glass column packed with 80/100 mesh chrom-Q
- *Stationary phase*: 15% QF-1 and 10% DC-200 (1:1)
- *Carrier gas*: Nitrogen
- *Flow rate*: 120 mL/min
- *Injection temperature*: 225°C
- *Column temperature*: 200°C
- *Detector*: ECD
- *Injection volume*: 1 µL

Carbamate Pesticides

GLC is also used for identification of carbamate compound such as propoxur, carbaryl, carbofuran, zineb, etc. NPD is the most suitable detector for analysis of carbamate insecticides. GLC conditions for carbamate insecticide are given below:
- *Column*: 15 m × 0.53 mm, DB-1 fused silica capillary column
- *Carrier gas*: Helium
- *Flow rate*: 10 mL/min
- *Initial temperature*: 50°C
- *Final temperature*: 235°C
- *Gradient to temperature*: 20°C/min
- *Duration*: 3.5 minutes
- *Detector*: NPD
- *Injection volume*: 1 µL

Pyrethroids

The pyrethroids have emerged as a major class of synthetic organic insecticides due to their commercial production for agricultural applications. These compounds are comparatively less toxic than other classes in respect of mammalian toxicity. ECD detector is more useful for halogen containing pyrethroids, viz., bifenthrin, cyfluthrin, cypermethrin, deltamethrin, etc. (detection limit nano- to picograms). The purified extract of sample may be subjected to GLC under following conditions:
- *Detector*: ECD
- *Column*: 15 m × 0.37 mm, DB-1 of film thickness 1.5 µm
- *Injection temperature*: 190°C
- *Column temperature*: 220°C
- *Detector temperature*: 270°C
- *Injection volume*: 1 µL

For other pyrethroids having no halogen atom, FID can be used. The stationary phases include OV-1, OV-101, SE-30, SP-2100, DC-200, etc. The purified extract of sample may be subjected to GLC under following conditions:
- *Detector*: FID
- *Packed column*: OV-17, OV-210, 1 m × 3 mm, Chromosorb WHP 80/100

- *Injection temperature*: 190°C
- *Column temperature*: 190°C
- *Detector temperature*: 250°C
- *Injection volume*: 1 µL

Identification and Quantification of Alcohol in Blood Sample

Ethanol is one of the most widely abused drugs all over the world. In India, total prohibition is in force in Gujarat state. The government has fixed the age limit for consuming alcohols as 21 years. As for the Motor Vehicles Act (1988, Amended) Section 185, the statutory limit is 30 mg of alcohol in blood. Driving under the influence of alcohol is punishable in the form of fine, which can extend up to Rupees 2,000 or imprisonment, which can extend up to 6 months or imposition of both. Alcohol intoxication is strongly associated with road traffic accidents, suicides, and homicides. Therefore, the estimation of alcohol in blood has become very necessary in medicolegal cases and GLC provides a sophisticated system for quantitative analysis of alcohol.

1 mL of blood is diluted with 4 mL of water and acidified with a few drops of 5% tartaric acid or dilute sulfuric acid and then distilled. 5 mL of distillate is collected in ice cold condition and 1–10 µL of it is injected to GLC under following conditions:
- *Column*: Porapak Q
- *Oven temperature*: 140°C
- *Injector temperature*: 140°C
- *Detector temperature*: 160°C
- *Carrier gas*: Nitrogen
- *Nitrogen flow*: 30 mL/min
- *Hydrogen flow*: 25 mL/min
- *Air flow*: 250 mL/min
- *Detector*: FID
- *Injection volume*: 1 µL

Chromatograms of sample and standard are given in **Figures 6.35** and **6.36**. Rt of sample and standard is same hence, we can say that sample has alcohol. The % of alcohol can be calculated by using peak area or peak height of the sample and standard.

Identification and Quantification of Narcotic Drugs

Gas-liquid chromatography is widely used for identification and quantification of narcotic drugs such as morphine, codeine, thebaine, papaverine, etc. The purified extract of biological material is injected in GLC under following conditions:
- *Column*: 2 m × 4 mm, glass column packed with 2.5% SE-30 on 80–100 mesh Chromosorb W
- *Column temperature*: 240°C
- *Injection temperature*: 270°C
- *Detector temperature*: 270°C

GAS CHROMATOGRAPHY AND ITS APPLICATIONS

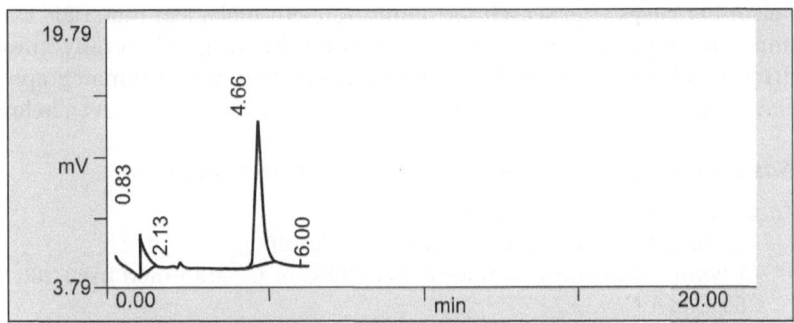

Rt	Ht	Area	Ht %	Area %	Pk Ty	Peak width
0.83	1345	304979	22.2572	14.9576	BB	0.145
2.13	150	30249	2.45822	1.4835	BB	0.137
4.66	4224	1696114	2.45822	83.1851	BB	0.246
6.00	324	7621	5.3616	0.3738	BB	0.011
	6e+03	2038963	100.0000	100.0000		

Fig. 6.35: Peak of alcohol in standard at Rt 4.66.

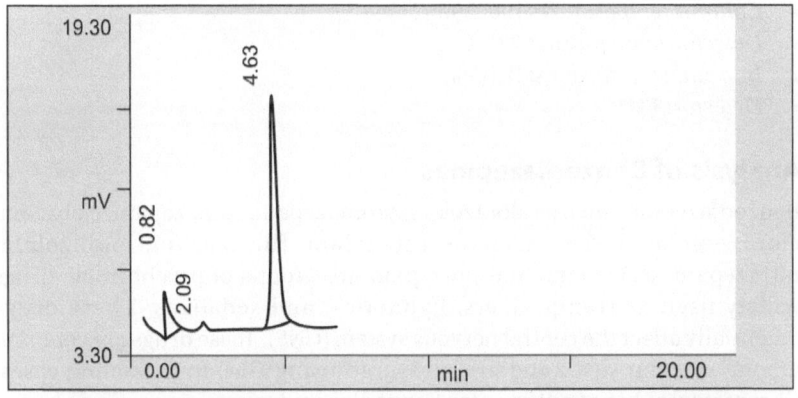

Rt	Ht	Area	Ht %	Area %	Pk Ty	Peak width
0.82	1334	292616	19.8789	12.0612	BB	0.134
2.09	174	33969	2.5924	1.4002	BB	0.126
4.63	5204	2099506	77.5328	86.5386	BB	0.251
	7e+03	2426091	100.0000	100.0000		

Fig. 6.36: Peak of alcohol in sample at Rt 4.63.

- *Carrier gas*: Nitrogen
- *Gas flow*: 45 mL/min
- *Detector*: FID

Identification and Quantification of Barbiturates

Barbiturates such as allobarbital, amobarbital, barbital, butalbital, butobarbital, cyclobarbital, methylphenobarbital, secbutabarbital, secobarbital, and vinylbital are the drugs that are associated with criminal poisoning cases. The search for barbiturates in biological materials is of importance in case of suspected poisoning by drugs. Generally, these drugs can be analyzed by GLC after derivatization. Gas chromatographic conditions without derivatization and with derivatization are given below.

Gas Chromatographic Conditions without Derivatization
- *Column*: SE-30 glass column
- *Carrier gas and flow rate*: Nitrogen 1 mL/min
- *Column temperature*: Isothermal at 200°C or programmed from 200 to 260°C at 4°C/min
- *Detector temperature*: 275°C
- *Internal standard*: n-alkanes
- *Detector*: FID

Gas Chromatographic Conditions with Derivatization
- *Column*: 6′ × 2–4 mm, glass column packed with 3% SE-30 on 80–100 mesh Chromosorb W
- *Carrier gas and flow rate*: Nitrogen 45–50 mL/min
- *Column temperature*: 190–200°C
- *Detector temperature*: 220°C
- *Internal standard*: n-alkanes
- *Detector*: FID

Analysis of Benzodiazepines

Benzodiazepines such as alprazolam, bromazepam, camazepam, clobazam, clorazepic acid, delorazepam, estazolam, flurazepam, loprazolam, nitrazepam, oxazepam, and prazepam are groups of psychotropic drugs widely used as tranquilizers, hypnotics, and sedatives. These drugs potentially affect the central nervous system (CNS). These drugs are common among suicidal cases and are measured using GLC in poisoning cases. Chromatographic conditions for benzodiazepines are:
- *Column*: 2 m × 4 mm glass column packed with 2.5% SE-30 on 80–100 mesh Chromosorb W
- *Column temperature*: 200–300°C
- *Injector temperature*: 290°C
- *Detector temperature*: 290°C
- *Carrier gas*: Nitrogen
- *Carrier gas flow*: 45 mL/min
- *Detector*: FID

Identification and Quantification of Antidepressants

Gas-liquid chromatography is very useful for antidepressants such as amitriptyline, butriptyline, clomipramine, desipramine, doxepin, iproniazid, nortriptyline, protriptyline, and trimipramine. Antidepressants are drugs generally used in psychiatric practices to treat endogenous

depressions. Amitriptyline is a tricyclic antidepressant commonly used in suicidal cases. Chromatographic conditions for antidepressants are:
- *Column*: 2 m × 4 mm glass column packed with 2.5% SE-30 on 80–100 mesh Chromosorb W
- *Column temperature*: 200–300°C
- *Injector temperature*: 260°C
- *Detector temperature*: 280°C
- *Carrier gas*: Nitrogen
- *Carrier gas flow*: 50 mL/min
- *Detector*: FID

Identification and Quantification of Stimulants and Amphetamines

Gas-liquid chromatography is very useful for stimulants such as amphetamine, benzphetamine, caffeine, chlorpheniramine, dimethylamphetamine, ephedrine, hydroxyamphetamine, mescaline, methoxyamphetamine, methylenedioxyamphetamine, methylephedrine, methylphenidate, phenmetrazine, phentermine, pseudoephedrine, and trimethoxyamphetamine. These are the drugs which stimulate the CNS and produce a false sense of euphoria, which is followed by depression. Amphetamines are employed for the abolition of fatigue and for the suppression of appetite. Chromatographic conditions for stimulants and amphetamines are:
- *Column*: 2 m × 4 mm glass column packed with 2.5% SE-30 on 80–100 mesh Chromosorb W
- *Column temperature*: 200–300°C
- *Injector temperature*: 290°C
- *Detector temperature*: 290°C
- *Carrier gas*: Nitrogen
- *Carrier gas flow*: 45 mL/min
- *Detector*: FID

Analysis of Basic Drugs

Quantitative work usually requires some form of sample preparation to isolate the drug from the bulk of material for interference-free analysis. For the purpose, some degree of concentration or dilution and purification is required. These steps or process will certainly invite some degree of analytical error. A wide range of basic drugs including alkaloids may be screened or detected by GC (sample concentration H" 1 μg/mL). The presence of one nitrogen atom in basic drugs will produce a signal in an alkali FID. The method of extraction of drugs and detector selected should insure minimum interference from other compounds, which do not contain nitrogen. Gas chromatographic conditions for basic drugs are:
- *Column*: 2.5% of dimethyldichlorosilane treated and acid washed 2 m × 4 mm glass column
- *Column temperature*: 200–300°C
- *Injector temperature*: 260°C
- *Detector temperature*: 280°C

- *Carrier gas*: Nitrogen
- *Carrier gas flow*: 45 mL/min
- *Detector*: FID

Identification and Quantification of Antihistamines

Gas-liquid chromatography is very useful for analysis of antihistamines such as brompheniramine, cyclizine, diphenhydramine, diphenylpyraline, pheniramine, promethazine, propiomazine, and trimeprazine. These drugs antagonize the action of histamine. Overdose leads to poisoning and it is commonly used for suicide. Chromatographic conditions for antihistamines are:

- *Column*: 2 m × 4 mm glass column packed with 2.5% SE-30 on 80–100 mesh Chromosorb W
- *Column temperature*: 200–300°C
- *Injector temperature*: 290°C
- *Detector temperature*: 290°C
- *Carrier gas*: Nitrogen
- *Carrier gas flow*: 45 mL/min
- *Detector*: FID

Identification and Quantification of Local Anesthetics

Most of local anesthetics such as amethocaine, benzocaine, butacaine, chloroprocaine, cocaine, hexylcaine, oxethazine, oxybuprocaine, pramoxine, prilocaine, procaine, propoxycaine, and proxymetacaine can be easily identified by GLC. Chromatographic conditions for local anesthetics are:

- *Column*: 2 m × 4 mm glass column packed with 2.5% SE-30 on 80–100 mesh Chromosorb W
- *Column temperature*: 200–300°C
- *Injector temperature*: 290°C
- *Detector temperature*: 290°C
- *Carrier gas*: Nitrogen
- *Carrier gas flow*: 50 mL/min
- *Detector*: FID

Analysis of Phenothiazines

Gas-liquid chromatography plays a very important role for identification and quantification of phenothiazines such as acepromazine, azacyclonol, benzocaine, carphenazine, chlorpromazine, dimethothiazine, ethopropazine, hydroxyzine, pericyazine, promazine, promethazine, propiomazine, thioridazine, trifluoperazine, and trimerazine. Chromatographic conditions for some phenothiazines are:

- *Column*: 2 m × 4 mm glass column packed with 2.5% SE-30 on 80–100 mesh Chromosorb W
- *Column temperature*: 200–300°C
- *Carrier gas*: Nitrogen
- *Carrier gas flow*: 45 mL/min

GAS CHROMATOGRAPHY AND ITS APPLICATIONS

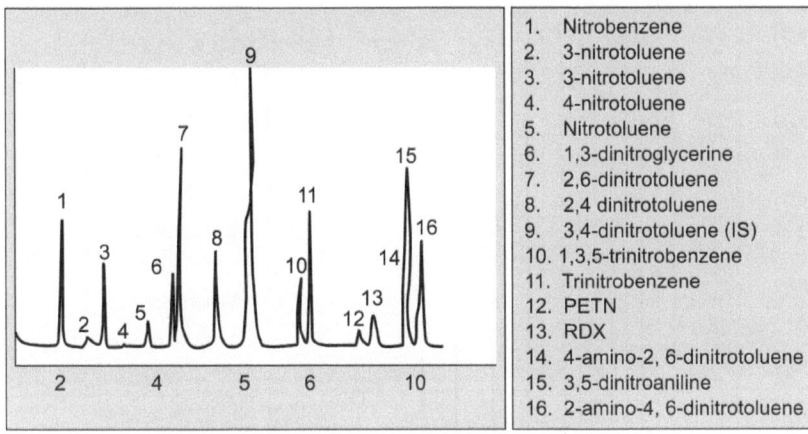

Fig. 6.37: Chromatogram of explosive compounds.

Analysis of Sulfonamides

Gas chromatography is an important analytical tool for the analysis of sulfonamides such as glymidine, sulfamerazine, sulfacetamide, sulfadiazine, sulfadimidine, sulfafurazole, sulfamethizole, sulfamethoxazole, sulfamethoxydiazine, sulfamethoxypyridazine, sulfamoxole, sulfaphenazole, sulfapyridine, and sulfathiazole.

The sulfonamides are separated as their methyl derivative (by injecting the samples mixed with 0.2 M trimethylanilinium hydroxide in methanol) as per the following chromatographic conditions.
- *Column*: 5% OV-17 on 80–100 mesh, 1.5 m × 2 mm glass column
- *Column temperature*: 250°C
- *Carrier gas*: Nitrogen
- *Carrier gas flow*: 30 mL/min

Analysis of Explosives

Gas chromatographic procedures have been well established for most common explosives. Nitroaromatic compounds pose no special problem under normal GC conditions. Certain difficulties are encountered with thermally labile compounds such as the nitrate esters and nitramines, which have now been overcome by the special columns and experimental conditions (**Fig. 6.37**).

Analysis of Petroleum Products

Simulated distillation (SimDist) is a temperature-programmed analysis that determines the boiling range distribution of petroleum samples using GC. ASTM test method is a commonly used method for petroleum products with a final boiling point < 380°C (excluding gasoline). This technique has been used for >25 years with packed columns. **Figure 6.38** shows the GLC graphs of petroleum products.

GAS CHROMATOGRAPHY AND ITS APPLICATIONS

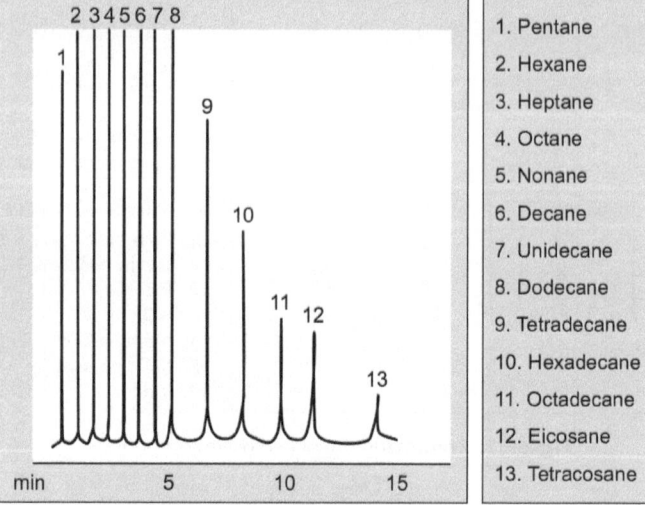

Fig. 6.38: Chromatogram of petroleum products.

■ COMPARISON OF GAS-LIQUID CHROMATOGRAPHY WITH HIGH-PERFORMANCE LIQUID CHROMATOGRAPHY

The GC is the most valuable separation technique in comparison to other chromatography techniques. Comparison between GLC and high-performance liquid chromatography (HPLC) is given in **Table 6.3**.

■ TROUBLESHOOTING IN GAS CHROMATOGRAPHY

When we are operating GC, we will come across various problems. It is necessary to diagnose the problem and set the machine right. Some of the problems with their causes and solutions are mentioned in **Table 6.4**.

■ **Table 6.3:** Comparison of GLC with HPLC.

S. No.	GLC	HPLC
1.	Mobile phase is gas	Mobile phase is liquid
2.	Sample may be solid, liquid, and gas	Sample should be solid and liquid
3.	Sample should be dissolved in volatile solvents	Sample should be dissolved in mobile phase
4.	Sample must be vaporized at the experimental temperature	Sample should be in dissolved state
5.	Not applicable for inorganic compounds	Applicable to both organic and inorganic compounds
6.	Unstable for thermolabile compounds	Thermolabile compounds can be analyzed

Continued

Continued

S. No.	GLC	HPLC
7.	GC detectors are: • Flame ionization detector (FID) • Electron capture detector (ECD) • Photoionization detector (PID) • Flame photometric detector (FPD) • Electrolytic conductivity detector (ECD)	HPLC detectors are: • Refractive index detector • UV-visible detector • Fluorescence detector • Electrochemical detector • Conductivity detector
8.	Only stationary phase and temperature have significant effect in altering retention time and resolution	Mobile phase has dramatic effect on retention time and resolution
9.	Destructive	Nondestructive
10.	Only limited compounds can be analyzed	Almost all compounds can be analyzed

(GLC: gas-liquid chromatography; HPLC: high-performance liquid chromatography; UV: ultraviolet).

Table 6.4: Troubleshooting in gas-liquid chromatography (GLC).

Probable symptoms	Possible causes	Required action
Spiking	1. Particulate matter passing through the detector 2. Loose connections on cables	1. Clean the detector 2. Repair the electrical connections
Noise	1. Contaminated injector or column 2. The column is inserted into the flame of an FID, NPD, or FPD 3. Air leak when using an ECD/TCD 4. Incorrect combustion or flow rates when using an FID/NPD/FPD 5. Physical defect in the detector 6. Defective detector board	1. Clean the injector and change column 2. Reinstall the column 3. Find and repair the leak 4. Check and reset the gases at their proper values 5. Consult service engineer
Wander	1. Contaminated carrier gas, if using isothermal conditions 2. Contaminated gas chromatograph 3. Poor control of the carrier gas or detector gas flow 4. Poor thermal control of the detector	1. Use carrier gas impurities traps or change the cylinder 2. Clean the injector/gas lines 3. Clean, repair, or change the flow controller 4. Contact the GLC engineer

Continued

GAS CHROMATOGRAPHY AND ITS APPLICATIONS

Continued

Probable symptoms	Possible causes	Required action
Drift (upward)	1. GC column contamination 2. Damage stationary phase	1. Rinse the column with solvent 2. Replace the column
Drift (downward)	1. Incomplete conditions of the column 2. Unequilibrated detector	1. Condition the column until a stable baseline is obtained 2. Allow the detector enough time to equilibrate
Offset	1. Injector or column contamination 2. Column is inserted into the flame of the FID, NPD, or FPD 3. Contaminated carrier or detector gas 4. Contaminated detector	1. Clean the injector and rinse the column 2. Reinstall the column 3. Change the gases 4. Clean the detector
No peaks appears	1. Plugged syringe 2. Broken columns 3. Injecting the sample into the wrong injector 4. Column installed into the wrong detector 5. Integrator or recording devices is connected to the wrong detector 6. Detector gases improperly set or not on 7. Very low or no carrier gas flow	1. Clean the syringe 2. Reinstall the column 3. Use the correct injector 4. Reinstall the column into correct detector 5. Connect the integrator into correct detector 6. Check and reset the detector gases 7. Immediately lower the column temperature to 30–35°C
All peaks reduced in size	1. Partially plugged syringe 2. Change in the injection technique 3. Large leaks in the injector 4. Split ratio is too high 5. Too short of purge activation time for splitless injections 6. Very high septum purge flow 7. Too low of an injector temperature	1. Clean the syringe or use a new syringe 2. Check the injection technique and verify that it is same as before 3. Find and repair the leak 4. Lower the split ratio 5. Increase the purge activation time 6. Decrease the septum purge flow

Continued

Continued

Probable symptoms	Possible causes	Required action
	1. High background signal caused by contaminations, excessive column damage, or autozero problems 2. Improperly operated detector. Impurities in the detector gas 3. Excessive attenuated integrator signal	1. Increase the injector temperature 2. Solvent rinse the column. Check the autozero function and setting 3. Consult the GLC engineer 4. Check and verify the attenuation signals
Select peaks reduced in size	1. Column and/or liner activity of contamination if the reduction or loss is for active compounds such as amines, carboxylic acids, alcohol, and diols 2. Leak in the injector 3. Mixed samples solvents for splitless or on-column injections 4. Decomposition or error in the sample	1. Clean or replace the injector liner. Solvent rinse or replace the column 2. Find and repair the leak 3. Use a single solvent for sample injection 4. Check and verify the sample integrity and concentration
Tailing peak	1. Active injector liner or column 2. Contaminated injector liner or column 3. Dead volume caused by a poorly installed column, liner, or union 4. Poorly cut column end 5. Polarity mismatch of the stationary phase, solute, or solvent 6. Cold spot in the flow path 7. Solid debris in the liner or column 8. Poor injection technique 9. Too low of split ratio 10. Overloading on a PLOT column	1. Clean or replace liner or column 2. Clean or replace the injector liner 3. Check and verify the installation of each fitting. Reinstall the column, if necessary 4. Recut or install the column 5. Change to solvent or phase that has a better polarity match 6. Check the flow path of the sample for possible cold spots or zones 7. Clean or replace liner. Cut the end of the column until the debris is removed 8. Change injection techniques 9. Increase the split ratio 10. Decrease the amount of sample reaching the column

Continued

Continued

Probable symptoms	Possible causes	Required action
Fronting	1. Poorly installed column 2. Leak in the injector 3. Too low of a split ratio 4. Too long of an injector temperature 5. Too long of a purge activation time for splitless injections 6. Large injections volume 7. Low column temperature and high boiling solvents 8. High column temperatures and higher boiling solvents	1. Recut and reinstall the column 2. Find and repair the peak 3. Use a higher split ratio 4. Use a higher injector temperature 5. Use a shorter purge activation time 6. Decrease the injection size 7. Use a higher initial column temperature or lower boiling solvent 8. Use a lower initial column temperature or a higher boiling solvent
Rounded or flat-topped peak	1. Overload detector 2. Exceeding the range of the integrator or recording device	1. Decrease the amount of sample reaching the detector 2. Reset the range of attenuation level on the recorder
Split peaks	1. Poor injection techniques 2. Poorly installed column in the injector 3. Column temperature fluctuations 4. Coelution of two or more compounds 5. Mixed sample solvents for splitless or on-column injections	1. Change injection techniques 2. Recut the column end 3. Check the oven temperature 4. Check for any changes in operational parameters 5. Use single solvent for single injections

Continued

GAS CHROMATOGRAPHY AND ITS APPLICATIONS

Continued

Probable symptoms	Possible causes	Required action
Negative peaks	1. All peaks are negative 2. Compound has greater thermal conductivity than a carrier gas 3. Dirty ECD cell	1. Check the polarity 2. Select peaks on a TCD 3. Clean or replace ECD cell
Retention time shifts	1. Different column temperature 2. Leak in injector, especially the septum 3. Contaminated septum 4. Change of sample solvent	1. Check and verify the column temperature 2. Find and repair the leak and change the septum 3. Solvent rinse the column 4. Use the same solvent for all samples and standards
Loss of separation or resolution	1. Contaminated column 2. Damage stationary phase (bleeding of column) 3. Large change in sample concentration 4. Improper injector operation	1. Rinse the column 2. Replace the column 3. Adjust or compensate for concentration change 4. Check the temperature, split ratio, purge time, and type of liner and leaks
Quantification difficulties	1. Injection techniques problems 2. Split discrimination 3. Using a different purge activation time for splitless injection 4. Baseline disturbance 5. Improper integration or recorder setting 6. Inconsistent detector gas flow 7. Column or liner activity	1. Use consistent injection techniques 2. Use consistent injection techniques 3. Use a consistent purge activation time 4. Remove baseline disturbances 5. Check and verify the integrator and recorder settings 6. Check and verify detector operation 7. Clean or replace the column liner

Continued

Continued

Probable symptoms	Possible causes	Required action
Rapid column deterioration	1. Exposure of the column to the air at elevated temperature 2. Exceeding temperature limit of the column for prolonged period 3. Chemical damage 4. Contamination of the column with high-molecular weight materials 5. Column breakage	1. Find and repair any leaks. Check the quality of the impurity traps and carrier gas 2. Replace the column. Do not exceed the upper temperature limit 3. Do not inject inorganic acids or bases 4. Use sample preparation techniques to remove the problem of contaminants. Use a guard column 5. Avoid abrading or scratching the column. Avoid sharp turns or bends in the tubing
Ghost peaks	1. Contamination in the injector of column 2. Septum bleed 3. Previous run terminated	1. Clean the injector liner. Solvent rinse of the column 2. Use a higher temperature septum. Lower the injector temperature 3. Prolong the run time to allow the complete elution of the sample

(ECD: electron capture detector; FPD: flame photometric detector; FID: flame ionization detector; NPD: nitrogen phosphorus detector; PLOT: porous layer open tubular; TCD: thermal conductivity detector)

■ CONCLUSION

Gas-liquid chromatography has proved a popular tool for the quantitative analysis of trace organics. The major reason for this, is probably, the fact that GLC was the first technique to combine a rapid, efficient separation step with detectors that could be used on line at high sensitivity and with wide applicability. A further advancement in column technology has been the introduction of capillary columns, which are much longer of narrower bore than traditional packed columns; capillary columns are particularly useful in the separation of complex mixtures. The sensitivity of a GLC assay depends to a large degree on the response evoked by a particular compound from the type of detector used. FID is probably the most widely used GLC detector since, most organic molecules cause a response. The comparatively high sensitivity, wide linear range of response, and excellent reliability, coupled with its wide range of applications, have made this type of detector popular for trace organic analysis including to a certain extent in the field of analytical toxicology. The combination of gas chromatography with mass spectrometry (GC-MS) results in a methodology, which is not only very specific, but also highly sensitive. In comparison to other technique, the range of compounds that can be handled by GLC is increased by the use of suitable derivatization procedures. The aim is often to prepare a derivative that is more stable than the parent compound, more volatile, less thermally labile, or less prone to an adsorption problem during the chromatographic process. A further reason for derivatization is to render a molecule more responsive to a particular type of detector. Headspace technique in GLC is another development in GLC, which is used for the analysis of volatile organics present in complex matrices such as blood and soil. These types of situation are encountered frequently in forensic analysis.

The sample to be analyzed is kept in the headspace chamber and a current of carrier gas is passed through it. The analyte is swept away along with the carrier gas to the GC instrument for analysis. The major disadvantage of GLC is that most of the samples received for forensic analysis are not amenable for injection directly in the GLC. The sample has to undergo suitable derivation technique. Overall, GLC is a sensitive and cheap technique for analysis of volatile compounds except few exceptions. Today, the GLC has proved to be a valuable method for analysis of forensic samples for alcohol, pesticides, drug of abuse, narcotics, etc. It has strengthened the criminal investigation by providing quick, reliable, and accurate scientific results, which forms strong evidence in the court of law. The rapid advancement in column technology and the development of suitable derivative techniques has increased the range of compounds that can be handled by GLC.

■ FURTHER READINGS

1. Aguilar C, Borrull F, Marce RM. Determination of pesticides in environmental waters by solid-phase extraction and gas chromatography with electron capture and mass-spectrometry detection. J Chromatogr A. 1997;771:221-31.
2. Amiss TJ, Smoak IW. Determination of chlorobutanol in mouse serum, urine and embryos by capillary gas-chromatography with electron-capture detection. J Chromatogr B. 1995;673:59-66.
3. Atkinson DA. Evaluation of gas chromatography coupled with ion mobility spectrometry for use as a field screening tool. Diss Abstr Int B. 1995;56:31-61.
4. Borgerding AD, Wilkerson CW. Cryogenically cooled microloop system for sampling and injection in fast GC. J Anal Chem. 1996;68:701-7.
5. Boswell SM, Smythe-Wright D. Dual-detector system for the shipboard analysis of halocarbons in sea-water and air for oceanographic tracer studies. Analyst. 1996;121:505-9.

6. Brtickner H, Hausch M. Gas chromatographic characterization of free D-amino acids in the blood serum of patients with renal disorders and of healthy volunteers. J Chromatogra. 1993;614:7-17.
7. Carlsson J. Simplified gas chromatographic procedure for identification of bacterial metabolic products. Appl Microbiol. 1973;25:287-9.
8. Chan L. The determination of tetra alkyl lead compounds in petrol using combined gas chromatography-atomic absorption spectrometry. For Sci Int. 1981;18:57-62.
9. Chivair G, Gandini N, Russo P, Fabbri D. Characterization of standard temperature painting layers containing proteinaceous binders by pyrolysis gas chromatography mass spectrometry. Chromatographia. 1998;47:420-6.
10. Dwarzanski JP, McClennen WH, Cole PA, Thornton SN, Meuzelaar HLC, Arnold N. Field-portable, automated pyrolysis-GC/IMS system for rapid biomarker detection in aerosols: a feasibility study. Field Anal Chem Tech. 1997;1:295-306.
11. Ehrmann EU, Dharmasena HP, Carney K, Overton EB. Novel column heater for fast capillary gas chromatography. J Chromatogr Sci. 1996;34:533-9.
12. Eiceman EA, Hill HH, Gardea-Torresday H. Gas Chromatography. Anal Chem Fundam Rev. 1998;70:321-39.
13. Gorbach SL, Mayhew JW, Bartlett JG. Rapid diagnosis of anaerobic infections by direct gas-liquid chromatography of clinical specimens. Clin Invest. 1976;57:478-84.
14. Haken JK. Pyrolysis gas chromatography of synthetic polymers: a bibliography. J Chromatogr A. 1998;825:171-87.
15. Handley PJ, Adlard EK. Gas Chromatographic Techniques and Applications. Sheffield: Sheffield Academic Press; 2001.
16. Harris W, Habgood H. Programmed Temperature Gas Chromatography. New York: J Wiley and Sons; 1966.
17. Hyver KJ, Sandra P. High-Resolution Gas Chromatography, 3rd edition. United States: Hewlett-Packard Corporation; 1989.
18. Jain V, Phillips JB. Fast temperature programming on fused-silica open-tubular capillary columns by direct resistive heating. J Chromatogr Sci. 1995;33:55-9.
19. Jaiswal AK. Do's and Don'ts for sophisticated analytical instruments. J Med Toxicol Legal Med. 2003;6:19-23.
20. James AT, Martin AJ. Gas-liquid partition chromatography: the separation and microestimation of volatile fatty acids from formic acid to dodecanoic acid. Biochem J. 1952;50:679.
21. Jeffery PG, Kipping PJ. Gas Analysis by Gas Chromatography. Pergamon, Oxford University Press; 1972.
22. Jennings W, Mittlefehldt E, Stremple P. Analytical Gas Chromatography. San Diego: Academic Press; 1997.
23. Cundy KV, Willard KE, Valeri LJ, Shanholtzer CJ, Singh J, Peterson LR. Comparison of traditional gas chromatography (GC), headspace GC, and the microbial identification library GC system for the identification of Clostridium difficile. J Clin Microbiol. 1991;29:260-3.
24. Keszler A, Heberger K, Gude M. Identification of volatile compounds in sunflower oil by headspace SPME and ion-trap GC/MS and HRC-J. High Res Chrom. 1988;21:368-70.
25. Klemp MA, Akard ML, Sacks RD. Cryofusing inlet with reverse flow sample collection for gas-chromatography. Anal Chem. 1993;65:2516-21.

26. Kongshaug KE, Pedersen S, Rasmussen KE, Krogh M. Solid-phase microextraction/ capillary gas chromatography for the profiling of confiscated ecstacy and amphetamine. Chromatographia. 1999;50:247-52.
27. Ladas S, Arapakis G, Malamou-Ladas, Palikaris G, Arseni A. Rapid diagnosis of anaerobic infections by gas liquid chromatography. J Clin Pathol. 1979;32:1163-7.
28. Larsson L, Mardh P, Odham G. Detection of alcohols and volatile fatty acids by headspace gas chromatography in identification of anaerobic bacteria. J Clin Microbiol. 1978;7:23-7.
29. Loffe BV, Viltenberg AG. Headspace Analysis and Related Methods in Gas Chromatography. New York: Wiley; 1984.
30. Loudon AG, Kolbe BJ, Adler J, Stach J. The use of on-site analysis for the protection of personnel. Analysis. 1995;23:22-4.
31. Mayhew JW, Gorbach SL. Internal standards for gas chromatographic analysis of metabolic end products from anaerobic bacteria. Appl Environ Microbiol. 1979;33:1002-3.
32. McKenzie SL, Tenaschuk D, Fortier G. Analysis of amino acids by gas liquid chromatography as tert-butyldimethylsilyl derivatives: preparation of derivatives in a single reaction. J Chromatogr. 1987;387:241-53.
33. Mortimer RD, Shields JB. Total, free, and glucose conjugated acid metabolites from permethrin and cypermethrin in foods by gas-chromatography electron-capture detection. J Assoc Off Anal Chem Int. 1995;78:102-7.
34. Olsavicky VM. A comparison of high temperature septa for gas chromatography. J Chromatogr Sci. 1978;2:197-200.
35. Ottenstein DM, Bartley DA. Separation of free acids C2-C5 in dilute aqueous solution column technology. J Chromatogr Sci. 1971;9:674-81.
36. Patterson PL. Recent advances in thermionic ionization detection for gas chromatography. J Chromatogr Sci. 1986;24:41-52.
37. Perrett RH, Purnell JH. Contribution of diffusion and mass transfer processes to efficiency of gas liquid chromatography columns. Anal Chem. 1963;35:430.
38. Phillips KD, Tearle PV, Willis AT. Rapid diagnosis of anaerobic infections by gas-liquid chromatography of clinical material. J Clin Pathol. 1971;29:428-32.
39. Piltingsrud HV. A field deployable gas chromatograph mass spectrometer for industrial hygiene applications. Am Ind Hyg Assoc J. 1997;58:564-77.
40. Reed PJ, Sanderson PJ. Detection of anaerobic wound infection by analysis of pus swabs for volatile fatty acids by gas-liquid chromatography. J Clin Pathol. 1979;32:1203-5.
41. Rogosa M, Love LL. Direct quantitative gas chromatographic separation of C2-C6 fatty acids, methanol, and ethyl alcohol in aqueous microbial fermentation media. Appl Microbiol. 1968;16:285-90.
42. Scarlata CJ, Ebeler SE. Headspace solid-phase microextraction for the analysis of dimethyl sulfide in beer. J Agric Food Chem. 1999;47:2505-8.
43. Sharma BK. Methods of Chemical Analysis, 16th edition. Uttar Pradesh: Krishna Prakashan Media (P) Ltd.; 1997.
44. Soulages NL. Determination of ethyl methyl lead alkyls and halide scavengers in petrol by gas chromatography and flame ionization detection. Analy Chem. 1967;39:1340-41.
45. Sullivan JJ. Detectors in Modern Practice of Gas Chromatography. New York: John Wiley and Sons; 1997. pp. 228-54.
46. Thadepalli H, Gangopadhyay PK. Rapid diagnosis of anaerobic empyema by direct gas-liquid chromatography. J Clin Microbiol. 1980;77:507-13.

47. van den Bogaard AE, Hazen MJ, Maes JH. The detection of obligate anaerobic bacteria in swine abscesses. A comparison between gas-liquid chromatography and bacteriological culturing methods. Vet Microbiol. 1983;8:389-96.
48. van Deursen M, Beens J, Cramers CA, Janssen HG. Possibilities and Limitations of Fast Temperature Programming as a Route towards Fast GC HRC-J. High Res Chrom. 1999;22:509-13.
49. Wang FCY, Burleson AD. The development of pyrolysis fast gas chromatography for analysis of synthetic polymers. J Chromatogr A. 1999;833:111-9.
50. Wang L, Ishida Y, Ohtani H, Tsuge S. Determination of fortified rosin glycerin ester sizing agents in paper by reactive pyrolysis gas chromatography in the presence of an organic alkali. Anal Sci. 1998;14:431-4.
51. Watt B, Geddes PA, Greenan OA, Napier SK, Mitchell A. Gas-liquid chromatography in the diagnosis of anaerobic infections: a three year experience. J Clin Pathol. 1982;35:709-14.
52. Yun H, Lee ML. Fast gas chromatography of light hydrocarbons and permanent gases on porous-layer open-tubular columns. Field Anal Chem Technol. 1996;1:60-4.
53. Zhang DN, Zhou ZP, Tang YZ, Wu CY, Zhan W, Xu Y. Analysis of organochlorine compounds in water by solid phase microextraction and gas chromatography. Chin J Anal Chem. 1999;27:768-72.
54. Zhu JY, Chai XS. Some recent developments in headspace gas chromatography. Curr Analy Chem. 2005;1:79-83.
55. Zijlstra JB, Beukema J, Wolthers BG, Byrne BM, Groen A, Dankert T. Pretreatment methods prior to gas chromatographic analysis of volatile fatty acids from faecal samples. Clin Chim Acta. 1977;78:243-50.

Chapter 7

High-performance Liquid Chromatography and its Applications

■ INTRODUCTION

High-performance liquid chromatography (HPLC) is a unique separation technique/analytical technique for separation of organic components of mixture, developed by Kirkland and Huber in 1969. Chromatography is defined as the separation technique involving mass transfer between stationary and mobile phase. It is conducted in the liquid phase in which mixture of compounds is separated into its constituent components by distributing between the mobile phase and a stationary phase held inside the chromatographic column. Depending on the mode of chromatography, the different types of adsorption forces are involved such as (i) hydrophobic interactions (RP-HPLC), (ii) dipole-dipole interaction (NP-HPLC), and ionic interactions (ion-exchange chromatography).

High-performance liquid chromatography is used for detection and quantification of separated organic compounds based on differential interaction of analytes between liquid phases passing through a column. Analyte molecules compete with the eluent molecules for the adsorption sites inside the column, so that stronger molecule interact with the surface, while weaker the eluent interaction, the longer the analyte will be retained on the surface. An online detector (types discussed later) monitors separated component in the column and generates analyte peaks, which is recorded as chromatogram. HPLC is widely used for the qualitative and quantitative analysis of pharmaceuticals, biomolecules, polymers, and many other organic compounds. HPLC provides a wide variety of operating variables that can be used to control and optimize a separation. Some important features of HPLC are:
- Pressure up to 4.14×10^7 Nm^2 (6,000 psi)
- Column-bonded phase selection with option of column switching
- Mobile phase changes with rapid re-equilibration
- Mobile phase polarity adjustment with gradient operation
- Column packing support selection for pH and temperature stability
- Temperature programming with gradient operation or inactive operation
- 100 times faster than by the use of conventional liquid chromatography.

HIGH-PERFORMANCE LIQUID CHROMATOGRAPHY AND ITS APPLICATIONS

■ THEORY OF HIGH-PERFORMANCE LIQUID CHROMATOGRAPHY

Partition chromatography is the fundamental principle of distribution mechanism in liquid–liquid chromatography, i.e., the solute has difference in solubility in two media, one is mobile phase and the other is stationary phase. The rate of partition of solute from mobile phase to stationary phase is referred as partition coefficient.

Thus, the components are separated because of the difference in their partition coefficient, as it passes through analytical column.

When a suitable column has been chosen for the separation, all components should pass through the analytical column, so as to elute as a peak at different times (**Fig. 7.1**). The time differential is due to the differences in the distribution of the various components between the mobile phase and stationary phase, which arise from the physical or chemical differences among the components of the mixture. Thus, with the difference in migration rates of the components through a stationary phase by a liquid mobile phase, each component passes through the detector to elute as a peak and it is recorded as a chromatogram. Separation of five components A, B, C, D, and E in HPLC using appropriate analytical column is shown in **Figure 7.2**.

■ TERMS USED IN HIGH-PERFORMANCE LIQUID CHROMATOGRAPHY

Distribution Constant

Distribution constant (K) of a compound for a chemical reaction between stationary phase and mobile phase in equilibrium is expressed as:

$$A_{mobile} \leftrightarrow A_{stationary}$$

$$K = \frac{C \text{ (stationary phase)}}{C \text{ (mobile phase)}}$$

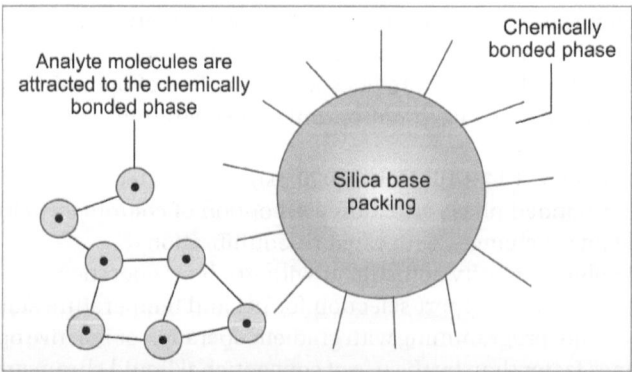

Fig. 7.1: Migration of analyte through column in high-performance liquid chromatography (HPLC).

HIGH-PERFORMANCE LIQUID CHROMATOGRAPHY AND ITS APPLICATIONS

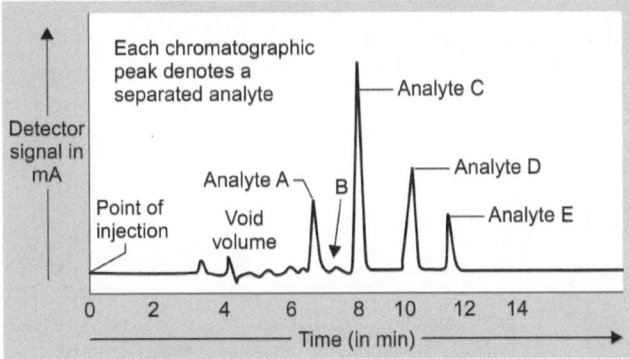

Fig. 7.2: Typical high-performance liquid chromatography (HPLC) chromatogram.

where, C is molar concentration and K is distribution constant and it is also termed as partition ratio.
- K would determine the time taken by a compound as adsorbed in the stationary phase and as solvated by mobile phase
- It also determines the time taken by a compound to travel through the length of the column

For example, if a compound adsorbs in more time in stationary phase, it takes more time to travel through the column and vice versa. The time taken for a compound to elute from a chromatographic column as peak from the point of injection is termed as the retention time (t_R) in a chromatographic separation. Analytes, while passing through the porous packing beads (silica base packing), are inclined to interact with the surface adsorption sites and thus, separated which are recorded as peak with the help of detector. Hydrophobic interactions are the principle function in reverse-phase separation, while dipole-dipole interactions for normal-phase separation.

Retention Time

It is defined as the time taken by an analyte peak reaching a detector at the end of the column from the point of injection. It is represented by t_R (**Fig. 7.3**).

Unretained Peak or Void Volume (t_m)

It is defined as the total volume of mobile phase, which is required to carry an unretained component in a given sample through a column. The time taken for the mobile phase to pass through the column is called t_m (**Fig. 7.3**).

Retention Factor or Capacity Factor (k′)

Retention factor, k', is often used to describe the migration rate of an analyte through a column. It is also called the capacity factor. The retention factor for analyte A is defined as:

$$k'_A = \frac{t_R - t_m}{t_m}$$

where, t_R is retention time and t_m is void volume.

HIGH-PERFORMANCE LIQUID CHROMATOGRAPHY AND ITS APPLICATIONS

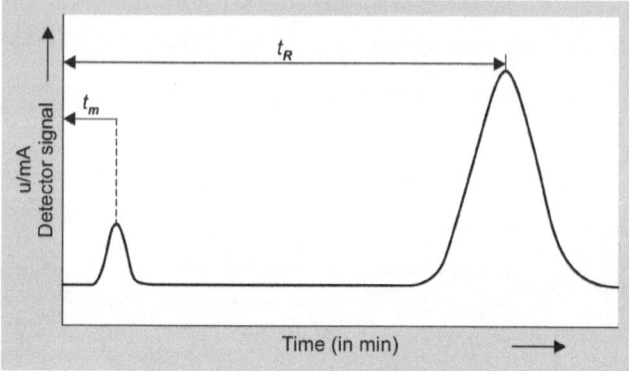

Fig. 7.3: Chromatogram showing t_m and t_R.

Band Broadening and Column Efficiency

The efficiency and optimum separation in chromatography are based on the number of theoretical plates of the column. Chromatographic column contains large number of separate imaginary layers called theoretical plates (**Fig. 7.4**), in which equilibrations of the sample between the stationary and mobile phase occur to move analyte from one plate to subsequent plate with the help of equilibrated mobile phase. Theoretical plate does not exist; it is a hypothetical plate by which we are able to calculate column's efficiency. This plate count is based on length and diameter of a given column. Different analytes have different dependencies of height equivalent to a theoretical plate (HETP) on the flow rate for the same column.

In a given chromatographic separation, the number of HETP is a measure of column efficiency, which is equivalent to the ratio of column length to the number of theoretical plates (**Table 7.1**).

$$HETP = \frac{L}{N}$$

where, L is length of the column and N is number of theoretical plates.

The efficiency of a column is reported as the number of theoretical plates (plate number). It is represented by N. Mathematically, it is defined as:

$$N = 16\left(\frac{t_R}{W_B}\right)^2$$

where, t_R is retention time for retained analyte and W_B is width of peak (**Fig. 7.5**).

For the optimization of separation efficiency, it is foremost to maximize the theoretical plates by reducing the plate height, which is related to flow rate of the mobile phase for a given separation. Therefore, separation efficiency can be maximized by optimizing flow rate for a fixed set of mobile

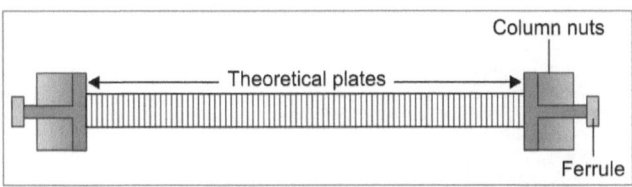

Fig. 7.4: Theoretical plates in a chromatographic column.

Table 7.1: Theoretical plates with column length and diameter.

Particle diameter (µ)	Column length (cm)	Number of plates (N)
3	15	17,000–20,000
10	25	8,000–10,000
5	10	7,000–9,000
5	15	10,000–12,000
5	25	17,000–20,000
3	5	6,000–7,000
3	7.5	9,000–11,000
3	10	12,000–14,000
10	15	6,000–7,000

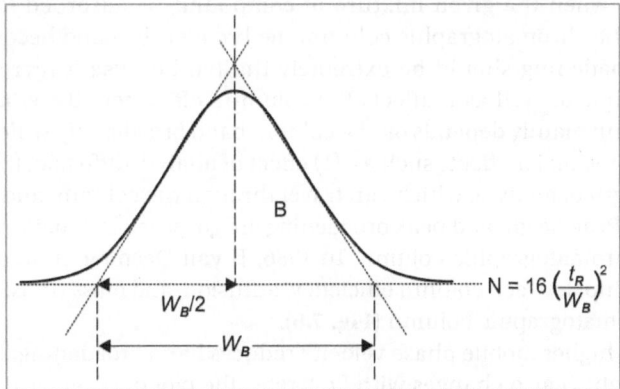

Fig. 7.5: Theoretical plate calculation.

phase, stationary phase, and analytes. The van Deemter equation explains graphically H/u curve, which is a plot of the plate height as a function of the mobile phase flow rate. The van Deemter equation for plate height is as follows:

$$\text{HETP} = A + B/u + Cu$$

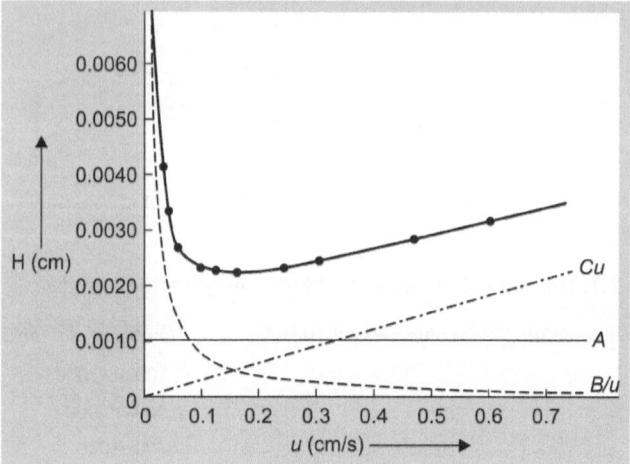

Fig. 7.6: van Deemter plot—H/u curve.

where,
  HETP = Height equivalent to a theoretical plate
  A = Eddy diffusion term
  B = Longitudinal diffusion term
  C = Resistance to mass transfer coefficient
  u = Linear velocity

Thus, when the given mixture of compounds is adsorbed for longer time in the chromatographic column, the broader the band becomes. The band broadening should be extremely limited because it increases the elution time as well as it affects the column's efficiency. The efficiency of the column mainly depends on the column band broadening, which occurs due to three major effects such as: (1) effect of analyte diffusion, (2) various path length of analyte, which can travel through the column, and (3) mass transfer. Peak height and peak broadening are governed by kinetic processes in the chromatographic column. In 1956, JJ van Deemter et al. proposed relationship between column efficiency, diffusion, and mass transfer effects in a chromatographic column (**Fig. 7.6**).

Thus, higher mobile phase velocity reduces band broadening; however, plate height H also changes with flow rate. The plot of H versus u is called van Deemter plot. The most significant result of the plot is the optimization of mobile phase flow rate, where the column efficiency will fit to the best. Some of the factors that can affect the efficiency of the column are:
- *Eddy diffusion or multiple paths*: Eddy diffusion describes when the molecules move through different paths with different length depending on the particles in which the analyte travels randomly through the stationary phase, which results in band broadening. Uniform packing with constant size of particles reduces eddy diffusion. Eddy diffusion band broadening is independent of the flow rate, i.e., at low flow rates, particles quickly switch paths, resulting in reduced transit time (**Fig. 7.7**).

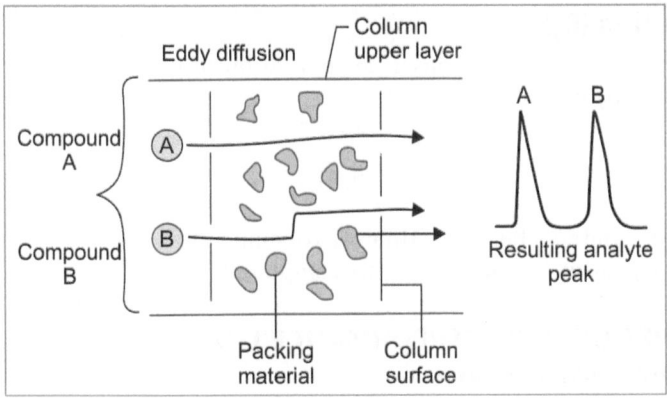

Fig. 7.7: Eddy diffusion.

- *Longitudinal diffusion*: Longitudinal diffusion occurs due to high concentration of analyte, which diffuses in the mobile phase, which is proportional to the mobile phase diffusion coefficient and inversely proportional to the flow rate. Longitudinal diffusion can be minimized by using tightly packed uniformly sized smaller diameter column for higher flow rates.
- *Mass transfer coefficient (C_S and C_M)*: Mass transfer (C) defines when the varying equilibration time of an analyte between stationary phase and mobile phase leads to band broadening. If two analytes passing through a chromatographic column, analyte (C_S) has the high affinity toward the stationary phase, then the analyte (C_M) in the mobile phase may move faster to cause band broadening. Mass transfer coefficient is proportional to flow rate, i.e., higher the flow rate of mobile phase, higher the broadening, although it can be reduced by using a thin uniform diameter stationary phase low flow rate of mobile phase.

Selectivity Factor

The selectivity factor refers to the ratio of partition coefficient of the two compounds A and B that retains in the stationary phase because they elute close together or nearly equal in a chromatographic separation. It is denoted by alpha (α).

$$\alpha = \frac{k'B}{k'A} = \frac{t_R(B) - t_m}{t_R(A) - t_m}$$

where,

t_m = Retention time of unretained peak

k'A and B = Partition coefficients of A and B

t_R A and B = Retention time of substance A and B

Selectivity factor is the ratio of the retention time factor and it is always greater than one when the compound B retains more time in the column than the compound A, which elutes later.

Resolution (R_S)

It refers to the extent of baseline separation of two components. It is calculated by formula as follows:

$$R_s = \frac{2(t_{R1}-t_{R2})}{W_1-W_2}$$

where,

t_{R1} and t_{R2} = Retention time of two compounds
w_1 and w_2 = Peak width of two compounds

■ TYPES OF HIGH-PERFORMANCE LIQUID CHROMATOGRAPHY

Normal Phase

It is called normal phase because the working principle and theory are same as in the earlier discovery of widely used column and thin-layer chromatography (TLC). Diagrammatic representation of normal phase is given in **Flowchart 7.1**. In normal-phase HPLC:
- The stationary phase is highly polar, e.g., silica gel
- Mobile phase is nonpolar, e.g., hexane
- Less polar compounds move faster (elute first) followed by more polar compounds
- Separation is based on difference in adsorption chromatography
- Stationary phase is solid

Reverse Phase

It is called reverse phase because it is opposite with respect to normal-phase HPLC. Mobile phase is more polar than stationary phase and selective for more nonpolar or weakly polar compounds. Stationary phase is either coated onto the support or chemically bonded to the support. Diagrammatic representation of reverse phase is given in **Flowchart 7.2**. In reverse-phase HPLC:
- The stationary phase is nonpolar or intermediate polar, e.g., octadecylsilane (ODS) C18-, C8-, C4-bonded phases

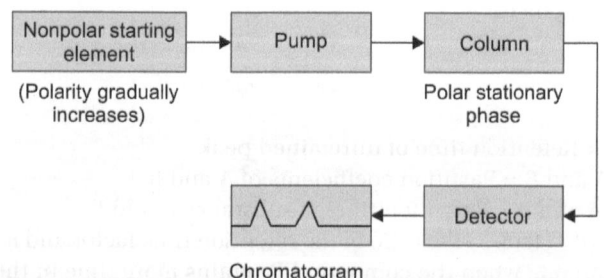

Flowchart 7.1: Diagrammatic representation of normal-phase high-performance liquid chromatography (HPLC).

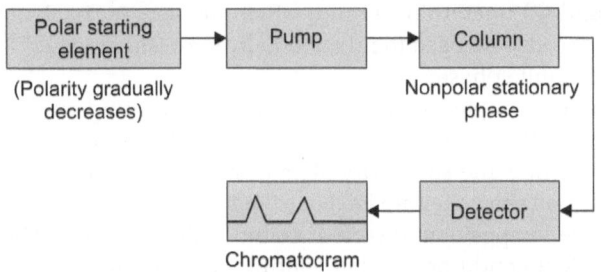

Flowchart 7.2: Diagrammatic representation of reverse-phase high-performance liquid chromatography (HPLC).

- Mobile phase is polar, e.g., methanol, acetonitrile, tetrahydrofuran, water
- Polar compounds are faster (elute first) followed by less polar compounds
- Separation is based on differences in partition coefficients (partition chromatography)
- Stationary phase is liquid and supported on silica

ELUTION TECHNIQUES IN HIGH-PERFORMANCE LIQUID CHROMATOGRAPHY

Isocratic Separation

Isocratic technique employs the same mobile phase throughout the elution process of the analytes in a chromatographic technique. In isocratic chromatography, the same polarity of the mobile phase or elution strength is maintained throughout the separation process with premixed mobile phase. Isocratic elution has the following disadvantages:

- Poor separation or late elution
- Limited peak capacity (the maximum number of peaks that can be accommodated in the chromatogram)
- Problems with samples containing analytes of diverse polarities
- Late eluters (such as dimers) are particularly difficult to quantitate due to excessive band broadening with long retention times
- Difficult in analyzing impurities or degradants for pharmaceutical with longer run time.

Gradient Separation

In gradient technique, the mobile phase combination of lower polarity or elution strength is gradually increased with programmed time, over the period of sample elution. In gradient elution, the desired solvent polarity in a desired period of time can be predetermined and programmed, e.g., if the elution is started with $H_2O:CH_3CN$ (10:0), it can be adjusted gradually and continually to $H_2O:CH_3CN$ (9:1) over a period of 35 minutes. Simply, it delivers variable mobile phase composition to the column. It can operate with two types of pumps: (1) binary gradient pump, which delivers two solvents and (2) quaternary pump, which delivers four solvents (mobile phase). It can also be used to mix and deliver an isocratic mobile phase or a gradient mobile phase.

It suits for complex samples and those containing analytes of wide polarities. Unlike isocratic analysis, flow rate has a dramatic influence on retention time and selectivity of analysis. Peaks have smaller width in gradient elution since they are forced to elute with by increasing the stronger mobile phase composition. Therefore, column efficiency cannot be measured under gradient conditions, as late eluting peaks would yield higher plate counts than early peaks in the same column. Gradient separation has the following disadvantages:
- The requirements for more complex instrumentation and greater skills in method development and difficulties in method transfer
- Gradient methods are more difficult to develop because the optimization of several additional parameters is also required

■ INSTRUMENTATION

High-performance liquid chromatography is a unique analytical technique for analysis of wide range of organic compounds. It is promising to observe many of the recent advances, focusing on improving chromatographic technique by simplifying instrumentation, and column efficiency to reduce analysis time with good robust analytical results making the HPLC technique significantly important, with respect to forensic toxicology applications. A typical diagrammatic scheme for HPLC is given in **Figure 7.8**.

There are several manufacturers of HPLC systems. Some of the commercial brands are shown in **Figures 7.9A** to **F**.

It is used for the analysis of wide range of substances such as pesticides, herbicides, insecticides, acidic drugs, basic drugs, narcotics, alcohols,

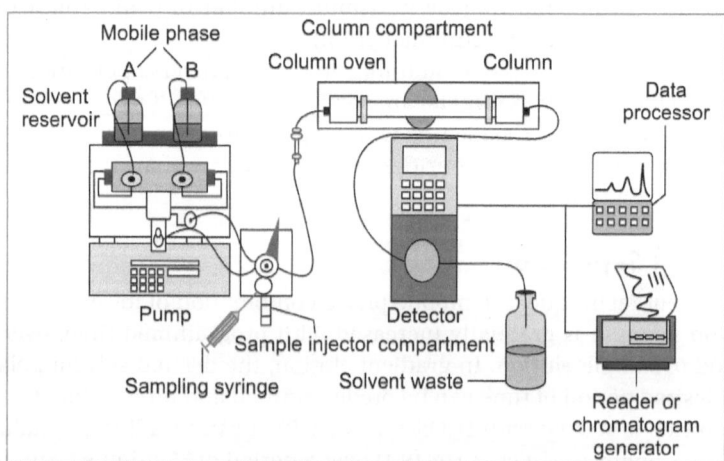

Fig. 7.8: Typical diagrammatic scheme for high-performance liquid chromatography (HPLC).

HIGH-PERFORMANCE LIQUID CHROMATOGRAPHY AND ITS APPLICATIONS

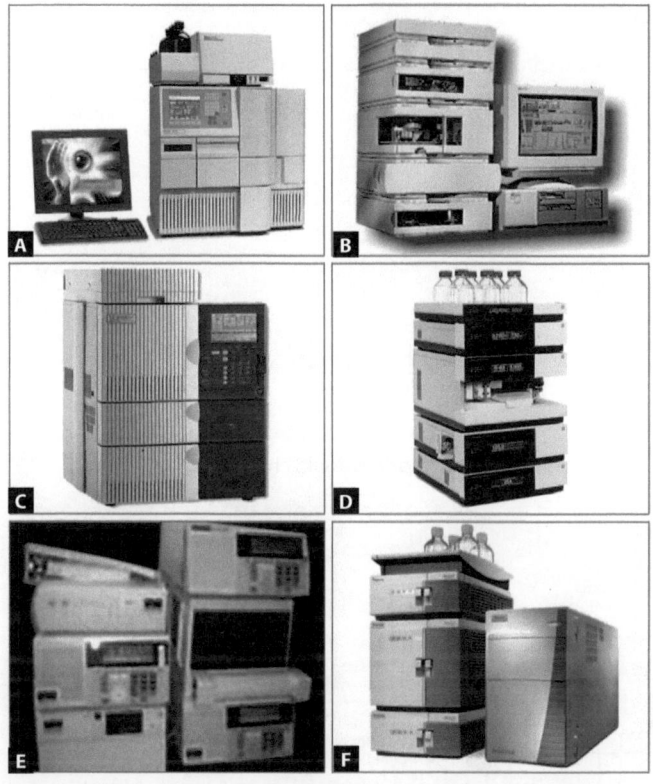

Figs. 7.9A to F: High-performance liquid chromatography (HPLC) system from different manufacturers. (A) Water Corporation Inc., HPLC; (B) Agilent Technologies HPLC; (C) Shimadzu Integrated HPLC; (D) Dionex HPLC; (E) PerkinElmer HPLC; and (F) Thermo Fisher Scientific HPLC.

analgesics, and inorganic samples explosives such as allergens, alkali bases, ballpoint pen inks, environmental poisons, natural and synthetic polymers, steroids, snake venom, and plant and animal poisons. Block diagram of modern HPLC is shown in **Figure 7.10**, which comprises of following systems:
1. Solvent reservoirs and mobile phase
2. Gradient device
3. Pump
4. Sample injector
5. Chromatographic column
6. Detector
7. Data processor
8. Recorder

Solvent Reservoir and Mobile Phase

Solvent reservoir is made up of glass containers, which can be used to store mobile phase for the chromatographic run. Mobile phase (column eluent)

HIGH-PERFORMANCE LIQUID CHROMATOGRAPHY AND ITS APPLICATIONS

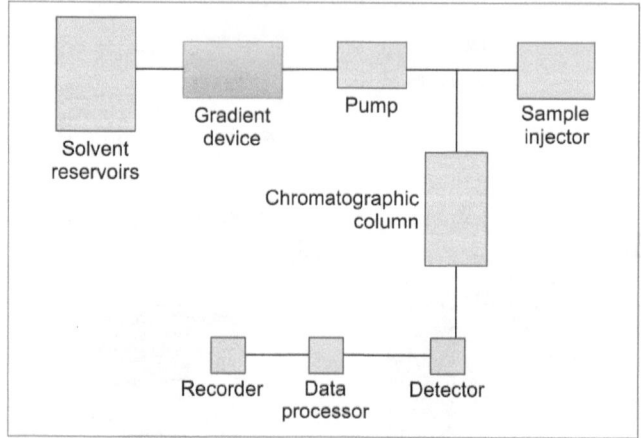

Fig. 7.10: Modern liquid chromatograph.

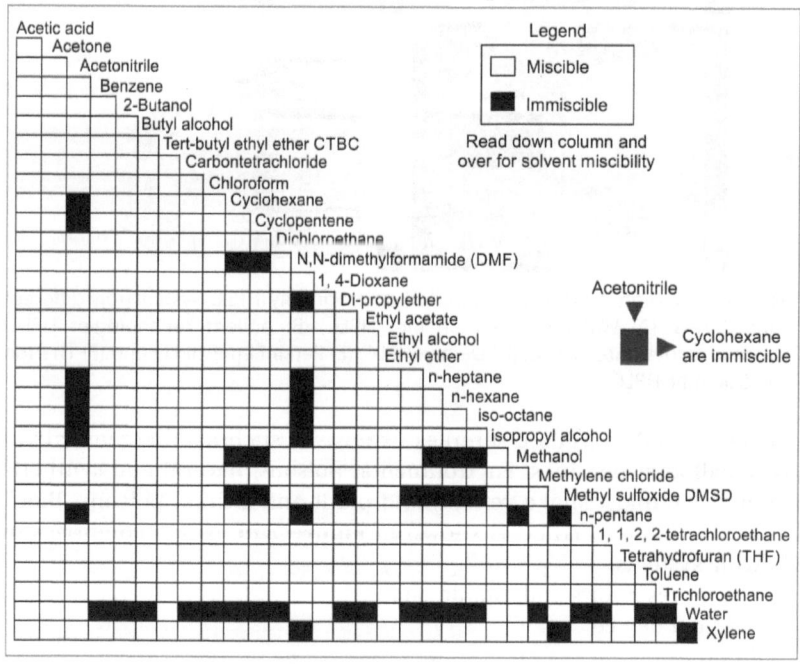

Fig. 7.11: Miscibility chart of mobile phase.

in HPLC is a liquid organic solvent such as acetonitrile, methanol, and chloroform, which is highly pure. The commonly used solvent mixtures are water, buffer solution, etc. Solvent miscibility chart is given in **Figure 7.11**. In normal-phase HPLC, the starting eluent is generally a nonpolar solvent such as n-hexane, n-octane, and $CHCl_3$. In reverse-phase HPLC, the starting eluent is highly polar such as CH_3OH or H_2O and solvent polarity gradually decreases. The mobile phase is pumped into the chromatography column at a very high pressure, so that it can travel through the packed column

with extremely small stationary phase particles. This technique in the early years of its discovery was called high-pressure liquid chromatography. Few points about mobile phase are:
- It is advisable to use deaerated mobile phase, which is thoroughly mixed
- Deaerating/degassing can be done by vacuum pump using inert gas such as helium or by ultrasonic stirring to suspend air or air bubbles
- The mobile phase is pumped under pressure from one or several reservoirs at a constant rate
- The choice of the mobile phase is highly dependent on nature of the compound to be separated
- The eluting power of the mobile phase is determined by its overall polarity
- For normal-phase separation, eluting power increases with increasing polarity of the solvent
- For reverse-phase separation, eluting power decreases with increasing solvent polarity
- Optimum separating conditions can often be achieved by making use of a mixture of two solvents
- Commercially available HPLC solvents should be adequately refined to eliminate ultraviolet (UV) absorbing impurities and particulate matter

Gradient Device

A gradient device may be operated in two modes either by binary mode or by quaternary mode depending on the chromatographic application. Gradient device helps to mix the solvents from each solvent reservoir to deliver the mobile phase into the analytical column at programmed time at a constant flow rate so as to enable the separation of analytes.

Mixing unit mixes the solvents to pass through the analytical column. When solvents are pumped under high pressure, the chances of gas bubble formation are expected to increase, which will interfere with the separation process with abnormal baseline and peak shape. Hence, degassing of solvent is important. Modern HPLC pumps have inbuilt low pressure mixing chamber, which uses helium for degassing and high pressure mixing chamber does not require degassing. Physical methods, such as vacuum filtration, helium purging, and ultrasonication, can also be employed for degassing the mobile phase.

Pumps

It helps to pass the mobile phase to the column at high pressure (1,000–6,000 psi) in controlled constant flow rate in reverse-phase HPLC and variable flow rate in normal-phase HPLC. The ideal characteristics of pump are it should be resistance to the flow of solvent, pulse-free output, and deliver flow rates ranging from 0.001 to 10 mL/min. The eluent is delivered from a pump at a constant rate, at a pressure sufficiently high to overcome the backpressure of the column. Operating pressure of 1,000–3,000 psi is essential for a chromatographic run, again it depends on the solvents used as mobile phase; however, an upper limit of 4,000 psi is manually feeded on the instrument. The solvents used must be HPLC grade and it should be filtered through 0.45 µ nylon filter. To get rid of small particulates, HPLC pumps carry check valves and pulse dampeners, which are used to control the flow rate and back pressure and pulses may be observed from the wavy baseline caused by the pumps. High pressures are required to force a liquid through a tightly-packed column filled with small particle material. There are different types of HPLC pumps such as:

1. *Direct gas-pressure system*: It comprises of cylinder gas pressure, which is applied directly to the eluent in a holding coil. It is economical, although solvent changing is found to be tedious
2. *Syringe-type pumps*: Fine volume of mobile phase pressurized by a piston with electrically driven lead screw. Solvent changing is found to be tedious
3. *Pneumatic intensifier (constant pressure) pumps*: It works basically with pressure when a large area piston drives a small area piston when acted on by pressure from a gasline. The gas pressure is, thus, amplified in the ratio of areas, as the forces of pistons result in a high pressure liquid at constant flow thus, introduced into the system
4. *Reciprocating (constant flow) pumps*: Functions with variable range of flow rates, driven by electrical motor, which moves back and forth within a hydraulic chamber. In the backward stroke, the piston sucks in eluent from the reservoir and in the forward stroke, the eluent is pushed onto the column. These pumps include a high output pressure with constant flow rates with the ability to be used for gradient elution.

Sample Injection System or Injector

The samples to be analyzed are introduced into the HPLC with the help of injector system, either by manual injection or by HPLC inbuilt autoinjection modes, which is commercially known as autosampler. Injector devices are meant for manual and autoinjection. The function of the injector is to introduce the sample into the column homogeneously to avoid the peak broadening. Syringe injection through an elastomeric septum is often used in HPLC although, it is not reproducible and is constricted to low pressures. The most widely used methods are those based on sampling valves and loops. Different types of sample injection system are:

1. *Septum injectors or column injection*: In column injection, a variable volume of sample is introduced by means of a syringe through a septum. This technique is not common
2. *Stop flow injectors or valve injection*: In valve injection, a variable volume of sample is introduced by making use of an injection valve. The sample is introduced in HPLC with variable volume through a septum to withstand such pressure. The flow of mobile phase is stopped for a while at the time of injection onto the head of the column by means of a syringe through a value device. The flow is then restarted again.
3. *Rheodyne injector (loop type) or fixed volume injection*: It is popular and widely used HPLC injector and it has a fixed volume loop of 10–200 µL.

HIGH-PERFORMANCE LIQUID CHROMATOGRAPHY AND ITS APPLICATIONS

Sample is loaded in the loop in load position mode and introduced onto the analytical column in the inject mode at a constant flow

High-performance Liquid Chromatography Column

Chromatographic column or analytical column (**Fig. 7.12**) is the most important part of HPLC technique. In other words, it is the heart of chromatography; since, it decides the efficiency of separation. Columns can be made up of glass, stainless steel, polyethylene, polyetheretherketone (PEEK), and plastic with solid support (backbone for bonded phases), usually 10 µ, 5 µ, or 3 µ silica or polymeric particles, which can withstand high pressures, and are, thus, used to manufacture HPLC columns with smooth tubing, precised bore internal diameter. The separation efficiency is inversely proportional to the particle size of the column packing material while packing irregularities would cause peak broadening and a decrease in efficiency. Bonded phases should be extremely stable and reproducible with functional groups firmly linked (chemical bound) to the solid support (**Tables 7.2** and **7.3**). Analytical column should also possess the ability to resist the chemical action of the mobile phase. Column connections are made with low dead-volume fittings, which prevent stagnant pockets of eluent. Standard column hardware is given in **Figure 7.13**.

Typical analytical column has the following configuration:
- *Bonded phase*: C_8 or C_{18} (reverse phase); CN or diol (normal phase)
- *Column length*: Varies from 5 to 30 cm
- *Column diameter*: 2–50 mm
- *Particle size*: 1–20 µ

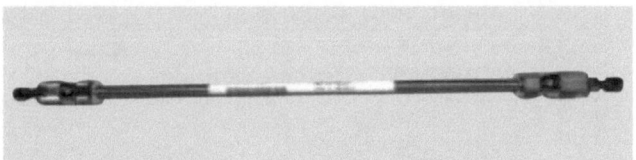

Fig. 7.12: High-performance liquid chromatography (HPLC) column.

Table 7.2: Reverse-phase (RP) and normal-phase (NP) column.

For RP		For NP	
Name	Functional groups	Name	Functional groups
C_{18} (octadecyl)	-$(CH_3)_{17}$-CH_3	Cyano	C_2H_6CNODS
C_8 (octyl)	-$(CH_2)_7$-CH_3	Diol	$C_3H_6OCH_2CHOHCH_2OH$
C_4	-$(CH_2)_3$-CH_3	Amino	$C_3H_6NH_2$
C_2	-CH_2-CH_3	Dimethylamino	$C_3H_6N(CH_3)_2$
C_3	-CH_2-CH_2-CH_3	Aminopropyl	-CH_2-CH_2-CH_2-NH_2
CN	-$(CH_2)_3$-CN	Silica	

HIGH-PERFORMANCE LIQUID CHROMATOGRAPHY AND ITS APPLICATIONS

Table 7.3: Commercially available columns and their applications.

Stationary material	Functional groups	Phase	Application
Si	Silica	Normal phase	Pesticides, steroid, aflatoxins, and alkaloids
C_{18}	Octadecyl	Reverse phase	Fatty acids, polycyclic aromatic hydrocarbons (PAH), fat-soluble vitamins, steroids, prostaglandins, amino acids, etc.
C_8	Octyl	Reverse phase and ion pair	Peptides, proteins, nucleotides, etc.
C_6H_5	Phenyl	Reverse phase	Polar aromatic fatty acids
CN	Cyano	Normal, reverse phase	Polar compounds
NO_2	Nitro	Normal, reverse phase	Polycyclic aromatic hydrocarbons
NH_2	Amino	Normal, reverse phase, and weak anion exchange	Carbohydrates, chlorinated pesticides, and organic acids
OH	Diol	Normal, reverse phase	Peptides and proteins
SA	Sulfonic acid	Cation exchange	Separation of cations, potassium, sodium, calcium, and magnesium
SB	Quaternary	Anionic exchange	Separation of anions, chlorides, fluorides, sulfate, etc.

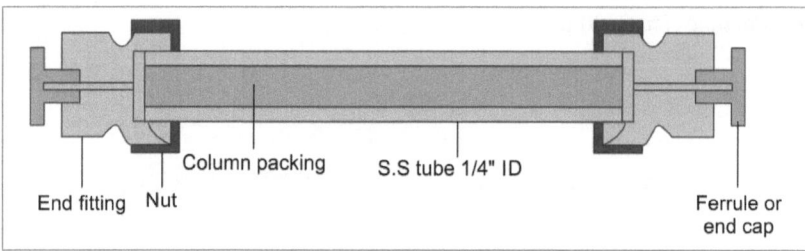

Fig. 7.13: Standard column hardware.

- *Particle nature*: Spherical, uniform sized, and porous materials are used
- *Surface area*: 1 g of stationary phase provides surface area ranging from 100 to 860 m² with an average of 400 m²
- *Pore size*: 80–100 Å (except for macromolecules)

Types of Chromatographic Column

1. *Polystyrene-/Divinylbenzene (DVB)-based resins*: It is relatively stable to pH. The rate of cross-linking is directly related to the extent to which DVB resin shrinks or swells in an aqueous media in the presence of organic solvents. These resin-based chromatographic columns are stable

to pH. There is loss of column efficiency, if resins shrink on the other hand. Swelling of the resins leads to higher column back pressures. It is of two types:
   a. Anion-exchange resin
   b. Cation-exchange resin
2. *Silica-based resins ion exchangers*:
   a. *Polymer coated*: Coated with polystyrene, silicone, or fluorocarbon and then derivatized with functional groups
   b. *Functionalized silica materials*: It is chemically bonded directly to silica particle with functional groups. Disadvantage of this type of column is at a pH below the covalent bond linking, the ion-exchange functionality to the silica substrate becomes unstable, which yields poor resolved analyte peaks
3. *Chelating resins*: It can be used to separate metal ions. It is made up of suitable ligand immobilized onto a stationary phase. The ligands are chemically bound to the stationary phase by an appropriate reaction

Maintenance of Column Lifetime and Performance

- Use well-packed columns
- Avoid environment exposure and make sure both ends are capped properly with ferrule
- Avoid mechanical and thermal shock
- Use a guard column
- Always flush the column frequently with strong solvent
- Pretreat dirty samples to minimize particulates and strongly retained components of no interest
- Use organic buffers when operating at intermediate pH 6–8
- Use column temperatures of <40°C
- Use mobile phase pH between 3.0 and 8.0 for most silica-based columns
- Always store the column with end cap when not in use

Guard Column

It is a short column which is placed between injector and analytical column, which has a small quantity of adsorbent, which helps to protect the analytical column by adsorbing any unwanted particles from the samples. Packing material of the guard column is same as the analytical column and it does not help for separation process. Pictorial view of guard column is given in **Figure 7.14**. Guard columns may be packed with microparticulate stationary phases or porous layer beds. Guard column has following advantages:

- The life of column can be increased by introducing a guard column
- Guard column protects the HPLC column from damage or loss of efficiency caused by particulate matter or strongly absorbed substances in sample or solvents

HIGH-PERFORMANCE LIQUID CHROMATOGRAPHY AND ITS APPLICATIONS

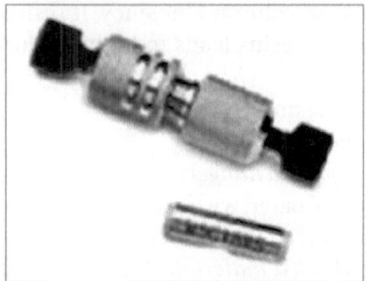

Fig. 7.14: High-performance liquid chromatography (HPLC) guard column.

Stationary Phase or Column Chemistry

Highly polar stationary phase materials are used for normal-phase HPLC. Nonpolar or intermediate polar stationary phase materials are used for reverse-phase HPLC. Both polar as well as nonpolar stationary phase materials are extremely small, spherical, and porous silica particles.

Polar stationary phase: The polar stationary phase (**Fig. 7.15**) silica particles have hydroxyl functional group on their surface.

Bonded stationary phase: Bonded stationary phase are of two types, one is intermediate polar and other is nonpolar stationary phase.
1. *Intermediate stationary phase*: Intermediate polar stationary phase silica particles have nitrile functional group, which is obtained by the reaction of silica with acetonitrile (**Fig. 7.16**)

Fig. 7.15: Polar stationary phase [normal-phase high-performance liquid chromatography (HPLC)]

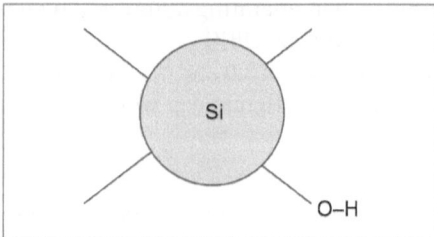

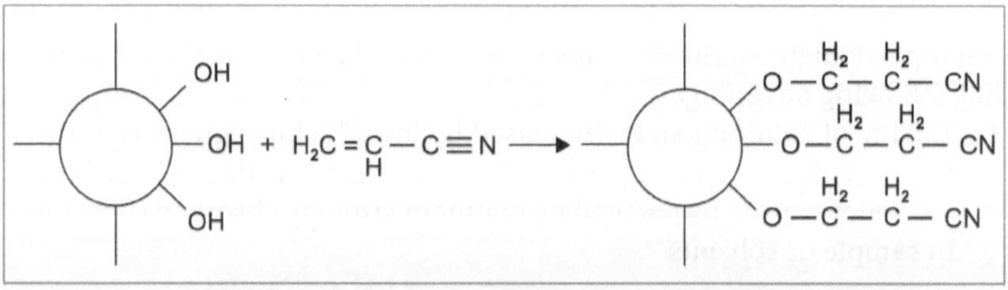

Fig. 7.16: Intermediate polar stationary phase.

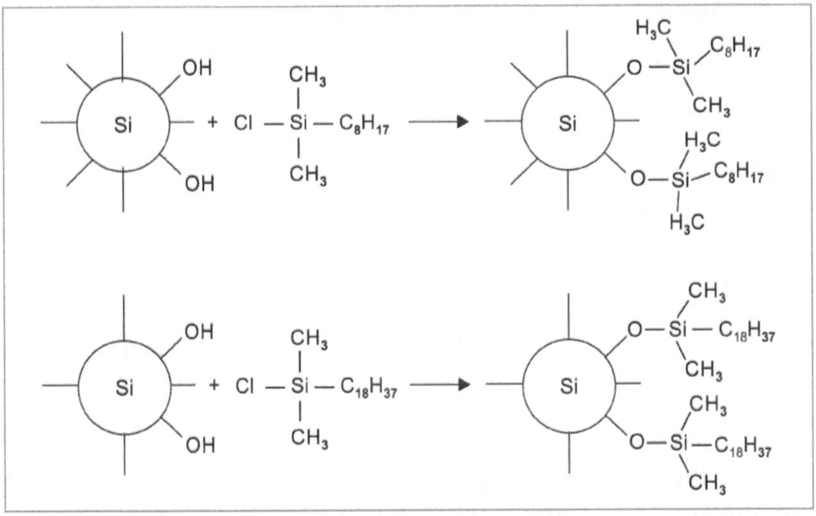

Fig. 7.17: Nonpolar stationary phase.

2. *Nonpolar stationary phase*: Nonpolar stationary phase silica particles have n-alkyl (C_8 or C_{18}) functional groups on their surface, which is obtained by silica with chlorosilanes (**Fig. 7.17**).

All these intermediate polar and nonpolar stationary phase particles are extremely small, spherical, and porous and provide large surface area of the stationary phase within small column. Therefore, complex mixtures as well as closely resembling compound get separated on these stationary phases. For this reason, these stationary phases are called high-performance materials and the technique is known as HPLC.

Column Packing

The packing material used in modern HPLC column consists of small, rigid particles having a narrow particle size distribution. Three main column packing are:

1. *Porous polymeric beds*:
   i. Based on styrene-divinyl benzene copolymers
   ii. These are used mainly in ion-exchange and size-exclusion chromatography
   iii. For many analytical purposes, these columns have now been replaced by silica-based packing, which are more efficient and mechanically more stable
2. *Porous layer beds*:
   i. It consists of a thin shell (1–3 μm) of silica or modified silica on a spherical inert core (e.g., glass beds)
   ii. It has not been used much in HPLC
3. *Totally porous silica particles*:
   i. These packings have widely been used for analytical HPLC in recent years

ii. The procedure chosen for column packing depends mainly on the mechanical strength of the packing and its particle size
iii. Particles of diameter > 20 µm are usually dry packed
iv. Particles of diameter < 20 µm are slurry packed

High-performance Liquid Chromatography Detectors

Detectors in HPLC are used to detect the molecules as a peak from the mobile phase that emerges from the column. The detector's results are presented as a record plotting of the components as peaks on a time scale, which is called as chromatogram. The detectors used in HPLC are classified on the basis of their properties here under. One of the functions of HPLC detector is to measure the concentration of eluting peak with respect to its molecular properties such as UV absorbance and refractive index. These detectors are selected depending on the nature of the compounds to be separated. Modern HPLC detectors equipped with wide linear, high sensitivity, and fast response, often allowing the detection range of nanograms (ng) and picogram (pg) levels of concentrated analyte normally found in biological samples with low drift and noise levels. Application comparison of HPLC detectors is given in **Table 7.4**. In addition, recent models are very flexible, allowing trace analysis even in femtograms (fg) on rapid conversion from one mobile phase to another and from one mode to another. The HPLC detectors are characterized by the following properties:

- *Sensitivity*: The detector must be highly sensitive for the compound to be tested and its reference
- *Linear response*: Importantly, detectors should have linear relationship in the sensitivity of solute particles at different concentrations
- *Type of response*: Whether the detector is universal, it is selective for certain particular compounds or certain components of solute
- *Response and detection limit*: The detector should be universal or selective for certain components of solute with extent of high sensitivity.

On the basis of physical properties, detectors are of two types:
1. *Bulk property detectors*: Based on overall changes in physical properties of mobile phase with or without an eluting solute, e.g., refractive index and conductivity detectors.
2. *Solute property detectors*: It is based on physical property of solute, which is not exhibited by the pure mobile phase. These are more sensitive and detect even a few nanograms of sample, e.g., UV detector, visible-absorption detector, fluorescent detector, and electron capture (EC) detector.

On the basis of above properties, there are several detectors which are coupled with HPLC such as:
1. Ultraviolet detector
2. Photodiode array (PDA) detector

Table 7.4: Application comparison of HPLC detectors.

Detectors	Analyte/Attributes	Sensitivity
UV-visible absorbance	Compounds with UV chromophores	ng-pg
Photodiode array (PDA)	Same as UV/visible detectors that also provide UV spectra	ng-pg
Fluorescence index (FI)	1. It is very specific 2. Used for compounds with native fluorescence or with fluorescent tag	fg-pg
Refractive index (RI)	1. Universal 2. Polymers, sugars, triglycerides, organic acids, etc.	0.1–10 µg
Evaporative light scattering detector (ELSD)	1. Universal 2. Nonvolatile or semivolatile compounds, compatible with radiant analysis	10 ng
Corona-charged aerosol detector (CAD)	1. Universal 2. Use nebulizer technology such as ELSD and detection of charges induced by a high voltage corona wire	Low ng
Chemiluminescent nitrogen detector (CLND)	Specific to nitrogen-containing compounds based on pyrochemiluminescence	Low ng
Electrochemical	1. It is very specific 2. Electroactive compounds (redox)	pg
Conductivity	Specific to anions and cations, organic acids, and surfactants	ng or ppm-ppb
Radioactivity	Specific, radioactive-labeled compounds	Low levels
Mass spectrometry (MS)	1. Both universal and specific, structural identification 2. Very sensitive and specific	pg-fg
Nuclear magnetic resonance (NMR)	Universal for structure elucidation and confirmation	µg-ng

(HPLC: high-performance liquid chromatography; UV: ultraviolet)

3. Refractive index (RI) detector
4. Fluorimetric detector
5. Atomic spectroscopic detector
6. Electrochemical detector (ECD)
7. Conductivity detector
8. Amperometric detector
9. Potentiometric detector
10. Nuclear magnetic resonance (NMR) detector
11. Chemiluminescent nitrogen detector (CLND)
12. Laser light scattering detector (LLSD)
13. Evaporative light scattering detector (ELSD)

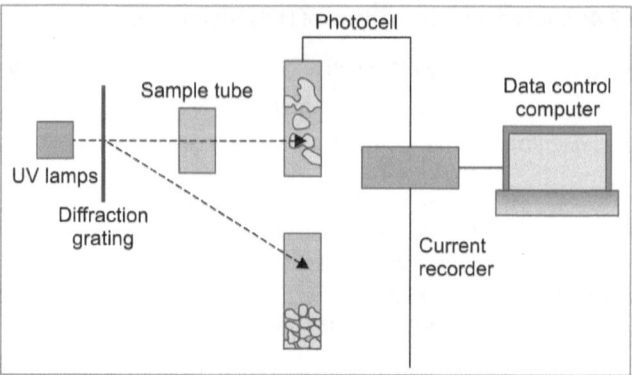

Fig. 7.18: Ultraviolet (UV) detector.

14. Corona detector
15. Chiral detectors
16. Radiometric detector

Ultraviolet detector: UV detectors (**Fig. 7.18**) have been one of the most widely used universal detectors in HPLC technique because most of the organic compounds absorb UV-visible light, as the effluent from the column is passed through a small flow, cell held in radiation beam. These are of two types:
1. Single beam UV detectors
2. Double-beam UV detectors

The only difference between these two detectors is of photocell, one for sample and one for reference in single-beam UV detector, while there are two different cells for sample and reference in double-beam UV detector. Each molecule at a particular wavelength (ë) absorbs UV light, which can be measured with UV detectors. It consists of deuterium lamp, a monochromator, and a small flow cell in which it measures the change in the UV absorption as the sample beam passes through the sample flow cell, which has typical volumes of 2–10 µL and path lengths of 2–10 mm, with quartz lenses. A monochromator consists of a movable prism that allows the selection of a specific wavelength (λmax) to pass through the exit slit for the samples that adsorb UV light in the range of 200–350 Å, including all substances having one or more double bonds and all substances that have unshared electrons, e.g., all olefins, all aromatics, and all substances containing >C=O, >C=S, -N=O, -N=N- groups. Based on the mechanism, there are two types of UV detector: (1) fixed wavelength detector and (2) the multiwavelength detector. In fixed wavelength detector, UV lamp passes through the cell and falls on a UV photoelectric cell, which operates at fixed 254 nm in which most of the drug compounds will absorb, e.g., mercury vapor lamp (253.7 nm), cadmium vapor lamp (228.8 and 346.6 nm). Variable wavelength detector can operate from 190 to 600 nm (**Fig. 7.19**).

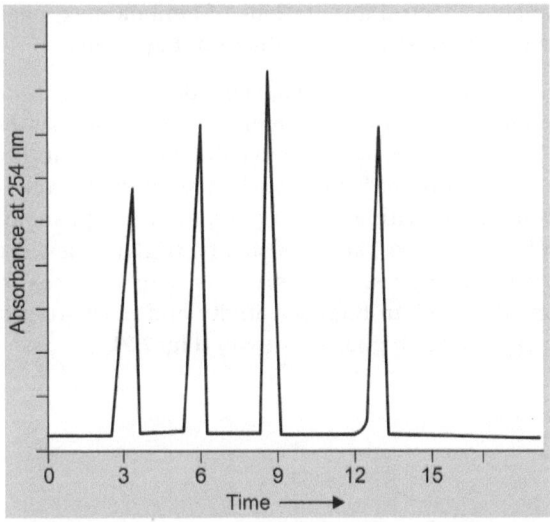

(HPLC: high-performance liquid chromatography; UV: ultraviolet)
Fig. 7.19: Typical HPLC chromatogram with UV absorbance.

Advantages and disadvantages of UV detector are given below:
- It is based on the principle of absorption of UV-visible light as the effluent from the column
- It is characterized by high sensitivity
- It is not sensitive to change in temperature and flow rate because it is a solute property detector
- It is suitable for gradient elution because many solvents used in HPLC do not absorb to any significant extent

Although it is the most popular detector, it has some definite limitations particularly, these detectors cannot be used for the nonpolar compounds that do not have a UV chromophore. But, this can be overwhelmed using derivatization method.

Photodiode array detector: The application of fixed and variable detectors was found to be somewhat limited. This urges the optional PDA detector in HPLC, which can operate by using a charge-coupled diode array with 512–1,024 diodes (or pixels) capable of spectral resolution of about 1 nm with wide range of wavelength simultaneously. The PDA detector generates a spectrum when a polychromatic beam from the source is irradiated onto the slit of polychromator after passing through the sample compartment. The polychromator disperses the narrow band of the spectrum onto the diode array, where it converts light into electrical signals to record as time-series signals. As the PDA acquires data at each wavelength by electrical scanning, the wavelength reproducibility of a PDA instrument is much better than the conventional mechanical scanning. UV-visible spectrophotometer, as the spectral evaluation software, allows the display of both chromatographic and spectral data in samples. The application of PDA detector is worth, since

HIGH-PERFORMANCE LIQUID CHROMATOGRAPHY AND ITS APPLICATIONS

it gives automated spectral annotations of lambda max, peak matching, library searches, and peak purity evaluation (**Fig. 7.20**).

Refractive index detector: It is a nonspecific detector, which measures the change in refractive index in the eluent as the solute passes through a sample cell. This detector is less used in HPLC because of its low sensitivity (0.01–0.1 µg) and poor reproducibility when temperature and flow change. It is also incompatible with gradient elution, although some analytes of low chromophoric samples, such as sugars, triglycerides, organic acids, pharmaceutical excipients, and polymers, can be measured without derivatization. They lack in high sensitivity and need strict temperature control to be operated at higher sensitivity (**Fig. 7.21**).

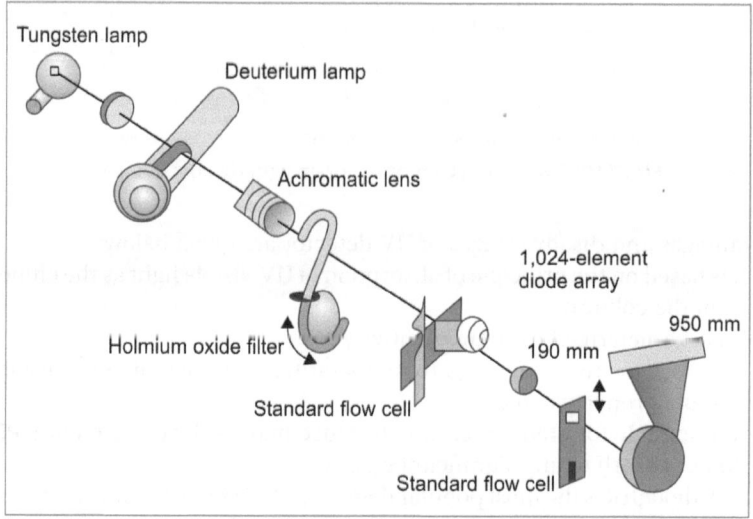

Fig. 7.20: Photodiode array detector.

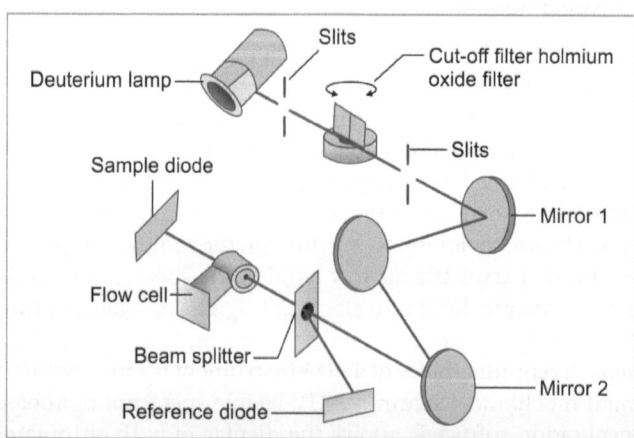

Fig. 7.21: Refractive index detector.

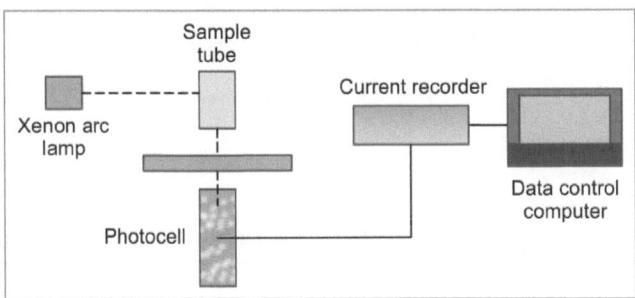

Fig. 7.22: Fluorimetric detector.

Fluorimetric detector: Fluorescence detector is selective and extremely sensitive, which is able to detect the analyte concentration of up to picogram and femtogram level. It works by monitoring the emitted fluorescent light of an analyte when passing through the flow cell at a particular wavelength with irradiation of an excitation light. It consists of a xenon source, an excitation monochromator, emission monochromator, a square flow cell optical slits, and a photomultiplier for amplifying the emitted photons. It can also measure phosphorescence, chemiluminescence, and bioluminescence (**Fig. 7.22**).

These are extensively used for polycyclic hydrocarbons, sulfa drugs, environmental contaminants, etc. Many organic and inorganic fluorescent materials can be detected with sensitivity with these detectors. Several biologically active compounds, drugs and environmental contaminants, e.g., polycyclic hydrocarbons (aromatic), can be detected with high sensitivity with these detectors.

Atomic spectroscopic detector: Atomic spectroscopy is the technique to determine the elemental composition of an analyte. Those levels have well-defined energies and electrons moving between them must absorb or emit energy equal to the difference between them. In this technique, the atomic species can only be performed on a gaseous medium in which the individual atoms are well separated from one another. Since every element has a unique electronic structure, the wavelength of light emitted is a unique property of each individual element. There are many electronic transitions which can occur, each transition resulting in the emission of a characteristic wavelength of light. The atomic spectroscopy has yielded three techniques for analytical use: (1) atomic absorption, (2) atomic emission, and (3) atomic fluorescence.

Electrochemical detector: ECD is used to measure the electric current generated by electroactive analytes in the eluent between electrodes in the flow cell. It has common electrode materials, such as carbon, silver, gold, or platinum, operated in oxidative or reductive mode. It is extremely sensitive in measuring sugars, glycoprotein, catecholamines, and neurotransmitters. Schematic diagram of ECD is given in **Figure 7.23**.

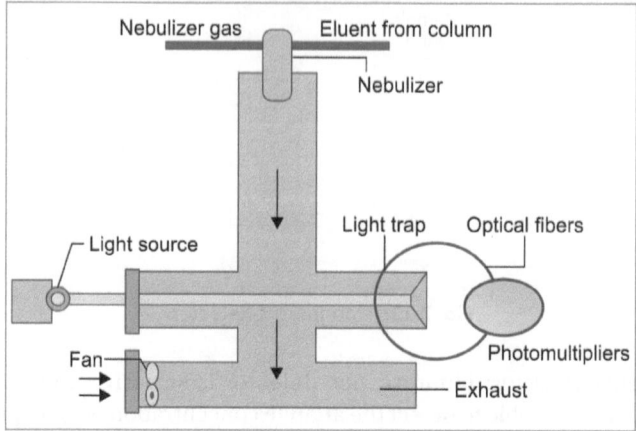

Fig. 7.23: Electrochemical detector (ECD).

Conductivity detector: Conductivity detectors are used to detect electrically conducting ions based on conductance of an eluent prior or during elution of any analyte. The detector actually measures the electrical resistance between the electrodes by suitable nonlinear amplification, an output that is linearly related to solute concentration. The sensitivity of the detector depends on the considerable difference of ionic conductance of the solute and eluent ions. The resulting difference can be positive or negative depending on whether the eluent ion is weakly or strongly conducting nature, resulting in direct or indirect detection, respectively. AC voltage is used across the electrodes with the frequency potential of 10 kHz.

Amperometric detector: Amperometry and potentiometry techniques have increased applications in recent years. Amperometric detection provides sensitive and selective detection for a limited range of anions such as cyanide sulfide, bromide, iodide nitrite, sulfite, and thiosulfate. Amperometric detection with HPLC is a very powerful combination for trace and ultratrace analysis of electrochemically active compounds. Some of electrochemical inactive compounds can also be chemically converted to oxidizable or reducible derivatives by precolumn derivatization and postcolumn derivatization. Amperometric detector functions with the current, which is in the pA to µA, amplified, and recorded as a function of the time flow of the mobile phase. The concentration-time profile or chromatogram of the analyte in the effluent can be measured by the rate of amplification. The potential of the working electrodes is set relative to the reference electrode and the current flowing through the working electrode is the measured signal. The current flowing from the electrode process is proportional to the analyte concentration (Faraday's law) under hydrodynamic conditions. Increasing the electrode surface area will increase the sensitivity in an amperometric detector. Carbon is the preferred electrode material. It is important that the HPLC column is a reverse-phase type, so that aqueous mixed solvent eluents, buffers, or supporting electrolyte salts, which are soluble, can be used. Detector cell is constructed from polychlorotrifluoroethylene, whereas indenoperylene, fluoranthene and benzopyrene give a maximum detection signal at potentials between +1.30 and +1.35 V. Detection limits are usually in the sub μg/liter range.

Potentiometric detector: Potentiometry is the process in which potential changes at an indicator electrode are measured with respect to a reference electrode under conditions of constant current flow. It is normally performed with an ion-selective electrode of some kind, typically a solid-state or coated wire electrode. The potential of the indicator electrode varies with the concentration of a particular ion (or ions) in the analyte solution contacting electrode, and thereby, provides a means for determining ion concentrations. This approach is generally used when high detection selectivity is required rather than good detection sensitivity. Potentiometry is commercially successful for determination of number of metal cations, halogen anions, and some other small inorganic anions such as S^{2-}, SCN^-, NO_3^-, NO_2^-, and ClO_4^-. Their application extends to larger ionic organics including organic acids, amines, and basic pharmaceutical drugs.

Nuclear magnetic resonance detector: The combination of HPLC with NMR is a powerful tool for analyzing and characterizing complex chemical mixtures. NMR spectroscopy technique is the study of spin change in the nuclear level of a molecule when radiofrequency energy is absorbed in the presence of magnetic field. When energy in the form of radiofrequency is applied and when it is equal to processional frequency, then absorption of energy occurs and a NMR signal is recorded. HPLC with NMR has various applications such as separation and characterization of peptide, separation and identification of drug metabolites in body fluids, lipoproteins from human serum, identification of drug impurities, and characterization of isomers of acid glucuronides and vitamin A derivatives.

Chemiluminescent nitrogen detector: Similar to mass spectroscopy, CLND can also be combined to HPLC for the structural analysis to interpretate the unknown compounds in the samples. The working principle of CLND is pyrochemiluminesence technology, where nitrogen-containing compounds are oxidized to nitric oxide, which will emit light at specific wavelength on reacting with ozone. Subsequently, CLND also responds to nitrogen content which may be present in the sample. CLND cannot be used with mobile phase containing acetonitrile or ammonium compounds, but it can be calibrated with compounds of known nitrogen content.

Laser light scattering detector: LLSD can approximately determine molecular weight of an analyte even without reference standard. However, the accuracy of LLSD for determining molecular weight is far below than that of measuring by LC-MS.

Evaporative light scattering detector: ELSD measures the scattered radiation of a laser beam of nonvolatile analytes by nebulizing the HPLC eluent. Unlike RI detector, it has an advantage of eminent sensitivity (~10 ng) with gradient elution compatibility, even with measurement of compounds of low UV absorbance, e.g. sugars, triglycerides.

Corona detector: A corona-charged aerosol detector is a new HPLC detector introduced by ESA in 2004. Unlike frequent techniques with other detectors, corona detector is used to determine the concentration of any compounds in a sample irrespective of their physiochemical characteristics, which include high-molecular weight, neutral, acidic, basic and Zwitter-ionic small molecules as well as proteins, carbohydrates in various types of sample matrices. Basically, corona detector operates by nebulizing the mobile phase using stream of nitrogen gas, positive-charged ions induced by a high voltage corona wire. It has high sensitivity in measuring concentration of an analyte even in nanogram level with high response factor relatively independent of chemical structure. Schematic diagram of corona detector is given in **Figure 7.24**.

Chiral detector: Combination of HPLC, with chiral detectors, commonly used to distinguish between the enantiomeric forms of an analyte or molecules to obtain the sign of rotation information. However, structural information of an analyte was not possible with this detector.

Radiometric detector: Radiometric detector operates with liquid scintillation technology to measure radioactivity of a radioactive compound passing

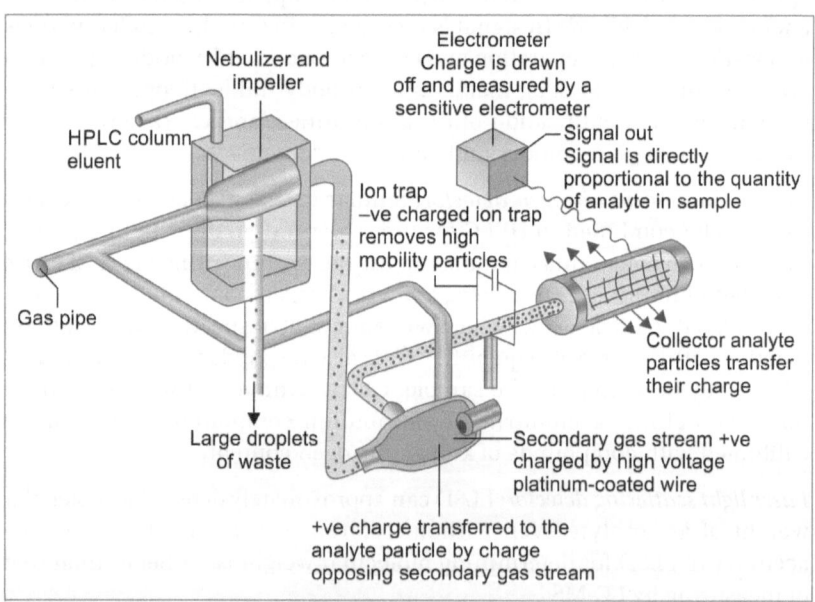

(HPLC: high-performance liquid chromatography)

Fig. 7.24: Corona detector.

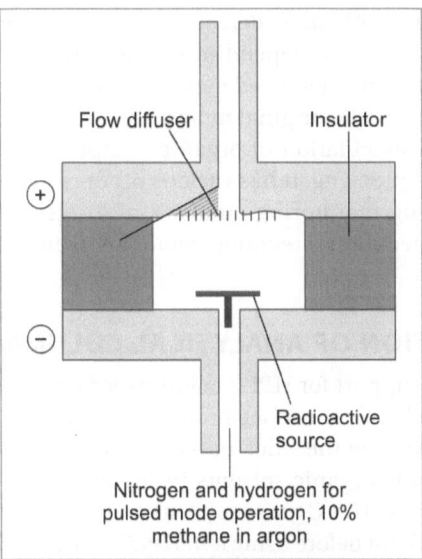

Fig. 7.25: Radiometric detector.

through a flow cell. These detectors are specific to radioactive compounds or tritium, C_{14} radiolabeled compounds in toxicology, metabolism, or degradation studies. It has the advantage of acquiring extremely sensitive detection by converting the analytes into more chromophoric forms by postcolumn derivatization. For example, amino acid analysis using ninhydrin (with visible detection) and carbamate pesticide analysis using o-phthalaldehyde (with fluorescence detection). Schematic diagram of radiometric detector is given in **Figure 7.25**.

All the above detectors have different sensitivity that is used for different analyte. Comparative statements of these are given in **Table 7.4**.

■ COMBINATION OF HIGH-PERFORMANCE LIQUID CHROMATOGRAPHY WITH OTHER TECHNIQUES

Liquid Chromatography-Fourier-transform Infrared Spectroscopy

The HPLC can be combined with Fourier-transform infrared spectroscopy (FTIR) to generate valuable structural information to interpretate the chemical structure of all unknown compounds, which may present in the complex samples. It is mostly used by trapping and evaporating aliquots of the column effluent, followed by spectroscopic measurement.

Liquid Chromatography-mass Spectroscopy

Mass spectrometry is an analytical tool used for measuring the molecular mass of a sample. Mass spectra are also called as positive ion spectra. Its work is based on the separation, detection, and recording of the ions formed by ionization of molecules. Depending on the nature of ionization and the molecular structure, intact ionized molecules or fragments were produced, which help to identify the original molecules. Mass spectrometry is useful for the structural elucidation of organic compounds and for peptide or oligonucleotide sequencing. It has various other clinical applications such as therapeutic drug monitoring, analysis of drugs abuse, poisons, toxic and illicit drugs, neonatal screening, hemoglobin analysis, and other drug testing.

■ REGENERATION OF ANALYTICAL COLUMN

Silica is the ideal support for HPLC columns for its stability; because of its excellent physicochemical surface properties, columns are stable within a pH range of 2–8. Most of the silica-based stationary phases are compatible with all HPLC grade organic solvents in the above pH range. Precaution should be taken to use HPLC grade solvents and also to filtered mobile phase buffer through 0.45 µm before using it in HPLC. The non-HPLC grade solvent will cause adsorption of impurities on the column head which leads to block the adsorption site, which can cause back pressure and "ghost peaks". It is ideal that a contaminated column must be cleaned and regenerated to return it to its original operating conditions with the help of a stronger solvent or series of solvents to get a steady baseline. Generally, these silica columns are always stored in aprotic solvents (acetonitrile), in which the water content should not be higher than 50%. Ideal column washing system for a typical bonded silica column is a mobile phase without buffer salts, 100% methanol, 100% acetonitrile, 75% acetonitrile, 25% isopropanol, 100% isopropanol, 100% methylene chloride, and 100% hexane. A minimum of 10 column volumes of each wash solvents should be passed with optimum flow rate. Using isopropanol as an intermediate solvent is recommended followed by mobile phase without buffer, finally with the starting mobile phase composition. Tetrahydrofuran is another popular solvent that can be used for cleaning contaminated columns. For severe fouling, mix dimethyl sulfoxide (DMSO) or dimethylformamide in 50:50 ratio with water and pass them at flow rates <0.5 mL/min. The regeneration of a reverse-phase column is a time-consuming process, so it can be programmed as an overnight process.

Regeneration process for columns, which is used for biological samples analysis, such as serum or plasma, is somewhat different. In most cases, organic solvents such as acetonitrile or methanol are ineffective for cleaning, since it does not dissolve peptides and proteins. However, mixtures of organic solvents with buffer, acids, sometimes, ion-pairing reagents can be effective. Some study suggests that up-and-down gradients between aqueous trifluoroacetic acid and trifluoroacetic acid-propanol can regenerate contaminated reverse-phase columns, which are used for biological samples. However, flushing a column with mobile phase that contains somewhat higher percentage of the stronger solvent should be attempted.

Strong eluents or solubilizing agents can be used to remove proteins. Certain polymer-based columns can swell or shrink with particular solvent combinations, but silica-based columns are usually compatible.

■ EFFECT OF TEMPERATURE IN HIGH-PERFORMANCE LIQUID CHROMATOGRAPHY

Advantages of an Increase in Temperature

1. An increase in temperature shortens the analysis time for most mobile phases
2. Peaks, which are normally hidden, suddenly appear as the temperature rises
3. The number of theoretical plates is also expected to increase on the temperature rise
4. The use of temperature increase as a means of improving resolution is very suitable in case of ion-exchange and ion-pair chromatography, but not for absorption method
5. High temperature is also required for highly viscous solvents or sample

Disadvantages of an Increase in Temperature

1. In HPLC, solvent or sample component is expected to decompose
2. In HPLC, the vapor pressure of solvent increases. It causes the risk of bubbles in the detector, which may then produce uneven baseline, ghost peaks, or even complete light absorption
3. In HPLC, reproducibility is expected to be poor, if proper thermostating is not made
4. The solubility of silica is greatly enhanced in all mobile phases as the temperature rises
5. In HPLC, the maximum temperature is around 120°C for silica columns and should not exceed 80°C in chemically bonded systems

■ TECHNICAL SPECIFICATIONS FOR HIGH-PERFORMANCE LIQUID CHROMATOGRAPHY SYSTEM

Thermostated Column Compartment

- *Temperature range*: 10°C below ambient to 80°C or more
- *Temperature stability*: ±0.15°C or better
- *Temperature accuracy*: ±0.8°C or better
- *Column capacity*: Three columns of 30 cm or more

Pump Quaternary Gradient

- Low pressure mixing quaternary gradient pump
- *Flow rate range*: 0.001–10.0 mL/min
- *Pressure*: 0–400 bar or more

- *Flow precision*: <0.1% RSD
- *Flow accuracy*: ±1% or more
- Rheodyne injector with different loop sizes

Vacuum Degasser (Four Channel Online)

Rapid degassing of up to four solvents including tubings, fittings, bottles, and organizer.

Ultraviolet Detector

- *Wavelength range*: 190–800 nm
- *Light source*: D2 and tungsten
- *Spectral bandwidth*: Programmable from 1 to 16 nm
- *Wavelength accuracy*: ±1 nm or more
- *Linearity*: >2 AU upper limit

Refractive Index Detector

- *RI range*: 1–1.75
- *Noise*: ±2.5 × 10^{-9} RIU
- *Temperature control*: Up to 50°C or more
- *Flow cell*: Approximately 7–9 μL volume
- *pH range*: 4.0–9.5

Photodiode Array Detector

- *Number of diodes*: 1,024
- *Light source*: D2 and tungsten
- *Wavelength range*: 190–800 nm
- *Spectral bandwidth*: Programmable from 1 to 16 nm
- *Noise*: ±0.9 × 10^{-5} AU at 254 nm and at 750 nm
- *Wavelength accuracy*: ±1 nm
- *Flow cell*: Approximately 10–15 μL volume and 8–10 mm path length
- *Linearity*: >2 AU upper limit or more

Accessories and Spares

- C-18, C-8, 250 × 4.6 mm, 5 μ—two each
- Si, amino, cyano 250 × 4.6 mm, 5 μ—one each
- Guard columns for the above columns
- *Syringes*: 10 μL, 25 μL—five each, and 100 μL, 500 μL—two each

Control Unit

- *Software*: 32 bit windows XP-based software for single point control of all the modules for data acquisition and procession. It should have the validation built in as per good laboratory practice (GLP), multilevel password protection, audit trail facility, and system suitability test (SST) for the validation of the column parameters

- *Computer*: Latest branded computer with all facility
- *Printer*: Laser jet printer

Others/Miscellaneous
- Online UPS for the system with 30-minute battery backup
- Solvent filtration kit
- High-performance liquid chromatography grade solvent—methanol, ethanol, acetonitrile, acetone, ethyl ether, benzene, and water, each 5 L

This is a general specification, which can be changed as per the laboratory requirement.

■ DERIVATIZATION TECHNIQUES IN HIGH-PERFORMANCE LIQUID CHROMATOGRAPHY

Derivatization is a technique in which a chemical compound is converted into a product of similar chemical structure to facilitate the sensitive detection with the available detection system in a laboratory. The resulted derivatized product is called as derivative. For example, compounds which have chromophore moiety in its chemical structure can be easily detected with UV light as a peak, whereas compounds with no chromophore cannot be detected by UV. Therefore, compounds can be derivatized so that it can absorb UV light to measure as a signal to record a chromatogram.

To overcome derivatization for UV, alternative detectors can also be used such as fluorescence and refractive index detectors for some organic compounds. In some cases, materials that show no or little UV absorbency, derivatization method is applied to improve detection specifically when determining traces of analytes in complex matrices such as biological samples such as blood, serum, and urine. For example, ninhydrin derivatizing agent is used to derivatize amino acid at the wavelength of 570 nm in UV light and dansyl chloride derivatizing agent is used to derivatize proteins, amines, and phenolic compounds in fluorescence detector at excited wavelength of 335 nm and emission wavelength of 365 nm.

There are two types of derivatization techniques:
1. Precolumn offline derivatization—requires no modification to the instrument
2. Postcolumn online derivatization—separation and detection process can be optimized individually.

■ BIOLOGICAL SAMPLE PREPARATION FOR HIGH-PERFORMANCE LIQUID CHROMATOGRAPHY ANALYSIS

Sample preparation is one of the key important procedures in bioanalytical techniques, which need a thorough understanding about the sample and its interference. The biological samples should not be injected as such into the analytical column in HPLC analysis, since proteins and other interferences can interact with bonded phase to alter the characteristic of the analytical column. Therefore, biological samples have to be deproteinized before an analytical injection into the column, which can be achieved by mixing equal volume of organic solvents, e.g., methanol, vortex and centrifuge to separate denatured proteins and inject the clear supernatant. In any toxicological testing, once the suspected toxin is found to be moderately lipophilic compound having methanol solubility with good UV absorption, then partition chromatography with reverse-phase column may be employed. In many cases of toxicological emergencies, screening the plasma drug concentration would be higher than the normal levels expected. In all poisoning cases, identification of the toxin itself is a successful task for their clinical management. Types of biological samples for toxicological examinations by HPLC are:

1. Whole blood/Plasma/Serum
2. Cerebrospinal fluid (CSF)
3. Saliva/Sweat/Vitreous humor
4. Hair/Nail
5. Bile
6. Urine/Feces
7. Tissues
8. Breast milk

Although for most of the bioanalytical techniques, plasma is the choice of matrix, but unfortunately, there may be interference from the unknown substance usually present in the plasma, which is also termed as matrix effect. If the sample contains known toxins, it can be easily quantified against a reference standard injection, whereas if unknown toxins are detected, it can be qualitatively determined against a group of reference standard injection available in the laboratory. On completion of the qualitative determination, subsequently, it can be quantified as well successfully.

■ QUALITATIVE AND QUANTITATIVE ANALYSIS IN HIGH-PERFORMANCE LIQUID CHROMATOGRAPHY

Qualitative Analysis

Qualitative analysis is a technique in HPLC widely used to identify unknown components in the sample by comparing against the reference standard. Generally, qualitative analysis is performed by comparing the peak retention time of unknown components with the reference standard peak retention time in chromatographic analysis. However, sometimes, retention time in HPLC is not fixed and is affected by many factors. If the components have the variable retention time against the reference standard retention times, one can identify by measuring relative retention time (RRT) and relative retention factor (RRF) in critical situations. For further confirmation, one can also spike the samples with reference standard to confirm the peak identity.

Quantitative Analysis

Quantification is a technique in HPLC in which the concentration of the unknown compounds can be estimated against the known concentration of reference standard. This is the most widely used technique in HPLC; it is performed by measuring peak area and peak height of both known and unknown sample to estimate the concentration. However, in bioanalytical procedures, standard calibration techniques are used routinely. It is of two types:
1. *External standard method*: Multiple concentrations of the standard mixtures containing known concentrations of analytes are analyzed and their peak response is recorded. A calibration graph of area versus concentration of drug is plotted to confirm a linear detector response, from which the amount of unknown analyte is determined by interpolation.
2. *Internal standard method*: It requires extensive sample preparation procedures. An internal standard is selected accordingly, so that it has the same retention time such that it is eluted close to the retention time of analytes. It is performed by adding known concentration of internal standard to the sample matrix. The calculation is based on peak area ratio of sample response and internal standard and the concentration of unknown solution is determined.

■ METHOD VALIDATION

It is essential for bioanalytical procedures, which require some form of validation so as to generate repeated reliable results from chromatographic techniques such as HPLC. The primary objective of method validation is to provide a high degree of assurance that the specified newly developed HPLC method consistently generates accurate test results. However, validation does help a method better or more efficient. It is a process to confirm that the method is suited for its intended purpose. The method validation parameters include:
1. *Specificity*: Specificity measures the analyte of interest in the presence of other components in the sample matrix
2. *Linearity*: Linearity measures the ability of the method to quantitate the compound over multiple concentrations
3. *Range*: Range measures the interval between the upper and lower levels of an analyte that has been determined with acceptable precision with accuracy and linearity
4. *Accuracy*: Accuracy is the measure of exactness of an analytical method
5. *Precision*: Precision is the measure of degree of repeatability of an analytical method

6. *Limit of detection (LOD) and limit of quantification (LOQ)*: LOD and LOQ are the measurement of lowest concentration of any analyte in a sample that can be detected and quantified
7. *Robustness*: Robustness is to measure the capacity of an analytical method to remain unaffected by small deliberate or accidental variations in specified method parameters

■ RECENT DEVELOPMENT IN HIGH-PERFORMANCE LIQUID CHROMATOGRAPHY IS ULTRA-PERFORMANCE LIQUID CHROMATOGRAPHY

In the year 2004, first commercial ACQUITY ultra-performance liquid chromatography (UPLC) (**Fig. 7.26**) was introduced by Waters Corporation, one of the pioneers in manufacturing of HPLC instruments. UPLC has the same working principle of HPLC, with the advantage of chromatographic separation using shorter columns with higher flow rates to benefit with good sensitive resolved peaks with increased speed of analysis by reduced running time. The speed of the analysis lies in prime technology of packing material of the UPLC shorter column [bridged ethylene hybrid (BEH) 1.7 µm technology]. The typical UPLC column packed with narrow particle size of high strength silica (HSS) particles is governed by the van Deemter equation, which describes the relationship between linear velocity (flow rate) and plate height (HETP) or column efficiency that allow separation to achieve with maximum speed with high quality, sensitivity, and resolution in contrast with normal HPLC. The comparison of HPLC and UPLC is discussed in **Fig. 7.27**.

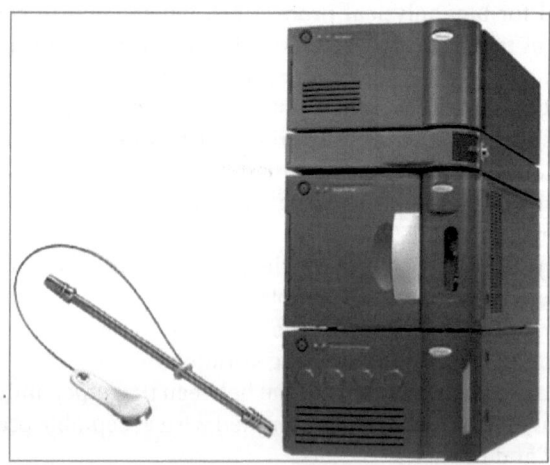

(BEH: bridged ethylene hybrid; UPLC: ultra-performance liquid chromatography)
Fig. 7.26: Waters ACQUITY UPLC with BEH column.

HIGH-PERFORMANCE LIQUID CHROMATOGRAPHY AND ITS APPLICATIONS

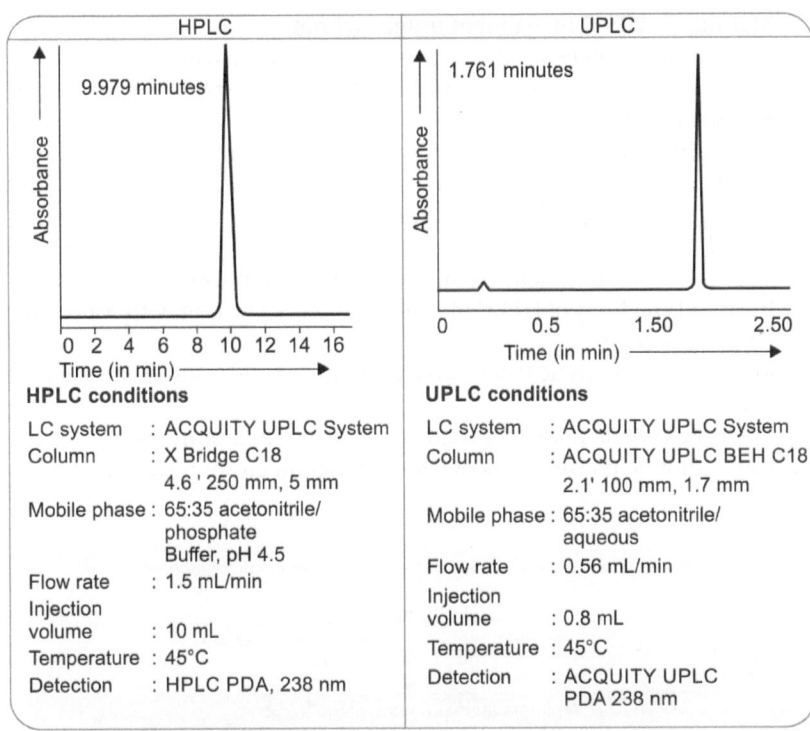

(HPLC: high-performance liquid chromatography; UPLC: ultra-performance liquid chromatography)

Fig. 7.27: Comparison of HPLC and UPLC chromatogram.

■ PERFORMANCE OF HIGH-PERFORMANCE LIQUID CHROMATOGRAPHY

A reference testing procedure should be performed periodically as a diagnostic test to insure that the overall HPLC system is functioning properly and the generated results were reliable enough. This test can be a system suitability test that can be performed with repeated injection of known concentration of reference standard routinely on the HPLC system or with the autosampler precision test used in HPLC calibration. This chromatogram documents the expected parameters under a set of standardized conditions when the system is functioning properly. It provides a powerful troubleshooting tool for diagnosing and fixing problems.

■ DO'S AND DON'TS FOR HIGH-PERFORMANCE LIQUID CHROMATOGRAPHY

Do's (Flowchart 7.3)

1. Maintain standard operating procedure (SOP) and follow GLP and good manufacturing practice (GMP) guidelines for handling HPLC

HIGH-PERFORMANCE LIQUID CHROMATOGRAPHY AND ITS APPLICATIONS

2. Maintain a HPLC instrument usage logbook
3. Trained personnel's should only operate HPLC instrument
4. Use manufacturer software to handle HPLC instrument instead of manual handling
5. Maintain a clean HPLC laboratory to avoid any cross-contamination
6. Calibrate the HPLC instrument periodically at least once in 6 months by authorized personnel or by a manufacturer and document the same as well
7. Leave the unit for at least 30 minutes ON for stabilization
8. Purge all the lines of HPLC instrument before starting with water and 50% acetonitrile
9. Maintain the analytical column with both the ends closed when not in use
10. Filter the mobile phase through 0.45 μ nylon membrane filter
11. Degas mobile phase with slow purged helium gas or ultrasonic bath

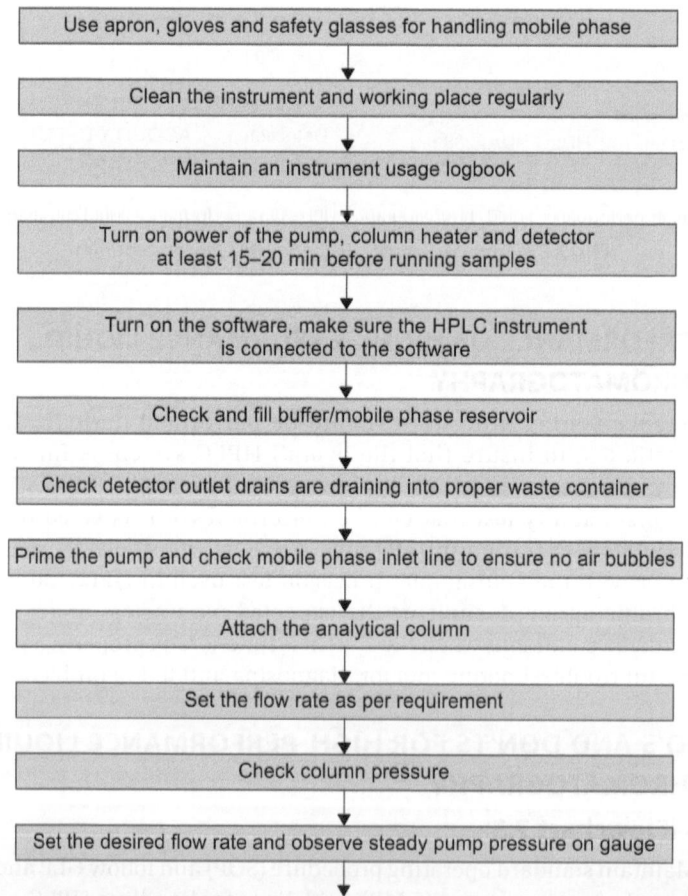

Continued

Continued

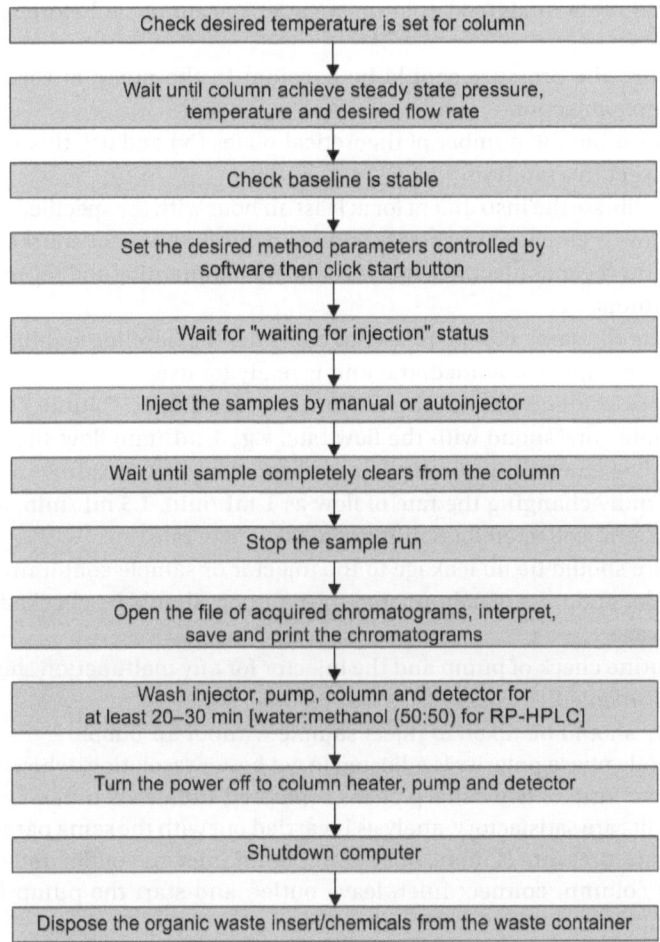

Flowchart 7.3: High-performance liquid chromatography (HPLC) instrument setup.

12. Equilibrate the analytical column with 50% of acetonitrile before using with 1.0 mL/min flow
13. Always use guard columns for any analysis to increase the life of analytical column
14. Monitor expected pressure in the pump and check for normal baseline
15. Monitor and replace or clean piston seals, check valves, and in filters regularly
16. Always clean and replace detector source such as deuterium lamp and flow cell, if contaminated
17. Switch off detector lamps when not in use to increase the life of lamp
18. Perform peak purity test before confirming a peak in PDA detector
19. Always clean the sample injection needle or autosampler with strong solvents

20. System suitability to be checked everyday before starting an analysis
21. Equilibrate analytical column with 50% acetonitrile before shutting down
22. Insure the pressure should be constant in the pump at the time of sample injection
23. Determine the number of theoretical plates (N) and use this value for consecutive analysis
24. Equilibrate the instrument for at least an hour with the specified method
25. Follow manufacturer specification to calibrate detector sources
26. Follow the manufacturer specification for maintaining and regenerating columns
27. Inject the same mobile phase for checking the baseline stability. Once the baseline is obtained, the unit is ready for use.
28. Check the flow rate of the eluent by collecting it. Volume collected should correspond with the flow rate, e.g., 1 mL/min flow should give 1 mL of eluent in 1 minute. For confirmation, three readings are to be taken by changing the rate of flow as 1 mL/min, 1.5 mL/min, and 2.0 mL/min, collected for 5 minutes at each flow rate
29. There should be no leakage to the injector or sample contamination
30. Outlet and inlet of column and injector port should be checked up for leakage
31. Routine check of pump and the injector for any malfunction should be documented
32. Care should be taken to inject sample without air bubble
33. Mobile phase polarity is adjusted to get better resolution, which will be in the form of good sharp peaks separated from each other. Once the results are satisfactory, analysis is carried out with the same parameters
34. If back pressure is more, open the column inlet and outlet and reverse the column, connect inlet, leave outlet, and start the pump for few minutes and then connect as usual
35. Flush mobile phase for 1 hour before and after the use of sample analysis for the column maintenance
36. Equilibrate instrument with 50% methanol when not in use
37. To attempt restitution of column performance, the column should be first flushed (reverse flow) with high aqueous content to wash out the buffer. This wash then should be followed by extensive flushing with 100% acetonitrile prior to equilibrating in the original mobile phase and retesting
38. System test—turn off all modules and power up to perform startup diagnostics. Perform static leak test of the pump and compression test of the autosampler as suggested by the manufacturer
39. For normal-phase separations, eluting power increases with increasing the polarity of the solvent, but for reverse-phase separations, eluting power decreases with increasing solvent polarity
40. Power supply should be given through UPS only

41. For manual injection, the sample is drawn into the syringe a number of times to remove any air bubble and injected very rapidly

Don'ts

1. Do not allow sample injection without complete tuning of the instrument
2. Do not inject biological samples directly into the HPLC instrument
3. Do not use contaminated, microbial growth, and precipitated buffers as mobile phase
4. Do not use expired HPLC grade solvents and reagents
5. Do not prepare samples near to HPLC instrument to avoid contamination
6. Do not open the column oven door in the mid of chromatographic run
7. Do not use RP-HPLC for NP-HPLC analysis as such, use after converting the phase
8. Do not overload the column with high concentrated samples
9. Do not store the column without end cap
10. Do not inject inorganic samples into the column
11. Do not use any mobile phase or sample without filtering. This can result in poor column efficiency and higher back pressure with poor peak shape
12. Do not allow any air bubbles either through syringe or line of mobile phase to the pump
13. Do not use mobile phase without degassing, since it may block the check valves of the pump
14. After injecting the sample, do not stop the analysis; wait till the assigned run time to complete, in order to avoid component deposition on column, which may lead carry over problems
15. Do not use any other grade solvent except HPLC grade for mobile phase as well as for preparation of standard and sample solution
16. Do not allow the temperature of the room to increase above 25°C. It causes risk of bubbles in the detector. This may then produce uneven baseline or short peak or even complete light absorption
17. Do not open sample cooler door at the run time of analysis
18. Do not switch off the instrument directly and use proper shutdown methods recommended by manufacturer
19. Do not use HPLC instrument computer for other works, besides, the HPLC analysis
20. Do not allow more viscous sample directly to the injector, dilute it, and then inject because lower viscosity usually gives greater chromatographic efficiency
21. Do not allow dust inside the HPLC room
22. Do not allow to operate the HPLC instrument by an unauthorized person
23. Do not inject sample in HPLC instrument, unless clear baseline is obtained
24. Do not allow any leakage on either side of the joints of the column
25. Do not use old solution for quantization and calibration
26. Do not use the HPLC instrument, unless it is calibrated properly

TROUBLESHOOTING IN HIGH-PERFORMANCE LIQUID CHROMATOGRAPHY

When we are operating HPLC, we will come across various problems. It is necessary to diagnose the problems and set the machine right. Some of the problems with their cause and solutions are mentioned in **Table 7.5**.

Table 7.5 Troubleshooting in high-performance liquid chromatography (HPLC).

Probable symptoms	Possible causes	Possible solution
Noisy baseline	1. Pump pulses 2. Bubbles in detector or mobile phase	1. Check and replace pump damper; purge air from pump; clean or replace check valves 2. Degas mobile phase
	3. Lack of solvent mixing	3. Monitor ultraviolet (UV) absorbance detector output and remix solvent
	4. External electrical interference	4. Use voltage stabilizer
	5. Continuous detector lamp problem or dry cell	5. Replace UV lamp, clean and flush flow cell
	6. Column contamination and column temperature	6. Flush column with strong solvent
Cyclic	1. Sensitivity too high	1. Adjust detector sensitivity
	2. Pump problem	2. Degas mobile phase and flush detector cell
Synchronous noise	1. Problem in pump	1. Clean and check valve or replace, mix the solvents, and degas
Spikes	1. Air bubbles in solvent or mobile phase	1. Degas mobile phase; use back pressure restrictor at detector outlet
	2. Storage of column without ferrules	2. Store column tightly capped; flush reverse-phase columns with degassed methanol and water
	3. Detector	3. Replace lamp
Asynchronous noise	1. Problem in pump bubble in the mobile phase	1. Mix the solvents, degas, flush detector, and change electric circuits

Continued

Continued

Probable symptoms	Possible causes	Possible solution
No peak	1. Detector off	1. Check detector
	2. Leakage	2. Check connections for leakage at detector end
	3. Wrong sample with wrong detector setting	3. Be sure, it is not deteriorated. Check for bubbles in the sample vial. Check attenuation
	4. Improper flow	4. Check the back pressure and rinse the pump
Drift	1. Negative direction absorbance of mobile phase	1. Use non-UV absorbing mobile phase solvents; use HPLC grade mobile phase solvents
	2. Positive direction	2. Use higher UV absorbance detector
Positive and negative peaks	1. Detector problem	1. Flush detector; change detector polarity, check attenuation
	2. Solvent	2. Change solvent
	3. Air bubble	3. Purge mobile phase or filter
	4. Pump problem	4. Filter and degas mobile phase
Tailing	1. Basic solutes—silanol interaction	1. Use peak modifier such as use base deactivated silica-based reverse-phase column
	2. Peak doubling	2. See peak doubling. Perform peak doubling test
	3. Contamination	3. Flush the column, detector, and pumping lines with ethanol and water thoroughly
	4. Void formation at head of column	4. Replace column or open top end fitting and clean and fill in void with glass beads or same column packing; rotate injection valve quickly
Fronting	1. Column overloaded	1. Use higher-capacity stationary phase; decrease sample amount; decrease injection volume
Poor separation	1. Blockage in frit	1. Replace or clean frit; eliminate sample contaminants
	2. Column overloaded	2. Decrease sample amount, possibly decrease column volume
	3. Carryover of interfering compound from previous injection	3. Flush column with strong solvent run
	4. Injection solvent too strong	4. Use weaker injection solvent or stronger mobile phase

Continued

HIGH-PERFORMANCE LIQUID CHROMATOGRAPHY AND ITS APPLICATIONS

Continued

Probable symptoms	Possible causes	Possible solution
Tailing on solvent peak	1. Contamination	1. Flush column and detector lines with HPLC gas solvent flush injector
	2. Carryover and previous injection	2. Flush column with strong solvent and ethanol gas run
	3. Void high back pressure	3. Check flow and clean pump seal and prime
Baseline separation	1. Contamination	1. Flush column occasionally
	2. Equilibrate	2. Condition column by injecting concentrated sample
	3. Buffer retention times	3. Use buffer with concentration greater than 20 mM
	4. Evaporation of mobile-phase component	4. Cover solvent reservoirs; use less vigorous helium purging; prepare fresh mobile phase
	5. Improper mixing	5. Check gradient system is delivering a constant composition; partially premix mobile phase
	6. Column temperature	6. Insure laboratory temperature is constant
Negative	1. UV-absorbance detection—absorbance of solute less than that of mobile phase	1. Use mobile phase with lower UV absorbance
	2. In RI detection—refractive index of solute is less than that of mobile phase	2. Reverse polarity to make peak positive
Broad	1. Overload	1. Dilute sample (1:10) and reinject
	2. Detector-cell volume too large	2. Use smallest possible cell volume consistent with sensitivity needs; use detector with no heat exchanger in the system
	3. Injection volume too large	3. Inject smaller volume
	4. Replace column	4. Use low or zero dead volume end fittings and connectors
	5. Mobile-phase solvent viscosity too high	5. Increase column temperature; change to lower viscosity solvent

Continued

Probable symptoms	Possible causes	Possible solution
	6. Peak dispersion in injector valve	6. Decrease injector sample loop size, introduce air bubble in front and back of sample in loop
	7. Poor column efficiency	7. Use smaller particle diameter packing; lower viscosity mobile phase; high column temperature; lower flow rate
	8. Retention time too long	8. Use gradient elution or stronger isocratic mobile phase
	9. Sampling rate of data system too low	9. Increase sampling frequency
	10. Slow detector time constant	10. Adjust time constant to match peak width
	11. Some peaks broad—late elution of analytes retained from previous injection	11. Flush column with strong solvent at end of run; end gradient at higher solvent concentration
Flat top	1. High concentration of sample	1. Reduce or dilute sample concentration
	2. High injection volume	2. Reduce injection volume
	3. Detector attenuation	3. Check for proper attenuator
Swinging baseline	1. Detector problem	1. Degas mobile phase, prime the pump
Jumping baseline	1. Detector problem	1. Adjust attenuation
Extraneous peak	1. Contamination or carryover	1. Clean sample syringe or prime autosampler; equilibrate the column in high proportion of organic solvents

■ RELEVANCE OF HIGH-PERFORMANCE LIQUID CHROMATOGRAPHY OVER GAS-LIQUID CHROMATOGRAPHY

1. Gas-liquid chromatography (GLC) is not applicable for inorganic compounds, while HPLC can detect inorganic compounds too
2. We can also analyze thermolabile compounds with HPLC, while with GLC, it is not possible

3. In GLC, only stationary phase and temperature effect the resolution and RT. But in HPLC, mobile phase also has a dramatic effect on RT and resolution
4. With GLC, we can analyze only 15–20% of all known compounds, whereas with HPLC, one can analyze almost all known compounds
5. If there is a small amount of sample with GLC, one cannot retain the sample. While, with HPLC, we retain the sample and this retained sample can be used for further analysis

■ FORENSIC APPLICATIONS OF HIGH-PERFORMANCE LIQUID CHROMATOGRAPHY

High-performance liquid chromatography is being extensively used nowadays in analysis of forensic investigations due to its high specificity and sensitivity. HPLC can detect large number of thermally labile molecules, which cannot be analyzed by GLC. HPLC is applied in detection and separation of substances on the basis of their chemical nature. Some common applications of HPLC are as follow:

Identification of Pesticides

Suicide by consuming pesticide is a common cause of death in India. Majority of the Indian population live in rural areas who are mostly farmers. There has been series of suicides by farmers in various parts of India due to tragedy of crop failure and financial burden of loan. Most of them have died due to pesticide poisoning, as it is easily available in their home. There has also been occupational disease due to chronic exposure to pesticides by contaminated groundwater. In the news, there were also allegations of detecting pesticides in soft drinks such as coca cola. In all these cases, HPLC plays a significant role in analyzing the pesticides content in the blood, tissues, and drinks.

Organophosphorus Insecticides

Organophosphorus insecticides such as dichlorvos, phosphamidon, parathion, methyl parathion, paraoxon, chlorothion, chlorpyrifos, malathion, dimethoate, morphothion, tetrathion, phosalone, edifenphos, trichlorfon, and EPN can be easily analyzed by HPLC. The chromatographic conditions for the organophosphorus compounds are given below:
- *Column*: 4.6 mm × 250 mm stainless steel tube slurry packed, 5 µm, cyno
- *Mobile phase*: 20% ethyl acetate in iso-octane
- *Flow rate*: 1 mL/min
- *Detector*: Refractive index detector
- *Injection volume*: 20 µL

Carbamate Pesticides

Carbamates such as propoxur, carbaryl, carbofuran, and zineb can be easily analyzed by HPLC. The chromatographic conditions for carbamates are given below:
- *Column*: 150 mm × 4.6 mm, 5 μm, C18
- *Mobile phase*: 18% methanol in water for 0.5 minute followed by linear gradient to 70% methanol in water over 28.5 minute and now 70–100% methanol for 1 minute finally, 100% methanol for 10 minute
- *Flow rate*: 1 mL/min
- *Detector*: Fluorescence detector
- *Excitation*: 330 nm
- *Injection volume*: 10–20 μL

Pyrethroids

The analysis of pyrethroids such as fenvalerate, permethrin, dichlorovinyl, cyfluthrin, deltamethrin, fenpropathrin, and bifenthrin in forensic samples can be done through HPLC using high-performance column, new detector, optimum methods, etc. The chromatographic conditions for pyrethroids are given below:

Condition I:
- *Column*: 200 mm × 4.6 mm, 5 μm, hypersil
- *Mobile phase*: Hexane: Dichloromethane (85:15)
- *Flow rate*: 15 mL/min
- *Detector*: UV
- *Excitation*: 212 nm

Condition II:
- *Column*: 150 mm × 7 mm LiChrosorb, RP-8
- *Mobile phase*: Hexane: Dipropyl ether (93:7)
- *Flow rate*: 1.33 mL/min
- *Detector*: UV
- *Excitation*: 230 nm

Identification of Common Drugs

High-performance liquid chromatography methods are used in screening, identification, and quantification of several drugs of forensic samples. These drugs may be basic, acidic, or neutral. HPLC techniques are especially applied for amphetamines, antidepressants, narcotics, etc.

Amphetamine

Amphetamine is a psychostimulant drug that is known to produce increased wakefulness and focus in association with decreased fatigue and appetite. Amphetamine is related to drugs, such as methamphetamine and lisdexamfetamine, which are a group of potent drugs that act by increasing levels of dopamine and norepinephrine in the brain, inducing euphoria. The chromatographic conditions for amphetamines are given below:

Condition I:
- *Column*: 4.9 mm × 125 mm, 5 µm, silica
- *Eluent*: A solution of 1.175 g (0.01 M) of ammonium perchlorate in 1,000 mL of methanol with adjustment of pH at 6.7 by adding 1 mL of sodium hydroxide in methanol
- *Detector*: UV detector with a wavelength 254 nm.

Condition II:
- *Column*: 5 mm × 250 mm, 5 µm, ODS-silica
- *Eluent*: 19.66 g (0.2 M) phosphoric acid and 7.314 g (0.1 M) diethylamine in 1,000 mL of 10% methanol with a pH 3.14 by addition of NaOH
- *Detector*: UV detector with a wavelength 254 nm

Antidepressants

An antidepressant is a psychiatric medication used for alleviating major depression or dysthymia. Drug groups known as monoamine oxidase inhibitors (MAOIs), tricyclics, and second-generation antidepressants, such as selective serotonin reuptake inhibitors (SSRIs) and serotonin-norepinephrine reuptake inhibitors (SNRIs), are particularly associated with the term. Antidepressants are often used in the treatment of other conditions including anxiety disorders, bipolar disorder, chronic pain, dysmenorrheal, etc. The chromatographic conditions for antidepressants are given below:

Condition I:
- *Column*: 4.9 mm × 125 mm, 5 µm, silica
- *Eluent*: A solution of 1.175 g of ammonium perchlorate in 1,000 mL of methanol with adjustment of pH at 6.7 by adding 1 mL of sodium hydroxide in methanol
- *Detector*: UV detector with a wavelength 254 nm

Condition II:
- *Column*: 5 mm × 125 m, 5 µm, ODS-silica
- *Eluent*: Acetonitrile: Phosphate buffer (30:70)
- *Detector*: UV with wavelength 254 nm

Antihistamines

These are the drugs, which are used to decrease the secretion of histamine in blood. They are also known as antiallergens, e.g. chlorphenamine, promethazine, cetirizine. The chromatographic conditions for antihistamines are given below:
- *Column*: Silica 5 µm, 125 mm × 4.9 mm
- *Eluent*: A solution of 1.175 g of ammonium perchlorate in 1,000 mL of methanol with adjustment of pH at 6.7 by adding 1 mL of sodium hydroxide in methanol
- *Detector*: UV detector with a wavelength 254 nm

Anesthetics

Local anesthetics are agents, which prevent transmission of nerve impulses without causing unconsciousness. Local anesthetics can be either ester or amide based. Inhaled general anesthetic agents are desflurane, xenon, and isoflurane. The chromatographic conditions for anesthetics are given below:

Condition I:
- *Column*: Silica 5 µm, 125 mm × 4.9 mm
- *Eluent*: A solution of 1.175 g of ammonium perchlorate in 1,000 mL of methanol with adjustment of pH at 6.7 by adding 1 mL of sodium hydroxide in methanol
- *Detector*: UV detector with a wavelength 254 nm

Condition II:
- *Column*: ODS-silica, 5 µm, 160 mm × 5 mm
- *Eluent*: Methanol: Water (30:70)
- *Detector*: UV detector with a wavelength 254 nm

Benzodiazepines

The benzodiazepines are a class of psychoactive drugs with varying hypnotic, sedative, anxiolytic, anticonvulsant, muscle relaxant, and amnesic properties, which are mediated by slowing down the central nervous system. They are useful in treating anxiety, insomnia, agitation, seizures, and muscle spasms as well as alcohol withdrawal. The chromatographic conditions for benzodiazepines are given below:

Condition I:
- *Column*: ODS-silica, 5 µm, 200 mm × 0.5 mm
- *Eluent*: Methanol: Water: Phosphate buffer (55:25:20)
- *Detector*: UV detector with a wavelength 254 nm

Condition II:
- *Column*: Silica, 5 µm, 250 mm × 5 mm
- *Eluent*: Methanol: Perchloric acid
- *Detector*: UV detector with a wavelength 254 nm

Phenothiazines

Phenothiazine is the organic compound with formula $S(C_6H_4)_2NH$. This yellow tricyclic compound is soluble in acetic acid, benzene, and ether. The compound is related to the thiazine class of heterocyclic compounds. Derivatives of the parent compound find wide use as drugs. The chromatographic conditions for phenothiazines are given below:
- *Column*: Silica, 5 mm, 125 mm × 4.9 mm
- *Eluent*: A solution of 1.175 g (0.01 M) of ammonium perchlorate in 1,000 mL of methanol with adjustment of pH at 6.7 by adding 1 mL of sodium hydroxide in methanol (0.1 M)
- *Detector*: UV detector with a wavelength 254 nm

Applied for Plant Poisons

Plant poisons are specially analyzed by HPLC techniques. The chromatographic conditions are mentioned here under.

Morphine and Other Alkaloids

Morphine is a highly potent opiate analgesic drug, is the principal active agent in opium, and is considered to be the prototypical opioid. Morphine was the first alkaloid isolated from plant source in 1803. It acts directly on central nervous system to relieve pains. Other alkaloids are quinine isolated from *Cinchona succirubra* and ergot alkaloids comes from *Claviceps purpurea*. The chromatographic conditions for morphine and other alkaloids are given below:
- *Column*: Alumina (250 mm × 4.6 mm)
- *Mobile phase*: Methanol: Acetonitrile: Citrate—TMS buffer (0.01 M) pH 6.0 (28:17:55)
- *Flow rate*: 1.0 mL/min
- *Detector*: UV detector with wavelength 260 nm and fluorescence detector with wavelength 260/400 nm

Strychnine

Strychnine nux-vomica or kuchila seed contains two main alkaloids: (1) strychnine and (2) brucine. The alkaloids are extracted from the tissues and other biological materials by organic solvents from alkaline aqueous solution. The chromatographic conditions for strychnine are given below:
- *Column*: Normal phase (normal silica gel 250 mm × 2.6 mm)
- *Mobile phase*: Ammonium hydroxide (28-30% NH_3): Methanol (0.75:99.25)
- *Flow rate*: 1.1 mL/min
- *Internal standard*: Quinine 10 mg/mL
- *Detector*: UV with wavelength 254 nm

Acidic Poisons

Acids such as hydroiodic acid, hydrobromic acid, hydrochloric acid, nitric acid, sulfuric acid, acetic acid, formic acid, hydrocyanic acid, oxalic acid, and nitrous acid can be analyzed by HPLC. The chromatographic conditions for various acidic poisons are given below:

Condition I:
- *Column*: 250 mm × 4.6 mm octadecyl silica (ODS) (media load of C18 on Partisil 5)
- *Mobile phase*: 0.02 ammonium sulfate [$(NH_3)_2SO_4$]:methanol (20:80)
- *Flow rate*: 2 mL/min
- *Internal standard*: Di-n-octyl phthalate (13 g/mL)
- *Detector*: UV with wavelength 220/254 nm

HIGH-PERFORMANCE LIQUID CHROMATOGRAPHY AND ITS APPLICATIONS

Condition II:
- *Column*: 150 mm × 4.6 mm, 5 μm, C18 column
- *Mobile phase*: 18% methanol in water for 0.5 minute followed by linear gradient to 70% methanol in water over 28.5 minutes and now 70–100% methanol for 1 minute finally 100% methanol for 10 minute
- *Flow rate*: 1 mL/min
- *Detector*: Fluorescence detector

Applied for Warfarin

High-performance liquid chromatography techniques are applied for separation and identification of warfarin for forensic interest. The chromatographic conditions are as follows:
- *Column*: SUPELCOSIL-ABZ 50 mm × 4.6 mm ID, 5 mm particles
- *Mobile phase*: Acetonitrile: 25 mM KH_2PO_4 (pH 2.3) with phosphoric acid (40:60)
- *Flow rate*: 2.0 mL/min
- *Detector*: UV detector with wavelength 230 nm

Explosives

High-performance liquid chromatography is very useful for the analysis of explosives such as trinitrotoluene (TNT), RDX, and pentaerythritol tetranitrate (PETN). The chromatographic conditions for explosives given above are as follows:
- *Column*: C8 (reverse-phase column)
- *Mobile phase*: Water: Acetonitrile (78:29)
- *Flow rate*: 1 mL/min
- *Detector*: UV detector with wavelength 254 nm

Miscellaneous Applications

High-performance liquid chromatography has several miscellaneous applications such as cardiac drugs and sedatives.

Applied for Cardiac Drugs
- *Column*: 150 mm × 4.6 mm ID, 5 μm
- *Mobile phase*: Methanol: Water (50:50)
- *Flow rate*: 2.0 mL/min
- *Detector*: UV detector with wavelength 220 nm

Applied for Sedatives and Barbiturates in Serum
- *Column*: Hisep, 150 mm × 4.6 mm ID, 5 mm particles
- *Mobile phase*: 50 mM KH_2PO_4/5 mM sodium dodecyl sulfate (SDS) pH 6.6
- *Flow rate*: 1.0 mL/min
- *Temperature*: 35°C
- *Detector*: UV detector with wavelength 220 nm

Applied in Chemical Criminology

High-performance liquid chromatography techniques are field of interest for investigations of chemical criminology.

- Heroin brown, lysergic acid diethylamide (LSD) green, amphetamine blue or yellow, tetrazine, etc. and many other chemicals are analyzed by HPLC techniques in forensic analysis
- High-performance liquid chromatography has been used to distinguish between the components of 25 blue ballpoint pen inks
- High-performance liquid chromatography has also been utilized in identification and comparison of lipstick smears. Small amount of lipstick is very helpful in investigation because lipstick smear can be found on clothing of man who has assaulted a woman.

■ CONCLUSION

A few glimpses have been discussed into the new developments and applications of HPLC, which will impact on the future progress in the modern area of forensic toxicology field. It is promising to observe that many of the recent advances are focusing on improving on chromatographic techniques by simplifying instrumentation, column efficiency to reduce analysis time with good robust analytical results making the HPLC technique significantly important for forensic toxicology. However, traditional FTIR, NMR, and mass spectral analysis can also be performed with sufficient sample. All these technical inventions and advances are giving a positive hope that the HPLC technique will answer various types of complex forensic toxicology questions by making a chromatographer even faster and more productive. Despite recent advances and scientific progress in analytical chemistry, toxicology, and poisons control, providing analytical services remain a difficult area. However, today HPLC has proved to be a valuable technique for forensic analysis. HPLC is very effective in almost all organic samples such as organic samples, pesticides, herbicides, insecticides, acidic drugs, basic drugs, narcotics, alcohols, analgesics, allergens, ballpoint pen inks, environmental poisons, natural and synthetic polymers, snake venom, and plant and animal poisons. The rapid advancements in technology and newly developed suitable derivatization techniques have increased the range of compounds that can be analyzed with HPLC, and thus, improving the results.

■ FURTHER READINGS

1. Chatwal DC, Anant QC. Instrumental Method of Chemical Analysis, 1st edition. New Delhi: Himalayan Publishing House; 1994.
2. Chatwal GR. Analytical Chromatography, 2nd edition. New Delhi: Himalayan Publishing House; 1998.
3. Doukas AG. Spectroscopic determination of skin viability: A predictor of postmortem interval. J Forensic Sci. 2000;45(2):36-41.

4. Fifield FW, Haines PJ. Environmental Analytical Chemistry. New York: Blackwell Publishing; 2000.
5. Hamilton RJ, Sewall PA. Introduction to High-performance Liquid Chromatography. London: Champion and Hall; 2004.
6. European Medicines Agency (EMA). (1995). ICH Topic Q2 (R1): Validation of Analytical Procedures: Text and Methodology. [online] Available from https://www.ema.europa.eu/en/documents/scientific-guideline/ich-q-2-r1-validation-analytical-procedures-text-methodology-step-5_en.pdf. [Last accessed March, 2021].
7. Ministry of Health and Family Welfare. (1996). Indian Pharmacopoeia. [online] Available from https://www.worldcat.org/title/indian-pharmacopoeia-1996/oclc/35742130. [Last accessed March, 2021].
8. Jaiswal AK, Millo T, Gupta M, Teotia AK, Tanwar TC. High-performance Liquid Chromatography and its Forensic Applications: A Review. J Forensic Med Toxicol. 2008;25(2):19-31.
9. Jaiswal AK. Do's and Don'ts for Sophisticated Analytical Instruments. Int J Med Toxicol Legal Med. 2003;6(1):13-23.
10. Khopkar SM. Basic Concepts of Analytical Chemistry. New York: Marcel Dekker; 1971.
11. Laboratory Procedure Manual Forensic Toxicology. New Delhi: Directorate Forensic Science, Ministry of Home Affairs; 2005.
12. Ira SL, Witter J, John D. High-performance Liquid Chromatography in Forensic Chemistry, 3rd edition. New York: Marcel Dekker Inc.; 1983.
13. Rana SVS. Biotechniques Theory and Practice, 2nd edition. Meerut: Rastogi Publications; 2006.
14. Sethi PD. Quantitative Analysis of Drugs in Pharmaceutical Formulations, 3rd edition. New Delhi: CBS Publishers and Distributors; 1997.
15. Sharma BK. Instrumental Methods of Chemical Analysis (Analytical Chemistry), 16th edition. Meerut: Krishna Prakashan Media (P) Ltd; 1997.
16. Sharma BK. Methods of Chemical Analysis, 16th edition. Meerut: Krishna Prakashan Media (P) Ltd.; 1996.
17. Skoog DA, Holler FJ, Nieman TA. Principle of Instrumental Analysis, 5th edition. New York: Thomson Brooks Cole; 2004.
18. Skoog DA, West DM, Holler FJ, Crouch SR. Fundamentals of Analytical chemistry, 8th edition. New York: Thomson Asia Pvt. Ltd.; 2006.
19. Skoog DA. Principles of Instrumental Analysis, 3rd edition. Philadelphia: CBS College Publishing; 1985.
20. Veerakumari L. Bioinstrumentations. Chennai: MJP Publishers; 2006.
21. Vissers JPC, Hulst WP, Chervet JP, Snijders HMJ, Kramers CA. Automated On-line Ionic Detergent Removal from Minute Protein/Peptide Samples Prior to Liquid Chromatography-Electrospray Mass Spectrometry. J Chromatogr B. 1996;686:119-28.
22. Willard HH. Instrumental Methods of Analysis, 6th edition. New Delhi: CBS Publishers and Distributors; 1986.
23. Willard HH. Instrumental Methods of Analysis, 7th edition. New Delhi: CBS Publishers and Distributors; 1987.
24. Wilson K, Walker J. Principle and Techniques of Biochemistry and Molecular Biology, 3rd edition. New York: Cambridge University Press; 2014.

Chapter 8

Ultraviolet-visible Spectroscopy and its Applications

■ INTRODUCTION

Electromagnetic spectrum covers a wide range of electromagnetic radiations from cosmic rays (wavelength in fractions of an angstrom) to radiowaves (wavelengths in meters or even kilometers). The arrangement of all types of electromagnetic radiations in order of their wavelengths or frequencies is known as the complete electromagnetic spectrum (**Fig. 8.1**). Few important points about electromagnetic spectrum are:
- Visible light is a form of electromagnetic wave, which lies in the wavelength range of 3,800–7,600 Å. If the wavelength is <3,800 Å, the radiation is called ultraviolet (UV) light and if the wavelength is >7,600 Å, the radiation is called infrared (IR) radiation.
- The radiowaves have the highest wavelength, while cosmic rays have the shortest wavelength. The energy of radiowaves is the least, while energy of cosmic rays is very large.

As energy is inversely proportional to wavelength, therefore cosmic rays have highest energy, whereas radiowaves have least energy.

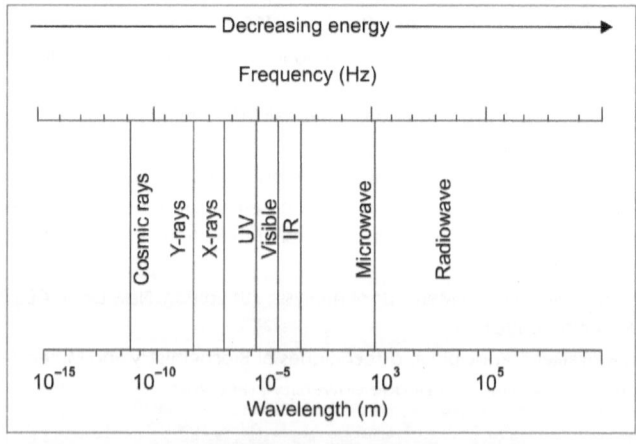

(IR: infrared; UV: ultraviolet)

Fig. 8.1: Electromagnetic spectrum.

ULTRAVIOLET-VISIBLE SPECTROSCOPY AND ITS APPLICATIONS

Table 8.1: Regions of electromagnetic spectrum.

Electromagnetic spectrum	Range	Frequency (in Hertz)
X-rays	10^{-2}–10^{2} Å	10^{20}–10^{16}
Far-UV	100–200 nm	10^{16}–10^{15}
Near-UV	200–400 nm	10^{15}–7.5×10^{14}
Visible	400–750 nm	7.5×10^{14}–40×10^{14}
Near-IR	0.750–2.2 μm	4.0×10^{14}–1.2×10^{14}
Mid-IR	2.50–50 μm	1.2×10^{14}–6×10^{12}
Far-IR	50–1,000 μm	6×10^{12}–10^{11}
Microwaves	0.10–100 cm	10^{11}–10^{8}
Radiowaves	10–1,000 m	10^{8}–10^{5}

(IR: infrared; UV: ultraviolet)

- Arrangement of different electromagnetic radiations with increasing order of their wavelength is:

    Cosmic rays < Gamma rays < X-rays < UV rays < Visible rays < IR rays < Microwaves < Radiowaves

- Arrangement of different electromagnetic radiations in increasing order of their frequency is:

    Radiowaves < Microwaves < IR rays < Visible rays < UV rays < X-rays < Gamma rays < Cosmic rays

The approximate wavelengths, wave numbers, and frequencies of various regions of the electromagnetic spectrum are given in **Table 8.1**. Except the visible region, various regions overlap. The regions of greatest interest to organic chemists are 200–400 nm (UV), 400–800 nm (visible), and 2.5–15 μm (IR).

SPECTROSCOPY

In spectroscopy, we study the interaction of electromagnetic radiation with matter. There are two types of spectroscopy:
1. *Atomic spectroscopy*: Interaction of electromagnetic radiation with atoms
2. *Molecular spectroscopy*: Interaction of electromagnetic radiation with molecules. When different types of electromagnetic radiations interact with matter, they give rise to different types of spectroscopy. For example:
    i. Absorption of electromagnetic radiation by the matter in the radiofrequency region gives rise to nuclear magnetic resonance (NMR) or electron spin resonance (ESR) spectroscopy
    ii. In microwave region, separation between rotational levels of molecule gives rise to rotational spectroscopy
    iii. In IR region, the absorption of radiation by organic compounds results into molecular vibrations and hence known as vibrational spectroscopy

iv. In visible and UV region, electronic transition is caused by atoms and molecules and known as electronic spectroscopy

ULTRAVIOLET-VISIBLE SPECTROSCOPY

The UV region extends from 1,000 to 4,000 Å or 100–400 nm. It is subdivided into far-UV region—below 200 nm (vacuum UV) and near-UV region—200–400 nm. The vacuum UV region is so named because the molecules of air absorb radiation in this region and thus, this region is accessible only with special vacuum equipment.

The region for visible spectroscopy is 400–750 nm. There are two main problems, which are encountered practically in visible spectrometry:
1. To prepare a colored solution
2. To measure the light absorptive capacity of the solution or to compare it with that of a colored solution of known concentration

Origin of Ultraviolet Absorption Spectra

1. Ultraviolet absorption spectra are attributed to a process in which the outer electrons of atoms or molecules absorb radiant energy and undergo transitions to higher energy level
2. Both organic and inorganic species exhibit electronic transitions in which outermost bonded electrons are promoted to higher energy level
3. The main function of the absorbed energy is to raise the molecule from the ground state energy E_0 to the higher excited state E_1

$$\Delta E = E_1 - E_0$$
$$= h\nu$$
$$\Delta E = \frac{hc}{\lambda}$$

where, h is Planck constant, c is velocity of light, and λ is wavelength of the absorbed radiation. ΔE depends upon how tightly the electrons are bound in the bonds and accordingly, the absorption will occur in UV or particular region of visible range

4. If the electrons of a molecule are tightly bound as in compounds containing sigma bonds, such as methane, ethane, etc., no light of visible region will be absorbed. The light of UV region will only be absorbed and hence, the compound will appear colorless
5. If the electrons of a molecule are loosely bound as in unsaturated compounds, such as ethene, ethyne, etc., the absorption may occur in the visible region and the substance will appear colored
6. Total energy of the molecule is the sum of electronic energy, vibrational energy, and rotational energy.

$$E_{total} = E_{electronic} + E_{vibrational} + E_{rotational}$$

7. It is observed that the electronic transitions require more energy in comparison to vibrational changes and the latter requires more energy than rotational changes inside the molecule.

$$E_{electronic} > E_{vibrational} > E_{rotational}$$

Because of this electronic excitation, UV spectroscopy is sometimes also known as electronic spectroscopy.

Basic Principle of Ultraviolet-visible Spectroscopy (Lambert–Beer Law)

A UV-visible spectrophotometer records a plot of wavelength versus absorbance (A) or optical density (OD) or molar absorptivity or molar extinction coefficient as defined by Lambert–Beer law.

Lambert's Law

According to Lambert's law, the fraction of incident radiation absorbed by homogeneous medium is independent of the intensity of the incident radiation.

Beer's Law

According to Beer's law, the fraction of incident radiation absorbed by homogeneous medium is proportional to the number of absorbing molecule or concentration.

On combining above two laws, we get:

$$\log\left(\frac{I}{I_0}\right) = A = abC$$

or $A = abC$
or $A = \varepsilon bC$

where, I_0 is the intensity of incident radiation, I is the intensity of radiation transmitted through sample solution, A is the absorbance or optical density, a or ε is the molar absorptivity or molar extinction coefficient, C is the concentration of solute (mol/L), and b is the path length of sample (in cm).

This is the fundamental equation of colorimetry and spectrophotometry and is often spoken as Beer–Lambert law or Lambert–Beer law. This equation indicates that the absorbance of a solution is directly proportional to the concentration of absorbing species when the length of the light path is fixed and directly proportional to the light path when the concentration is fixed.

The molar absorptivity of an organic compound is constant at a given wavelength. The intensity of an absorption band in the UV-visible spectrum is usually expressed as the molar absorptivity at maximum absorption a_{max}. The wavelength of the maximum absorption is denoted by λ_{max}.

When the molecular weight of a sample is unknown or when a mixture is being examined, the intensity of absorption is expressed as $E_{1cm}^{1\%}$ or $A_{1cm}^{\%}$ value.

$$E_{1cm}^{1\%} = \frac{A}{bC}$$

where, c is the concentration (in g/100 mL), b is the path length of the sample (in cm), and $E_{1cm}^{1\%}$ is easily related to ε by the expression.

$$\varepsilon = \frac{E_{1cm}^{1\%} \times \text{molecular weight}}{10}$$

Terms and Symbols Used in Ultraviolet-visible Spectrophotometry

Transmittance (T)
The ratio of transmitted light and incident light is called transmittance and is denoted by T. The obsolete or alternate of transmittance is the name transmission.

$$T = I/I_0$$

Absorbance (A)
It is logarithm of the reciprocal of the transmittance. It is represented by A. The obsolete or alternative of this term is OD.

$$A = \text{Log}_{10}(1/T) = -\text{Log } T$$

or

$$A = \text{Log} I_0/I$$

or

$$A = abC$$

Absorptivity (a)
It is the ratio of the absorbance to the product of concentration and length of optical path. It is a constant characteristic of substance and wavelength. It is represented by a or å. The obsolete or alternative of this term is extinction coefficient or absorbency index.

$$a = \frac{A}{bC}$$

Molar Absorptivity (Molar Extinction Coefficient)
Molar absorptivity is absorptivity for a concentration of 1 mol/dm³, a path length of 1 cm. This obsolete or alternate term for molar absorptivity is molar extinction coefficient or molar absorption coefficient or molar absorbency index.

$$\varepsilon = \frac{A}{bC}$$

Path Length (b)
It is the internal cell length expressed in centimeters. It is represented by b or l.

Spectral Bandwidth

The range of wavelength of radiant energy emerging from the exit slit of the monochromator.

Slit Width

The slit width is the mechanical distance (nm) between the sides of the narrow apparatus, which permits radiant energy to enter and leave the monochromator.

Application of Lambert–Beer's Law

The concentration of the unknown may be established by mathematical as well as by graphical procedures.

For any one of the standard solution, Beer's law applies:

$$A_{standard} = abC_{standard} \quad (1)$$

where,
$A_{standard}$ = absorbance of standard
a = absorptivity
b = path length
$C_{standard}$ = concentration of standard

Similarly, for unknown solution:

$$A_{unknown} = abC_{unknown} \quad (2)$$

where,
$C_{unknown}$ = concentration of unknown

Dividing equations 1 and 2, we will get:

$$\frac{A_{Standard}}{A_{unknown}} = \frac{C_{Standard}}{C_{unknown}} \quad (3)$$

By putting the values of absorbance of standard ($A_{standard}$), absorbance of unknown ($A_{unknown}$), and concentration of standard ($C_{standard}$), we can calculate the concentration of the unknown, i.e., $C_{unknown}$.

Deviation from Lambert–Beer's Law

If graph between absorbance and concentration is straight line, then Lambert–Beer's law holds good. If it is not a straight line, this law does not hold good (**Fig. 8.2**). Deviation from Lambert–Beer's law is due to:
1. When solute ionizes, dissociates, or associates in solution

$$4C_6H_5CH_2OH \longrightarrow (C_6H_5CH_2OH)_4$$

2. When the color solute forms complex, the composition of which depends upon the concentration
3. When the monochromatic light is not used
4. Another most important chemical deviation from the absorption law is the change of color, e.g., dichromate ion to chromate ion on dilution with water

$$Cr_2O_7^{2-} + H_2O \longrightarrow 2H^+ + 2CrO_4^{1-}$$
$$\text{Orange} \qquad\qquad \text{Yellow}$$

ULTRAVIOLET-VISIBLE SPECTROSCOPY AND ITS APPLICATIONS

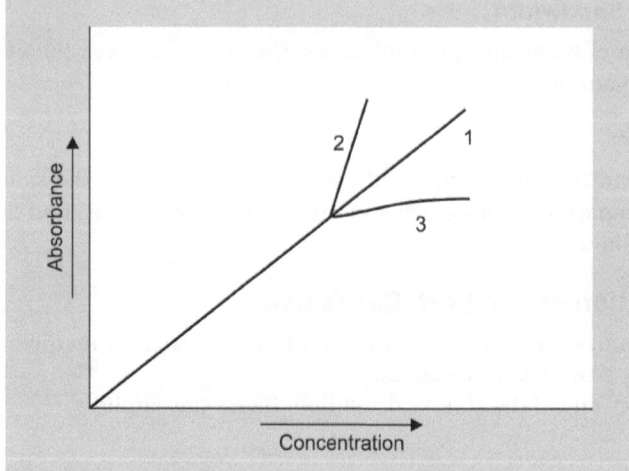

Fig. 8.2: Beer's law. (1) Obeyed; (2) Positive deviation; and (3) Negative deviation.

5. Beer's law is also not valid in case the absorbing material is coagulated
6. The presence of impurities may also cause deviation from the Beer's law
7. Beer's law is not applicable in case of suspension.

Absorption Bands in UV-visible Spectroscopy

Designation of Absorption Bands

In UV-visible spectroscopy, bands may be designated by the type of electronic transitions from which they originate, e.g., $\sigma \rightarrow \sigma^*$ band and $\pi \rightarrow \pi^*$ band by the letter designation. The following letter designations were proposed.

K-bands: These bands originate from $\pi \rightarrow \pi^*$ transitions in compounds having a $\pi \rightarrow \pi$ conjugated system, e.g., 1,3-butadiene shows K-band at λ_{max} 217 nm, ϵ_{max} 21,000 and acrolein at λ_{max} 210 nm, ϵ_{max} 11,500. Aromatic compounds also exhibit K-band in their UV spectra, e.g., acetophenone shows K-band at λ_{max} 240 nm, ϵ_{max} 13,000 and styrene at λ_{max} 244 nm, ϵ_{max} 12,000.

R-bands: These bands originate from n $\rightarrow \pi^*$ transitions of a single chromophoric group, e.g., carbonyl or nitro group. R-bands are also called forbidden bands. For example, acetone shows an R-band at λ_{max} 279 nm, ϵ_{max} 15 and acetophenone at λ_{max} 319 nm, ϵ_{max} 50.

B-bands: It is also known as benzenoid bands. These bands originate from $\pi \rightarrow \pi^*$ transitions in aromatic or heteroaromatic compounds. For example, benzene shows a B-band at λ_{max} 256 nm, ϵ_{max} 200 and acetophenone at λ_{max} 278 nm, ϵ_{max} 100.

E-bands: It is also called ethylene bands. Similar to B-band, these are characteristics of aromatic and heteroaromatic compounds and originate

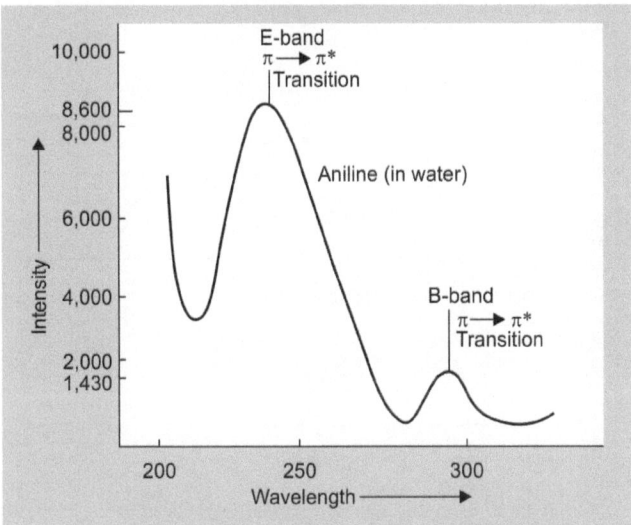

Fig. 8.3: E- and B-bands of aniline.

from $\pi \rightarrow \pi^*$ transitions of the ethylenic bonds present in the aromatic ring (**Fig. 8.3**).

Absorption by Organic Molecules

Electrons Present in Organic Molecules

Organic molecules have the following types of electrons:
1. Sigma (σ) electrons—C-C, C-H, -OH, etc.
2. Pi (π) electrons—>C=C<, -C≡C-, >C=N<, etc.
3. Nonbonding (n) electrons—>C=O<, R-O-R, R-CO-R, etc.

According to molecular orbital theory, the exclusion of a molecule by the absorption of radiation in the UV-visible region involves promotion of its electrons from a bonding or nonbonding (n) orbital to an antibonding orbital. There are σ and π bonding orbitals associated with σ^* and π^* antibonding orbitals, respectively (**Fig. 8.4**).

Types of Electronic Transitions

Following electronic transitions are involved in the UV-visible region. These transitions are shown in **Figure 8.5**.
1. $\sigma \rightarrow \sigma^*$ transition
2. $n \rightarrow \sigma^*$ transition
3. $\pi \rightarrow \pi^*$ transition
4. $n \rightarrow \pi^*$ transition

The energy required for various transitions obey the following order:

$$\sigma \rightarrow \sigma^* > n \rightarrow \sigma^* > \pi \rightarrow \pi^* > n \rightarrow \pi^*$$

ULTRAVIOLET-VISIBLE SPECTROSCOPY AND ITS APPLICATIONS

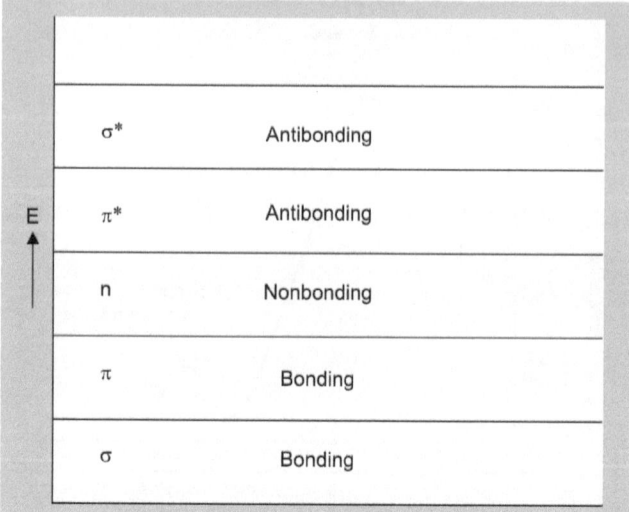

Fig. 8.4: Various electronic energy levels.

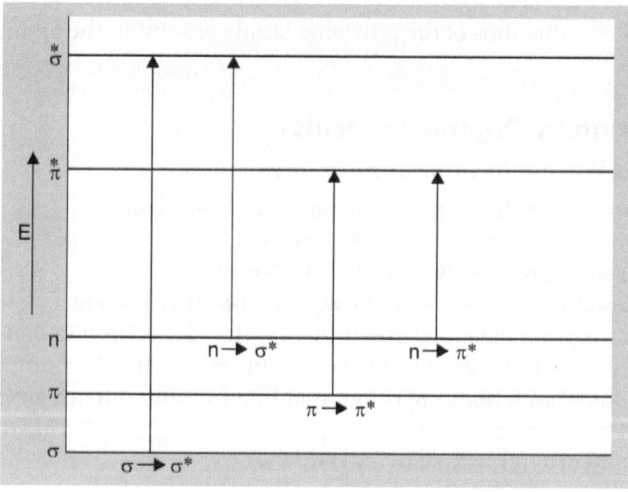

Fig. 8.5: Different types of electronic transitions.

$\sigma \rightarrow \sigma^*$ *transition (Fig. 8.6)*: The transition or promotion of an electron from a bonding sigma orbital to the antibonding sigma orbital is $\sigma \rightarrow \sigma^*$ transition. Few important points about $\sigma \rightarrow \sigma^*$ transition are given below:
1. It is high energy process, since bonding in general is very strong
2. Organic compounds, in which all valence shell electrons are involved in the formation of bond, do not show absorption in the normal UV region, i.e., 180 nm
3. For saturated hydrocarbons such as methane and propane, absorption occurs near 150 nm

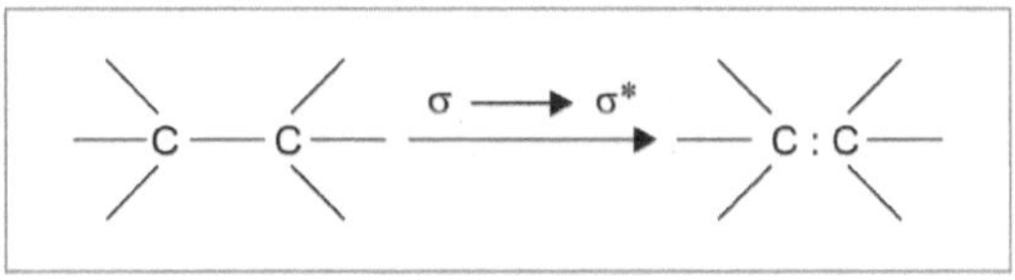

ULTRAVIOLET-VISIBLE SPECTROSCOPY AND ITS APPLICATIONS

Fig. 8.6: $\sigma \rightarrow \sigma^*$ transition.

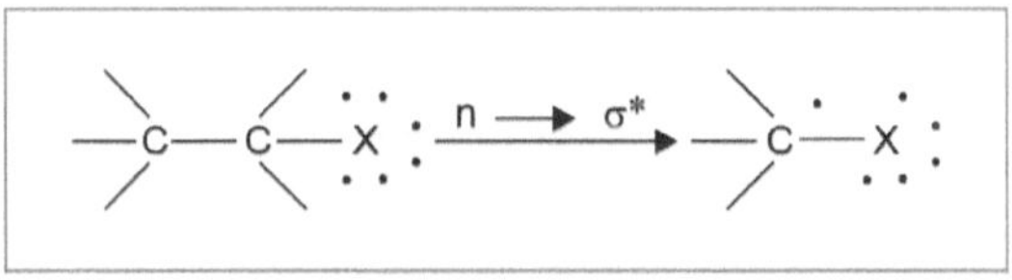

Fig. 8.7: $n \rightarrow \sigma^*$ transition.

4. The usual spectroscopic technique cannot be below 200 nm, since O_2 (present in air) begins to absorb. Thus, the region below 200 nm is commonly called vacuum UV region

$n \rightarrow \sigma^*$ transition (Fig. 8.7): The transition or promotion of an electron from a nonbonding orbital to an antibonding sigma orbital, which is designated as $n \rightarrow \sigma^*$ transition. Few important points about $n \rightarrow \sigma^*$ are given below:
1. This type of transition takes place in saturated compounds containing one heteroatom
2. Some compounds undergoing this type of transition are saturated halides, alcohols, ethers, aldehydes, ketones, etc.
3. Such transition requires comparatively less energy than required for $n \rightarrow \sigma^*$ transition
4. In alkyl halides, the energy required for such a transition changes with the increase in the size of the halogen atom (or decreases with electronegativity of the atom)
5. For example, the absorption maximum for methyl chloride is 172–175 nm, whereas that for methyl iodide is 258 nm
6. Similarly, amines absorb at higher wavelength as compared to alcohol and hence, the extinction coefficients for amines will be larger.
7. $n \rightarrow \sigma^*$ transitions are very sensitive to hydrogen bonding
8. Association occurs due to the presence of nonbonding electron in the heteroatom and thus, transitions require greater energy. Hydrogen bonding shifts the UV absorption to shorter wavelengths

$n \rightarrow \pi^*$ transition (Fig. 8.8): The transition or promotion of an electron from a nonbonding orbital to a pi antibonding orbital is designated as $n \rightarrow \pi^*$ transition. Few important points about $n \rightarrow \pi^*$ are given below:
1. This type of transition requires least amount of energy out of all transitions and hence, occurs at longer wavelengths
2. Saturated aldehyde shows both the type of transitions, i.e., low energy $n \rightarrow \pi^*$ and high energy $\pi \rightarrow \pi^*$ occurring around 290 nm and 180 nm, respectively. Absorption occurring at lower wavelength is usually intense

ULTRAVIOLET-VISIBLE SPECTROSCOPY AND ITS APPLICATIONS

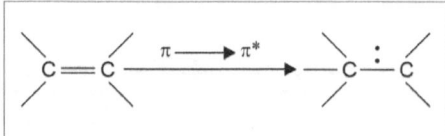

Fig. 8.8: n → π* transition.

Fig. 8.9: π → π* transition.

3. In simple cases, it is quite easy to tell whether the transition is n → σ* or π → π*, since the extinction coefficient of former is quite low as compared to that of the latter.
4. In saturated carbonyl compounds, two types of transitions take place which can be classified as:
   i. *High-energy transition*:
      a. n → σ* (intense)
      b. π → π* (intense)
   ii. *Low-energy transition*:
      a. n → π* (weak)

π → π* transition (Fig. 8.9): The transition or promotion of an electron from a bonding pi orbital to the associated antibonding pi orbital is π → π* transition. Few important points are given below:
1. π → π* transition occurs in the unsaturated electrons of the molecule, i.e., compounds containing double or triple bonds and also in aromatics
2. The excitation of electron requires smaller energy and hence, transition of this type occurs at longer wavelength
3. This transition requires still lesser energy as compared to n → σ* transition
4. In carbonyl compounds, the band due to π → π* transition appears around 180 nm and most intense, i.e., the value of extinction coefficient is high

■ CHROMOPHORE

It is defined as any group, which has characteristic absorptions in the UV or the visible region. For example, C=C, C=O, R-NO$_2$, -COOH, -CHO, -N=N-, -CONH$_2$. There are two types of chromophores (**Table 8.2**):
1. In which the group contains π electrons. They undergo π → π* transitions, e.g., ethane and ethyne
2. In which the group contain both π and bonding electrons. They undergo π → π* and n → π* transition, e.g., nitrile, azo, and carbonyl

Table 8.2: Common unconjugated chromophores.

Chromophores	Examples	λ_{max} (nm)	Transition
>C=C<	Ethylene	171	$\pi \rightarrow \pi^*$
-C≡C-	Acetylene	150	$\pi \rightarrow \pi^*$
		173	$\pi \rightarrow \pi^*$
-CHO	Acetaldehyde	160	$n \rightarrow \sigma^*$
		180	$\pi \rightarrow \pi^*$
		290	$n \rightarrow \pi^*$
>C=O	Acetone	166	$n \rightarrow \sigma^*$
		188	$\pi \rightarrow \pi^*$
		279	$n \rightarrow \pi^*$
-COOH	Acetic acid	204	$n \rightarrow \pi^*$
-CONH$_2$	Acetamide	178	$\pi \rightarrow \pi^*$
		220	$n \rightarrow \pi^*$
-COOR	Ethyl acetate	211	$n \rightarrow \pi^*$
-NO$_2$	Nitromethane	201	$\pi \rightarrow \pi^*$
		274	$n \rightarrow \pi^*$
C=N-OH	Acetoxime	190	$n \rightarrow \pi^*$
-C≡N	Acetonitrile	160	$\pi \rightarrow \pi^*$
-N=N-	Azomethane	338	$n \rightarrow \pi^*$

AUXOCHROME

An auxochrome can be defined as any group which does not itself acts as chromophore, but whose presence brings about a shift of the absorption band toward the longer wavelength λ, e.g., -OH, -OR, -NH$_2$, -NHR, -NR$_2$, and -SH. Auxochromes generally increase the value of λ_{max} as well as ϵ_{max} hence, it is also called color enhancing group. For example:

1. Benzene shows λ_{max} 256 nm, ϵ_{max} 200, whereas aniline shows λ_{max} 280 nm, ϵ_{max} 1,430. Hence, amino (NH$_2$) group is an auxochrome
2. C$_6$H$_5$O$^-$ is colorless, whereas, p-NO$_2$C$_6$H$_4$O$^-$ is yellow color. Here, nitro group (-NO$_2$) acts as auxochrome
3. (C$_6$H$_5$)$_3$C$^+$ is colorless, whereas, (p-OHC$_6$H$_4$)3C$^+$ is deep red. Here, hydroxyl group (-OH) acts as auxochrome

ABSORPTION AND INTENSITY SHIFTS

Bathochromic Shift or Red Shift

It is an effect by virtue of which the absorption maximum is shifted toward longer wavelength due to the presence of auxochrome or by the change of solvent. Such an absorption shift toward longer wavelength is called red shift or bathochromic shift (**Fig. 8.10**). The transition for n $\rightarrow \pi^*$ experiences bathochromic shift. For example, benzene shows appreciable absorption in the near-UV. The introduction of conjugated unsaturated side chain causes a shift to longer wavelengths. Hence, stilbene is colorless, whereas diphenyl polyenes are colored.

Hypsochromic Shift or Blue Shift

It is an effect by virtue of which the absorption maximum is shifted toward shorter wavelength. The absorption shift toward shorter wavelength is called blue shift or hypsochromic shift (**Fig. 8.10**). It is caused by the removal of conjugation and also by changing the polarity of solvent. For example:
1. $C_6H_5(CH=CH)_4C_6H_5$ is colored, whereas $C_6H_5\text{-}(CH=CH)\text{-}C_6H_5$ is colorless
2. The conjugation is destroyed by an introduction of a $-CH_2$ group in the unsaturated chain and hence, it causes a shift of the absorption band to shorter wavelengths. For example, $C_6H_5(CH=CH)_4C_6H_5$ is greenish-yellow color, whereas $C_6H_5CH_2(CH=CH)_4C_6H_5$ is colorless

Hyperchromic Effect

It is an effect due to which the intensity of absorption maximum increases, i.e., ϵ_{max} increases. The introduction of an auxochrome usually causes hyperchromic shift (**Fig. 8.10**). For example, benzene shows B-band at 256 nm, ϵ_{max} 200, whereas aniline shows B-band at 280 nm, ϵ_{max} 1,430.

Hypochromic Effect

It is an effect due to which intensity of absorption maximum decreases, i.e., extinction coefficient ϵ_{max} decreases. The introduction of groups which distorts the geometry of the molecule causes hypochromic effect (**Fig. 8.10**). For example, biphenyl shows λ_{max} 252 nm, ϵ_{max} 19,000, whereas 2, 2'-dimethylbiphenyl shows λ_{max} 270 nm, ϵ_{max} 800.

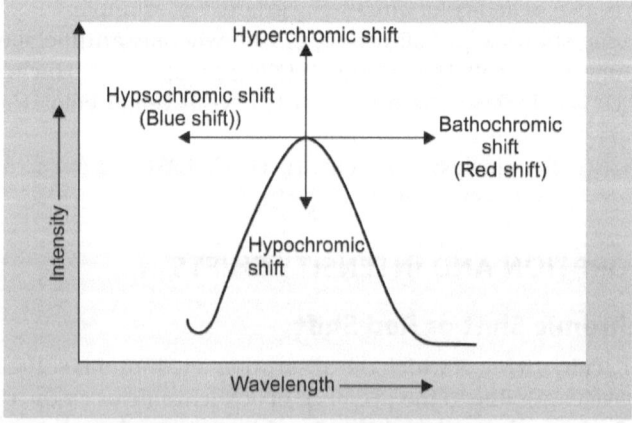

Fig. 8.10: Absorption and intensity shift.

ULTRAVIOLET-VISIBLE SPECTROSCOPY AND ITS APPLICATIONS

■ BASIS OF COLOR IN ORGANIC COMPOUNDS

1. Colored substances can be studied in the visible region. Colorless substances do not absorb white light appreciably and they must be investigated in the UV region
2. The electrons are tightly bound in completely saturated aliphatic compounds. Hence, in order to raise the molecule to an excited state, a large amount of energy would be needed. Such substances exhibit absorption in the far-UV region of the spectrum
3. The electrons are loosely bound in unsaturated compounds such as -C=C-, -N=N-C, -C=O-, and -N=O-. Hence, in order to raise the molecule to an excited state, a small amount of energy would be needed. Such substances exhibit absorption in the near-UV and sometimes in visible spectrum
4. Benzene shows appreciable absorption in the near-UV. The introduction of conjugated unsaturated side chain causes a shift to longer wavelengths. For example, stilbene $C_6H_5CH=CHC_6H_5$ is colorless, whereas diphenyl polyenes $C_6H_5(CH=CH)_nC_6H_5$ is colored. As the number of -CH=CH- group increases, the color passes through yellow to green and orange and when n = 8, $(-CH=CH-)_8$, the compound has a bluish-copper red color
5. The conjugation is destroyed by an introduction of a $-CH_2$ group in the unsaturated chain and hence, it causes a shift of the absorption band to shorter wavelengths. For example, $C_6H_5(CH=CH)_4C_6H_5$ is greenish yellow, whereas $C_6H_5CH_2(CH=CH)_4C_6H_5$ is colorless
6. The -N=N- also behaves almost to the -CH=CH- group. For example:
   - CH_3-N=N-CH_3—appears at higher wavelength region
   - CH_3-CH_2-N=N-CH_3—appears at shorter wavelength region
   - C_6H_5-N=N-C_6H_5—lower wavelength
   - C_6H_5-N=N-N=N-C_6H_5—higher wavelength
7. Free radicals and odd electron molecules are usually associated with absorption bands in the visible region, perhaps because of the fact that one of the electrons is loosely bound.
8. In case of dyes, the intense color is due to the presence of a chromophoric structure such as conjugated chain or one or more benzene rings and of an auxochrome group. For example, $C_6H_5O^-$ ion is colorless, whereas p-$NO_2C_6H_5O^-$ ion is yellow colored
9. Basic or positive groups such as -OH, -OR, -NR_2, -NHPh, and -NH_2 are effective generally in acidic solutions. Acidic or negative groups such as -NO_2, -NO, -CO, and -CN are effective in alkaline solutions. These auxochromes refer particularly to dyes in which the benzene ring is a part of choromophore. Substitution in the ortho and para positions, especially the latter, gives the greatest intensification of color, but metasubstitution has little or no influence

VARIOUS TYPES OF DOUBLE IN CONJUGATION

Alicyclic Dienes

Dienes containing an open chain system is called alicyclic dienes. Basic unit of alicyclic dienes is butadienes.

$$CH_2=CH-CH=CH_2$$
Butadienes

Homoannular Dienes

In homoannular dienes, conjugated double bonds are present in the same ring and having cisoid configuration. Few examples of homoannular dienes are given below:

Heteroannular Dienes

In heteroannular dienes, conjugated double bonds are not present in the same ring and these have transoid configuration. Few examples of heteroannular dienes are given below:

Exocyclic and Endocyclic Conjugated

The carbon-carbon double bonds projecting outside a ring are called exocyclic double bonds. For example:

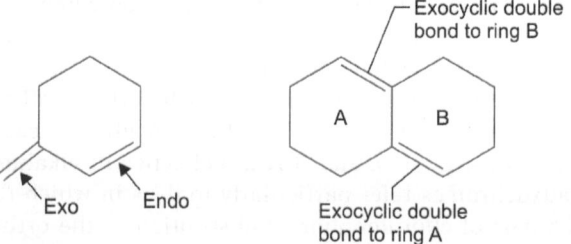

Alkyl Substituents and Ring Residues

Only the alkyl substituents and ring residues attached to the carbon atoms constituting the conjugated system of the compound are taken into account.

Few examples for alkyl substituents and ring residues are:

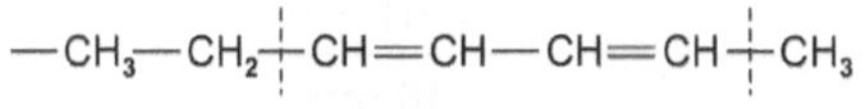

—CH₃—CH₂—CH=CH—CH=CH—CH₃   ⟨ ⟩=CH—CH=CH₂
Two alkyl substituents 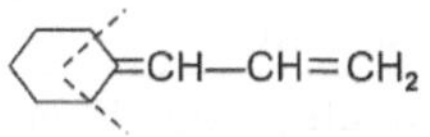   Two ring residues

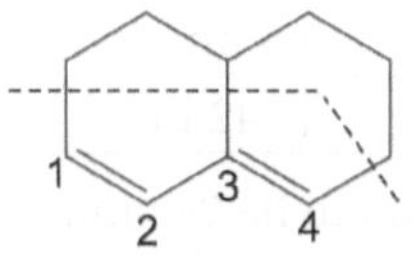

Three ring residues

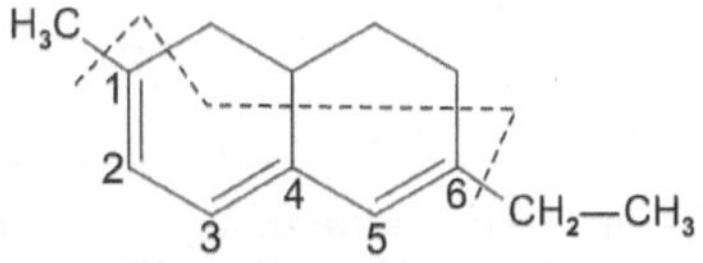

Three ring residues and two alkyl substituents

■ WOODWARD–FIESER RULES FOR CALCULATING λ_{max} FOR CONJUGATED DIENES AND TRIENES

Woodward in 1941 formulated a set of empirical rules for calculating or predicting λ_{max} in conjugated acyclic/cyclic systems. These rules, modified by Fieser and hence called Woodward-Fieser rules, are summarized below:
1. Parent value for conjugated dienes—217 nm
2. Homoannular conjugated dienes—253 nm
3. Heteroannular conjugated dienes—214 nm
4. *Increment for each substituent*:
   - Alkyl substituent or ring residue—5 nm
   - Exocyclic double bond—5 nm
   - Double bond extending conjugation—30 nm
5. *Auxochrome*:
   - -OR—6 nm
   - -SR—30 nm
   - -Cl and -Br—5 nm
   - -NR₂—60 nm
   - -OCOCH₃—0 nm

Some examples illustrating the above rules are as follows:
1. *2,4-hexadiene*:

$$CH_3-CH=CH-CH=CH-CH_3$$

Basic value	217 nm
Two alkyl substituents (2 × 5)	10 nm
Calculated value of λ_{max}	227 nm

The observed value of λ_{max} is also found to be 227 nm.
2.

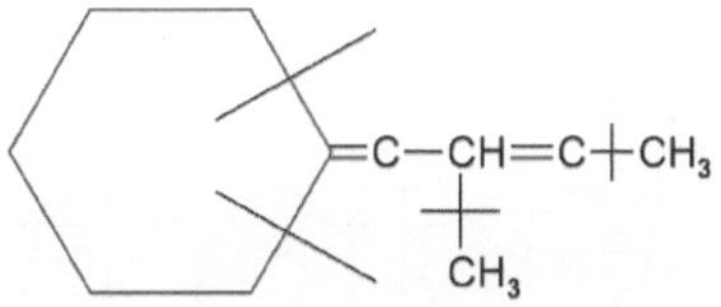

The value of absorption maximum is calculated as follows:

Basic value	217 nm
Two alkyl substituents (2 × 5)	10 nm
Two ring residues (2 × 5)	10 nm
One exocyclic double bond	5 nm
Calculated value of λ_{max}	242 nm

The observed value of λ_{max} is also found to be 242 nm.

3. *Heteroannular diene*:

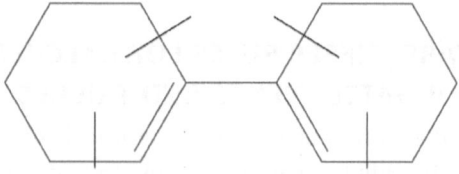

Basic value	214 nm
Four ring residues (4 × 5)	20 nm
Calculated value of λ_{max}	234 nm

The observed value of λ_{max} is also found to be 234 nm.

4.

Basic value	253 nm
Three ring residues (3 × 5)	15 nm
One exocyclic double bond	5 nm
Calculated value of λ_{max}	273nm

The observed value of λ_{max} is also found to be 273 nm.

5.

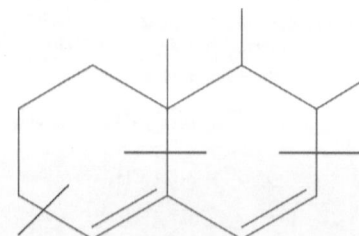

ULTRAVIOLET-VISIBLE SPECTROSCOPY AND ITS APPLICATIONS

Basic value	214 nm
Three ring residues (3 × 5)	15 nm
One exocyclic double bond	5 nm
Calculated value of λ_{max}	234 nm

The observed value of λ_{max} is also found to be 235 nm.

6.

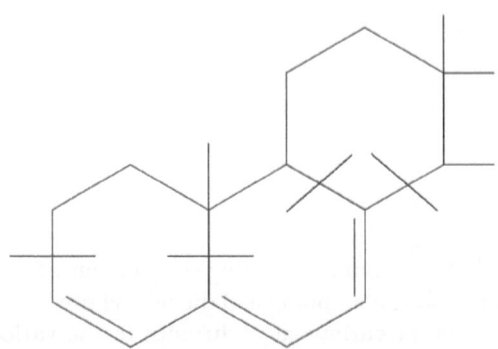

Basic value	253 nm
One double bond extending conjugation	30 nm
Four ring residues	20 nm
One exocyclic double bond	10 nm
Calculated value of λ_{max}	313 nm

The observed value of λ_{max} is also found to be 312 nm.

■ WOODWARD–FIESER RULES FOR CALCULATING ABSORPTION MAXIMUM IN α, β-UNSATURATED CARBONYL COMPOUNDS

Similar to trienes and dienes, there are set rules for α, β-unsaturated aldehydes and ketones called Woodward-Fieser rules for calculating λ_{max} in α, β-unsaturated carbonyl compounds which are given below:
- Basic value for acyclic α, β-unsaturated ketones = 215 nm
- Basic value for six-membered cyclic α, β-unsaturated ketones = 215 nm
- Basic value for five-membered cyclic α, β-unsaturated ketones = 202 nm
- Basic value for α, β-unsaturated aldehydes = 207 nm
- The structural increments for estimating maximum for a given α, β-unsaturated carbonyl compound are as follows:
  - For each exocyclic double bond + 5 nm
  - For each double bond endocyclic in five- or seven-membered ring, except 2-cyclopentenone + 5 nm
  - *For each alkyl substituent or ring residue at the*:
    - α-position + 10 nm

ULTRAVIOLET-VISIBLE SPECTROSCOPY AND ITS APPLICATIONS

Table 8.3: Auxochromes increment (in nm) for position with respect to the carbonyl group.

	α	β	λ	Higher
-OH	+35	+30	+50	+50
-OAc	+6	+6	+6	+6
-Cl	+15	+12	-	-
-Br	+23	+35	-	-
-OR	+35	+30	17	31
-SR	-	+85	-	-
-NR$_2$	-	+95	-	-

- β-position + 12 nm
- λ, δ, or higher position + 18 nm
- For each double bond extending conjugation + 30 nm
- For a homoannular conjugated diene + 39 nm
- Increments for various auxochromes in the various α, β, λ, etc., positions are given in **Table 8.3**.

Few examples are:
1.

Basic value	215 nm
Two alkyl substituents (2 × 12)	24 nm
Calculated value of λ_{max}	239 nm

The observed value of λ_{max} is also found to be 237 nm.

2.

ULTRAVIOLET-VISIBLE SPECTROSCOPY AND ITS APPLICATIONS

Basic value	215 nm
Two ring residues (2 × 12)	24 nm
One exocyclic double bond	5 nm
Calculated value of λ_{max}	244 nm

The observed value of λ_{max} is also found to be 342 nm.

3.

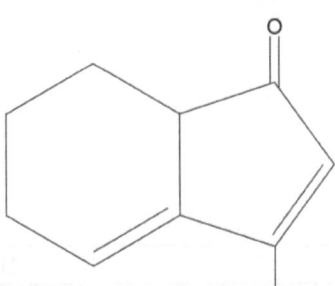

Basic value	215 nm
OH substitution at α position	35 nm
Two substituents (one alkyl and one ring residue)	24 nm
Calculated value of λ_{max}	274 nm

The observed value of λ_{max} is also found to be 274 nm.

4.

Basic value	202 nm
One alkyl ring substitution	12 nm
One exocyclic double bond	5 nm
One double bond extending conjugation	30 nm
One gamma ring residue	18 nm
One ring residue	18 nm
Calculated value of λ_{max}	285 nm

Observed value of λ_{max} is also found to be 287 nm.

5.

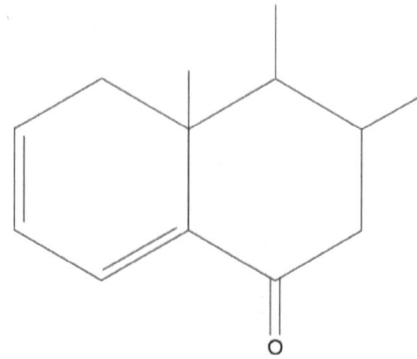

Basic value	215 nm
Alpha ring residue	10 nm
Ring residue	18 nm
One exocyclic double bond	5 nm
Homoannular conjugated diene	39 nm
One double bond extending conjugation	30 nm
Calculated value of λ_{max}	317 nm

Observed value of λ_{max} is also found to be 319 nm.

6.

Basic value	215 nm
One ring residue	12 nm
One (+2) ring residue	18 nm
One (+2) ring residue (2 × 18)	36 nm
Two double bond extending conjugation (2 × 30)	60 nm
Two exocyclic double bonds (2 × 5)	10 nm
Calculated value of λ_{max}	351 nm

The observed value of λ_{max} is also found to be 354 nm.

RULES FOR CALCULATING ABSORPTION MAXIMUM FOR DERIVATIVES OF ACYL BENZENES

Similar to Woodward–Fieser rules, Scott formulated a set rule for calculating the absorption maximum of substituted benzene derivatives of the type $C_6H_5-\overset{\overset{O}{\|}}{C}-X$ which is given below:

- The basic value if X is an alkyl group or alicyclic residues = 246 nm
- If X is a hydrogen atom, the basic value = 250 nm
- If X is -OH or -OR, the basic value = 230 μ
  Increment for each substituents are given in **Table 8.4**.

Examples are:
1.

Basic value	246 nm
Cl substitution at para position	10 nm
Calculated value of λ_{max}	256 nm

The observed value of λ_{max} is found to be 254 nm.

Table 8.4: Increment for each substituent.

Auxochrome	Increments (in nm) according to the position of substituent		
	Ortho	Meta	Para
Alkyl	+3	+3	+10
OH and OR	+7	+7	+25
Cl	0	0	+10
Br	+2	+2	+15
NH_2	+13	+13	+58
NHAc	+20	+20	+45
XR_2	+20	+20	+85
O	+11	+20	+75

2.

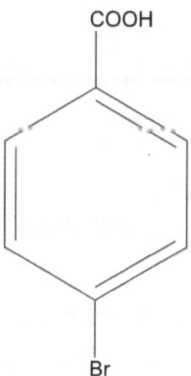

Basic value	246 nm
OH substitution at meta	7 nm
OH substitution at para	25 nm
Calculated value of λ_{max}	278 nm

Observed value of λ_{max} is found out to be 281 nm.

3.

Basic value	230 nm
Br substitution at para	15 nm
Calculated value of λ_{max}	245 nm

Observed value of λ_{max} is found out to be 245 nm.

■ INSTRUMENTATION

A UV-visible spectrophotometer compares the intensity of the transmitted radiation with that of the incident UV-visible radiation. There are two types of UV-visible spectrophotometer. One is single-beam spectrophotometer and another is double-beam spectrophotometer. Block diagrams of single-beam and double-beam spectrophotometer are given in **Figures 8.11** and **8.12**, respectively.

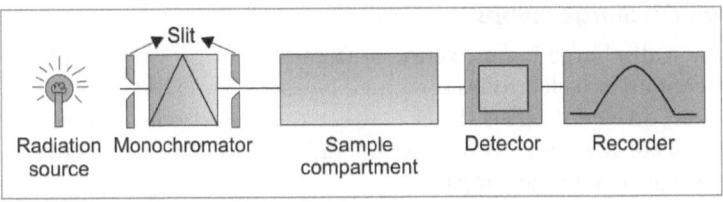

Fig. 8.11: Single-beam ultraviolet (UV)-visible spectrophotometer.

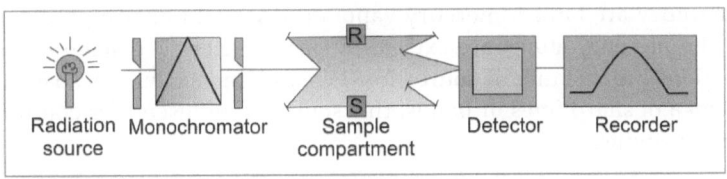

Fig. 8.12: Double-beam ultraviolet (UV)-visible spectrophotometer.

Different components such as radiation sources, monochromator, sample compartment, detector, and recorder of modern spectrophotometer are described below.

Radiation Sources

The hydrogen discharge lamp is the most commonly used source of radiation in the UV region (180–400 nm). Deuterium lamps are more intense than those of hydrogen discharge lamp and cover the same wavelength. A tungsten filament lamp is the most common source for visible region (400–800 nm). Some other radiation sources for UV are xenon discharge lamp, mercury arc, etc. Basic requirements of radiation source are:
- It must be stable
- It must be of sufficient intensity for the transmitted energy
- It must supply continuous radiation

Hydrogen Discharge Lamps

In hydrogen discharge lamps, hydrogen is stored under pressure and an electric discharge is passed through them. This excites hydrogen molecule, which emits UV radiations. As the pressure is high, we get a continuous hydrogen spectrum. Hydrogen discharge lamps are used in the range of 350–120 nm. Such lamps are found to be robust and stable, which are widely used.

Deuterium Lamps

In deuterium lamps, deuterium is used instead of ordinary hydrogen. The intensity of radiation emitted by such lamps is found to be 3–5 times more as compared to that in hydrogen discharge lamps. Deuterium lamps are more expensive than hydrogen discharge lamps and are used when more intensity is required.

Xenon Discharge Lamps

In xenon discharge lamps, xenon is stored under pressure of 10–30 atm. They contain two electrodes separated by about 8 mm. When a low voltage is passed, an electric arc is struck between these electrodes and the UV light is produced. The intensity of these UV radiations is much more than those of hydrogen discharge lamps.

Mercury Arc Lamps

In mercury arc lamps, mercury vapors are stored under high pressure and the mercury atoms are excited by passing electric discharge. These radiations are a standard source for UV experiments, but because of the presence of sharp lines or bands, this source is not useful for continuous spectral studies.

Monochromator

It will allow passing radiant energy of particular wavelength. It contains two parts:
1. Slit (entrance and exit)
2. Dispersion media (prism or grating)

In older types of instruments, fused silica prism was used to disperse the light. However, in modern instruments, diffraction gratings are used except when the highest accuracy is required then prism dispersion remains the method of choice. The most widely used dispersing element is a prism or grating made up of quartz because quartz is transparent throughout the UV range. Glass absorbs UV radiation hence, it cannot be used in this region. Glass can be used in the visible region.

The dispersed radiation is divided by the beam into two parallel beams of equal intensity; one of which passes through a cuvette containing the sample solution and the other through an identical cuvette containing the solvent. The former is called sample beam and the latter reference beam in case of double-beam spectrophotometer.

Sample Compartment (Sample Cells)

Sample and reference are kept in sample cells simply called cuvettes. Glass cuvettes are used for visible region and silica or quartz cuvettes are used for UV region in sample compartment. Cuvettes either are rectangular or cylindrical. Cuvette thickness of 1, 2, and 5 cm is used in which 1 cm thickness is quite common. Such cells/cuvettes are generally available in matched pairs, so that one of these is used as reference cell. Basic requirement of a cuvette is:
- They should be uniform and surfaces that face the incident radiation must be flat
- They should be made of such a material that is inert to solvent
- They must transmit light of the wavelength used

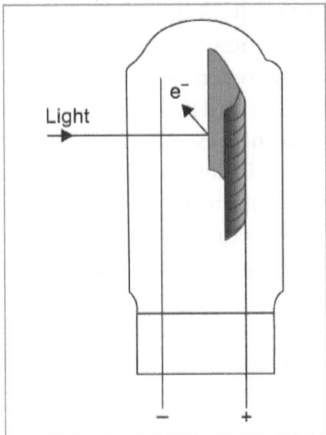

Fig. 8.13: Photomultiplier tube.

Detector

Light may or may not be absorbed by passage through the sample. This is determined by a quantitative measurement of light passing through the instrument by means of detector such as barrier layer cell, photovoltaic cell, photomultiplier tube, and photoconductive cell. Basic requirements of detectors are:
1. It must respond to radiant energy over a broad wavelength range
2. It should be sensitive to low levels of radiant power
3. It should rapidly respond to the radiation and produce an electrical signal
4. It should have relatively low noise level
5. The signal produced is directly proportional to the power of beam striking it

Photomultiplier Tube

Photomultiplier tube is generally used in a photospectrometer. A photomultiplier tube is shown in **Figure 8.13**. It consists of an evacuated tube containing one photocathode and 9–16 electrodes known as dynodes. The surface of each dynode is of Be-Cu, Cs-Sb, or some such similar material. When incident radiation falls on the metal surface of cathode, electrons gets emitted, which are attracted toward the first dynode. These are attracted by second dynode and electrons are emitted by second dynode. Hence, the process is repeated at all dynodes, until a shower of electrons reach the collector. The number of electrons that reach the collector is a measure of incident radiations on the detector. For steady signal, dynodes are operated at optimum voltage. Photomultiplier tube is quite sensitive and responds quickly.

Photovoltaic Cell

Photovoltaic cell consists of a semiconductor, such as selenium, which is deposited on a strong metal base such as iron. A thin layer of gold or silver is then sputtered over the semiconductor, which then acts as a second collector electrode. When radiations fall on the surface, it produces electrons at the selenium-silver interface. Since, a barrier exists between selenium and iron, the flow of electrons is prevented, which results in an accumulation of electrons on the silver surface and produces an electrical voltage difference between silver surface and the base of cell. If the external circuit has a low resistance, a photocurrent will flow, which is directly proportional to the intensity of the incident radiation. The sensitivity of the photovoltaic cell is not very high, which allows wide bands of radiation to strike the detector. This type of cell is used in photometers. Schematic diagram of photovoltaic cell is given in **Figure 8.14**.

This cell is simple in design and requires no supply of power. It can be hooked directly to a micrometer or galvanometer to read its output. As the time passes, such cell becomes useless due to transformation of selenium layer.

Photocell

It consists of a light-sensitive cathode in the form of a half cylinder of metal contained in an evacuated tube. The anode is also present in the tube and is fixed roughly. Schematic diagram of photocell is given in **Figure 8.15**.

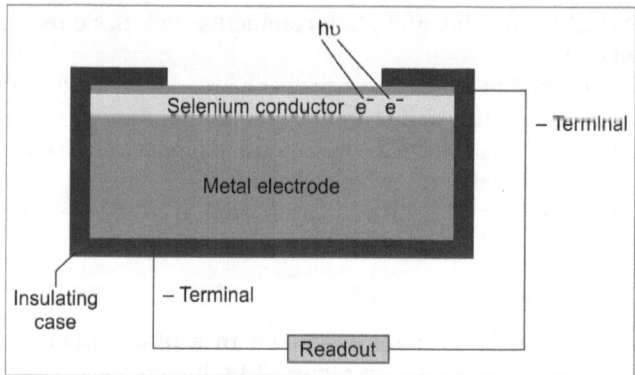

Fig. 8.14: Photovoltaic cell.

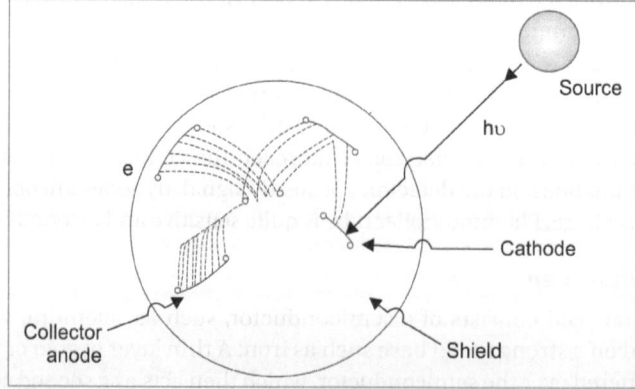

Fig. 8.15: Photocell.

When the incident light falls on a cell, electrons are emitted by the surface. These electrons are attracted and collected by anode. The current so produced is the measure of incident radiations. This type of cell is more sensitive because high degree of amplification can be used. In case of quartz or silica, windows are used, then the range of such a cell can be increased to cover both UV and far-UV region.

Recorder

The output of detector may be displayed or recorded in several ways. In many instruments, chart recorder is used. Alternatively, modern instruments are equipped with a digital output accessory, which enables a numerical printout of the absorbance and wavelength variation to be obtained.

Ultraviolet-visible spectrophotometer from different manufacturer is given in **Figures 8.16A** to **L**.

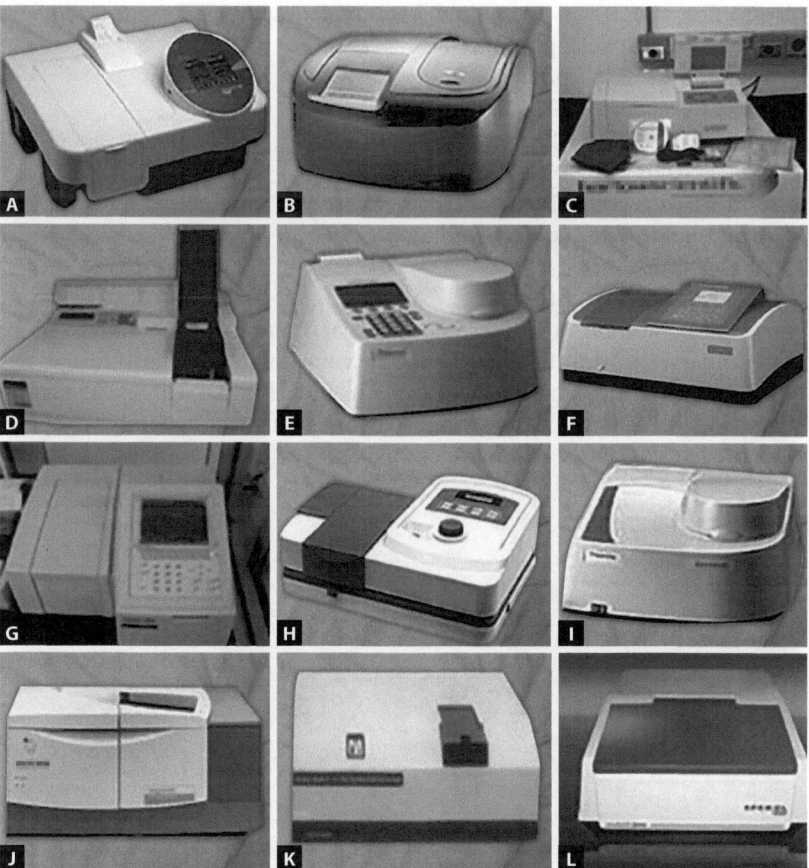

Figs. 8.16A to L: Ultraviolet (UV)-visible spectrophotometer by different manufacturers. (A) Biochrom Libra; (B) Hach-DR 5000; (C) Harlow Scientific; (D) PerkinElmer; (E) Preiser Scientific; (F) Tomos Biotools Co. Ltd.; (G) Shimadzu; (H) Aurora Instruments; (I) Thermo Scientific; (J) Varian Agilent; (K) Electronic Corporation of India Ltd.; and (L) Analytik Jena.

CALIBRATION OF ULTRAVIOLET-VISIBLE SPECTROPHOTOMETER

Calibration of an instrument used for analytical purpose is a necessary prerequisite for any sample analysis using UV-visible spectrophotometer. Any shortcoming in the functioning of the instrumental components can cause systematic errors of measurement. In all such cases, the error is removed by calibration of the spectrophotometer. For example, instability of a radiation source would cause errors in the observed signal. Hence, to maintain a constant intensity of source, the voltage stabilizer is necessary. Calibration of the various components of a spectrophotometer can be carried out systematically as follows.

Baseline Flatness

Baseline flatness is defined by the amount of baseline drift, excluding electronic noise. It can be studied, keeping following parameters constant in a UV-visible spectrophotometer:
- *Data mode*: Absorbance
- *Start wavelength*: 200 nm
- *Stop wavelength*: 1,100 nm
- *Upper scale*: (+)0.005
- *Lower scale*: (–)0.005
- *Beam mode*: Double beam/Single beam
- *Scan step*: 0.2 nm
- *Lamp switch*: 340 nm

Keeping sample and reference compartment empty, the system on scanning determines the absorbance in the whole wavelength range. The baseline is said to be flat if it is within ± 0.005 AU in the whole wavelength range (**Fig. 8.17**). If not, then warm up the instrument sufficiently (~2 h) and then proceed by setting up wavelength scan variables as above.

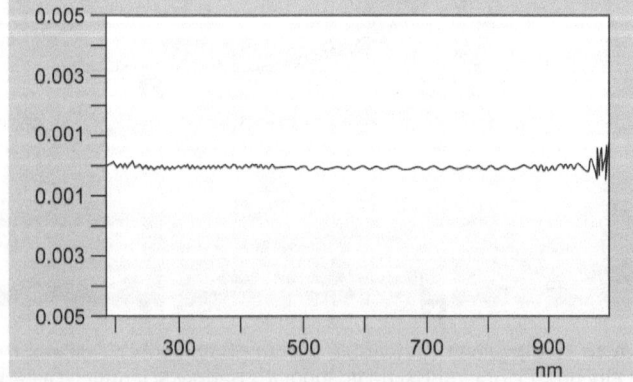

Fig. 8.17: A test for baseline flatness.

Spectrum Bandwidth

Bandwidth of a segment of spectrum is the wavelength between the points at which the transmittance is equal to one-half of the peak. It is expressed in nanometers. Spectrum bandwidth can be studied, keeping following parameters constant in a UV-visible spectrophotometer:
- *Data mode*: %Transmittance
- *Start wavelength*: 652 nm
- *Stop wavelength*: 657 nm
- *Integration time*: 31 s
- *Beam mode*: Double beam/Single beam
- D_2 *on*: Always

Keeping sample and reference cuvettes empty in transmittance mode, the instrument automatically scan the deuterium lamp energy, around its emission peak at 656.1 nm. Measure the peak width in nm at half height; if the value is below 2 nm, the bandwidth is considered to be normal (**Fig. 8.18**).

Resolution Power

The resolution is defined as the separation factor, yielding relative positions of peaks to each other, measured as the distance between the apexes of the two consecutive peaks. To carry out a test for resolution power, dissolve 28 µL toluene in 100 mL of hexane in a volumetric flask to prepare 0.028% toluene in hexane (v/v). Take this toluene solution as sample and hexane as reference. Resolution of toluene in hexane can be studied, keeping following parameters constant:
- *Measurement mode*: Absorbance
- *Upper wavelength*: 275 nm
- *Lower wavelength*: 265 nm
- *Scan speed*: 240 nm/min
- *Wavelength step*: 0.10 nm
- *Lamp change*: 350 nm

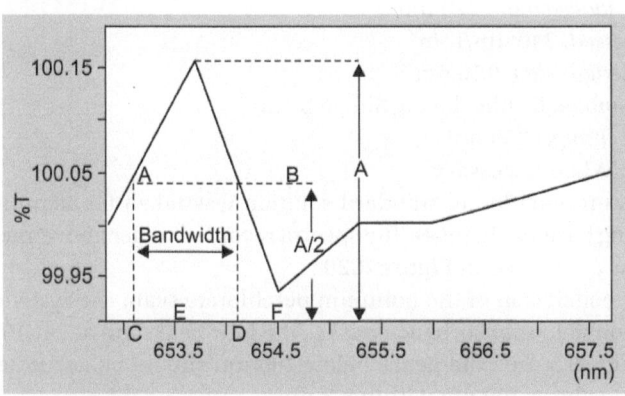

Fig. 8.18: Spectrum for determination of bandwidth.

ULTRAVIOLET-VISIBLE SPECTROSCOPY AND ITS APPLICATIONS

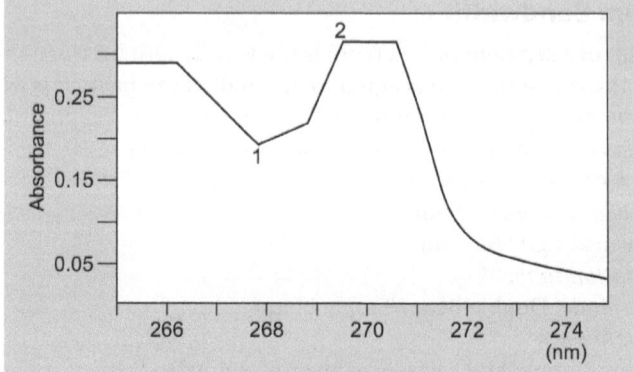

Fig. 8.19: Resolution of toluene in hexane.

- *Beam mode*: Double beam/Single beam
- D_2 *on*: When necessary

On scanning, the system determines the ratio of the absorbance at the maxima and minima at about 269.11 nm and 267.45 nm (**Fig. 8.19**). To ascertain that the resolution is okay, this ratio should not be <1.5:1.

Wavelength Accuracy

The wavelength accuracy is the difference between the true wavelength and the average observed wavelength. There are two wavelength tests that may be performed: (1) Holmium perchlorate solution test; and (2) Deuterium lamp test.

Holmium Perchlorate Solution Test

The wavelength accuracy can be studied, keeping following parameters constant in a UV-visible spectrophotometer:
- *Measurement mode*: Absorbance
- *Upper wavelength*: 570 nm
- *Lower wavelength*: 220 nm
- *Scan speed*: 240 nm/min
- *Wavelength step*: 0.10 nm
- *Beam mode*: Double beam/Single beam
- *Lamp change*: 350 nm
- D_2 *on*: When necessary

Holmium perchlorate standard solution was taken for scanning after conforming baseline flatness. The spectra recorded under above-mentioned conditions are shown in **Figure 8.20**.

At the conclusion of the holmium perchlorate scan, the system checks the location of four absorbance peaks. The four peaks are at 241.15, 287.15, 361.5, and 536.3 nm. The peaks below 400 nm should be accurate within ± 1 nm and above 400 nm within ± 3 nm.

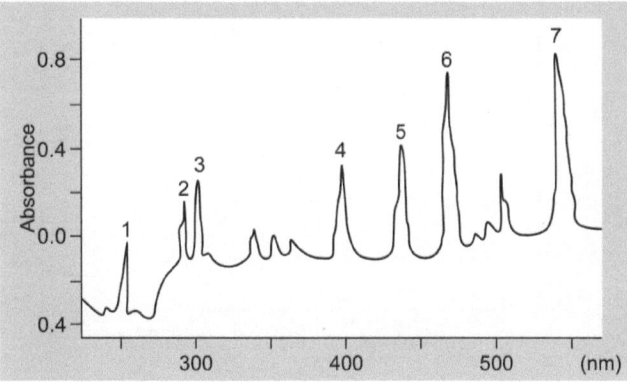

Fig. 8.20: A test of wavelength accuracy using holmium perchlorate solution.

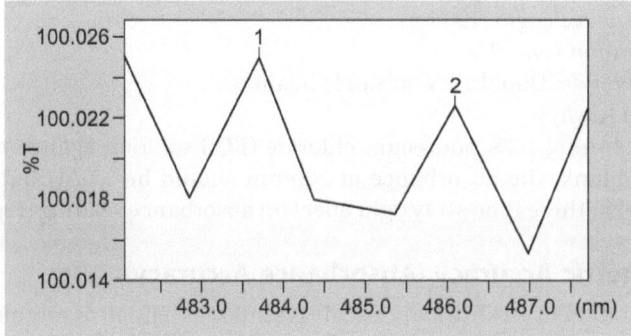

Fig. 8.21: A test of wavelength accuracy using deuterium lamp test.

Deuterium Lamp Test

The wavelength accuracy can be studied, keeping following parameters constant:
- *Measurement mode*: %Transmittance
- *Upper wavelength*: 488 nm
- *Lower wavelength*: 482 nm
- *Scan speed*: 20 nm/min
- *Wavelength step*: 0.1 nm
- *Beam mode*: Single beam
- D_2 *on*: Always

At conclusion of the scan, the system checks the location of the deuterium emission line. The peak should be at 486 nm and accurate within ± 3 nm. Spectra obtained are shown in **Figure 8.21**.

Stray Light Interference Test

Stray light interference test can be studied, keeping following parameters constant:
- *Measurement mode*: Absorbance
- *Upper wavelength*: 230 nm

ULTRAVIOLET-VISIBLE SPECTROSCOPY AND ITS APPLICATIONS

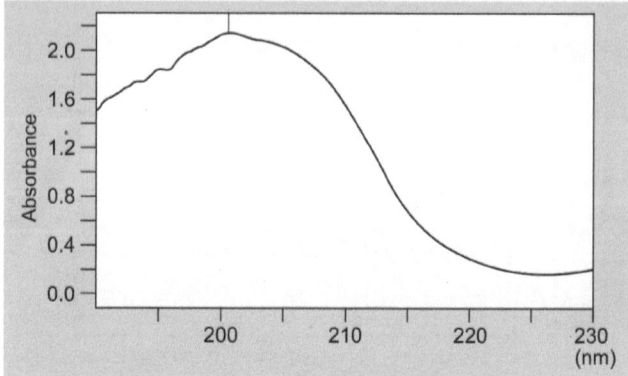

Fig. 8.22: Showing no effect of stray light interference.

- *Lower wavelength*: 190 nm
- *Integration time*: 2 s
- *Beam mode*: Double beam/Single beam
- *D_2 on*: Always

On scanning 1.2% potassium chloride (KCl) solution against distilled water as blank, the absorbance at 200 nm should be >2 AU indicating, thereby, that there is no stray light effect on absorbance reading (**Fig. 8.22**).

Photometric Accuracy (Absorbance Accuracy)

The calibration of an absorbance scale is almost essential, as any alteration in slit width either reduces the spectral resolution or lowers down the value of absorbance. It may also lead to a reduction in sensitivity and a low signal-to-noise ratio, resulting, thereby, errors in absorbance readings. There are two tests that can be performed: (1) Using absorption filter; and (2) Using potassium dichromate solution or potassium nitrate solution

Potassium Dichromate Solution Test

The absorbance accuracy can be studied, keeping following parameters constant:
- *Measurement mode*: Absorbance
- *Upper wavelength*: 400 nm
- *Lower wavelength*: 200 nm
- *Integration time*: 2 s
- *Beam mode*: Double beam/Single beam
- *D_2 on*: When necessary

On scanning potassium dichromate ($K_2Cr_2O_7$) solution [60.06 mg $K_2Cr_2O_7$ in 1 L of 0.01 N sulfuric acid (H_2SO_4)] against 0.01 N H_2SO_4, the system checks the absorbance readings against expected at 235, 257, 313, and 350 nm, respectively. The observed absorbance should not differ from the expected values by >0.01 AU (**Fig. 8.23**).

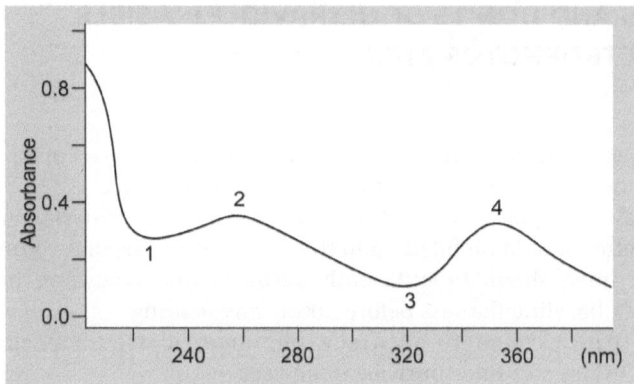

Fig. 8.23: A test of photometric accuracy using potassium dichromate.

Potassium Nitrate Solution Test

The photometric accuracy (absorbance accuracy) can be studied, keeping following parameters constant:
- *Measurement mode*: Absorbance
- *Lower wavelength*: 250 nm
- *Upper wavelength*: 350 nm
- *Integration time*: 2 s
- *Beam mode*: Double beam/Single beam

On scanning potassium nitrate (KNO_3) solution (14.207% w/v) and diluting it to the concentrations of 1.065%, 0.710%, and 0.355% w/v, the spectra are recorded at 302 nm. The system checks the absorbance readings against expected. The observed absorbance should not differ the expected values by >0.01 AU. The spectra obtained for all the above concentrations of KNO_3 are shown in **Figure 8.24**.

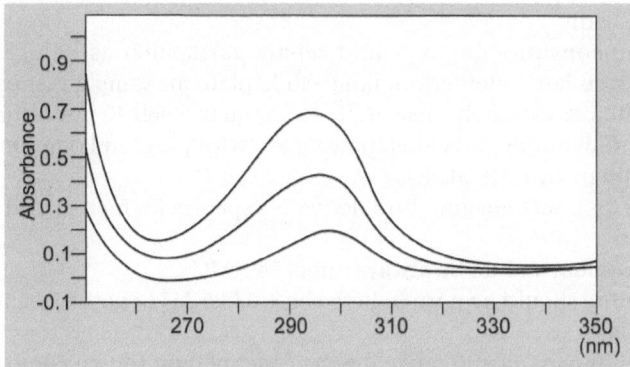

Fig. 8.24: A test of photometric accuracy using potassium nitrate.

■ DO'S AND DON'TS OF ULTRAVIOLET-VISIBLE SPECTROPHOTOMETER

Do's

1. Inspect both the cuvettes daily for any foreign material before use
2. Use similar cuvettes for both standard and reference
3. Always use quartz cuvettes not silica or any other material cuvettes
4. Cuvettes should be filled up to third-fourths of the total volume
5. Instrument should be sufficiently warmed before analyzing the sample
6. Check baseline flatness before taking any reading
7. Confirm wavelength accuracy, photometric accuracy, slit width, resolution, etc., once or twice in an year
8. Check once a week or more frequently whether or not the quartz window plate located at the entrance and the exit of the optical path of the sample compartment are smeared with fingerprint or other substances. If any smear is detected, remove it by using tissue paper or clean cloth soaked with alcohol
9. Absorbance should always be <2
10. Inspect the bottom of the sample compartment for any split samples before and after operation. Such split samples be left accumulated there, may evaporate, and evaporated atoms or molecules may fill the optical path of the sample compartment, thereby, resulting in errorless measurements in some cases
11. For calibration, use only spectroscopy grade solvents
12. Both the light source compartments are considerably heated
13. Prior to replacing the light sources, turn off the power source and confirm that the light source has been cooled down
14. Handle a new lamp with the hand wearing gloves so that the light flux window of the new lamp may not be smeared with fingerprint. Otherwise, the portion smeared with fingerprint may get burnt when the lamp wall is heated, thereby, resulting in poor optical transmission
15. Power supply should be given through uninterruptible power supply (UPS) only
16. Some consumable parts and repair parts such as halogen lamp, tungsten lamp, deuterium lamp, slide plate for sample compartment, cell holder assembly, fuse 5A, fuse 3A, quartz cell 10 mm square (four Pcs), didymium glass filter, power card with plug, and photomultiplier should be in stock always
17. Take first, second, and third derivative spectra for memorized spectral data
18. Instrument should be always under in AMC
19. Baseline should be normal between ± 0.005 AU in both UV and visible regions
20. When removing and replacing the cover of light source compartment, be careful not to hit the protrusion of the deuterium lamp end with the cover rear side, vacuum leakage of the lamp may result

Don'ts

1. Do not touch the optical surface of cuvettes during handling
2. Do not allow the solution in cuvettes for long time
3. Do not use glass cuvettes for R and D purpose
4. Do not disturb the adjustment of sample holder or slit width
5. Do not open the instrument in absence of engineer for any problem
6. Do not take more concentrated solution in cuvettes. Dilute it first then fill and take reading
7. Do not put D_2 lamp always on.
8. Do not switch off the spectrophotometer directly, first switch off D_2 lamp, then PC, and finally main plug.
9. Do not disturb the position of the sources such as D_2 and tungsten lamp
10. Do not use old solution for quantitation, prepare always fresh solution

■ TECHNICAL SPECIFICATIONS OF DOUBLE-BEAM ULTRAVIOLET-VISIBLE SPECTROPHOTOMETER

Optics

PC-based double beam ratio recording spectrophotometer having wavelength range of 190–1,100 nm.

- *Scan mode*: Absorbance or transmittance
- *Source changeover*: Automatic
- *Wavelength calibration*: Automatic using deuterium emission lines
- *Slow speed*: 10,000 rm/min or better
- *Band pass*: 2 nm or better
- *Wavelength accuracy*: ± 0.3 nm
- *Photometric drift*: 0.0003 ABS units/h at 340 nm or better
- *Lamp*: Tungsten halogen lamp for visible and near-IR region and deuterium lamp for UV region

Software and Data Station

1. %T/Absorbance and concentration calculation using linear and quadratic regression with multistandard derivative calculation
2. Window-based friendly and fills in front type, the spectrum is reported either in %T or absorbance as mode selected
3. The peak value and their wavelength are displayed. Any portion of peak can be zoomed for minute details
4. Branded PC with all accessories and software

Kinetic Function

Kinetic functions display the change in photometric data over a period of time.

Performance Validation

Program allows wavelength accuracy verification and reproducibility, baseline flatness, etc.

Accessories

1. Dust cover and manual
2. 1 KVA UPS with 30 minutes backup
3. 3.5 mL quartz cuvette 10 mm path length (set of two pairs)
4. Rectangular glass cuvette 10 mm path length (set of two pairs)

This is a general specification of UV-visible spectrophotometer, which can be changed as per the laboratory requirement.

■ SOLVENTS FOR ULTRAVIOLET-VISIBLE SPECTROSCOPY

The choice of solvent to be used in UV-visible spectroscopy is quite important. The first criterion for a good solvent is that it should not absorb UV radiation in the same region as the substance whose spectrum is being determined. Usually, solvents which do not contain conjugated system are the most suitable for this purpose, although they vary as to shortest wavelengths at which they remain transparent to UV radiation. **Table 8.5** lists some common UV spectroscopy solvents and their cutoff points.

■ GENERAL APPLICATIONS OF ULTRAVIOLET-VISIBLE SPECTROSCOPY

Detection of Functional Group

The presence or absence of a particular group may be indicated by the presence or absence of an absorption band in the expected wavelength region. For example, the presence of a low intensity band in the region 270–300 nm indicates the presence of a carbonyl group. If the spectrum is transparent above 200 nm, it shows the absence of carbonyl group, a conjugated system, an aromatic ring, and a bromine or iodine atom in the molecule. However, an unconjugated C=C bond or some other atoms or groups may be present in the molecule, if it does not absorb above 200 nm. Thus, no definite conclusion can be drawn regarding the structure of the molecule, if it absorbs below 200 nm.

■ **Table 8.5:** Cutoff points for different solvents.

Solvents	Cutoffs (nm)	Solvents	Cutoffs (nm)
Acetonitrile	190	n-hexane	201
Chloroform	240	Methanol	205
Cyclohexane	195	Iso-octane	195
1,4-Dioxane	215	Water	190
95% ethanol	205	TMP	210

Qualitative Analysis

Qualitative matching of spectra can be done by comparison of an unknown against known sample in the laboratory or alternatively by matching the unknown spectra with standard (**Fig. 8.25**).

Quantitative Analysis

Prepare a series of standard solution in the concentration range desired. A blank must be prepared, which acts as a reference, set the λ_{max}. Calibrate the 0% transmittance with the shutter closed and the 100% transmittance with the shutter open and the blank in the optical path, obtain the absorbance at various concentrations of the standards, and plot absorbance versus concentration.

Ideal calibration curve is a straight line, which intersects the origin (**Fig. 26A**). Sometimes, the calibration curve is a straight line but not passing through origin (**Fig. 8.26B**). The concentration of unknown is obtained by reading its absorbance and determining corresponding concentration. In dotted line in **Figure 8.26A**, the absorbance of 0.55 corresponds to the unknown concentration of 4.5 mg/mL.

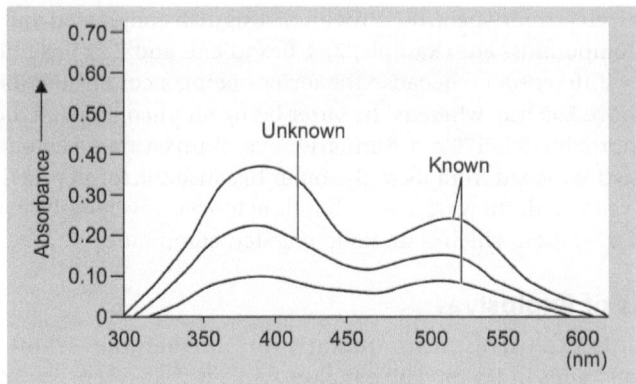

Fig. 8.25: Comparison of spectra of unknown and known substances.

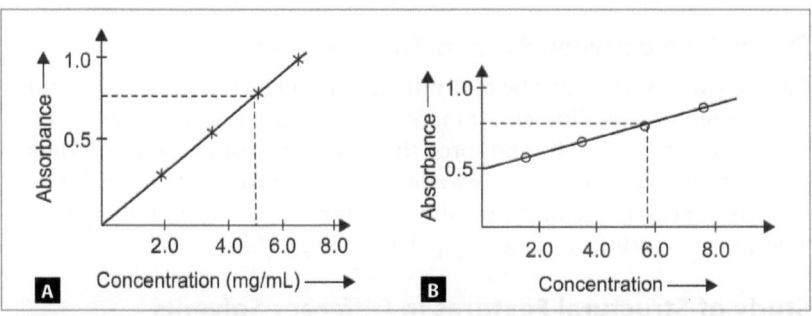

Figs. 8.26A and B: Calibration graph of absorbance versus concentration. (A) Passing through origin; and (B) Not passing through origin.

Detection of Conjugation and Elucidation of its Nature

Compounds containing a conjugated system including aromatics are characterized by their absorption above 200 nm. The longer the conjugated system, the longer is the wavelength of absorption. Also, substitutions on a conjugated system generally cause bathochromic and hyperchromic effects. Thus, we can elucidate the nature of conjugation by comparing the values of λ_{max} and ϵ_{max} for the compound under study.

Study of Extent of Conjugation

The values of λ_{max} increase as the number of conjugated multiple bonds increases thus, the extent of conjugation can be estimated. It has been found that the absorption occurs in the visible region if a polyene has eight or more conjugated double bonds. A polyene with such a sufficient conjugation becomes colored, e.g., β-carotene (orange) and lycopene (red) having 11 conjugated double bonds are colored and absorb in the visible region at 450 nm and 474 nm, respectively.

Distinction between Conjugated and Unconjugated Compounds

In general, electronic spectroscopy can distinguish conjugated and unconjugated compounds. For example, 2, 4-hexadiene and 2, 5-hexadiene can be readily differentiated because the former being a conjugated diene will absorb above 200 nm, whereas the latter being an unconjugated diene will absorb approximately 170 nm. Similarly, an α, β-unsaturated ketone can be readily distinguished from its α, β-isomer because the former having conjugated system will show transition bands at longer wavelengths compared to that of the latter, which is an unconjugated compound.

Analysis of Explosives

The organic explosives, nitroaromatic and nitroamines, show typical absorption bands in UV or visible region, while nitrate esters do not absorb in this region. **Table 8.6** shows the values of absorption maxima (λ_{max}) for a series of explosives and related compounds in different solvents.

Distinction between Cis and Trans Isomers

Cis and trans isomers can be easily distinguished on the basis of UV-visible spectrophotometer. The *cis*-isomers in which groups are closer to each other cause steric strain and force the groups out of coplanarity. Hence, *cis*-isomers absorb at shorter wavelengths and have lower intensity than *trans*-isomers, For example, *cis*-stilbene shows λ_{max} 283 nm, ϵ_{max} 12,300, whereas *trans*-stilbene shows λ_{max} 295 nm, ϵ_{max} 25,000.

Study of Structural Features in Different Solvents

In certain cases, the structure of a compound changes with the change in the solvent. For example, chloral hydrate shows an absorption maximum at

Table 8.6: UV absorption maxima in different solvent coefficients of some explosives.

Solvent compound	Ethanol λ_{max} (nm)	Methanol λ_{max} (nm)	Water λ_{max} (nm)
Nitrobenzene	260	267	259.5
1,3-DNB	232	245	234
1,3,5-TNB	233	229	224
2,4-DNT	227	-	-
2,5-DNT	267	-	-
2,4,6-TNT	224	233	227
Nitroguanidine	265	264	-

(DNB: dinitrobenzene; DNT: dinitrotoluene; TNB: trinitrobenzene; TNT: trinitrotoluene; UV: ultraviolet)

290 nm in hexane, but this band disappears when the spectrum is recorded in aqueous solution. This shows that the compound has a structure CCl_3CHO in hexane, whereas in aqueous medium, it changes to $Cl_3CCH(OH)_2$.

FORENSIC APPLICATIONS OF ULTRAVIOLET-VISIBLE SPECTROPHOTOMETER

Analysis of Drugs of Benzodiazepines

A majority of drug samples from benzodiazepine exhibit high molar absorbtivities in UV region. Specific UV absorption is listed in **Table 8.7**.

Characterization of the Material

Ultraviolet-visible spectroscopy is often used as a quick and inexpensive method for identification of certain classes of materials. Substances containing choromophores absorb the UV-visible radiation. Molecules may be identified by the position and height of the absorption bands. In some cases, absorption maxima can be predicted by increment rules. In these cases, identification is easier by UV-visible spectroscopy than by NMR and other techniques.

Table 8.7: Specific absorption of benzodiazepines derivatives.

Benzodiazepines	Major wavelength (in nm)
Chlorodiazepoxide	248 and 310
Clonazepam	279 and 350
Clorazepate	240, 283, and 362
Diazepam	242, 285, and 360
Flurazepam	235, 283, and 362
Lorazepam	236, 283, and 366
Oxazepam	239, 282, and 359
Prazepam	244, 289, and 358

ULTRAVIOLET-VISIBLE SPECTROSCOPY AND ITS APPLICATIONS

Table 8.8: Specific absorption of tranquilizers.

Name of tranquilizers	λ_{max} (nm)
Promazine hydrochloride	252
Chloropromazine hydrochloride	255
Thioridazine	263
Chlordiazepoxide	245
Imipramine	251
Phenothiazines	255

Analysis of Morphine

The substances to be tested are purified by thin-layer chromatographic method. The residue, thus, obtained is dissolved in 2 mL of 0.1 N H_2SO_4 and absorption is measured from 220 to 320 nm wavelength in UV spectrophotometer using 1 cm cell. For morphine, the wavelength at maximum absorption (λ_{max}) is 284 nm.

Analysis of Tranquilizers

The residue obtained by purification by thin-layer chromatography (TLC) is dissolved in 2 mL of 0.1 N H_2SO_4 and subjected to UV spectrophotometry and absorption spectra are recorded. Wavelength at maximum absorbance for different tranquilizers is given in **Table 8.8**.

Analysis of Dichlorodiphenyltrichloroethane

The extracted residue is purified by thin-layer chromatographic method. The purified residue is dissolved in 2.5 mL of 0.1 N H_2SO_4 and its absorption spectrum is measured with the help of UV-visible spectrophotometer from 220 to 320 nm. The major wavelengths for dichlorodiphenyltrichloroethane (DDT) are 236 nm, 266 nm, and 276 nm.

Analysis of Parathion

A portion of the purified extracted residue is dissolved in 5 mL of n-hexane. It is filtered, if necessary, and the absorption spectrum is studied in a spectrophotometer from 220 to 320 nm. The λ_{max} for parathion is 274 nm.

Analysis of Strychnine

After purification by TLC, the elution is made with 2 mL chloroform and it is evaporated to dryness. The residue is dissolved in 2 mL of 0.1 N H_2SO_4 and studied in a UV-visible spectrophotometer using 1 cm cell from 220 to 320 nm. Wavelength at maximum absorption (λ_{max}) is observed at 253 nm.

Analysis of Aconitine

After purification and elution from TLC plate, the elute is evaporated to dryness. The residue is taken into 2 mL of 0.1 N H_2SO_4 and absorption spectrum is recorded with the help of a UV-visible spectrophotometer. Wavelength at maximum absorption (λ_{max}) is absorbed at 234 nm.

■ CONCLUSION

Spectroscopy is the measurement and interpretation of electromagnetic radiation absorbed or emitted when the molecules or atoms or ions moves from one energy state to another energy state. UV-visible spectroscopy is routinely used in analytical chemistry for the qualitative/quantitative determination of different analytes, such as transition metal ions, conjugated organic compounds, and biological macromolecules. Spectroscopic analysis is commonly carried out in solutions but solids and gases may also be studied.

Using a UV-visible spectrophotometer and carrying out absorption/transmission measurements we can determine the concentration of a known chemical substance simply, by studying the number of photons (light intensity) that reach the detector. The more a material absorbs light at a particular wavelength, the higher the concentration of the known substance. In the present chapter different aspects of UV-visible spectrophotometer with different application is explained in a very simple manner.

■ FURTHER READINGS

1. Aruldhas G. Molecular Structure and Spectroscopy. New Delhi: Prentice Hall of India (P) Ltd; 2005.
2. DFS Manual of Toxicology, 1st edition. New Delhi: Selective and Scientific Publishers; 2005.
3. Doukas AG. Spectroscopic determination of skin viability: a predictor of postmortem interval. J Forensic Sci. 2000;45(2):36-41.
4. Jaffe HH, Orchin M. Theory and Applications of UV Spectroscopy. New York: John Wiley and Sons; 1962.
5. Jaiswal AK, Millo T. Do's and Don'ts for Forensic Sophisticated Analytical Instruments Vol–II. Int J Med Toxicol Legal Med. 2006;9(1):6-8.
6. Jaiswal AK, Ramteke VB, Millo T, Murthy OP. Forensic application of UV-visible spectrophotometer—a review. J Forensic Med Toxicol. 2009;26(2):47-60.
7. Jaiswal AK. Determination of Chlorpyriphos by UV-Visible Spectrophotometer. Indian J Criminol Criminal. 2004;1-3:90-5.
8. Jaiswal AK. Determination of TNT by UV-visible Spectrophotometer. Indian Police J. 2002;3:40-3.
9. Kalsi PS. Spectroscopy of Organic Compounds, 3rd edition. New Delhi: New Age International (P) Ltd; 1998.
10. Landeira AC. A new spectrophotometric method for the toxicological diagnosis of cyanide poisoning. J Anal Toxicol. 2000;24(4):266-70.
11. Lshaut H, Schwack W. Selective trace determination of dithiocarbamate fungicides in fruits and vegetables by reversed phase ion-pair liquid chromatography with UV and electrochemical detector. AOAC. 2000;83(3):720-7.
12. Rajvanshi AC, Jaiswal AK, Usha J. UV-VIS Spectrophotometer-Calibration. J Criminol Criminal. 2002;23(3):234-47.

13. Rao CN. Ultraviolet and Visible Spectroscopy. London: Butterworth; 1961.
14. Sharma BK. Instrumental Methods of Chemical Analysis (Analytical Chemistry), 16th edition. Meerut: Krishna Prakashan Media (P) Ltd; 1997.
15. Sharma YR, Vig OP. Elementary Organic Spectroscopy. New Delhi: S Chand and Company (P) Ltd; 1993.
16. Skoog DA, Holler FJ, Nieman TA. Principles of Instrumental Analysis. Singapore: Thomson Asia (P) Ltd; 2004.
17. Tiwari SN. Analytical Toxicology, 1st edition. Agra: Forensic Science Laboratory; 1976.
18. Tyagi OD, Yadav M. Textbook of Spectroscopy. New Delhi: Anmol Publications; 2002.
19. Vogel Al. A Textbook of Quantitative Inorganic Analysis, 4th edition. London: Longman Group Ltd; 1978.
20. West W. Chemical Applications of Spectroscopy, 2nd edition. New Delhi: John Wiley and Sons; 1968.
21. Willard HH, Merriff LL, Dean JA, Settle FA. Instrumental Method of Analysis. New Delhi: CBS Publishers and Distributors; 1986.
22. Yadav LDS. Organic Spectroscopy. New Delhi: Anamaya Publishers; 2005.

Chapter 9

Atomic Absorption Spectroscopy and its Applications

■ INTRODUCTION

Since its introduction by Alan Walsh in the mid-1950, atomic absorption spectroscopy (AAS) has proved itself to be the most powerful instrumental technique for the qualitative/quantitative determination of metals in any substance. This method provides a total metal content of the sample and is almost independent of molecular form of the metal in the liquid. The importance of this instrument can be realized from the fact that nearly >70 elements including most of the common rare earth metals have been determined in concentrations that ranges from traces to macro quantities. In this method, one can determine metal concentration in the presence of many other elements. AAS is not only used for aqueous solutions, but also for nonaqueous solutions. The metallurgical engineer, nonchemist, biologist or clinician can handle this instrument very conveniently.

■ PRINCIPLE OF ATOMIC ABSORPTION SPECTROSCOPY

This technique involves the study of absorption of radiation (usually in the ultraviolet visible region) by neutral atoms in the gaseous state. Thus in AAS, the sample is first converted into an atomic vapor and the absorption of atomic vapor is measured at a selected wavelength, which is characteristic of each individual element. So, when a light of this wavelength is allowed to pass through a flame having atoms of the metallic species, part of that light will be absorbed and the absorption will be proportional to the density of the atoms in the flame. Thus, in AAS one determines the amount of light absorbed. Once this value of absorption is known, the concentration of metallic element can be calculated, because the absorption is directly proportional to the concentration of the atoms in the flame. Here, the absorption is independent of the wavelength of absorption and the temperature of the atoms. The process of excitation and decay is given in **Figure 9.1**.

In AAS, the signal is obtained from the difference between the intensity of the source in the absence of metallic elements present in the liquid and the decreased intensity obtained when metallic elements

ATOMIC ABSORPTION SPECTROSCOPY AND ITS APPLICATIONS

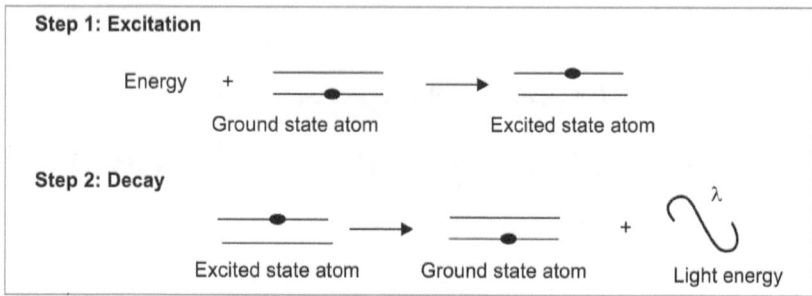

Fig. 9.1: Process of excitation and decay.

are present in the optical path. In this technique, atomic absorption depends upon the number of unexcited and the absorption intensity does not depend on the temperature of the flame. The relation between the absorbance and the concentration is nearly linear.

Advantages of Atomic Absorption Spectroscopy over Flame Emission Spectroscopy

- The atomic absorption technique is specific, because the atoms of a particular element can only absorb radiation of their own characteristic wavelength. Spectral interferences which occur in flame emission spectroscopy, whereas, in AAS occur rarely.
- Because of the much larger number of metal atoms that contribute to an atomic absorption signal, variation in flame temperatures has shown relatively less effect in AAS than flame emission spectroscopy in which the smaller numbers of atom are producing an emission signal.
- It is more sensitive than flame emission.
- This technique is quite independent of flame temperature.
- It is rapid and requires only small amount of materials.

Disadvantages of Atomic Absorption Spectroscopy

- A separate lamp for each element to be determined is required. Nowadays to overcome this, multielement lamp are developed with a high resolution monochromator.
- This technique cannot be used very successfully for the estimation of refractory metals such as Al, Mo, V, and Si, etc.
- The use of this technique is limited to metals only.

Atomic Absorption Process

The atomic absorption process is given in the **Figure 9.2**. Light at the resonance wavelength of initial intensity I_0 is focused on the flame cell containing ground state atoms. The initial light intensity is decreased by an amount determined by the atom concentration in the flame cell. The light is then directed on to the detector where the reduced intensity I is

ATOMIC ABSORPTION SPECTROSCOPY AND ITS APPLICATIONS

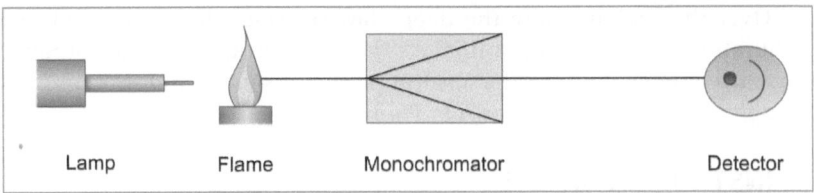

Fig. 9.2: Atomic absorption process.

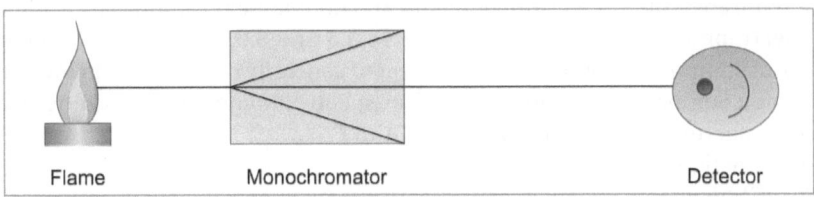

Fig. 9.3: Atomic emission process.

measured. The amount of light absorbed is determined by comparing I to I_0. The process of atomic emission and absorption is given in **Figures 9.2** and **9.3**, respectively.

The "transmittance (T)" is defined as the ratio of the final intensity to the initial intensity. Transmittance is an indication of the fraction of initial light which passes through the flame cell to fall on the detector.

$$T = I/I_0$$
$$\%T = 100 \times I/I_0$$
$$A = 100 - T$$
$$\%A = 100 - \%T$$

There is another term "absorbance (A)", which is purely a mathematical quantity.

$$A = \log(I/I_0)$$

Absorbance is the most commonly used term for characterizing light absorption in absorption spectrophotometry, as this quantity follows a linear relationship with concentration. As per Beer's law:

$$A = abc$$

where;
- A = Absorbance
- a = Absorption coefficient, a constant which is characteristic of the absorbing species
- b = Path length
- c = Concentration of the absorbing species in the absorption cell

This equation states that the absorbance is directly proportional to the concentration of the absorbing species for a given set of instrumental conditions. When the absorbance of standard solutions of known concentration of analyte is measured and the absorbance data are plotted against concentration, a calibration relationship similar to that in **Figure 9.4** is obtained.

ATOMIC ABSORPTION SPECTROSCOPY AND ITS APPLICATIONS

Over the region where the Beer's law relationship is observed, the calibration yields a straight line. As the concentration and absorbance increase, nonidealities in the absorption process cause a deviation from straight line behavior, as shown in **Figure 9.4**.

■ INSTRUMENTATION

There are two basic types of atomic absorption instruments, one is single-beam, and the other is double-beam. Schematic diagram of single beam atomic absorption spectrophotometer and double-beam atomic absorption spectrophotometer are given in **Figures 9.5** and **9.6**, respectively. Atomic absorption spectrophotometer instrument generally contains the following basic components. Atomic absorption spectrophotometer from different manufacturers is given in **Figures 9.7A to F**.

1. The light source
2. Chopper
3. Absorption cell
4. Monochromator
5. Detector
6. Readout system

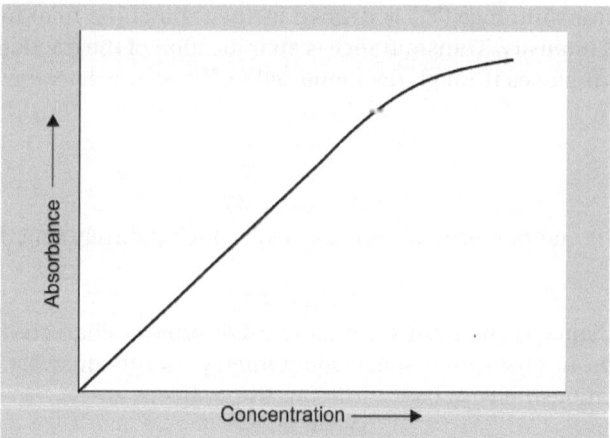

Fig. 9.4: Graphical representation of Beer's law.

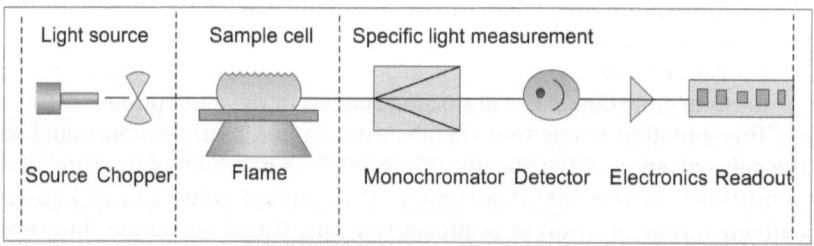

Fig. 9.5: Single-beam atomic absorption spectrophotometer.

ATOMIC ABSORPTION SPECTROSCOPY AND ITS APPLICATIONS

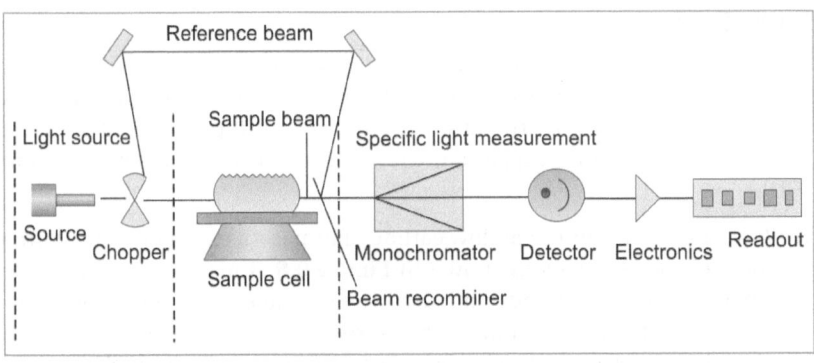

Fig. 9.6: Double-beam atomic absorption spectrophotometer.

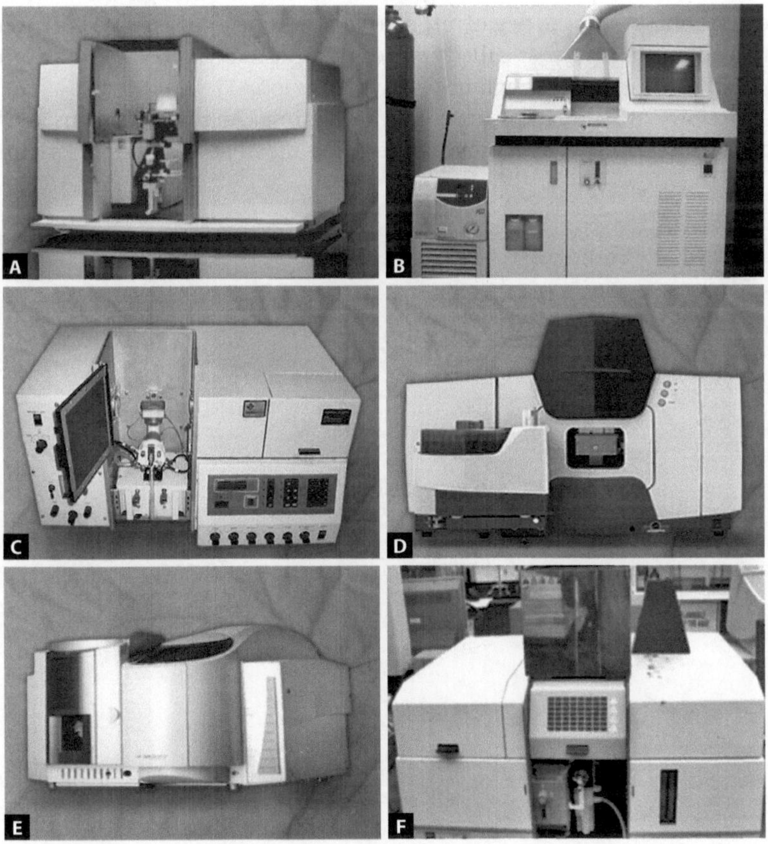

Figs. 9.7A to F: Atomic absorption spectrophotometer by different manufacturers. (A) Analytik Jena; (B) Hitachi; (C) PerkinElmer®; (D) Shimadzu; (E) Varian; (F) Thermofisher.

ATOMIC ABSORPTION SPECTROSCOPY AND ITS APPLICATIONS

Light Sources

In order to measure this narrow light absorption with maximum sensitivity, it is necessary to use a light source, which emits the very specific wavelengths that can be absorbed by the atom. There are two types of light sources, one is hollow cathode lamp, and the other is electrodeless discharge lamp (EDL).

Hollow cathode lamp: The hollow cathode lamp is an excellent light source for most of the elements as shown in **Figure 9.8**. The anode and cathode are sealed in a glass cylinder filled with either neon or argon. A window transparent to the emitted radiation is fused to the end of the cylinder. The anode is in the form of a thick wire, generally of tungsten or nickel.

The emission process is illustrated in **Figure 9.9**. When an electrical potential is applied between anode and cathode, some of the filled gas atoms are ionized. The positively charged ions accelerate through the electrical field to collide with the negatively charged cathode and dislodge individual metal atoms in a process called sputtering. Sputtered metal atoms are then excited to emission through impact with gas ions.

Hollow cathode lamps have a finite lifetime. As the lamp is used, the sputtering process may remove some of the metal atoms from the vicinity

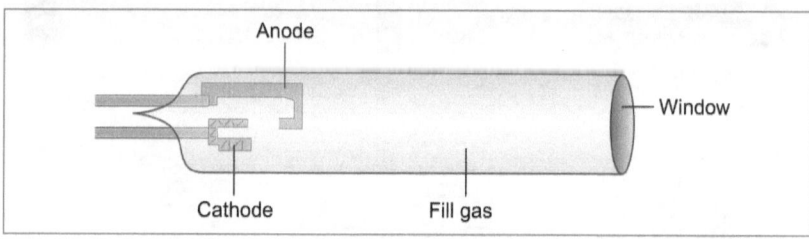

Fig. 9.8: Hollow cathode lamp.

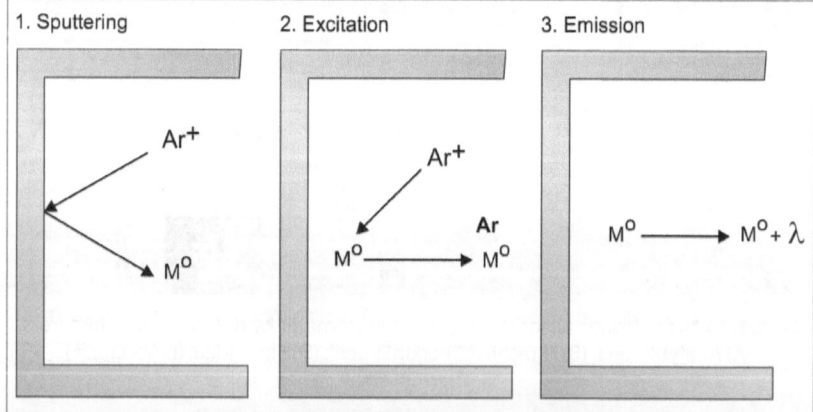

Fig. 9.9: Hollow cathode lamp process.

of the cathode to be deposited elsewhere. Lamps for volatile metals such as arsenic, selenium, and cadmium damage faster due to rapid vaporization of the cathode during use. Adsorption of fill gas atoms onto the inside surface of the lamp housing is a primary cause of this type of lamp failure.

Electrodeless discharge lamps: Another light source is EDL. EDLs offer better spectral output, longer life, for better precision and lower detection limits. A small amount of the element or salt of the element for which the source is to be used is sealed inside a quartz bulb. This bulb is placed inside a ceramic cylinder on which the antenna from a radiofrequency (RF) generator is coiled. When an RF field of sufficient power is applied, the coupled energy will vaporize and excite the atoms inside the bulb into emitting their characteristic spectrum. EDLs are available for aluminum, antimony, arsenic, bismuth, cadmium, cesium, germanium, mercury, potassium, phosphorus, rubidium, selenium, tellurium, thallium, tin, titanium, etc. Hollow cathode lamps also exist for these elements.

Chopper

A rotating wheel is placed in between the hollow cathode lamp and the flame. This rotating wheel is called chopper and is imposed to break the steady light from the lamp into pulsating light. Chopper gives a pulsating current in the photocell. There is also a steady current caused by light which is emitted by a flame, but only the pulsating current is amplified and recorded and, thus the absorption of light will be measured without interference from the light emitted by the flame itself.

Absorption Cell

In order to achieve absorption by atoms, it becomes necessary to bring the sample to the atomic state. The most common way is to use a flame (Burner system) which is used for converting the liquid sample into the gaseous state and also for conversion of the molecular entities into an atomic vapor. Cutaway view of an atomic absorption burner system is shown in **Figure 9.10**. Generally, there are two types of burners in use.

Total Consumption Burner

Total consumption burner is noisy and hard to use. The efficiency of this burner is not very good. In this burner, the sample solution, the fuel and oxidizing gas are passed through separate passages and meet at an opening at the base of the flame.

Premixed Burner

Most of the AAS instruments have the premixed burners. In this, a mixture of the sample solution and premixed gases say acetylene and oxygen is allowed to enter the burner. In this premix system, sample solution is aspirated through a nebulizer and sprayed as a fine aerosol into the mixing chamber. Here, the sample aerosol is mixed with fuel and oxidant gases

ATOMIC ABSORPTION SPECTROSCOPY AND ITS APPLICATIONS

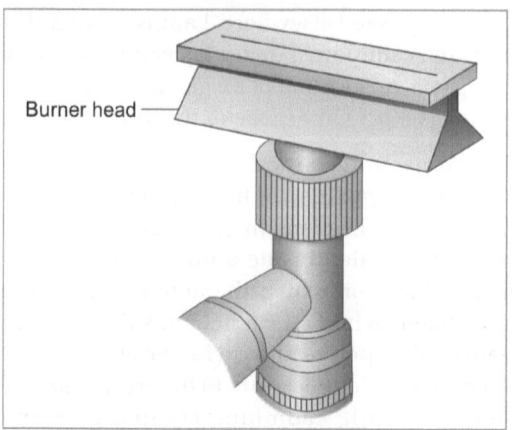

Fig. 9.10: Cutaway view of an atomic absorption burner system.

and carried to the burner head, where combustion and sample atomization occur. Fuel gas is introduced into the mixing chamber through the fuel inlet, and oxidant enters through the nebulizer side arm.

Stainless steel has been the most common material used for construction of the nebulizer, but this has the disadvantage of corrosion from samples. For such cases, nebulizers constructed of a corrosion resistant material, such as an inert plastic or platinum-rhodium alloy can be used.

Parts of Absorption Burner System

Burner heads: Burners are designed specifically for the various combustion gas mixtures employed. They are all made of solid titanium which is corrosion resistant and free of most of the elements commonly determined by atomic absorption. There are three burner heads available for use with the dual option burner system.
1. The 10 cm burner head is designed to be used with the air-acetylene flame. Because of its long burner path length, it provides the best sensitivity for air-acetylene elements.
2. The 5 cm burner head or nitrous oxide burner head is required for nitrous oxide-acetylene operation. It can also be used with air-acetylene or air-hydrogen. It can be rotated 90 degrees to provide reduced sensitivity.
3. The three slot burner head can be used for air-acetylene and argon-hydrogen-entrained air flames. It is designed to be used when analyzing samples with high concentrations of dissolved solids. With a fuel-rich, chemically reducing flame, free analyte atoms persist up to 4 cm above the burner tip.

Flames: Major function of the flame is to convert the sample to the atomic state. The process of flame is expressed in **Figure 9.11**. The two most

ATOMIC ABSORPTION SPECTROSCOPY AND ITS APPLICATIONS

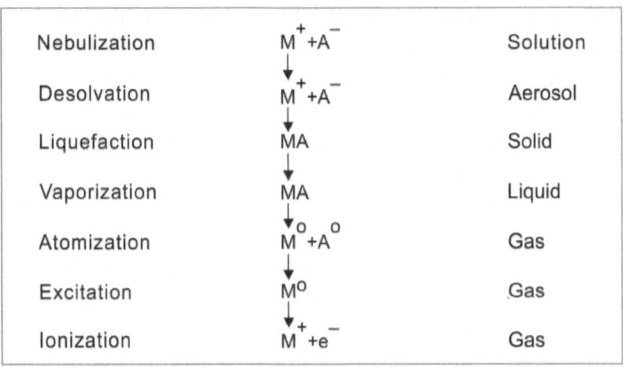

Fig. 9.11: Flame process.

common oxidant/fuel combinations used in atomic absorption are air-acetylene and nitrous oxide-acetylene. Other flames that can be used for atomic absorption are the air-hydrogen flame and the argon-hydrogen-entrained air flame.

1. *Air-acetylene flame*: Air-acetylene is the preferred flame for the determination of marked elements by atomic absorption. The temperature of the air-acetylene flame is about 2300°C. For the air-acetylene flame, the acetylene flow is about 4 L/min. Following precautions should be taken during handling of air-acetylene flame.
    - Normally, welding grade acetylene is supplied dissolved in acetone. As tank pressure falls, the concentration of acetone entering the flame increases. This increase may produce erratic results when determining elements that require a fuel-rich flame or elements with analytical wavelengths in the lower UV range.
    - Acetone passing into the gas control box may damage valve and tubing. For these reasons, acetylene cylinders should be replaced when the tank pressure falls below 75 psi (520 kPa).
    - Cylinders should always be used in a vertical position to minimize liquid acetone entering the gas line.
    - Acetylene line pressure from the cylinder to the instrument should never be allowed to exceed 100 kPa (15 psi). At higher pressures, acetylene can spontaneously decompose or explode.
    - Acetylene and copper form an explosive combination. So copper tubing or fittings for acetylene gas must, be strictly avoided.
    - Both fuel and oxidant pressure in all gas lines should be relieved at the end of the experiment.
    - Compressed air is needed for air-acetylene flame. The air supply should provide a minimum of 28 L/min at a minimum pressure of 275 kPa.
    - It is essential to have water and oil traps or filter between the compressor and the instrument gas control system to keep oil and water droplets out of the flow-metering stem.

2. *Nitrous oxide–acetylene* flame: The nitrous oxide–acetylene flame has a maximum temperature of about 2900°C and is used for the determination of elements which form refractory oxides. It is also used to overcome chemical interferences that may be present in flames of lower temperature. The use of nitrous oxide requires a number of accessories and precautions. Some of them are discussed as:
    - When nitrous oxide is rapidly removed from the cylinder, the expanding gas causes cooling of the cylinder pressure regulator and the regulator diaphragm so that it sometimes freezes. This can create erratic flame conditions. It is therefore, advisable to heat the regulator, using either a built-in heater or an externally supplied source of heat, such as an electrical resistance heating tape.
    - Only the nitrous oxide burner head can be used with the nitrous oxide-acetylene flame.
    - All lines carrying nitrous oxide should be free of grease, oil or other organic material, as it is possible for spontaneous combustion to occur.
    - Care should be taken with nitrous oxide on cold and humid days in that the flow of gas through the regulator forms ice and under extreme conditions can freeze-up the regulator causing erratic results.

Monochromator

The function of the monochromator is to isolate that resonance line from nonabsorbing lines situated close to it in the source system. A general purpose monochromator should be able to separate two lines 0.1 nm apart or less when operating with minimum slit width. The better the monochromator, the smaller is the slit width.

Pictorial view of monochromator is given in **Figure 9.12**. Light from the source enters the monochromator at the entrance slit and is directed to the grating where dispersion takes place. The diverging wavelengths of light are directed toward the exit slit. By adjusting the angle of the grating, a selected emission line from the source can be allowed to pass through the exit slit and fall onto the detector. All other lines are blocked from exiting. The useful atomic absorption wavelength ranges from 200 to 900 nm.

Detectors

Photomultiplier tubes are used for conversion of the radiant energy signal to an electrical one. Photomultiplier tube consists of a vacuum photocell with an anode, a radiation sensitive electrode, and a number of emission cathodes which have increasing positive potential with respect to the photocathode. Photomultipliers with a total of 10–15 electrodes are frequently used. Photons entering the detector through a window strike a photocathode, electrons are ejected from the photocathode and accelerated by a voltage potential to the first dynode, where more electrons

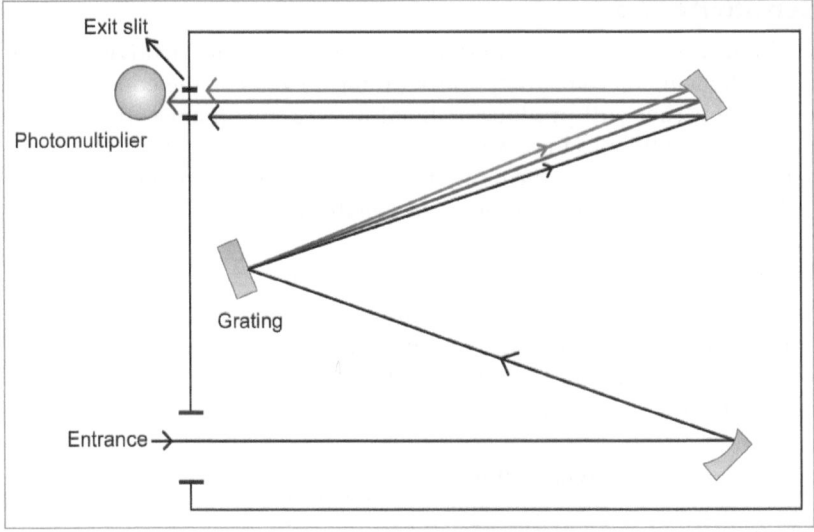

Fig. 9.12: Monochromator.

are released. These are accelerated to the second dynode, repeating the electron multiplication step. The process repeats with each dynode stage, until finally, the stream of electrons reaches the anode, amplified as much as a hundred million times. The resulting electrical signal then goes to the main amplifier.

Readout System

The readout system of an atomic absorption spectrophotometer is simply the means whereby, amplified electrical signals from the photomultiplier are translated into instrumental readings corresponding to the analytical result. In most of the atomic absorption measurement, simple meters, digital displays, printers, chart recorders, and of course computers are used.

■ SENSITIVITY, DETECTION LIMIT AND WORKING RANGE

Sensitivity

Sensitivity is the concentration of an element that will produce a transmittance of 99% (absorbance of 0.0044), also known as reciprocal sensitivity or characteristic concentration. As long as measurements are made in the linear working range, the sensitivity of an element can be determined by reading the absorbance produced by a known concentration of the element, and solving the proportional equation below:

$$\text{Sensitivity} = \frac{\text{Concentration of standard} \times 0.0044}{\text{Measured absorbance}}$$

Sensitivity Check

Different instruments will produce different values of sensitivity for the same element. The sensitivity check (in mg/L) value is the concentration of element that will produce a signal of ~0.2 absorbance units under optimum conditions at the wavelength listed. Using the sensitivity check, the operator can determine if instrumental parameters are optimized and if the instrument is performing up to specifications.

Detection Limit

The detection limit is defined as the minimum concentration of an element which can be detected with 95% certainty. This is that quantity of the element which gives a reading equal to twice the standard deviation of a series of at least 10 determinations at or near blank level.

$$\text{Detection limit} = \frac{2 \text{ Std Dev} \times \text{Conc.}}{\text{Mean Abs.}}$$

where,
Std Dev = standard deviation
Conc. = concentration
Abs. = absorbance

Working Range

This is the range of concentration of analyte element which will produce suitable absorbance values for practical analysis. Generally, however, the working range should lie between 0.1 and 0.8 absorbance since this is usually the region of optimum optical precision. Specifically, the % relative error is minimum in the absorbance range from 0.1 to 0.8. Useful measurements can be made at lower absorbance, and the overall working range can extend to a lower limit that is about ten times the detection limit.

The working range can be extended by either diluting all the solutions or altering the instrumental sensitivity. In flame analysis, selecting alternative (less sensitivity) wavelengths, rotating the burner across the optical path, or doing both will allow determinations to be carried out at significantly higher concentrations.

■ INTERFERENCE IN ATOMIC ABSORPTION

Following types of interferences are generally encountered in AAS.

Spectral Interferences

This type of interference may be caused by overlapping of any radiation with that of characteristic radiation of the test element to be estimated. The interfering radiation may be an emission line of another element radical or molecule, unresolved band spectra or general background radiation from the flame, solvent.

1. In this case, the lines will be read together in proportion to the degree of overlap, if the resolving power and spectral bandpass of the monochromator permit the undesired radiation to reach the photoreceptor. For example, the overlapping of manganese triplet (4031, 4033, and 4035 A), the gallium line (4033 A) and potassium doublet (4044 and 4047 A).
 2. This type of overlapping can be overcome by selecting other spectral lines.
 3. Suppose, the spectral interferences are due to sample matrices or flame components, one can overcome this problem by working with AC amplifiers, tuned to the frequency at which the source is chopped or modulated.

Matrix Interferences

 1. Matrix interferences are due to the number of free atoms reaching the optical path to be absorbed.
 2. Factors such as precipitation of the sample before its entry into the nebulizer are critical, as are the physical characteristics of solutions, such as viscosity, surface tension, density, pH and solvent vapor pressure, since all these parameters influence nebulization.
 3. For accurate results, the standards and samples should be matched as closely as possible with respect to the above physical parameters.
 4. Other forms of matrix interference are stable compound formation and ionization.

Chemical Interferences

 1. Stable compound formation is responsible for many of the depressive effects that are observed, both in atomic absorption and flame emission spectrometry.
 2. It arises because the element forms a stable compound either with a species in the matrix or with a species in the flame, such as aluminum, vanadium, boron, etc., which forms stable refractory oxides not broken down in the cooler air-acetylene flame.
 3. Using high temperatures in the nitrous oxide-acetylene flame, dissociates the refractory compounds into atoms.
 4. Alternatively, a releasing agent, such as lanthanum or strontium, will help to prevent the formation of the refractory compounds.
 5. Lanthanum works as an agent by forming more stable compounds.
 6. It is added in a sufficiently large quantity to complex the interference. The use of such releasing agents should be added to match standards also.

Interference due to Ionization

 1. The temperatures of the acetylene or nitrous oxide-acetylene flames may cause considerable ionization of the analyte.

2. To overcome this problem, an easily ionizable element, such as potassium, sodium or cesium is added sufficiently to produce an excess of electrons in the flame, thus inhibiting ionization of the analyte.

■ TECHNIQUES FOR OPTIMIZATION

Choice of Wavelength

Use a wavelength that does not require excessive dilution of the sample. Use of line free from spectral interference also produces a large linear range of the calibration curve.

Lamp Current Optimization

The use of as low an operating current as possible, is better to increase the life of the lamp and to minimize curvature due to self-absorption. However, if the signal is noisy, a higher lamp current will have to be used, taking care not to exceed the maximum lamp current.

Sample Introduction System

The sample introduction system comprises nebulization, spray chamber burner and flame conditions. After optimizing the wavelength and zeroing the absorbance reading, the burner is adjusted by using the horizontal vertical rotational controls. The main aim in adjusting these controls is to locate the optimum position of the flame in the light beam. Generally, an uptake of 3–6 mL/min is optimum for pneumatic nebulizers. In the case of nitrous oxide-acetylene flame, an uptake of 2–4 mL/min is good. Only nebulization should be done in air-acetylene flame. Optimization of the nebulizer is normally carried out with 5 ppm copper standard solution. Usually, three standards and a blank are used to cover the range of 0.1–0.8 Abs. The calibration is performed by using the blank solution to zero. The standards should be aspirated in ascending order and blank run between standards to insure the baseline has not changed. A graph of absorbance versus concentration is plotted for linearity (**Figs. 9.13** and **9.14**).

■ APPLICATIONS OF THE ATOMIC ABSORPTION SPECTROSCOPY

Analysis of Metallic Elements in Biological Samples

The AAS is becoming a very important instrument for the measurement of trace metals in biological materials. The procedure which has been developed recently for decomposition of the organic material, is the use of hydrogen peroxide. We can get good results with the digestion of blood, liver and meat products with combination of acids such as concentrated H_2SO_4, HNO_3, etc.

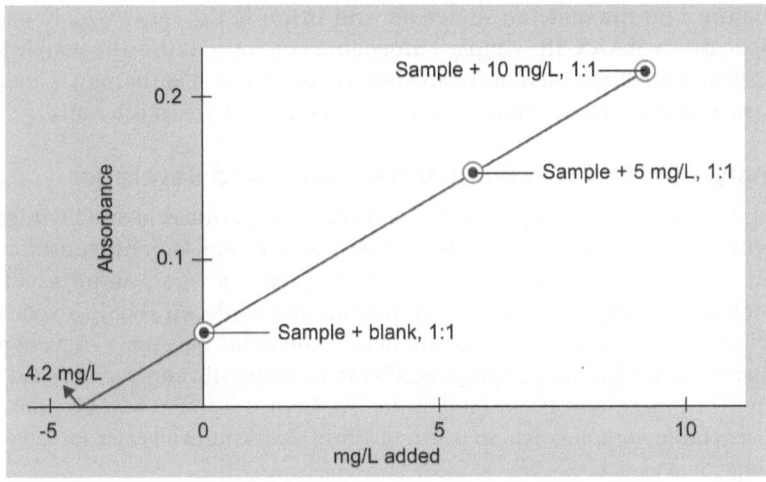

Fig. 9.13: Standard addition method.

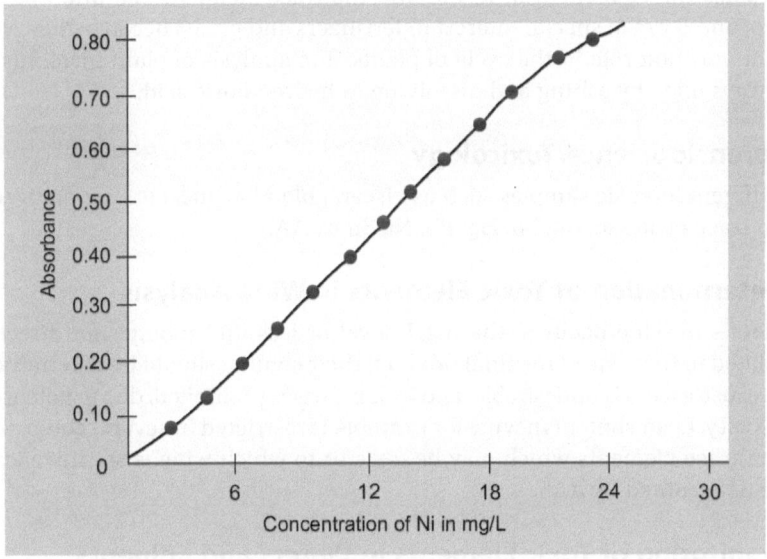

Fig. 9.14: Calibration method.

Analysis of Calcium, Magnesium in Blood Serum for Clinical Diagnosis

The determination of these elements in blood serum is of vital importance in diagnosing many pathological conditions, like diabetes, and primary aldosteronism. AAS is regarded as the most suitable instrument for the determination of these elements in blood serum. The determination of calcium and magnesium in serum and urine is the most widely used applications of AAS. The simplest procedure employed is the direct analysis of 1:20 to 1:50 diluted sample in an air-acetylene flame. Lanthanum is added to the diluted serum sample to suppress the phosphate interference.

Analysis of Metal in Foodstuffs, Drinks and Beverages

Combinations of nitric, perchloric, sulfuric, phosphoric acid and hydrogen peroxide can be used to bring the sample into solution. Organic substances can also be decomposed with oxidizing agents, such as potassium perchlorate, hydrogen peroxide, vanadium pentoxide, etc. For less volatile elements, ashing is advantageous before the acid digestions. Beverages must be degassed before spraying. Elements generally analyzed are Cd in fish, Al in milk, and Pb in food stuffs, Al, Ca, Cd, Cu, Fe, Mg, Pb and Zn in vegetable samples. As, Se, Hg and Pb in drinking water, Cr in sewage sludge, leaves, etc.

Different Elements in Agricultural Samples

Besides the elements Na, K, Ca, Mn, the trace elements Cu, Mn, Zn, Fe, Mo, and B are of special interest in fertilizers and plants because they play an important role in the cycle of plants. The analysis of plant materials is always done by ashing and dissolving in hydrochloric acid.

Forensic Science/Toxicology

Different forensic samples such as viscera, blood, urine, etc., are analyzed for trace elements Cu, Sb, Hg, Pb, Ni, Sn by AAS.

Determination of Toxic Elements in Wine Analysis

Metals in wine occur at the mg/L level or less and though not directly related to the taste of the final product, their content should be determined because excess is undesirable, and in some cases prohibited, due to potential toxicity. Lead content in wine for example is restricted in several countries. Ten trace elements which may be toxic or to which wine is sensitive, can be determined by AAS.

Monitoring of Toxic Elements in Waters and Effluents

Monitoring toxic elements in effluents or sludge, leachate from waste material. Drinking water from ground, waste water, and sludge samples are analyzed for nearly 33 elements using AAS. The preconcentration of the water sample, i.e., 250:10 after acidification by either hydrochloric acid or nitric acid is the best technique for analysis by AAS.

Analysis of Metals in Geochemical, Mineralogical Samples

Rock samples received during exploration and mining activities are normally determined by digesting with the combinations of either nitric acid (HNO_3) and hydrofluoric acid (HF), HF and hydrochloric acid (HCl) or HF, HNO_3, sulfuric acid (H_2SO_4) and preparing the clear solution in diluted acid, usually, HCl. For mineralogical samples, depending on the nature of the sample, several fusion techniques are suggested. After fusion, the samples are brought into solution using H_2SO_4 or HCl. This solution can be introduced to flame for the elemental analysis by AAS.

Determination of Lead, Barium, and Tin in Forensic Sample

Determination of lead (Pb), barium (Ba), and tin (Sn) is very important in forensic samples especially in gunshot residue for identification of the shooter in a gunshot case. A simple and fast method of determination of Pb, Ba and Sn by atomic absorption spectrophotometer has got many advantages over other methods, e.g., colorimetric method in terms of reliability and accuracy of results. Swabs can be taken from hands with a suitable acid, such as HCl or HNO_3 and the sample solution can be aspirated into the flame of an atomic absorption spectrophotometer for determination of Pb, Ba, and Sn content.

■ DO'S AND DON'TS FOR ATOMIC ABSORPTION SPECTROMETRY

Do's

1. After the analysis is over, immediately switch off the gas flow and lamps.
2. Always keep the sample inlet in the deionized or double distilled or ultrapure water.
3. In order to prevent the matrix interference due to the surface tension and viscosity of a test solution which is different from that of the standards, always simulate the test solution with that of the standard.
4. Whenever a new method is doped in determining trace levels of elements in media that contain appreciable loadings of foreign ions, a check for nonspecific background absorption should be made.
5. Optimum and uniform flame conditions must be maintained in order to obtain the good and high degree of results. It is normally attained by selecting a burner height, setting the oxidizing gas to a fixed flow rate, and then regulating the fuel so that peak absorption is obtained when a suitable standard solution is aspirated into the flame.
6. The depression effect caused by phosphate upon the absorption of calcium in the air-ethylene flame, can be overcome either by using the nitrous oxide-acetylene flame or diluting the sample with which it ties upon the phosphate ions.
7. Depression effect of phosphate on calcium in the air-acetylene flame can be overcome with the addition of lanthanum chloride or EDTA disodium salt. Lanthanum chloride ties up the phosphate, thereby, releasing the calcium ions for absorption in the flame. EDTA exerts more affinity toward calcium and the so formed calcium-EDTA complex then breaks up in the flame to yield calcium.

8. Cylinders should be placed in a secure, weather proof, adequately ventilated and fire resistant room. It should always be turned off at the end of analysis from cylinder.
9. When the instrument is switched on, do not forget to on the fume extraction system, i.e., exhaust hood.
10. If cyanide solution is used, always insure that contents of the waste reservoir are distinctly alkaline.
11. Nitrous oxide-acetylene flame should never be viewed directly with the naked eye as it emits strongly in the UV-region of the spectra.
12. Flame should be viewed through the protection screen supplied by the manufacturer.
13. Liquid samples, such as beer, mineral water, etc., must be degassed before aspiration to the instrument.
14. Samples that have high concentration of salt, such as sea water, urine and other body fluids may cause decrease in absorption signal, decrease in sample flow rate and loss of signal by clogging the burner and the small residue may be introduced into the flame which can scatter the light. This problem can be overcome by diluting the sample or by using absorption background correction or by solvent extraction method in which either metal of interest or salt may be extracted, leaving the metal of interest in an analyzable solution.
15. Blood sample should run with dilute ammonia.
16. At the start and end, instrument must be run in double distilled water.

Don'ts

1. Do not use low lamp flames such as air-hydrogen or air-propane flame because chemical interferences are much more likely to occur even though some elements may be of higher sensitivity and better stability in the low temperature flames.
2. The waste liquid from the spray chamber should never be collected in a glass container, always use a suitable plastic container.
3. In case of carbon build up in the burner slot, it should be carefully cleaned and never attempt to scrape off the carbon deposits with the flame.
4. Do not use ordinary water or tape water or mineral water for dilution.

■ TECHNICAL SPECIFICATIONS FOR PURCHASE OF DOUBLE BEAM ATOMIC ABSORPTION SPECTROPHOTOMETER (AAS)

General

- AAS should be fully computer controlled with flame, graphite furnace and hydride generation (VGA) system with:
    - 8 lamp positions
    - Motorized lamp turret

ATOMIC ABSORPTION SPECTROSCOPY AND ITS APPLICATIONS

- Auto lamp selection
- Auto high speed deuterium and self-reversal or Zeeman background correction system.
- Automated monochromator and slits selection.
* Optics: Double beam optics, beams should be as narrow as possible.
* Detectors: Photo multiplier (PMT)/solid state detector covering the full range of wavelength.
* Burner heads: About 10 cm (100 mm) long or more single slot/three slot air acetylene burner. Burner head should be PC controlled auto setting and auto height adjustable. Burner adjustment should be computer controlled with external rotation facility.
* Spray chamber: It should be made up of corrosion resistant material unaffected by corrosive acids like $HF/HClO_4$ and organic solvents.
* Nebulizer: High precision inert nebulizer, adjustable and should be made of platinum/iridium. It should be compatible to highly corrosive acid solutions, strong electrolytes, organic solvents.
* Fully automatic PC controlled lamp/slit selection/wavelength selection/gas flow/gas monitoring.
* Instrument should work for elemental analysis from biological samples such as blood, urine, tissue, serum, etc.

Monochromator

* Czerny turner configuration with 1800 lines/mm, blaze wavelength of 230 nm/236 nm or better.
* Wavelength coverage: 190 nm ~ 900 nm or better
* Spectral bandwidth: Auto-selection and variable

Flame System

* RSD (Cu): <2% or better
* Detection limit (Cu): <0.006 µg/mL or better

Graphite Furnace System

* Temperature control range: Room temperature to 2500°C or better
* Heating rate: 2000°C/s or better
* RSD (Cd): ≤2% (for auto sampling) or better
* Detection limit (Cd): ≤2pg
* Autosampler for graphite furnace
* Autosampler capacity: 50 or more
* The internal and external gas of graphite furnace is automatically controlled by computer based on software heating procedures.

Vapour Generation Accessory (VGA) System

* Automatic software control continues hydride vapour generation system for analysis of metals such as As, Hg, Se, Sb, Sn, Bi at trace level.

- Hydride System should be modular continuous flow vapor generation accessory for determination of As, Hg, Se, Sb, Te, Bi.
- Detection limit for VGA elements should be 1 p pb

Software

- Fully compatible, licensed Windows 7 operating software with external PC with mouse or keyboard control.
- Report should be printable during run or post run by users selectable sequential or multi element format.
- All the facilities for fully instruments parameters selection, controlling, peak, valley, zooming, curve plotting, signals, and method stored, auto calculations, data and standards management, via software and external PC with printer.
- All the facilities for fully instruments parameters selection, controlling, peak, valley, zooming, curve plotting, signals, and method stored, auto calculations, data and standards management, via software and external PC with printer.
- Software shall be compatible with Windows 7 and above.

Computer and Printer

- Branded computer with branded laser colour printer with compatible software.
- The computer should possess the latest minimum configuration. Such as intel Core i5, 1 TB hard disc, 4GB RAM, DVDRW, 19" LCD/TFT color monitor, optical mouse, branded UPS 1 KVA with minimum 20 min backup.
- Genuine software: Windows 10 O.S, MS-Office and antivirus with one external hard disk of 1TB.

Accessories

- Hollow cathode lamp/for elements Cu, Al, As, Hg, Se, Sb,Sn B, Ba, Bi, Cd, Co, Cr, Fe, Zn, Tl,Pb Mg, Mn, Ni (one each).
- Oil-free air compressor.
- Water cooling system (chiller).
- Pyrolytically graphite tubes approx 50 pcs.
- C_2H_2 and argon gas cylinders along with double stage regulators and gas purification panel.
- Supply and Installation of suitable fume hood (exhaust system) should also be quoted.
- System must be supplied along with all necessary accessory required for smooth functioning.

Safety Features

- Cooling water flow monitoring.
- Carrier gas pressure monitoring.

- Graphite tube temperature monitoring.
- Graphite furnace temperature monitoring.
- C_2H_2 leaking preventive measure.
- C_2H_2 pressure monitoring.
- Air pressure monitoring.
- Burner monitoring.
- Flaming burning monitoring.
- Water seal monitoring.
- Ignition of flame should be prevented by fully interlocked operation.
- Provision should be there for separate flame ignition and emergency flame off button.
- At the end of analysis the flame should be automatically extinguished.

Chemical and Reagent

- NIST traceable standard solution of 1,000 ppm (minimum 100 mL) for element Cu, Al, As, Hg, Se, Sb, Sn, B, Ba, Bi, Cd, Co, Cr, Fe, Zn, Tl, Pb Mg, Mn, Ni (one each) must be supplied.
- NIST traceable multy element standard solution of 1,000 ppm (minimum 100 mL) must be supplied.

Warranty and CMC

05 years warranty from date of installation followed by 05 years CAMC.

This is a generalized specification which can be modified according the ureses of laboratories.

■ CONCLUSION

Atomic absorption spectrometry can be used in qualitative and quantitative analysis of metals. Atomic absorption spectroscopy is a procedure for the qualitative and quantitative determination of elements using the absorption of optical radiation by free atoms in the gaseous state. Atomic absorption spectroscopy is based on absorption of light by free metallic ions. This technique is used for determining the concentration of a particular element (metals) in a sample to be analyzed. AAS can be used to determine >70 different elements in solution, or directly in solid samples via electrothermal, vaporization and is used in chemistry, pharmacology, biophysics toxicology etc. Atomic absorption spectrometry has many uses in different areas of forensic chemistry and toxicology such as analysis of metals in biological fluids and tissues such as whole blood, plasma, urine, saliva, brain tissue, liver, hair, muscle tissue, etc.

■ FURTHER READINGS

1. Elwell WT. Atomic Absorption Spectrophotometry, 2nd edition. Oxford: Pengamon Press; 1966.
2. Furman NH. Standard Methods of Chemical Analysis. In: The Elements, 6th edition. Florida: Robert E Krieger Publications; 1985.

3. Mavrodineanu R. Analytical Flame Spectroscopy. Selected topics, 1st edition. London: Macmillan and Co. Ltd.; 1970.
4. Mendham J, Denney RC, Barnes JD, Thomas M, Sivasankar B. VOGEL'S text book of quantitative analysis, 6th edition. Delhi: Pearson Education (Singapore) Pvt. Ltd.; 2004.
5. Skoog DA. Principles of Instrumental Analysis, 3rd edition. Philadelphia: CBS College Publishing; 1985.
6. Slavin M. Atomic Absorption Spectroscopy, 2nd edition. New York: John Wiley and Sons; 1978.
7. Welz B. Atomic Absorption Spectrometry, 2nd edition. Weinheim, Germany: VCH Verlagsgesellschaft mbH; 1985.
8. Willard HH, Merritt LL, Dean JA, Settle FA Jr, et al. Instrumental Methods of Analysis, 6th edition. Delhi: CBS Publishers and Distributors; 1986.

Chapter 10

Voltammetry/Polarography Trace Metal Analyzer and its Applications

■ INTRODUCTION

Monitoring of heavy metals is of great importance. Contamination by these metals is indeed widespread all over the world. Due to their toxicity, even at low concentrations, Pb, Cd, As, Hg, Al, and Cr are key elements, while Cu, Zn, Ni, Co, Se, and Bi are important because they may play a vital or a toxic role, depending on their concentrations and the nature of organisms. The determination of trace metals in biological fluids and tissues is important for managing metal poisoning. Electroanalytical methods, such as stripping voltammetric techniques, are not only capable of determining trace amounts of an electroactive drug compounds, but also supply useful information concerning its physical and chemical properties. Anodic stripping voltammetry, coupled with easy accessible procedure, provides a sensitive and reliable method for analyzing biological material for trace metals. Electrochemistry has always provided analytical techniques characterized by instrumental simplicity, moderate cost, and portability. The basic aim of this chapter is to provide some brief information about trace metal analyzer and to outline some of its applications for the determination of heavy metals in biological fluids.

■ PRINCIPLE OF TRACE METAL ANALYZER

Trace metal analyzer (TMA) is based on principle of polarography and voltammetry. Polarography and voltammetry are the names of analytical methods based on current potential measurements in electrochemical cells. The analytical signal is the current, normally a Faradic current which flows through the cell during the reaction of the analyte at the working electrode with a small surface. The analyte may be a cation, an anion, or a molecule. Voltammetry includes all methods in which the current potential measurements are made at stationary and fixed working electrodes. These include:
- Hanging mercury drop electrode (HMDE)
- Thin mercury film electrode (TMFE)

- Glass carbon electrodes (GCEs) and carbon paste electrodes (CPEs)
- Platinum electrode, e.g., gold, platinum

Polarographic is related to the current and potential curve, which is recorded by using a liquid working electrode whose surface can be renewed periodically or continuously. This includes:
- Dropping mercury drop electrode (DMDE)
- Static mercury drop electrode (SMDE)

■ STRIPPING METHODS

The term stripping stands for the fact that during the determination, the accumulated product is removed from the working electrode. Stripping voltammetry methods are the most efficient electrochemical techniques for trace analysis. A few points about the stripping methods are:

1. The unusually high sensitivity and selectivity are based on the fact that the analyte is accumulated before it is determined and that both accumulation and determination are electrochemical processes whose progress can be controlled
2. Electrochemical stripping analysis techniques incorporate a variety of electrochemical procedures based on following two steps:
    - The electrochemical deposition or accumulation of the investigated analyte at the electrode surface under the controlled potential
    - The stripping or dissolution of the investigated analyte from the electrode surface by the voltammetric techniques
3. The sensitivity of voltammetric methods can be greatly enhanced by the use of a preconcentration or accumulation step in which the compound is accumulated at the electrode by either a Faradic such as anodic, cathodic, or potentiometric or nonfaradic such as adsorption process
4. Stripping voltammetry is generally more sensitive by a factor of 10^3–10^5, so that the detection limits are between 10^{-9} and 10^{-11} mol/L and in some cases even 10^{-12} mol/L
5. Stripping methods are among the most sensitive instrumental analysis methods of all, they are also superior to other trace analysis techniques as regard the correctness of the measured values obtained
6. Accumulation and the determination take place at the same electrode without needing to change vessels; this means that the occurrence of systematic errors by contamination or evaporation can be kept at a very low level
7. Accumulation always takes place at constant potential at a stationary mercury drop, mercury film, graphite, or noble metal electrode and for a controlled period. The analyte is deposited electrolytically as a metal, as a sparingly soluble mercury compound, or adsorptively as a complex compound.
8. The removal of the accumulated analyte species from the working electrode and the real determination step is based on an oxidation or reduction reaction. In the classical case, where the analyte is accumulated at the mercury drop or mercury film electrode as an

amalgam, the determination is the reverse process to accumulation, this is where the name inverse voltammetry originated from.
9. Stripping techniques have several advantages such as low detection and determination limits, high sensitivity, relative simplicity, rapidity, wide spectrum of the analyte, and insignificant effect of the matrix
10. There are several types of stripping voltammetry method such as anodic stripping voltammetry (ASV), cathodic stripping voltammetry (CSV), and adsorptive stripping voltammetry (AdSV).

Anodic Stripping Voltammetry

Anodic stripping voltammetry can be used to determine all metals, which are soluble in mercury with the formation of amalgams or which can be deposited electrolytically at carbon or noble metal electrodes.

$$Me^{n+} + n e^- + Hg \xleftarrow{\text{Deposition (cathodic)}} Me^\circ(Hg)$$

Accuracy is proportionate to the way we calibrate our sample, 5% when calibrated directly via the method of standard additions. In ASV, the determination is based on the anodic dissolution of the accumulated analyte. Such process is followed voltammetrically and produces a current peak, which (when the HMDE is used) is proportional to the potential and radius of drop.

Cathodic Stripping Voltammetry

Cathodic stripping voltammetry is similar to ASV; the only difference lies in the determination process and the accumulation procedure, except that for the plating step, the CSV is used to determine substances that form insoluble salts with the mercurous ion. The simplest and most frequent process is accumulation as the mercury (I) salt Hg_2A_2. The Hg^{2+} from the electrode mercury, which is oxidized at even slightly negative potentials, depending on the base solution, the solubility product of the compound, and the concentration of the analyte in sample solution. During the analysis, the Hg_2A_2 of the accumulated Hg_2A_2 is cathodically reduced and mechanism can be described as follows:

Deposition: $2 Hg \longrightarrow Hg_2^{2+} + 2e^-$
$Hg_2^{2+} + 2 A^- \longrightarrow Hg_2A_2$
Determination: $Hg_2A_2 + 2e^- \longrightarrow 2 Hg + 2 A^-$

Some important points about CSV are:
1. Cathodic stripping voltammetry is best suited for the determination of a wide range of organic sulfur compounds such as penicillin, thiols and inorganic anions, halides, and sulfides that form insoluble salts with the electrode material
2. Organic compounds, such as nucleic acid bases, also form insoluble salts and can be determined using this technique

3. Cathodic stripping voltammetry is also used for the determination of several elements, for example, arsenic, selenium, and tellurium are sparingly soluble in mercury, but can be accumulated together with an added solution partner copper (II) salt on the electrode surface as an intermetallic compound.
4. Potential range for the accumulation of anions lies between −0.2 and +0.4 V (Ag/AgCl, 3 M KCl)

Adsorptive Stripping Voltammetry

It is one of the important techniques according to the drug analysis point of view because of the low limit of determination, such as ng/mL or ppb. AdSV is a sensitive and selective electroanalytical technique comprising following two steps:
1. First, metal ions are electrodeposited on the mercury electrode, which is held at a suitable potential
2. Then, the (amalgamated) metal deposits are anodically stripped from the mercury electrode by scanning the potential

Combination of accumulation and voltammetric determination is known as AdSV, if the analyte can be accumulated in a suitable form by adsorption on the electrode surface and then voltammetrically determined by oxidation or reduction. Few points about AdSV are:
1. Adsorptive accumulation makes stripping voltammetry interesting even for those elements that cannot be accumulated or determined owing to irreversible electrode reactions or lack of amalgam formation at mercury electrodes
2. Metals which can be determined by AdSV are aluminium, iron, cobalt, nickel, titanium, chromium, molybdenum, tungsten, antimony, vanadium, uranium, and the platinum metals
3. Adsorptive stripping voltammetry is also suitable for the trace analysis of numerous organic compounds
4. Adsorptive stripping voltammetry method differs in the complex formation and in the accumulation mechanism, which can be described as follows:
    - In case, the analyte M^{n+} forms the absorbable complex with the ligand L in the solution, this is then adsorbed on the surface of the working electrode
    - In other cases, the complexing agent is adsorbed on the electrode, so that complex formation takes place on the electrode surface
    - In case, Mn^+ does not form a surface-active compound with the complexing agent, the analyte will be electrochemically reduced or oxidized and transformed into a suitable oxidation state for complex formation which can take placed either in the solution or on the electrode surface.
5. Adsorptive stripping voltammetry is even more efficient than ASV

6. The higher sensitivity of AdSV is based on the fact that the adsorbed compound remains on the electrode surface, whereas in ASV, the deposited metal diffuses into the mercury drop. As a result, after adsorptive accumulation, the local accumulation factor is larger than that after electrolysis and amalgam formation.

■ INSTRUMENTATION

The basic instruments are given in **Figure 10.1**. The basic instrument consists of the following parts:

Voltammetric/Polarographic Vessel

It is a vessel in which sample, buffer, and standard are taken for the analysis. The polarographic vessel is a glass or teflon vessel in which three electrodes and a tube for bubbling of nitrogen gas are placed. Diagram of polarographic vessel is given in **Figure 10.2**.

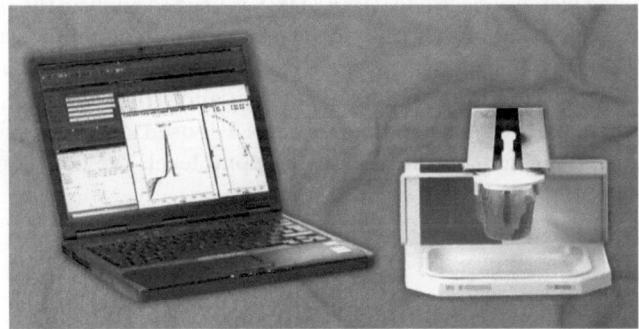

Fig. 10.1: Metrohm trace metal analyzer (model 797 VA Computrace).

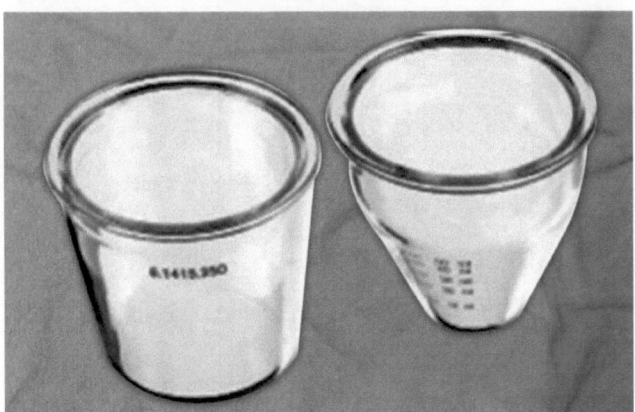

Fig. 10.2: Voltammetric/Polarographic vessel (from Metrohm).

Electrodes

The proper choice of the working electrode is very important for the success of the stripping techniques. It is three electrode system namely working electrode, reference electrode, and auxiliary electrode.

Working Electrode

The most important types of working electrodes are the valve controlled mercury electrodes. These consist of relatively narrow capillary connected to the mercury reservoirs. The mercury flow is controlled by a valve and is connected with a mercury container or a solid electrode. There are two types of working electrodes, one is multi-mode electrode (MME) and another is rotating disk electrode (RDE).

Multi-mode electrode: MME is most commonly used working electrode. It is used for the analysis of several metals such as Pb, Cu, Cd, As, and Zn. There are three different modes of MMEs, which are given below. Schematic diagram of MME is given in **Figure 10.3**.

- *Dropping mercury electrode (DME)*: DME is used to analyze the metals in higher concentrations and is also used for organic compounds analysis, e.g., vitamins. In this system, there is a continuous flow of the mercury from the electrode followed by deposition and stripping.
- *Static mercury drop electrode (SMDE)*: SMDE is used to analyze the metals in mid-level of concentrations (10–100 ppm) level. The flow of mercury is noncontinuous in this system.

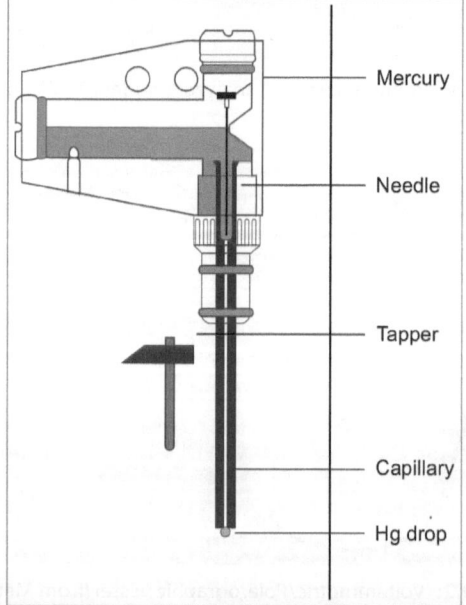

Fig. 10.3: Multi-mode electrode (from Metrohm).

- *Hanging mercury drop electrode*: HMDE is used to analyze the metals in lower concentrations such as ppm, ppb, and ppt level. It is most commonly used mode for the trace metal analysis. Unlike, DME and SMDE, in HMDE, only one drop of mercury is sufficient for the analysis.

Rotating disk electrode: RDE is used to analyze Hg and other elements, which are not possible by MME. This is basically a stirrer connected with different electrode tips such as gold, glassy carbon, and ultratrace electrode. Schematic diagram of RDE is given in **Figure 10.4**.

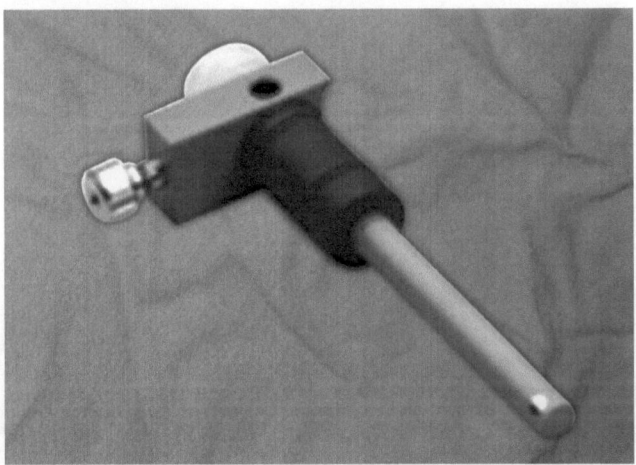

Fig. 10.4: Rotating disk electrode (from Metrohm).

Reference Electrode

Ag/AgCl filled with 3 M KCl solution is used as reference electrode when MME is used as working electrode. Ag/AgCl filled with mercury buffer is used as reference electrode when RDE is used (**Fig. 10.5**). Potential for the analysis is applied between working and reference electrode. So, reference electrode is used to apply the necessary potential along with working electrode. This electrode provides a standard voltage that stabilizes the application and measurement of cell voltages.

Auxiliary Electrode

Current is measured between working and auxiliary electrode and that is proportional to the concentration of the analyte. There are two types of auxiliary electrodes:
1. *Platinum electrode*: A platinum wire is inserted on a teflon rod. Pt electrode is most widely used auxiliary electrode for the analysis of trace metals such as Pb, Cu, Cd, As, and Zn. Schematic diagram of Pt electrode is given in **Figure 10.6A**.
2. *Glassy carbon electrode*: A glassy carbon wire is inserted on a teflon rod. It is used to analyze mercury. Schematic diagram of glassy carbon electrode is given in **Figure 10.6B**.

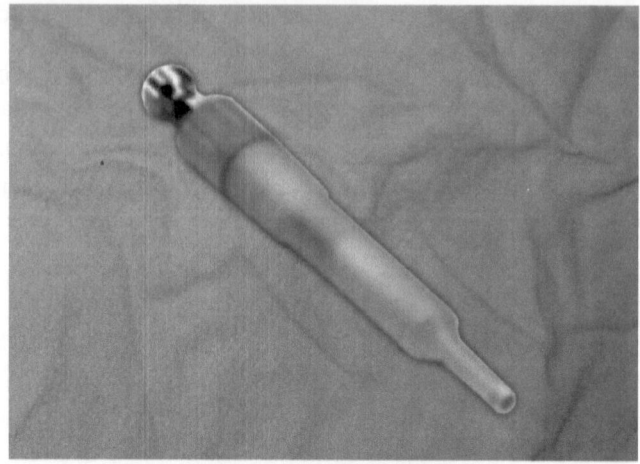

Fig. 10.5: Reference electrode (from Metrohm).

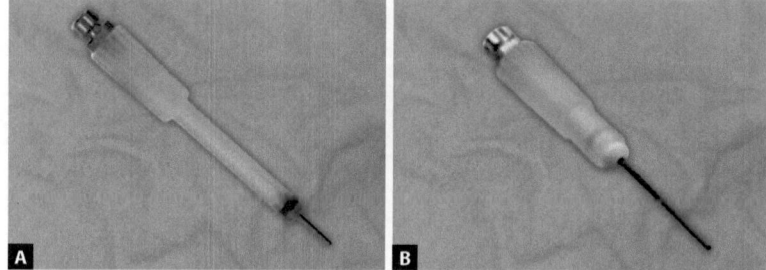

Figs. 10.6A and B: Auxiliary electrodes (from Metrohm). (A) Pt electrode and (B) Glassy carbon electrode.

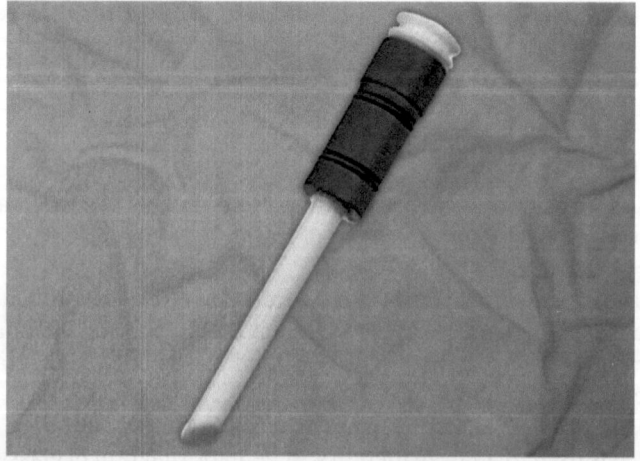

Fig. 10.7: Stirrer (from Metrohm).

Stirrer VA Stand

Stirrer is used to mix the sample solution for homogeneity. The diagram of stirrer is given in **Figure 10.7**.

Capillary

Mercury is flowing from the Hg reservoir through the capillary and forms the Hg dropper measurement. There are two types of capillary used:
1. *Nonsilanized capillary*: The pH working range of this capillary is 0–14 (**Fig. 10.8A**)
2. *Silanized capillary*: It is most commonly used capillary. The pH working range of this capillary is up to 10 (**Fig. 10.8B**).

Driving Belt

It is used to operate the stirrer. Schematic diagram of driving belt is given in **Figure 10.9**.

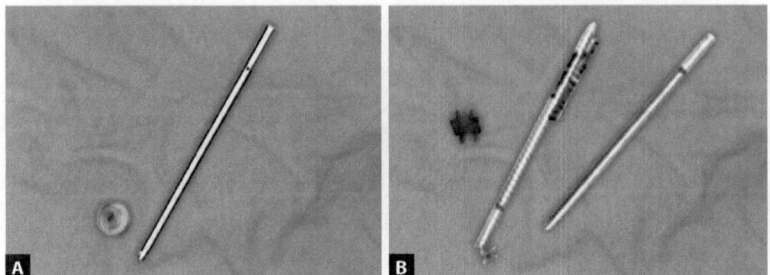

Figs. 10.8A and B: (A) Nonsilanized capillary and (B) Silanized capillary (from Metrohm).

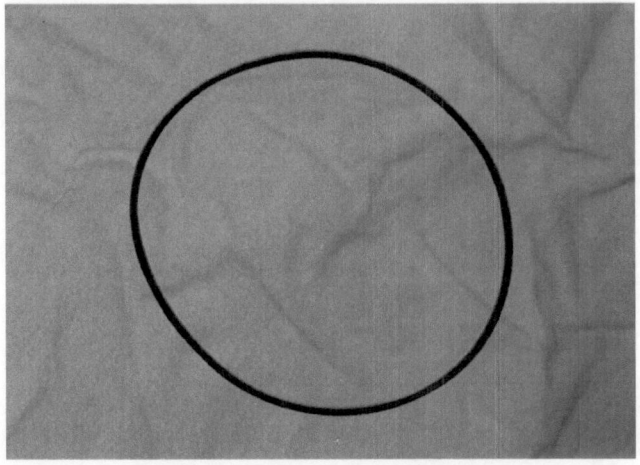

Fig. 10.9: Driving belt (from Metrohm).

Mercury Drop Catcher

This is used to collect the waste mercury after the analysis. Schematic diagram of Hg drop catcher is given in **Figure 10.10**.

Dummy Stopper

It is located in place of MME when RDE is used. Schematic diagram of dummy stopper is given in **Figure 10.11**.

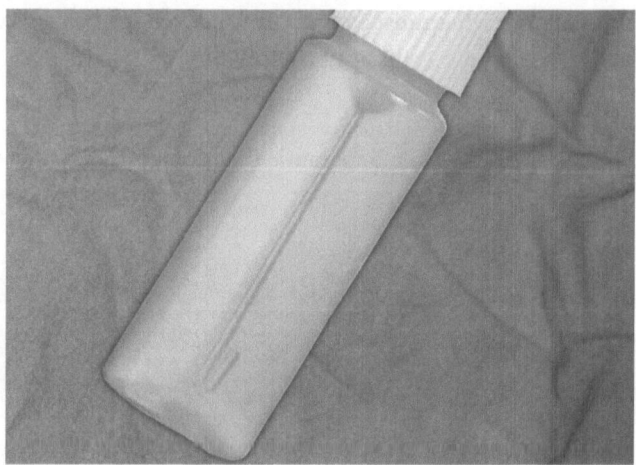

Fig. 10.10: Hg drop catcher (from Metrohm).

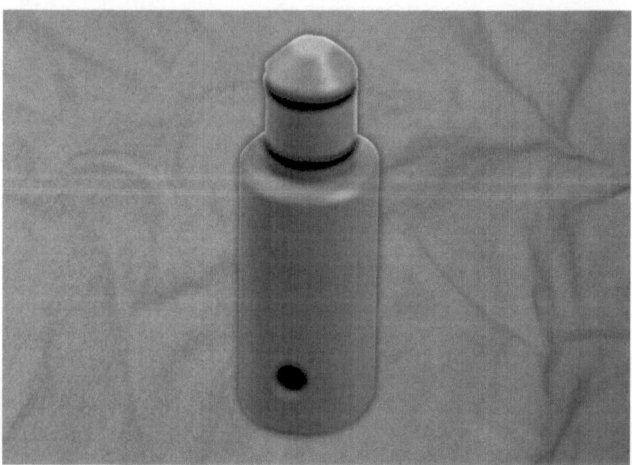

Fig. 10.11: Dummy stopper (from Metrohm).

DO'S AND DON'TS FOR VOLTAMMETRIC TRACE METAL ANALYSIS

Do's

1. Before starting the analysis, prepare all the necessary solutions and check the pH, if necessary
2. Always freshly prepared solutions should be used
3. Wash the electrode before analysis
4. Check the solution, i.e., 3 M KCl is filled in the reference electrode. It should be always filled up to appropriate mark
5. Vessel has to be cleaned with dilute nitric acid (HNO_3), if it is contaminated with impurities
6. Purge the instrument properly, if it is contaminated
7. Use only highly pure N_2 gas to avoid any contamination
8. Pressure should be under check (1 bar or 1 kg/m^3)
9. Collect the waste mercury using mercury catcher
10. Suprapur chemicals should be used for the better results
11. Be careful while using the glassy carbon electrode during mercury analysis

Don'ts

1. Do not take used pipette tips for buffer, standard, and sample analysis
2. Do not touch the electrode; otherwise, it can be a source of impurities
3. Do not abrupt the running operation, except in emergency
4. Do not use old buffer
5. Do not use old standard
6. Do not keep the sample vessel in the dry conditions, always keep some water
7. Do not keep the mercury in open condition
8. Do not use the normal grade chemicals or reagents for the buffer preparation, always use suprapur or GR-grade reagents or ultrapure
9. Do not wear gold items when working with mercury electrode
10. Do not change the default parameters

CHARACTERISTICS OF VOLTAMMETRIC TRACE METAL ANALYZER

1. Wide variety of voltammetry analyzer (VA) techniques available including DP, DC, potentiometric stripping analysis (PSA), cyclic voltammetric stripping (CVS), CV, etc.
2. Stripping voltammetry for voltammetric trace analysis of metal ions and other substances
3. Cyclic voltammetric stripping for the determination of additives in plating solutions

4. It is helpful in tracing the metals from the sample even at the lower concentration
5. Analysis of many metals can be done simultaneously
6. Powerful data handling and evaluation with report generator
7. More than 220 important analysis methods are pre-installed
8. Results available in a wide variety of formats as well as customizable formats
9. Integrated quality assurance with the good laboratory practice (GLP) wizard, access rights for each user, and the automatic electrode test
10. Simple and easy Windows XP/Vista/Windows 7-based program with simple user interface

■ BASIC STEPS INVOLVED IN THE ANALYSIS OF DIFFERENT METALS

It varies greatly with the particular samples involved and the desired type of measurement. If the total metal content is desired, the sample must first be digested to extract all metals from the sample matrix. Basic steps involved in the analysis of different metals are:

Digestion of Sample

Vessels are cleaned with HNO_3: water (1:1) mixture followed by water and dried. The weighed sample is taken into the liner vessel. 15 mL HNO_3 (concentration/dilute depending on the sample) is added to each vessel inside the fume hood to allow the sample to outgas and then the vessels are sealed. In the reference vessel, 1 mL of water (instead of sample) is added along with 15 mL HNO_3 for sample blank. Vessel carousels are loaded in the microwave digestion oven and the microwave is run with various programs specific for different substances. After digestion, the samples are allowed to cool down and then each vessel is opened in the fume hood. Digested sample is transferred to suitable volumetric flask and then the volume is made up to the mark with the help of ultrapure water.

Preparation of Standard

1,000 ppm of required metal is prepared by dissolving the suitable amount of the salt in water. 1 ppm standard is prepared by diluting 0.1 mL of 1,000 ppm stock of that particular metal in 100 mL of ultrapure water.

Electrode Test

The electrodes used are automatically checked before each determination. If problem occurs, the faulty electrodes are identified and fault will be shown on the screen. Working of electrodes can be checked by following path:

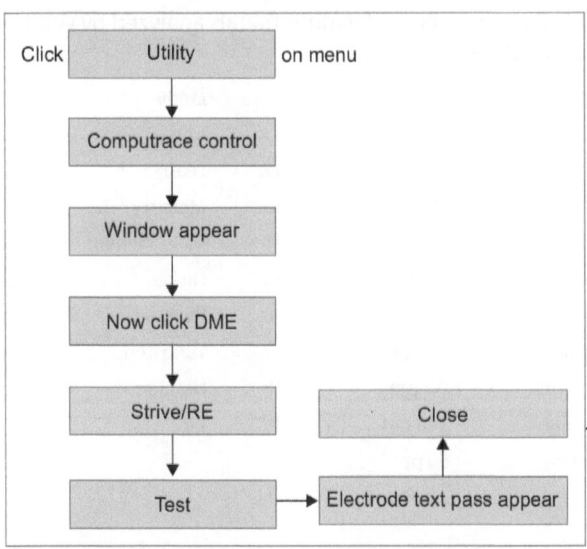

Washing of Electrode

All sample containers and electrodes should be cleaned in HNO_3/hydrochloric acid (HCl) solution. Generally used solution includes addition of 0.5 mL concentrated HNO_3 and 1.5 mL concentrated HCl to 100 mL of deionized or distilled water.

Loading of Required Method

Methods for the metals are already installed in the system. Combined methods are there for many metals simultaneously or individual method is also there for other metals also.

Blank Analysis

Addition of 10 mL distilled water followed by the integration of 1 mL of buffer for blank analysis.

Addition of Standard

0.1 mL of standard is added twice after the blank and sample analysis.

Result

Results are easily available as stored in the system.

■ DETECTION LIMIT OF VOLTAMMETRIC TRACE METAL ANALYZER

In voltammetric technique, the measurement plating time is proportionate to the detection limit and, as such, longer plate times will increase the

Table 10.1: Detection limit of various metals analyzed by voltammetric trace metal analyzer.

S. No.	Metals	Limit	S. No.	Metals	Limit
1.	Antimony	200 ppt	11.	Iron	50 ppt
2.	Arsenic	100 ppt	12.	Lead	50 ppt
3.	Bismuth	500 ppt	13.	Mercury	100 ppt
4.	Cadmium	50 ppt	14.	Molybdenum	50 ppt
5.	Chromium	25 ppt	15.	Nickel	50 ppt
6.	Copper	50 ppt	16.	Platinum	0.1 ppt
7.	Cobalt	50 ppt	17.	Tungsten	200 ppt
8.	Rhodium	0.1 ppt	18.	Uranium	25 ppt
9.	Selenium	300 ppt	19.	Zinc	50 ppt
10.	Thallium	50 ppt			

detection limit. Detection up to part per million is instantaneous, part per billion in 20 seconds or less, and part per trillion takes 1–3 minutes. Detection limit of various metals analyzed under voltammetric technique is given in **Table 10.1**.

ADVANTAGES OF VOLTAMMETRIC TRACE METAL ANALYZER OVER OTHER TECHNIQUES

1. Sample analysis is quick and easy
2. Allows for simultaneous detection of several elements
3. Exceptional detection limits
4. No expensive flammable gases and no specially constructed fume hoods in the laboratory
5. No problems with high salt concentration
6. Cr^{3+} and Cr^{6+} can be easily measured
7. No extensive laboratory infrastructure

LIMITATIONS OF VOLTAMMETRIC TRACE METAL ANALYZER

1. Sample has to be digested before the analysis and extraorganic material has to be removed, which makes the process more complicated
2. Since, the instrument is more sensitive, even the small impurities in the carrier gas can introduce a wrong signal or peak value
3. Some precious metals, such as mercury, are used in the electrodes, which sometime on contamination becomes useless
4. Accurate detection depends upon the purity of the chemical that is addition of suprapur chemicals make the result more confident

5. Since, the method is based upon 'hit and trial', exactly do not know that metal of interest is actually present or not. So, some preidentification test must be there to minimize the wastage of time and money
6. Suprapur chemicals are used, which are very costly.

■ TECHNICAL SPECIFICATIONS OF TRACE METAL ANALYZER

1. PC-controlled voltammetric metal analyzer for analysis of transition and heavy metals, including mercury, arsenic, lead, and organic ions in low ppm levels, on principle of voltammetry/polarographic system
2. *Modes for quantitative analysis*: Sampled DC voltammetry, differential pulse voltammetry, square wave voltammetry, AC voltammetry of first and second harmonic, CV, and potentiometric analysis
3. *Potentiostat*:
   - *Voltage range*: Approximately ±12 V
   - *Current amplification range*: Approximately ±35 mA
   - *Sweep rate*: Approximately 35 V/s maximum
4. *Working electrode*: Hg electrode, pneumatically operated electrode, and mercury reservoir capacity: 5–6 mL
5. *Operating modes*: Dropping mercury electrode, hanging mercury drop electrode, and static mercury drop electrode
6. *Auxiliary electrodes*: Glassy carbon and platinum
7. *Reference electrode*: Ag/AgCl
8. *Measuring vessel*: 4 No's or more
9. *Stirrer*: One
10. *Needles for mercury electrode*: 3 No's
11. *Capillary for mercury electrode*: 10 No's
12. *Polishing set and cutter for electrodes*
13. *Control unit*:
    - *Software*: Windows-based software for system control, data acquisition, and processing
    - *Computer*: Latest branded computer with all modern facility
    - *Printer*: Color—black and white
14. Branded online UPS with inbuilt battery
15. Minimum chemicals required for installation

■ STANDARD OPERATING PROCEDURE FOR VOLTAMMETRIC TRACE METAL ANALYZER (797 VA COMPUTRACE)

Cold Start

1. Switch on the nitrogen from the control panel and check the pressure which should be 1 bar

2. Switch on electric mains
3. Switch on the UPS
4. Plug the power cable of the instrument and turn power switch on of the 797V computrace
5. Switch on the computer
6. Go to the 797 VA computrace software icon on desktop and double click on it, 797 VA computrace metro-data will appear
7. Double click on start measurement, a beep sound will come that means instrument is on and connected properly. 797VA computrace window will appear.

Load Method

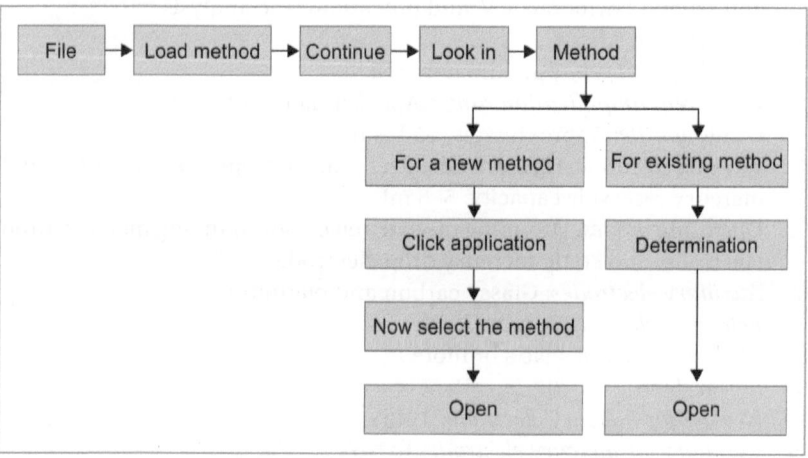

Analysis of Sample

1. Wash the sample vessel and electrodes properly with ultrapure water three to four times
2. Click on method, which is situated on the 13th position on top of the menu bar. Then, working method specification will appear as:

Bulletin of Arsenic (Metal to be Determined)

1. Select the addition either manual or automatic, which is generally manual
2. Select electrode DME, SMDE, HMDE, and RDE, which is generally HMDE
3. Read the remark 1 of working method specification and add the chemical according to it in the sample vessel

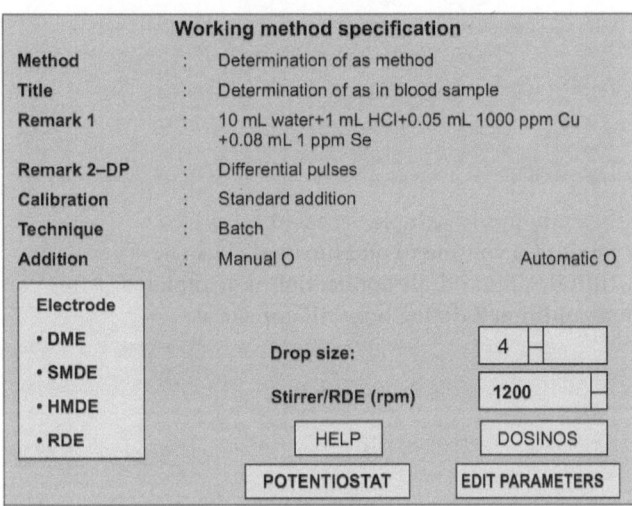

4. Close the working method specification window
5. Click on start, the following window will appear

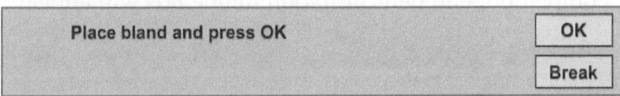

6. Wait till purging and all application is completed. After completion, following dialog box will appear.

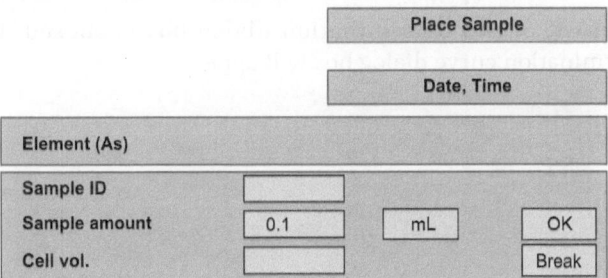

7. Enter the sample ID which is the distinguished file name (by this file name, we can see the result at any time in future)
8. Put the amount of sample in the sample vessel (0.1–1 mL)
9. Put the value of sample in sample amount box
10. Put the total volume (10 mL water + buffer + sample amount, etc.) in cell volume box and then click on OK
11. Wait till purging and all application is completed. After completion, manual addition dialog box will appear

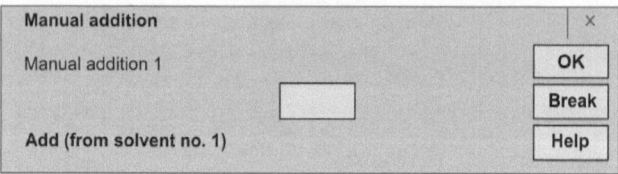

12. Add the standard in sample vessel (0.1-1 mL)
13. Now input this volume in add box and click OK
14. Wait till purging and all application is completed. After completion, manual addition 2 dialog box will appear as:

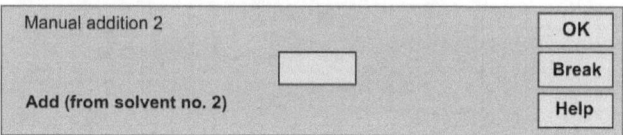

15. Add the standard in sample vessel (0.1-1 mL)
16. Now input this volume in add box and click OK
17. Wait till purging and all application is completed
18. After completion, end determination dialog box will appear

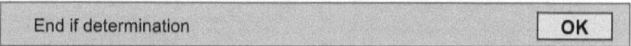

19. Now click on OK

Calculations/Interpretation

1. When OK of end determination dialog box is clicked, following determination curve dialog box will appear

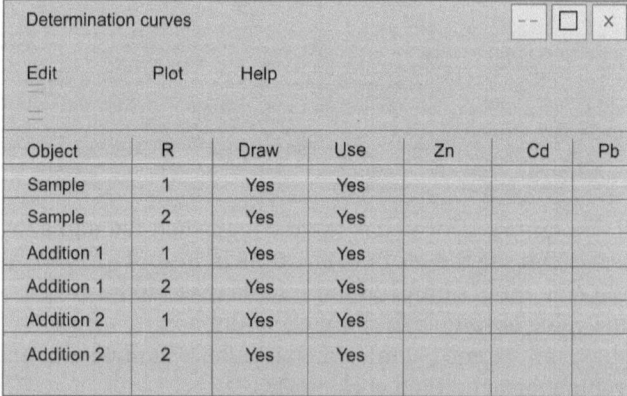

2. If you do not want to use any value, then right click on sample or addition

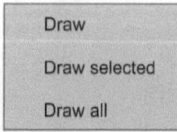

3. Now go to edit option and click on it (in determination curve window), following dialog box will appear:

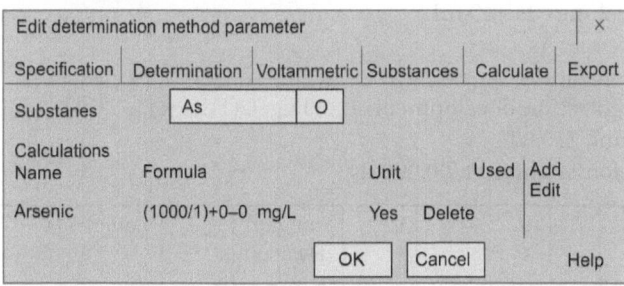

4. Change the element, i.e., as per the requirement and click on OK, following dialog box will appear.

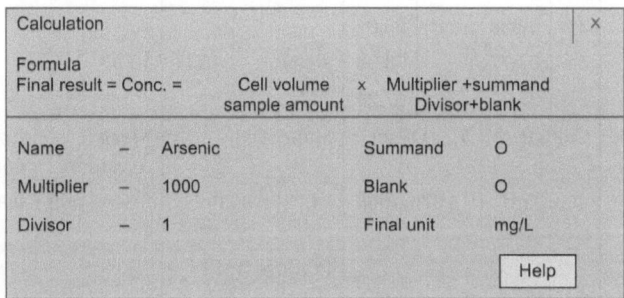

5. Change the final unit mg/L for ppm and µg/L for ppb
6. Apply multiplier which should be 1,000 × all dilution value
7. Apply divisor which should be actual sample volume
8. After applying multiplier, divisor, click on OK
9. Again click OK on edit determination parameter

Results

1. Go to the menu bar
2. Click on the result icon on the 16th position of the menu bar, result will come in the following form:
   == METROHM 797 VA COMPUTRACE (Version 1.3.1.84)
   (Serial No. 14253) ==
   Determination: 0910201048_20 Oct As1.dth
   Sample ID: 20 Oct As1
   Creator method: Date: 2009-09-08 and Time: 15:18:33
   Creator determination: Date: 2009-10-20 and Time: 10:48:57
   Modified by: Date: _____ and Time: _____
   Method: Determination of As method
   Title: Determination of As in blood sample
   Remark 1: 10 mL water + 1 mL HCl + 0.05 mL 1,000 ppm Cu + 0.08 mL 1 ppm Se

Remark 2: _____
Sample amount: 0.010 mL
Cell volume: 11.140 mL
Substance: As
Concentration: 10.399 µg/L
Concentration development: 1.229 µg/L (11.82%)
Amount: 115.848 ng
Addition of amount: 50.000 ng

VR	V	nA	I_{mean}	Standard deviation	I_{delta}	Comments
1	1	0.668	39.79	38.38	1.996	0.00
1	2	0.668	36.97			
2	1	0.677	57.95	56.91	1.470	18.53
2	2	0.668	55.87			
3	1	0.677	73.33	70.29	4.311	13.38
3	2	0.677	67.24			

Substance	Caliber	Y_{reg}/Offset	Slope	Mean deviation	Correlation coefficient	
As	Standard addition	-3.876e-008	-3.727e-003	3.509e-009	0.98454	
No. of content			Predose (mL)			
Final results	±Res dev		%		Comments	
As:						
Arsenic	289.620 mg/L		34.230		11.819	

Electrode test: Passed

Precautions/Trouble-shooting

1. N_2 gas should be on position and pressure should be 1 bar or 1 kg/m^3
2. Electrode should be dipped in the solution before any operation in software window
3. Vessel should not be empty
4. Vessel should be filled with 1 M HNO_3
5. After adding buffer, pH value should be 4.6 for Zn, Pb, Cd, and Cu
6. Maximum current value is 1 µA or 1,000 nA
7. If peak is not integrated or detected, then click on edit parameters, then on substances, after clicking on substances ± V option will appear, where we can increase the value from 0.05 to 0.1. This value can be changed to a maximum value of 0.2.
8. Compared to the sample current, the addition 1 current should be more, so that this peak is higher than the sample peak. If the peak is not higher than the sample peak then during addition 2, add more amount of standard

9. Sample vessel should contain sufficient amount of ultrapure water when system is not in use
10. If instrument is not in use for more than 1 week, vessel should be filled with 1 M HNO_3
11. Sample vessel has to be cleaned with HNO_3 once a week to remove any unwanted deposition
12. Freshly prepared buffer should be used for analysis
13. The baseline should be adjusted to get accurate results
14. The sample to be analyzed by this instrument should be properly digested, so that the instrument can perfectly analyze the metal present in the sample
15. The instrument should be switched on before switching on the software
16. For mercury analysis, separate vessel must be used
17. Freshly prepared standard must be used and it should be <1,000 ppm
18. The tip used, each time, for adding buffer, sample, and standard should be new to avoid contamination
19. Only suprapur chemical should be used for analysis
20. Reference electrode should be properly filled with electrolyte solution, i.e., 3 M KCl

■ FORENSIC APPLICATIONS OF VOLTAMMETRIC/POLAROGRAPHIC TRACE METAL ANALYZER

Determination of Lead (Pb), Copper (Cu), Zinc (Zn), and Cadmium (Cd) in Blood and Urine

Reagents/Chemicals/Apparatus

Reagents/chemicals/apparatus such as acetic acid, HNO_3, ammonia, sodium hydroxide (NaOH), buffer, ultrapure water, salts of Pb, Cd, Zn, and Cu for preparation of standard solution, TMA, pH meter, and micropipette. All reagents and chemicals must be of purest quality such as GR, ultrapure, and suprapur grade.

Sample Preparation

Vessel of microwave digester is cleaned up by HNO_3 and water mixture (1:1) and dried. 1 mL of blood or urine sample is transferred into the liner vessels. 15 mL of 35% HNO_3 is added into each vessel and the mixture is left for few minutes for autogas. In the reference vessel, 1 mL of water is added along with 15 mL of 35% HNO_3 for sample blank. Vessel carrousel is loaded in the microwave digestion oven and run the digestion machine according to program given in **Table 10.2**.

After completion of run, microwave digestion is kept for cooling. After cooling, the vessels are opened and digestion material is completely transferred in 50 mL volumetric flask with the help of ultrapure water and finally, volume is made up to 50 mL with ultrapure water.

Table 10.2: Programming conditions for the microwave digester.

Step	Time (s)	Starting temperature (°C)	Ending temperature (°C)
1.	210	28	100
2.	600	100	160
3.	600	160	170

Preparation of Standard

1,000 ppm of lead, 1,000 ppm of copper, 1,000 ppm of zinc, and 1,000 ppm of cadmium are prepared by dissolving the suitable amount of the salt in water. 1 ppm standard is prepared by diluting 1,000 ppm of lead, copper, zinc, and cadmium in 100 mL with ultrapure water.

Preparation of Ammonium Acetate Buffer

A 55.5 mL of suprapur acetic acid is taken in a 500 mL volumetric flask. To this amount, 100 mL of water is added. 37 mL of suprapur ammonia is added slowly to the volumetric flask. After this addition, the solution is diluted to 500 mL with ultrapure water. The pH of the buffer should be adjusted up to 4.6.

Analysis

The electrode is washed well with ultrapure water. 10 mL ultrapure water and 1 mL ammonium acetate buffer are taken in voltammetric vessel and voltammogram of blank is recorded under the voltammetric conditions given in **Table 10.3**. After completion of blank voltammogram, 0.1 mL of digested sample is added in voltammetric vessel and voltammogram is recorded. After completion of sample voltammogram, 0.1 mL of 1 ppm standard solution of Pb, Cu, Zn, or Cd is added and voltammogram is recorded. Again, 0.1 mL of 1 ppm standard solution is added in same vessel and voltammogram is recorded second time. The voltammogram of sample and standard for Pb, Cu, Zn, and Cd are given in **Figures 10.12, 10.14, 10.16** and **10.18**. Extrapolation graphs, which give the value of amount for Pb, Cu, Zn, and Cd, are given in **Figures 10.13, 10.15, 10.17** and **10.19**.

Results and Calculations

Software is automatically calculate the final results by taking dilution factor and sample size entered by user. It is calculated by the formula given below:

$$\text{Final result} = \text{concentration} \times \frac{\text{Cell volume}}{\text{Sample amount}} \times \frac{\text{Multiplier}}{\text{Divisor}}$$

where, divisor is sample amount taken for preparation and multiplier is dilution.

VOLTAMMETRY/POLAROGRAPHY TRACE METAL ANALYZER AND ITS APPLICATIONS

Table 10.3: Voltammetric conditions for the analysis of Pb, Cu, Zn, and Cd.

S. No.	Parameters	Description	S. No.	Parameters	Description
1.	Auxiliary electrode	Pt	14.	Sweep rate	60 mV/s
2.	Reference electrode	Ag/AgCl, 3 M KCl	15.	Deposition time	90 s
3.	Working electrode	MME (HMDE)	16.	Equilibration time	10 s
4.	Calibration method	Standard addition	17.	Pulse amplitude	50 mV
5.	Deposition potential	−1,150 mV	18.	Start potential	−1,150 mV
6.	Drop size	4	19.	End potential	50 mV
7.	Stirrer speed	2,000 rpm	20.	Voltage step	6 mV
8.	Mode	Differential pulse (DP)	21.	Peak potential of Pb^{2+}	−380 mV
9.	Initial purge time	300 s	22.	Peak potential of Zn^{2+}	−980 mV
10.	Addition purge time	10 s	23.	Peak potential of Cu^{2+}	−100 mV
11.	Voltage step time	0.1 s	24.	Peak potential of Cd^{2+}	−560 mV
12.	Stripping	Anodic	25.	No. of standard addition	2
13.	No. of replications	2			

(AgCl: silver chloride; HMDE: hanging mercury drop electrode; KCl: potassium chloride; MME: multi-mode electrode)

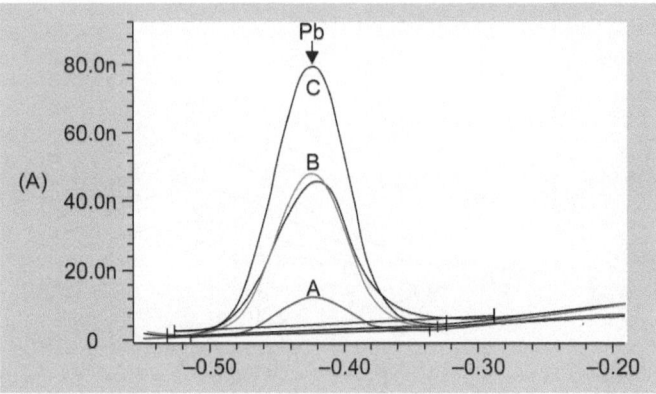

Fig. 10.12: Voltammogram of Pb. (A) 0.1 mL sample in 1 mL acetate buffer + 10 mL ultrapure water, (B) A + 0.1 mL standard solution of Pb (1 ppm), and (C) B + 0.1 mL standard solution of Pb (1 ppm).

427

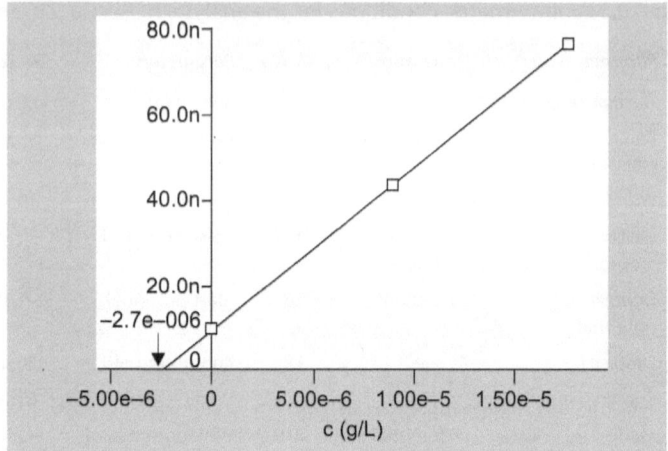

Fig. 10.13: Extrapolation curve of Pb obtained from standard addition technique.

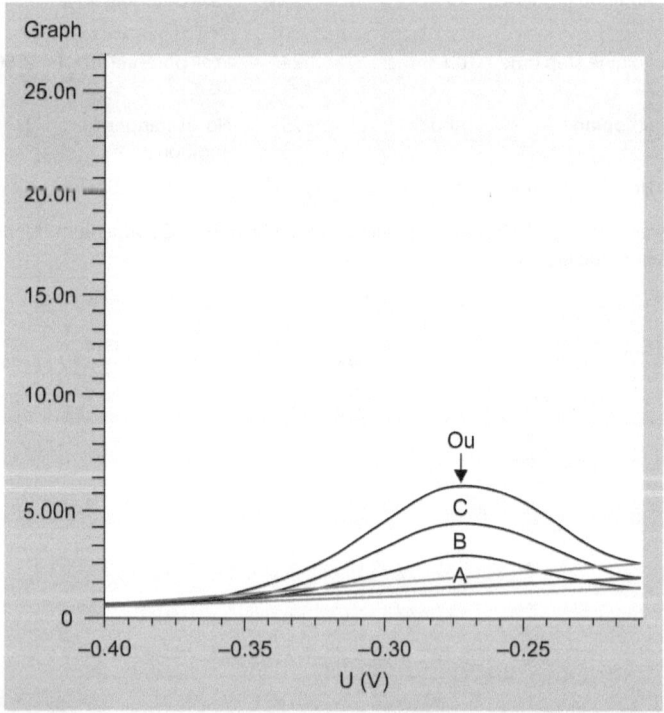

Fig. 10.14: Voltammogram of Cu. (A) 0.1 mL sample in 1 mL acetate buffer (pH 4.6) + 10 mL ultrapure water, (B) A + 0.1 mL standard solution of Cu (1 ppm), and (C) B + 0.1 mL standard solution of Cu (1 ppm).

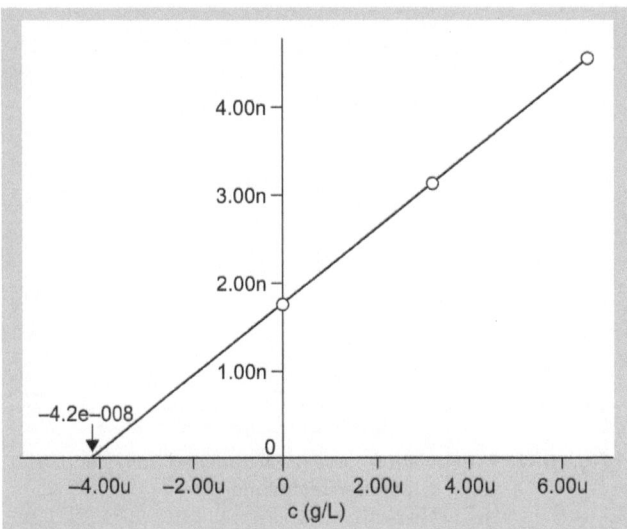

Fig. 10.15: Extrapolation curve of Cu obtained from standard addition technique.

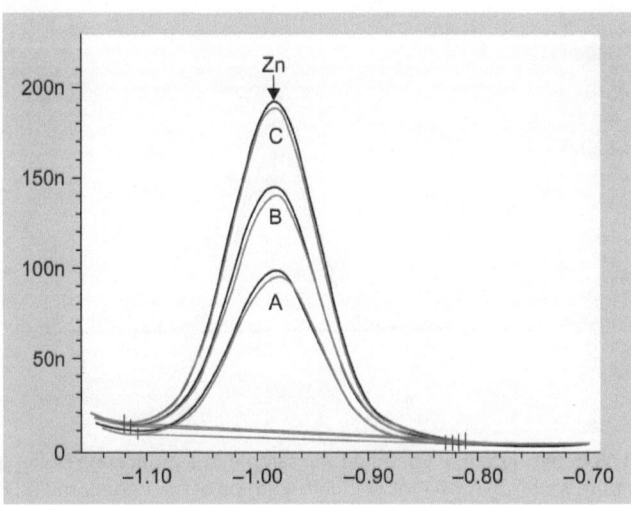

Fig. 10.16: Voltammogram of Zn. (A) 0.1 mL sample in 1 mL acetate buffer (pH 4.6) + 10 mL ultrapure water, (B) A + 0.1 mL standard solution of Zn (1 ppm), and (C) B + 0.1 mL standard solution of Zn (1 ppm).

Determination of Thallium (Tl) in Blood and Urine
Reagents/Chemicals/Apparatus
Reagents/chemicals/apparatus such as acetic acid, HNO_3, ammonia, NaOH, buffer, ultrapure water, salts of Tl for preparation of standard solution, TMA,

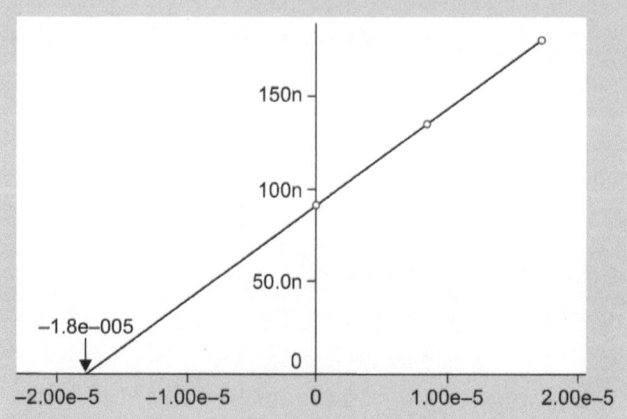

Fig. 10.17: Extrapolation curve of Zn obtained from standard addition technique.

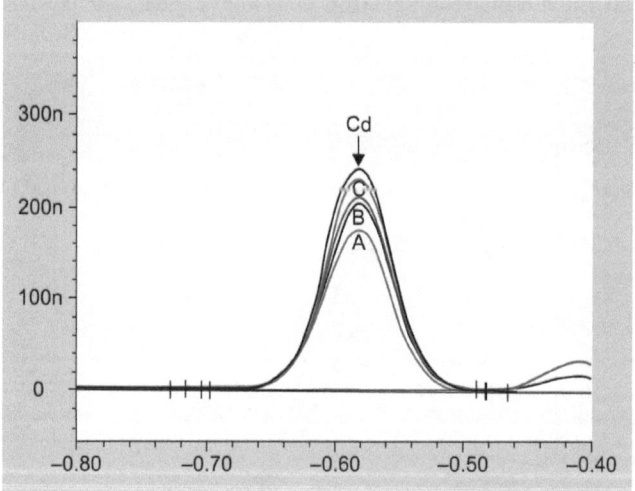

Fig. 10.18: Voltammogram of Cd. (A) 0.1 mL sample in 1 mL acetate buffer (pH 4.6) + 10 mL ultrapure water, (B) A + 0.1 mL standard solution of Cd (1 ppm), and (C) B + 0.1 mL standard solution of Cd (1 ppm).

pH meter, and micropipette. All reagents and chemicals must be of purest quality such as GR, ultrapure, and suprapur grade.

Sample Preparation

Sample preparation will be same as in case of determination of Pb, Cu, Zn, and Cd in blood and urine.

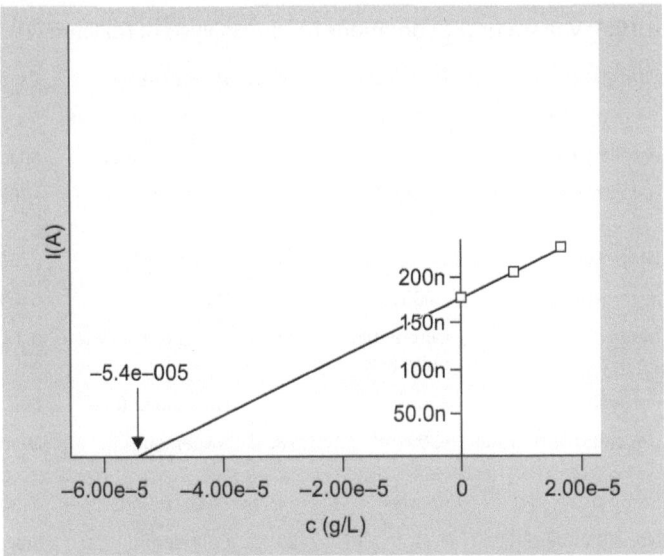

Fig. 10.19: Extrapolation curve of Cd obtained from standard addition technique.

Preparation of Standard

1,000 ppm of Tl is prepared by dissolving the suitable amount of the thallium salt in ultrapure water. 1 ppm standard is prepared by diluting 0.1 mL of 1,000 ppm of Tl in 100 mL of ultrapure water.

Preparation of Ammonium Acetate Buffer

Preparation will be same as discussed in case of determination of Pb, Cu, Zn, and Cd in blood and urine.

Analysis

The electrode is washed well with ultrapure water. 10 mL ultrapure water and 1 mL ammonium acetate are taken in voltammetric vessel and voltammogram of blank is recorded under the voltammetric conditions given in **Table 10.4**. After completion of blank voltammogram, 0.1 mL of digested sample is added in voltammetric vessel and voltammogram is recorded. After completion of sample voltammogram, 0.1 mL of 1 ppm standard solution of Tl is added and voltammogram is recorded. Again, 0.1 mL of 1 ppm standard solution is added in same vessel and voltammogram is recorded second time. Voltammogram of Tl obtained from standard addition technique with number of replications being two is given in **Figure 10.20**. The extrapolation graph, which gives the value of Tl present in sample, is shown in **Figure 10.21**.

Table 10.4: Voltammetric conditions for the analysis of thallium (Tl).

S. No.	Parameters	Description	S. No.	Parameters	Description
1.	Working electrode	MME (HMDE)	11.	Equilibration time	5 s
2.	Auxiliary electrode	Pt	12.	Pulse amplitude	50 mV
3.	Reference electrode	Ag/AgCl, 3 M KCl	13.	Start potential	−700 mV
4.	Drop size	7	14.	End potential	−250 mV
5.	Stirrer speed	2,000 rpm	15.	Voltage step	6 mV
6.	Mode	Differential pulse (DP)	16.	Voltage step time	0.3 s
7.	Purge time	300 s	17.	Deposition time	60 s
8.	Deposition potential	−700 mV	18.	Sweep rate	20 mV/s
9.	Stripping	Anodic	19.	Peak potential	−430 mV
10.	No. of standard addition	2	20.	Calibration method	Standard addition

(AgCl: silver chloride; HMDE: hanging mercury drop electrode; KCl: potassium chloride; MME: multi-mode electrode)

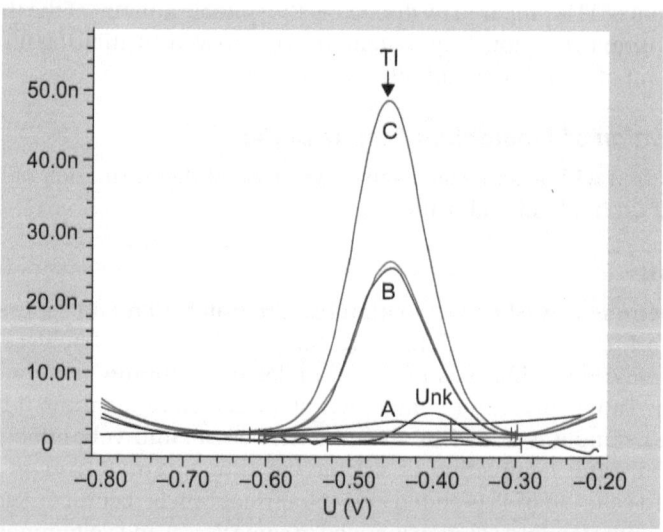

Fig. 10.20: Voltammogram of Tl obtained from standard addition technique with number of replications being two. (A) 0.1 mL sample in 1 mL acetate buffer (pH 4.6) + 10 mL ultrapure water; (B) A + 0.1 mL standard solution of Tl (1 ppm), and (C) B + 0.1 mL standard solution of Tl (1 ppm).

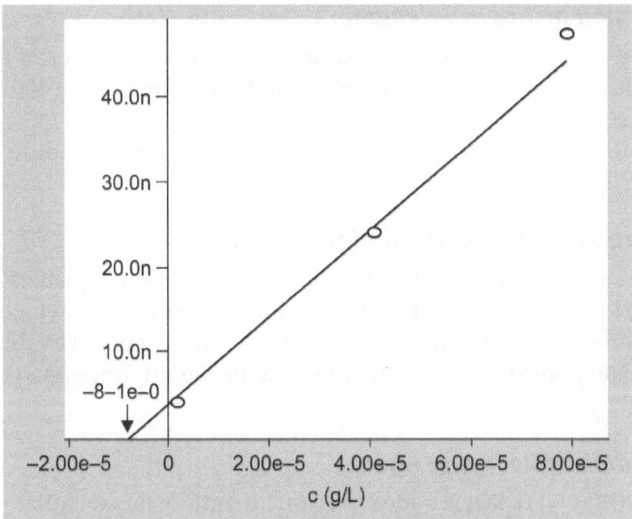

Fig. 10.21: Extrapolation curve of Tl obtained from standard addition technique.

Results and Calculations

The concentration of the heavy metal in blood and urine can be calculated by the formula as discussed in case of determination of Pb, Cu, Zn, and Cd in blood and urine.

Analysis of Arsenic (As) in Blood and Urine

Reagents/Chemicals/Apparatus

Reagents/chemicals/apparatus such as copper nitrate, selenium dioxide, arsenic, L-ascorbic acid, NaOH, arsenous oxide (As_2O_3), sodium metabisulfate, HCl, sulfuric acid (H_2SO_4), sodium thiosulfate, ultrapure water, TMA, pH meter, and micropipette. All reagents and chemicals must be of purest quality such as GR, ultrapure, and suprapur grade.

Sample Preparation

Sample preparation will be same as in case of determination of Pb, Cu, Zn, and Cd in blood and urine.

Preparation of 1,000 ppm Copper

0.3968 g of copper nitrate of high purity is taken in a 100 mL volumetric flask and make up to mark with ultrapure water.

Preparation of 1 ppm Selenium

0.14196 g of selenium dioxide is taken in a 100 mL volumetric flask and two to three drops of NaOH are added to it and made up to 100 mL with ultrapure water.

0.1 mL of this solution is diluted with 100 mL with ultrapure water in volumetric flask.

Preparation of Standard Solution

0.132 g As_2O_3 is taken in a 100 mL volumetric flask and two pellets of NaOH is added to it and made up to 100 mL with ultrapure water, which is 1,000 ppm arsenic. 1 ppm standard solution of arsenic is prepared by diluting 0.1 mL of 1,000 ppm stock solution of arsenic to 100 mL water. As (V) is also prepared by suitable method.

Preparation of Reducing Agent

5 mL of 10% (v/v) H_2SO_4 is added to 10 mL of sodium metabisulfate solution (14% w/v), with vigorous shaking, followed by the addition of 10 mL sodium thiosulfate solution (1.4% w/v) and 0.2 g solid L-ascorbic acid.

Analysis

The electrode is washed well with distilled water. 10 mL ultrapure water, 1 mL HCl, 0.05 mL 1,000 ppm Cu, 0.08 mL 1 ppm Se, and 0.35 mL reducing agent are taken in voltammetric vessel and voltammogram is recorded for blank under the conditions given in **Table 10.5**. After completion of blank voltammogram, 0.1 mL of digested sample is added in volumetric vessel and voltammogram is recorded under same condition. After completion of sample voltammogram, 0.1 mL of 1 ppm standard solution of As is added and voltammogram is recorded. Again, 0.1 mL of 1 ppm standard solution is added in same vessel and voltammogram is recorded second time. Voltammogram of As obtained from standard addition technique with number of replications being two is given in **Figure 10.22**. The extrapolation graph, which gives the value of As present in sample, is shown in **Figure 10.23**.

Results and Calculations

The concentration of the heavy metal in blood and urine can be calculated by the formula as discussed in case of determination of Pb, Cu, Zn, and Cd in blood and urine.

Analysis of Cyanide (CN) in Blood and Urine
Reagents/Chemicals/Apparatus

Reagents/chemical/apparatus such as potassium cyanide, potassium hydroxide, HNO_3, boric acid, ultrapure water, TMA, pH meter, and micropipette. All reagents and chemicals must be of purest quality such as GR, ultrapure, and suprapur grade.

Table 10.5: Voltammetric conditions for the analysis of arsenic (As).

S. No.	Parameters	Description	S. No.	Parameters	Description
1.	Working electrode	MME (HDME)	12.	Stirrer speed	2,000 rpm
2.	Auxiliary electrode	Pt	13.	Initial purge time	300 s
3.	Reference electrode	Ag/AgCl, 3 M KCl	14.	Addition purge time	10 s
4.	Calibration method	Standard addition	15.	Deposition potential	−440 mV
5.	Stripping	Cathodic	16.	Deposition time	60 s
6.	Mode	Differential pulse (DP)	17.	Equilibration time	10 s
7.	No. of standard addition	2	18.	Pulse amplitude	50 mV
8.	No. of replications	1	19.	Drop size	4
9.	Start potential	−400 mV	20.	Voltage step time	0.4 s
10.	End potential	−900 mV	21.	Sweep rate	25 mV/s
11.	Voltage step	10 mV	22.	Peak potential As^{5+}	−650 mV

(AgCl: silver chloride; HMDE: hanging mercury drop electrode; KCl: potassium chloride; MME: multi-mode electrode)

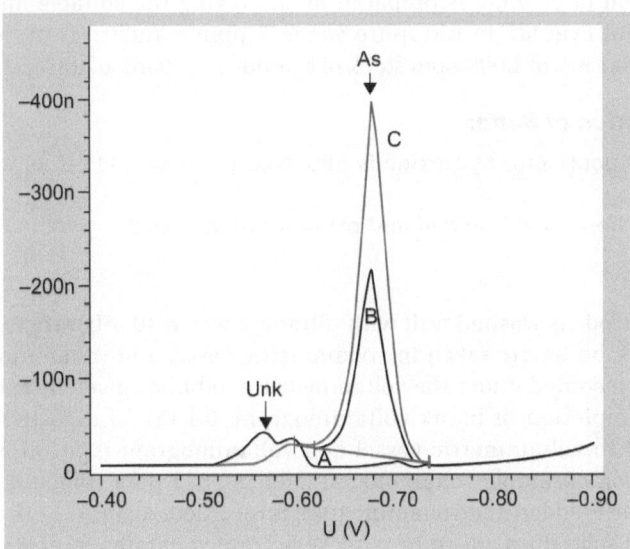

Fig. 10.22: Extrapolation of As obtained from standard addition technique with number of replications being one. (A) 10 mL water, 1 mL hydrochloric acid (HCl), 0.05 mL 1,000 ppm Cu, 0.08 mL 1 ppm Se, and 0.35 mL reducing agent, (B) A + 0.1 mL standard solution of As (1 ppm), and (C) B + 0.1 mL standard solution of As (1 ppm).

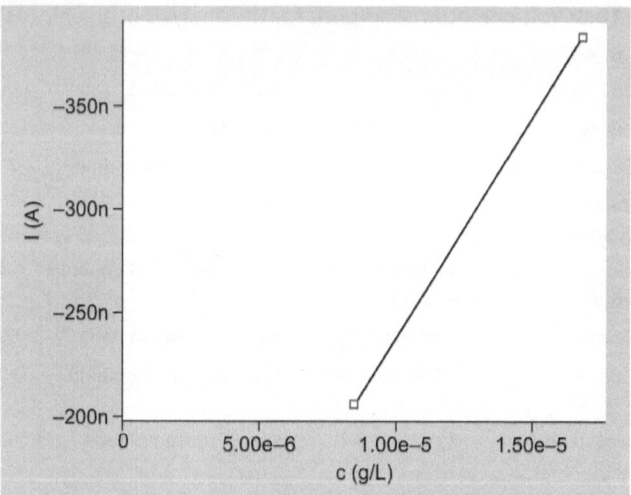

Fig. 10.23: The extrapolation curve of arsenic obtained from standard addition technique.

Sample Preparation
Sample preparation will be same as in case of thallium.

Preparation of Standard
1,000 ppm of cyanide is prepared by dissolving the suitable amount of potassium cyanide in ultrapure water. 1 ppm standard is prepared by diluting 0.1 mL of 1,000 ppm stock of cyanide in 100 mL of ultrapure water.

Preparation of Buffer
11.2 g of potassium hydroxide is dissolved in about 800 mL of ultrapure water.
12.4 g of boric acid is added and pH is adjusted to 10.2.

Analysis
The electrode is washed well with ultrapure water. 10 mL ultrapure water and 1 mL buffer are taken in voltammetric vessel and voltammogram of blank is recorded under the voltammetric conditions given in **Table 10.6**. After completion of blank voltammogram, 0.1 mL of digested sample is added in voltammetric vessel and voltammogram is recorded. After completion of sample voltammogram, 0.1 mL of 1 ppm standard solution of cyanide is added and voltammogram is recorded. Again, 0.1 mL of 1 ppm standard solution is added in same vessel and voltammogram is recorded second time. Voltammogram of cyanide obtained from standard addition technique with number of replications being two is given in **Figure 10.24**. The extrapolation graph, which gives the value of cyanide present in sample, is shown in **Figure 10.25**.

Table 10.6: Voltammetric conditions for the analysis of cyanide (CN).

S. No.	Parameters	Description	S. No.	Parameters	Description
1.	Working electrode	MME (HDME)	12.	Deposition potential	−900 mV
2.	Auxiliary electrode	Pt	13.	Deposition time	60 s
3.	Reference electrode	Ag/AgCl, 3 M KCl	14.	Equilibration time	5 s
4.	Stirrer speed	2,000 rpm	15.	Start potential	−900 mV
5.	Measurement mode	DP	16.	End potential	−100 mV
6.	Purge time	300 s	17.	Voltage step	6 mV
7.	Sweep rate	150 mV/s	18.	Peak potential (Ag)	250 mV
8.	Pulse amplitude	50 mV	19.	Voltage step time	0.4 s
9.	Calibration method	Standard addition	20.	No. of replications	2
10.	Stripping	Polarographic	21.	No. of standard addition	2
11.	Drop size	4	22.	No. of cycles	0

(AgCl: silver chloride; DE: differential pulse; HMDE: hanging mercury drop electrode; KCl: potassium chloride; MME: multi-mode electrode)

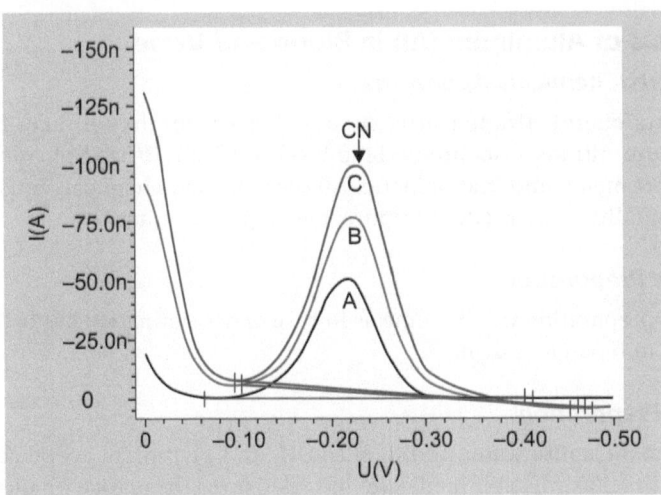

Fig. 10.24: Voltammogram of CN obtained from standard addition technique with number of replications being two. (A) 0.1 mL sample in 1 mL buffer (pH 10.2) + 10 mL ultrapure water, (B) A + 0.1 mL standard solution of CN (1 ppm), and (C) B + 0.1 mL standard solution of CN (1 ppm).

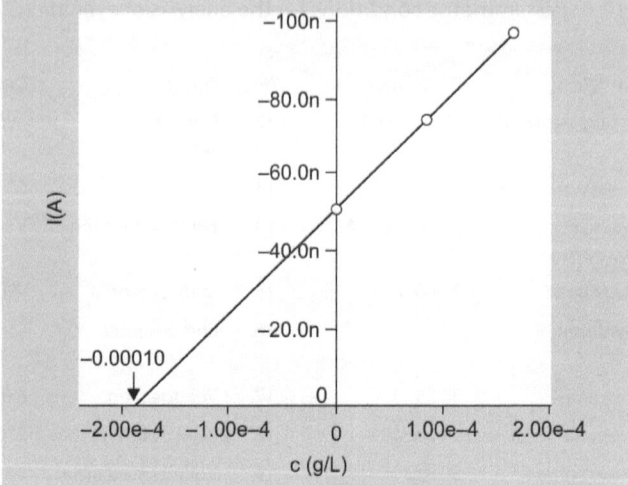

Fig. 10.25: Extrapolation curve of CN obtained from standard addition technique.

Results and Calculations

The concentration of the heavy metal in blood and urine can be calculated by the formula as discussed in case of determination of Pb, Cu, Zn, and Cd in blood and urine.

Analysis of Aluminum (Al) in Blood and Urine
Reagents/Chemicals/Apparatus

Reagents/chemical/apparatus such as NaOH, methanol, acetic acid, aluminum nitrate, Eriochrome blue-black B (EBB), HCl, TMA, ultrapure water, pH meter, and micropipette. All reagents and chemicals must be of purest quality such as GR, ultrapure, and suprapur grade.

Sample Preparation

Sample preparation will be same as in case of determination of Pb, Cu, Zn, and Cd in blood and urine.

Buffer Preparation

50 mL of ultrapure water, 10 mL of NaOH, and 11.4 mL of acetic acid are poured in a 100 mL calibrated flask and filled up to the mark with ultrapure water.

Preparation of Standard

1,000 ppm of Al is prepared by dissolving the suitable amount of aluminum nitrate in ultrapure water. 1 ppm standard is prepared by diluting 0.1 mL of 1,000 ppm stock of Al in 100 mL of ultrapure water.

Complexing Reagent

0.05 g of Eriochrome Blue Black is dissolved in 100 mL of methanol. This solution has to be prepared freshly everyday.

Analysis

The electrode is washed well with ultrapure water. 10 mL ultrapure hot water, 1 mL sodium acetate buffer, and 0.1 mL of EBB (indicator solution) are taken in voltammetric vessel and voltammogram of blank is recorded under the conditions given in **Table 10.7**. After completion of blank voltammogram, 0.1 mL of digested sample is added in voltammetric vessel and voltammogram is recorded. After completion of sample voltammogram, 0.1 mL of 1 ppm standard solution of Al is added and voltammogram is recorded. Again, 0.1 mL of 1 ppm standard solution is added in same vessel and voltammogram is recorded second time. The reason to use hot water for our analysis is to favor the complex formation. Voltammogram of Al obtained from standard addition technique with number of replications being two is given in **Figure 10.26**. The extrapolation graph, which gives the value of Al present in sample, is shown in **Figure 10.27**.

Results and Calculations

The concentration of the heavy metal in blood and urine can be calculated by the formula as discussed in case of determination of Pb, Cu, Zn, and Cd in blood and urine.

Table 10.7: Voltammetric conditions for the analysis of Al.

S. No.	Parameters	Description	S. No.	Parameters	Description
1.	Working electrode	MME (HMDE)	12.	Addition purge time	180 s
2.	Auxiliary electrode	Pt	13.	Deposition potential	−350 mV
3.	Reference electrode	Ag/AgCl, 3 M KCl	14.	Deposition time	30 s
4.	Calibration method	Standard addition	15.	Equilibration time	10 s
5.	No. of replications	2	16.	Pulse amplitude	50 mV
6.	Drop size	7	17.	Start potential	−300 mV
7.	Stirrer speed	1,200 rpm	18.	End potential	−650 mV
8.	Mode	Differential pulse	19.	Voltage step	6 mV
9.	No. of standard additions	2	20.	Voltage step time	0.4 s
10.	Stripping	Adsorptive	21.	Sweep rate	15 mV/s
11.	Initial purge time	300 s	22.	Peak potential	−420 mV

(AgCl: silver chloride; HMDE: hanging mercury drop electrode; KCl: potassium chloride; MME: multi-mode electrode)

VOLTAMMETRY/POLAROGRAPHY TRACE METAL ANALYZER AND ITS APPLICATIONS

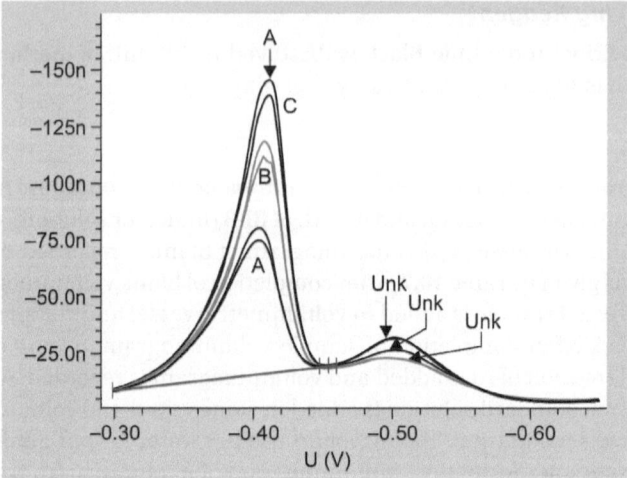

Fig. 10.26: Voltammogram of Al obtained from standard addition technique with number of replications being two. (A) 1 mL sodium acetate buffer + 0.1 mL of indicator solution + 10 mL ultrapure water, (B) A + 0.1 mL standard solution of Al (1 ppm), and (C) B + 0.1 mL standard solution of Al (1 ppm).

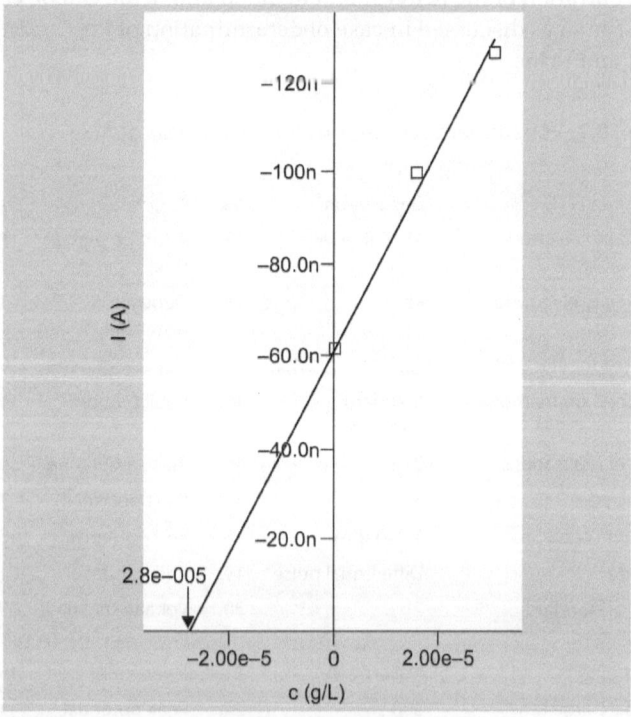

Fig. 10.27: Extrapolation curve of Al obtained from standard addition technique.

Simultaneous Analysis of Pb, Cu, Zn, and Cd in Blood and Urine
Reagents/Chemicals/Apparatus
Reagents/chemicals/apparatus such as acetic acid, ammonia, NaOH, ammonium acetate, buffer, standard solutions of Pb, Cd, Zn, and Cu, TMA, pH meter, and micropipette. All reagents and chemicals must be of purest quality such as GR, ultrapure, and suprapur grade.

Sample Preparation
Sample preparation will be same as in case of Pb, Cu, Zn, and Cd.

Preparation of Mix Standard for Pb, Cu, Zn, and Cd
1,000 ppm of lead, copper, zinc, and cadmium are prepared by dissolving the suitable amount of the metal salts in ultrapure water. 0.1 mL of 1,000 ppm of Pb, 0.1 mL of 1,000 ppm of Cu, 0.1 mL of 1,000 ppm of Zn, and 0.1 mL of 1,000 ppm of Cd are taken in 100 mL volumetric flask and volume is made up to mark with ultrapure water.

Preparation of Buffer
Same as discussed in determination of Pb, Cu, Zn, and Cd in blood and urine.

Analysis
The electrode is washed well with ultrapure water. 10 mL ultrapure water and 1 mL ammonium acetate are taken in voltammetric vessel and voltammogram of blank is recorded under the voltammetric conditions given in **Table 10.8**. After completion of blank voltammogram, 0.1 mL of digested sample is added in voltammetric vessel and voltammogram is recorded. After completion of sample voltammogram, 0.1 mL of 1 ppm standard solution is added and voltammogram is recorded. Again, 0.1 mL of 1 ppm standard solution is added in same vessel and voltammogram is recorded. Voltamogram of Zn, Cd, Pb, and Cu obtained from standard addition technique with number of replications being two is given in **Figure 10.28**.

Results and Calculations
The concentration of the heavy metal in blood and urine can be calculated by the formula as discussed in case of Tl.

Analysis of Mercury (Hg) in Blood and Urine
Reagents/Chemicals/Apparatus
Reagents/chemicals/apparatus such as mercury salt, HNO_3, mercuric oxide, sodium chloride (NaCl), disodium hydrogen ethylenediaminetetraacetic acid (EDTA), perchloric acid, buffer, ultrapure water, TMA, pH meter, and micropipette. All reagents and chemicals must be of purest quality such as GR, ultrapure, and suprapur grade.

VOLTAMMETRY/POLAROGRAPHY TRACE METAL ANALYZER AND ITS APPLICATIONS

Table 10.8: Voltammetric conditions for the simultaneous analysis of Pb, Cu, Zn, and Cd.

S. No.	Parameters	Description	S. No.	Parameters	Description
1.	Auxiliary electrode	Pt	13.	Equilibration time	10 s
2.	Reference electrode	Ag/AgCl, 3 M KCl	14.	Pulse amplitude	50 mV
3.	Working electrode	MME (HMDE)	15.	Start potential	−1,150 mV
4.	Calibration method	Standard addition	16.	End potential	50 mV
5.	No. of replications	2	17.	Voltage step	6 mV
6.	Drop size	4	18.	Voltage step time	0.1 s
7.	Stirrer speed	2,000 rpm	19.	Peak potential Pb^{2+}	−380 mV
8.	Mode	Differential pulse	20.	Peak potential Cu^{2+}	−100 mV
9.	Initial purge time	300 s	21.	Peak potential Zn^{2+}	−980 mV
10.	Addition purge time	10 s	22.	Peak potential Cd^{2+}	−560 mV
11.	Sweep rate	60 mV/s	23.	Deposition potential	−1,150 mV
12.	Stripping	Anodic	24.	No. of standard addition	2

(AgCl: silver chloride; HMDE: hanging mercury drop electrode; KCl: potassium chloride; MME: multi-mode electrode)

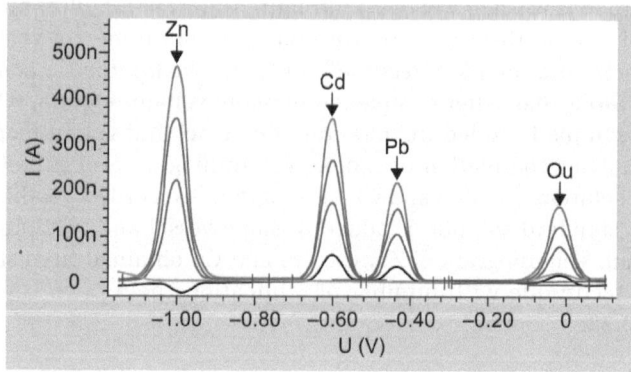

Fig. 10.28: Voltammogram of simultaneous analysis of Pb, Cd, Zn, and Cu.

Sample Preparation

Sample preparation will be same as in case of determination of Pb, Cu, Zn, and Cd in blood and urine.

Preparation of Standard

1,000 ppm of Hg is prepared by dissolving the suitable amount of mercuric chloride in HNO_3. 1 ppm standard is prepared by diluting 0.1 mL of 1,000 ppm stock of Hg in 100 mL of ultrapure water.

Preparation of Buffer

0.351 g NaCl and 1.50 g of $Na_2H_2EDTA.2H_2O$ are dissolved in 500 mL of ultrapure water. 22 mL of 60% $HClO_4$ (or 18.8 mL 70% $HClO_4$) is added to it and volume is made up to the 1 L with ultrapure water. This solution is stable up to 1 week.

Analysis

The electrode is washed well with ultrapure water. 10 mL ultrapure water and 1 mL buffer are taken in voltammetric vessel and voltammogram of blank is recorded under the voltammetric conditions given in **Table 10.9**. After completion of blank voltammogram, 0.1 mL of digested sample is added in voltammetric vessel and voltammogram is recorded. After completion of sample voltammogram, 0.1 mL of 1 ppm standard solution of Hg is added and voltammogram is recorded. Again, 0.1 mL of 1 ppm standard solution is added in same vessel and voltammogram is recorded second time. Voltammogram of Hg obtained from standard addition technique with number of replication being two is given in **Figure 10.29**. The extrapolation graph, which gives the value of Hg present in sample, is shown in **Figure 10.30**.

Results and Calculations

The concentration of the heavy metal in blood and urine can be calculated by the formula as discussed in case of determination of Pb, Cu, Zn, and Cd in blood and urine.

Table 10.9: Voltammetric conditions for the analysis of Hg.

S. No.	Parameters	Description	S. No.	Parameters	Description
1.	Working electrode	Gold electrode	11.	Start potential	0.5 V
2.	Auxiliary electrode	Glassy carbon	12.	End potential	0.85 V
3.	Reference electrode	Ag/AgCl	13.	Voltage step	2 mV
4.	Measurement mode	DP	14.	Voltage step time	0.1 s
5.	Pulse amplitude	0.05 V	15.	Sweep rate	20 mV/s
6.	Deposition potential	0.37 V	16.	Peak potential (Hg)	0.64 V
7.	Deposition time	60s	17.	No. of replications	2
8.	No. of cycles	2	18.	Purge time	300 s
9.	Stirrer speed	2,000 rpm	19.	Additional purge time	20 s
10.	Equilibration time	10 s	20.	Calibration method	Standard addition

(AgCl: silver chloride; DP: differential pulse)

VOLTAMMETRY/POLAROGRAPHY TRACE METAL ANALYZER AND ITS APPLICATIONS

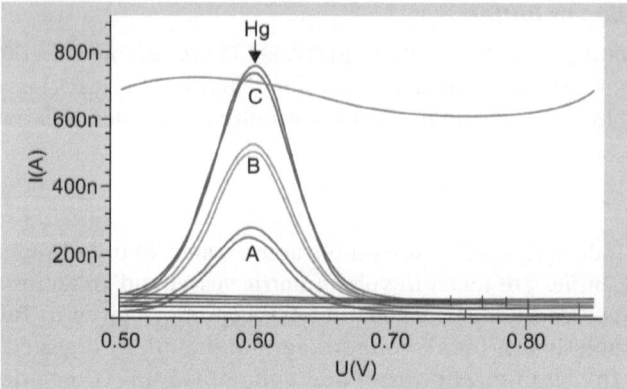

Fig. 10.29: Voltammogram of Hg obtained from standard addition technique with number of replications being two. (A) 0.1 mL sample in 1 mL buffer + 10 mL ultrapure water, (B) A + 0.1 mL standard solution of Hg (1 ppm), and (C) B + 0.1 mL standard solution of Hg (1 ppm).

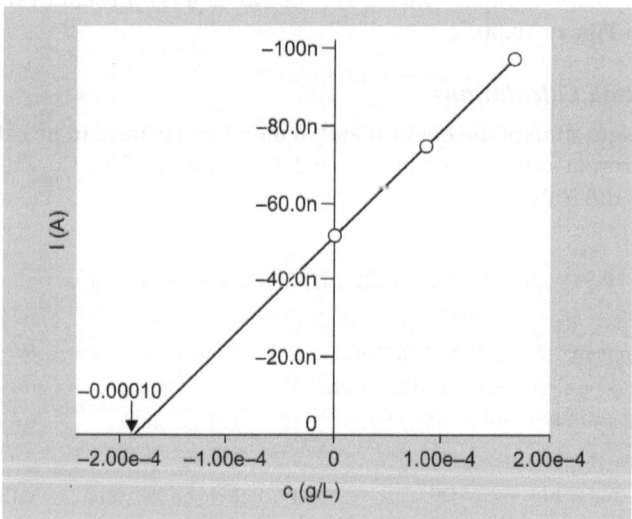

Fig. 10.30: Extrapolation curve of Hg obtained from standard addition technique.

■ CONCLUSION

Trace metal analysis plays an important role in many disciplines of quantitative analysis (**Table 10.10**). In drug analysis, stripping voltammetric techniques are very popular because of the low quantification limit, its accuracy and precision, and low cost of equipment compared to other analytical technique. Disadvantage is that it uses liquid mercury as

Table 10.10: Application of voltammetric/polarographic trace metal analyzer.

Application	Samples	Elements	Electrolytes	Auxiliary electrode	Reference electrode	Working electrode [multimode electrode (MME)]	Striping method (pulse amplitude)	Scan range (mV)	Peak potential (mV)
Determination of iron, cadmium, lead, and copper in cobalt acetate solution	Co(AC)$_2$	Fe	Catechol, pipes buffer, and pH = 7.0	pt	Ag/AgCl/3M KCl	HMDE	DPCSV (−50 mV)	−100 to −700	Fe = −405
		Cd Pb Cu	None	pt	Ag/AgCl/3M KCl	HMDE	DPASV (+50 mV)	−800 to +200	Cd = −500 Pb = −320 Cu = +100
Determination of chromium, manganese, and titanium in a polyterephthalic acid (PTA) solution	PTA in hydrochloric acid (HCl)	Cr	NaAC, DTPA, and pH = 6.2 with NaOH	pt	Ag/AgCl/3M KCl	HMDE	DPASV (−50 mV)	−1,000 to −1,500	Cr = −1,250
		Mn	NH$_4$Cl/NH$_3$ buffer, borate buffer, and Zn standard	pt	Ag/AgCl/3M KCl	HMDE	DPCSV (−75 mV)	−1,620 to −1,250	Mn = −1,400
		Ti	Mandelic acid and pH = 3 with NH$_3$ 25%	pt	Ag/AgCl/3M KCl	HMDE	DPCSV (−50 mV)	−100 to −900	Ti = −750
Determination of nickel, cobalt, and iron in a PTA solution	PTA in HCl	Ni and Co	Dimethylglyoxime in ethanol and NH$_4$Cl/NH$_3$ buffer	pt	Ag/AgCl/3M KCl	HMDE	DPCSV (−50 mV)	−700 to −1,200	Ni = −935 Co = −1,050
		Fe	Catechol, pipes buffer, and pH = 7.0	pt	Ag/AgCl/3M KCl	HMDE	DPCSV (−50 mV)	−100 to −700	Fe = −405
Determination of zinc, cadmium, lead, copper, and chromium in triglycerides	Triglycerides	Zn, Cd, Pb, and Cu	pH = 3 with NaOH	pt	Ag/AgCl/3M KCl	HMDE	DPASV (+50 mV)	−1,150 to +50	Zn = −940 Cd = −560 Pb = −340
		Cr	NaAC, DTPA, NaNO$_3$, and pH = 6.2 with NaOH	pt	Ag/AgCl/3M KCl	HMDE	DPCSV (−50 mV)	−1,000 to −1,500	Cu = −95 Cr = −1,260
Determination of selenium in standard	10 ppm standard	Se	EDTA and (NH$_4$)$_2$SO$_4$, Cu standard	pt	Ag/AgCl/3M KCl	HMDE	DPCSV (−30 mV)	−550 to −800	Se = −710

Continued

VOLTAMMETRY/POLAROGRAPHY TRACE METAL ANALYZER AND ITS APPLICATIONS

Continued

Application	Samples	Elements	Electrolytes	Auxiliary electrode	Reference electrode	Working electrode [multimode electrode (MME)]	Striping method (pulse amplitude)	Scan range (mV)	Peak potential (mV)
Determination of chromium, lead, and antimony in acetic acid (CH_3COOH)	CH_3COOH	Cd and Pb	$NaCH_3COO$	pt	Ag/AgCl/3M KCl	HMDE	DPASV (+50 mV)	−800 to −200	Cd = −560 Pb = −400
		Sb detection in the same vessel	HCl 30%	pt	Ag/AgCl/3M KCl	HMDE	DPASV (+50 mV)	−450 to −70	Sb = −150
Determination of total arsenic in brine	Saturated NaCl solution	As	HCl 30%	pt	Ag/AgCl/3M KCl	RDE	DPASV (+50 mV)	−200 to +300	As = −150
Determination of mercury in brine	Brine	Hg	Primary solution consists of NaCl, $HClO_4$, suprapur, and EDTA	Gc	Ag/AgCl/3M KCl	Au-RDE	DPASV (+50 mV)	+540 to +840	Hg = −640
Determination of cadmium, lead, and copper in brine and NaOH	Brine 300 mg/L	Cd, Pb, and Cu	Acetate buffer, pH = 4.6	pt	Ag/AgCl/3M KCl	HMDE	DPASV (+50 mV)	−700 to +30	Cd = −600 Pb = −380 Cu = −120
Determination of zinc, cadmium, lead, copper, iron, nickel, and cobalt in NaOH in one run	NaOH 50%	Zn, Cd, Pb, and Cu	Acetate buffer, pH = 4.6 with CH_3COOH, NH_3, and HCl	pt	Ag/AgCl/3M KCl	SMDE	Zn	−700 to +30	Zn = −960 Cd = −600 Pb = −380 Cu = −120
		Fe determination in the same vessel	Add catechol crystal and pipes buffer, pH = 7.0	pt	Ag/AgCl/3M KCl	HMDE	DPCSV (−50 mV)	−200 to −600	Fe = −450
		Ni and Co determination in the same vessel	Add dimethylglyoxime and NH_4Cl/NH_3 buffer	pt	Ag/AgCl/3M KCl	HMDE	DPCSV (−50 mV)	−800 to −1,300	Ni = −975 Co = −1,100

Continued

Continued

Application	Samples	Elements	Electrolytes	Auxiliary electrode	Reference electrode	Working electrode [multimode electrode (MME)]	Striping method (pulse amplitude)	Scan range (mV)	Peak potential (mV)
Determination of chromium in brine with MME and the graphite electrode	Brine 300 mg/L	Cr at MME	Acetic acid, ethylenediamine, and NH$_3$	pt	Ag/AgCl/3M KCl	SMDE	Differential pulse polaro-graphy (–50 mV)	+80 to –170	Cr = –50
		Cr at the ultra-trace graphite electrode (UTGE)	H$_2$SO$_4$ and diphenylcarbazide	Gc	Ag/AgCl/3M KCl	UTGE	DCCSV	+350 to –50	Cr = +100
Determination of zinc, cadmium, lead, copper, iron, nickel, and cobalt in elementary sulfur	Sulfur in the solid state	Zn, Cd, and Pb	KCl/NaCH$_3$COOH buffer	pt	Ag/AgCl/3M KCl	HMDE	DPASV (+50 mV)	–1,150 to –150	Zn = –960 Cd = –580 Pb = –375
		Fe and Cu	Catechol and pipes buffer	pt	Ag/AgCl/3M KCl	HMDE	DPCSV (–50 mV)	–50 to –600	Fe = –350 Cu = –190
		Ni and Co	Dimethylglyoxime and NH$_4$Cl buffer	pt	Ag/AgCl/3M KCl	HMDE	DPCSV (–50 mV)	–700 to –1,200	Ni = –985 Co = –1,110
Determination of cadmium, lead, and mercury in dissolved recycled glass	Acidic solution of recycled glass 20 g/L	Cd and Pb	pH = 3.0 ± 0.1 adjusted with NaOH 2 mol/L	pt	Ag/AgCl/3M KCl	HMDE and SMDE	Cd: DPASV (+50 mV) Pb: POL (–50 mV)	–800 to –450 +500 to +640	Cd = –560 Pb = –360
		Hg	NaCl, EDTA, and HClO$_4$	pt	Ag/AgCl/3M KCl	Au-RDE	DPASV (+50 mV)	+500 to +840	Hg = +640
Determination of iron and manganese in MgCl$_2$ brine	MgCl$_2$ brine	Fe	Phosphate buffer and catechol pH = 6.5	pt	Ag/AgCl/3M KCl	HMDE	DPCSV (–50 mV)	–180 to –650	Fe = –290
		Mn	pH = 6.5, borate buffer, and Zn standard	pt	Ag/AgCl/3M KCl	HMDE	DPASV (–75 mV)	–1,600 to –1,250	Mn = –1,480

Continued

VOLTAMMETRY/POLAROGRAPHY TRACE METAL ANALYZER AND ITS APPLICATIONS

Continued

Application	Samples	Elements	Electrolytes	Auxiliary electrode	Reference electrode	Working electrode [multimode electrode (MME)]	Striping method (pulse amplitude)	Scan range (mV)	Peak potential (mV)
Determination of nickel, antimony, cadmium, thallium, and copper in a neutral, highly concentrated Zn solution	Zn electrolyte	Ni	Dimethylglyoxime, NH_4Cl buffer, ascorbic acid, NH_3, and pH = 9.9	pt	Ag/AgCl/3M KCl	HMDE	DPCSV (−50 mV)	−750 to −1,100	Ni = −1,000
		Sb	HCl	pt	Ag/AgCl/3M KCl	HMDE	DPASV (+50 mV)	−250 to −80	Sb = −150
		Cd Tl Cu	HCl, $KMnO_4$, and ascorbic acid	pt	Ag/AgCl/3M KCl	HMDE	DPASV (+50 mV)	−800 to 0	Cd = −580 Cu = −120 Tl = −450
Determination of nickel, iron, and copper in a silver plating bath	Strongly alkaline silver bath containing 2.5 g/L CN− and 60 g/L Ag	Ni	Dimethylglyoxime NH_4Cl buffer	pt	Ag/AgCl/3M KCl	HMDE	DPCSV (−50 mV)	−700 to −1,200	Ni = −985
		Fe and Cu	Catechol and pipes buffer	pt	Ag/AgCl/3M KCl	HMDE	DPCSV (−50 mV)	0 to −600	Fe = −325 Cu = −175
Determination of chromium and selenium in a silver plating bath	Strongly alkaline silver bath containing 2.5 g/L CN− and 60 g/L Ag	Cr	Sodium acetate, dietriamine-pentaacetic acid, and $NaNO_3$	pt	Ag/AgCl/3M KCl	HMDE	DPCSV (−50 mV)	−1,000 to −1,500	Cr = −1,280
		Se	$NaNO_3$, EDTA, Cu standard, and $(NH_4)_2SO_4$	pt	Ag/AgCl/3M KCl	HMDE	SQWCSV (40 mV)	−550 to −900	Se = −650
Determination of tin and lead in organo plating bath	Organo plating bath	Sn	HCl and ammonium	pt	Ag/AgCl/3M KCl	HMDE	DPASV (−50 mV)	−800 to −430	Sn = −550
		Pb	HCl, ammonium oxalate, ammonium chloride, and methylene blue solution	pt	Ag/AgCl/3M KCl	HMDE	DPASV (+50 mV)	−530 to −200	Pb = −410

Continued

VOLTAMMETRY/POLAROGRAPHY TRACE METAL ANALYZER AND ITS APPLICATIONS

Continued

Application	Samples	Elements	Electrolytes	Auxiliary electrode	Reference electrode	Working electrode [multimode electrode (MME)]	Striping method (pulse amplitude)	Scan range (mV)	Peak potential (mV)
Determination of lead in electroless nickel plating baths	Electroless Ni bath	Analysis of Pb	C(HNO$_3$) 2 mol/L	pt	Ag/AgCl/3M KCl	HMDE	DP	−0.8 V to −0.2 V	Pb 0.8 mg/L
Determination of zinc, lead, and iron in NH$_4$Cl and CuSO$_4$	Solid NH$_4$Cl and solid CuSO$_4$	Zn and Pb	KCl/NaAC	pt	Ag/AgCl/3M KCl	HMDE	DPASV (+50 mV)	−1,100 to −100	Zn = −940 Pb = −360
		Fe	HCl, catechol and, pipes buffer	pt	Ag/AgCl/3M KCl	HMDE	DPCSV (−50 mV)	−250 to −600	Fe = −400
Determination of chromium and nickel in NH$_4$Cl and CuSO$_4$	NH$_4$Cl and CuSO$_4$	Cr	NaAC, diethylenediaminepentaacetic acid, and NaNO$_3$	pt	Ag/AgCl/3M KCl	HMDE	DPCSV (−50 mV)	−1,000 to −1,500	Cr = −1,250
		Ni	NaNO$_3$, dimethylglyoxime, and NH$_4$Cl/NH$_3$ buffer	pt	Ag/AgCl/3M KCl	HMDE	DPCSV (−50 mV)	−700 to −1,200	Ni = −970
Determination of antimony and bismuth in alkaline ZNO solution in one run	Alkaline ZNO solution	Bi	Digested solution	Pt	Ag/AgCl/3M KCl	HMDE	Bi: DPASV (+10 mV) and HMDE	−100 to −40	Bi = −60
		Sb	Digested solution	pt	Ag/AgCl/3M KCl	HMDE	Sb: DPASV (+10 mV) and HMDE	−300 to −70	Sb = −130
Determination of aluminum in alkaline ZNO solution	Alkaline ZNO solution	Al	Acetate buffer and Eriochrome Blue Black R	pt	Ag/AgCl/3M KCl	HMDE	DPCSV (−50 mV)	−300 to −600	Al = −450
Determination of copper and chromium in etching bath	Etching bath solution	Cu	EDTA and NH$_4$AC	pt	Ag/AgCl/3M KCl	HMDE	DPASV (+50 mV)	−300 to −100	Cu = +20

Continued

Chapter 10
VOLTAMMETRY/POLAROGRAPHY TRACE METAL ANALYZER AND ITS APPLICATIONS

Continued

Application	Samples	Elements	Electrolytes	Auxiliary electrode	Reference electrode	Working electrode [multimode electrode (MME)]	Striping method (pulse amplitude)	Scan range (mV)	Peak potential (mV)
		Cr	NaCH$_3$COO, NaNO$_3$ and diethylenetriamine tetraacetic acid pH = 6.2	pt	Ag/AgCl/3M KCl	HMDE	DPCSV (−50 mV)	−1,000 to −1,450	Cr = −1,230
Determination of iron in a nickel sulfonate bath containing surfactants	Nickel sulfonate plating bath	Fe	Catechol and pipes buffer and pH = 7.0 ± 0.1	pt	Ag/AgCl/3M KCl	HMDE	DPCSV (−50 mV)	−300 to −600	Fe = −450
Determination of iron and zinc in a nickel sulfate bath containing surfactants	Nickel sulfonate plating bath	Fe	Catechol and pipes buffer	pt	Ag/AgCl/3M KCl	HMDE	DPCSV (−50 mV)	−300 to −600	Fe = −480
		Zn	pH = 7.0 ± 0.1, EDTA, NH$_3$, and Ca(NO$_3$)$_2$	pt	Ag/AgCl/3M KCl	SMDE	DPPOL (−50 mV)	−600 to −14	Zn = −1,280
Determination of copper in nickel sulfate plating bath containing surfactants	Nickel sulfate plating bath	Cu	EDTA and NH$_4$AC	pt	Ag/AgCl/3M KCl	HMDE	DPASV (+50 mV)	−500 to 0	Cu = −120
Determination of zinc, cadmium, lead, nickel, and cobalt in HCl	HCl 37.8%	Zn, Cd, and Pb	Buffer NH$_4$AC	pt	Ag/AgCl/3M KCl	HMDE	DPASV (+50 mV)	−1,150 to −300	Zn = −960 Cd = −580 Pb = −380
		Ni and Co in the same vessel	Addition of dimethylglyoxime in triethanolamine and NH$_4$Cl buffer	pt	Ag/AgCl/3M KCl	HMDE	DPCSV (−75 mV)	−800 to −1,000	Ni = −960 Co = −1,050
Determination of zinc, cadmium, lead, nickel, and cobalt in Javelle water	Javelle water	Zn, Cd, and Pb	NH$_4$AC buffer	pt	Ag/AgCl/3M KCl	HMDE	DPCSV (−75 mV)	−1,150 to −250	Zn = −960 Cd = −580 Pb = −380
		Ni and Co in the same vessel	Addition of dimethylglyoxime in triethanolamine and NH$_4$Cl buffer	pt	Ag/AgCl/3M KCl	HMDE	DPASV (+50 mV)	−800 to −1,000	Ni = −920 Co = −1,050

Continued

Continued

Application	Samples	Elements	Electrolytes	Auxiliary electrode	Reference electrode	Working electrode [multimode electrode (MME)]	Stripping method (pulse amplitude)	Scan range (mV)	Peak potential (mV)
Determination of zinc, cadmium, lead, nickel, and cobalt in 40% FeCl$_3$ solution	40% FeCl$_3$ solution	Zn, Cd, and Pb	NH$_4$AC buffer, ascorbic acid, dimethylglyoxime in triethanolamine, and NH$_4$Cl buffer	pt	Ag/AgCl/3M KCl	HMDE	DPASV (+50 mV)	−1,150 to −200	Zn = −960 Cd = −580 Pb = −380
		Ni and Co		pt	Ag/AgCl/3M KCl	HMDE	DPCSV (−75 mV)	−800 to −1,000	Ni = −940 Co = −1,050
Determination of coumarin and tartrazine in vodka	Vodka sample	Coumarin	NH$_4$Cl/NH$_3$	pt	Ag/AgCl/3M KCl	HMDE	DPLSV (−50 mV)	−50 to −800	Ep = −400
		Tartrazine	Concentrate H$_2$SO$_4$	pt	Ag/AgCl/3M KCl	HMDE	DPLSV (−50mV)	+100 to −300	Ep = −108
Determination of zinc, cadmium, lead, copper, iron, nickel, and cobalt in freeze-dried hop	Freeze-dried hop samples	Fe	Catechol and pipes buffer, pH = 7.0 ± 0.1 with NH$_3$	pt	Ag/AgCl/3M KCl	HMDE	DPCSV (−50 mV)	−100 to −600	Fe = −310
		Ni and Co	Dimethylglyoxime, methanol, and NH$_4$Cl buffer	pt	Ag/AgCl/3M KCl	HMDE	DPCSV (−50 mV)	−700 to −1,200	Ni = −970 Co = −1,100
		Zn, Cd, Pb, and Cu	NH$_4$AC buffer pH = 4.6	pt	Ag/AgCl/3M KCl	HMDE	DPASV (+50 mV)	−1,150 to +200	Zn = −960 Cd = −550 Pb = −395 Cu = +55
Determination of zinc, lead, copper, and iron in sugar	Crystal sugar sample	Zn, Pb, and Cu	NH$_4$AC buffer pH = 4.6	pt	Ag/AgCl/3M KCl	HMDE	DPASV (50 mV)	−1,150 to +50	Zn = −980 Pb = −385 Cu = −100
		Fe	Catechol and pipes buffer	pt	Ag/AgCl/3M KCl	HMDE	DPCSV (−50 mV)	−100 to −600	Fe = −340

Continued

VOLTAMMETRY/POLAROGRAPHY TRACE METAL ANALYZER AND ITS APPLICATIONS

Continued

Application	Samples	Elements	Electrolytes	Auxiliary electrode	Reference electrode	Working electrode [multimode electrode (MME)]	Striping method (pulse amplitude)	Scan range (mV)	Peak potential (mV)
Determination of cadmium, lead, and copper in wine with EDTA after UV digestion	White coin	Cd, Pb, and Cu with EDTA cell	NH_4AC buffer	pt	Ag/AgCl/3M KCl	HMDE	DPASV (+50 mV)	−1,150 to +50	Cd = −980 Pb = −385 Cu = −100
Determination of zinc, cadmium, lead, and copper in chilli sauce after digestion	Chilli sauce powder	Zn, Cd, Pb, and Cu	NH_4AC buffer	pt	Ag/AgCl/3M KCl	HMDE	DPASV (50 mV)	−1,150 to +50	Zn = −960 Cd = −560 Pb = −385 Cu = −100
Determination of mercury in chilli sauce after digestion	Chilli sauce powder	Hg	EDTA, NaCl, and $HClO_4$	Gc	Ag/AgCl/LiCl	Au-RDE	DPASV (50 mV)	+500 to +840	Hg = +500
Determination of arsenic in chilli sauce	Chilli sauce powder	As	HCl 30%	pt with special electrolyte vessel	Ag/AgCl/3M KCl	HMDE special side and Au-RPE	DPASV (+50 mV)	−200 to +300	As = +130
Determination of aluminum in albumin lyophilisate after digestion	Albumin lyophilisate	Al	NaAC buffer pH = 4.64, NaOH, and CH_3COOH	pt	Ag/AgCl/3M KCl	HMDE	DPCSV (−50 mV)	−330 to −600	Al = −420
Determination of zinc, cadmium, lead, and copper in whisky after digestion	Whisky 40% v/v	Zn, Cd, Pb, and Cu	NH_4AC buffer pH = 4.6	pt	Ag/AgCl/3M KCl	pH = 4.6	HMDE (50 mV)	−1,100 to +100	Zn = −960 Cd = −560 Pb = −360 Cu = −80
Determination of aluminum and chromium in whisky after digestion	Whisky 40% v/v	Al	DASA BES. NaOH pH = 7.1	pt	Ag/AgCl/3M KCl	HMDE	DPCSV (50 mV)	−800 to −1,200	Al = −930
		Cr	NaAc, DTPA + $NaNO_3$	pt	Ag/AgCl/3M KCl	HMDE	DPCSV (−50 mV)	−1,000 to −1,550	Cr = −1,320

Continued

VOLTAMMETRY/POLAROGRAPHY TRACE METAL ANALYZER AND ITS APPLICATIONS

Continued

Application	Samples	Elements	Electrolytes	Auxiliary electrode	Reference electrode	Working electrode [multimode electrode (MME)]	Striping method (pulse amplitude)	Scan range (mV)	Peak potential (mV)
Determination of cadmium, lead, copper, nickel, and cobalt in soybean oil after digestion	Soybean oil	Cd, Pb, and Cu	Merck reagent cocktail KCl/NaAC	pt	Ag/AgCl/3M KCl	HMDE	DPASV (+50 mV)	−800 to 0	Cd = −650 Pb = −450 Cu = −135
		Ni and Co	Dimethylglyoxime in ethanol and NH$_4$Cl buffer	pt	Ag/AgCl/3M KCl	HMDE	DPCSV (−75 mV)	−800 to −1,250	Ni = −980 Co = −1,080
Determination of mercury in soybean oil after digestion	Soybean oil	Hg	EDTA, NaCl, and HClO$_4$	GC	Ag/AgCl/LiCl	AU-RDE	DPASV (+50 mV)	+500 to +800	Hg = +500
Determination of zinc in herbal pharmaceutical drug	Pharmaceutical product (drops)	Zn	DIN buffer based on KCl/NaCH$_3$COO	pt	Ag/AgCl/3M KCl	HMDE	DPASV (+50 mV)	−1,150 to −800	Zn = −950
Determination of boron in human plasma using Beryllon III as a ligand	Plasma samples	B	Suprapure HOAC/NH$_4$OAC buffer	pt	Ag/AgCl/KCl sat	HMDE	DPCSV (−50 mV)	−200 to −900	Ep = −342
Determination of uranium in water as an uranium(VI)-chloranilic acid complex	Water sample	U(VI)	Chloranilic acid	pt	Ag/AgCl/3M KCl	HMDE	DPCSV (−50 mV)	+150 to −200	Ep = −60
Determination of zinc, cadmium, lead, copper, nickel, and cobalt in vitamin tablets	Powder for vitamin tablet fabrication	Zn, Cd, Pb, and Cu	NH$_4$AC buffer and NH$_3$/CH$_3$COOH pH = 4.6	pt	Ag/AgCl/3M KCl	HMDE	DPASV (+50 mV)	−1,150 to +150	Zn = −900 Cd = −545 Pb = −400 Cu = −80
		Ni and Co	Dimethylglyoxime in ethanol and NH$_4$Cl buffer	pt	Ag/AgCl/3M KCl	HMDE	DPCSV (−50 mV)	−700 to −1,200	Ni = −970 Co = −1,080
Determination of manganese, iron, and molybdenum in vitamin tablets	Powder for vitamin tablets	Mn	NH$_4$Cl buffer, borate buffer, and Zn standard	pt	Ag/AgCl/3M KCl	HMDE	DPASV (−75 mV)	−1,620 to −1,250	Mn = −1,430

Continued

VOLTAMMETRY/POLAROGRAPHY TRACE METAL ANALYZER AND ITS APPLICATIONS

Continued

Application	Samples	Elements	Electrolytes	Auxiliary electrode	Reference electrode	Working electrode [multimode electrode (MME)]	Striping method (pulse amplitude)	Scan range (mV)	Peak potential (mV)
		Fe	Pipes buffer and catechol	pt	Ag/AgCl/3M KCl	HMDE	DPCSV (−50 mV)	−100 to −600	Fe = −310
		Mo	8-hydroxy-7-iodo-5-quinolinesulfonic acid in H_2SO_4 + KCl	pt	Ag/AgCl/3M KCl	SMDE	DPPOL (−50 mV)	−680 to −1,180	Mo = −1,040
Determination of clothiapine in standard	Clothiapine sample	Clothiapine	Pipes buffer	pt	Ag/AgCl/3M KCl	HMDE	DPCSV (−50 mV)	−900 to −1,400	Ep = −1,225
Determination of cadmium and lead in herbicide	Herbicide powder containing Cu and Zn N,N'-ethylenebisdi-thiocarbamate	Cd and Pb	NaAC buffer	pt	Ag/AgCl/3M KCl	HMDE	DPASV (+50 mV)	−700 to −250	Ep = −380
Determination of vanadium, nickel, cobalt, and chromium in solvent	Linear alkyl benzene	V	Pipes buffer and catechol	pt	Ag/AgCl/3M KCl	HDME	DPCSV (−50 mV)	−350 to −800	V = −630
		Ni and Co in same vessel	Dimethylglyoxime in ethanol, NH_4Cl buffer, NaAC + Na-DTPA, and $NaNO_3$	pt	Ag/AgCl/3M KCl	HDME	DPCSV (−50 mV)	−700 to −1,200	Ni = −970 CO = −1,080
		Cr		pt	Ag/AgCl/3M KCl	HDME	DPCSV (−50 mV)	−1,000 to −1,500	Cr = −1,250
Determination of artemisinin and artesunate in standard	Water standard	Artemisinin	Ammonium sulfate and methanol	pt	Ag/AgCl/LiCl	DME	DPPOL (−50 mV)	+150 to −150	As = −50
		Artesunate	Ammonium sulfate and methanol	pt	Ag/AgCl/LiCl	DME	DPPOL (−50 mV)	+200 to −500	Ar = +20
Determination of palladium in pharmaceutical products	Drug against high blood pressure	Analysis of Pd	Ammonium buffer and NaOH solution		Ag/AgCl/KCl (3 mol/L)	DME	DP	−0.4V to −1.0V	Pd = −0.77

Continued

Continued

Application	Samples	Elements	Electrolytes	Auxiliary electrode	Reference electrode	Working electrode [multimode electrode (MME)]	Striping method (pulse amplitude)	Scan range (mV)	Peak potential (mV)
Determination of β-propiolactone in vaccine	Vaccine sample	β-propio-lactone	$KH_2PO_4 + Na_2HPO_4$	pt	Ag/AgCl/KCl (3 mol/L)	SMDE	DPPOL (−50 mV)	0 to −950	β-propio-lactone = −375
Determination of ascorbic acid in vitamin capsules	Vitamin capsules samples	$C_6H_8O_6$	Oxalic acid and $NaOOCH_3/CH_3COOH$ buffer	pt	Ag/AgCl/KCl (3 mol/L)	DME	DPPOL (50 mV)	−50 to +200	$C_6H_8O_6$ = +100
Determination of thiomersal in eye drops	Eye drop containing NaCl, KCl, KH_2PO_4, surfactant, and chloro-acetamide	Thiomersal	Metrohm buffer	pt	Ag/AgCl/3M KCl	DME	DPPOL (50 mV)	−300 to −900	Thiomersal = −635
Determination of cysteine and cystine in infusion solution	Sample containing cysteine and cystine	Cysteine and cystine	$HClO_4$	pt	Ag/AgCl/3M NaCl	DME	DPPOL (50 mV)	+150 to −900	Cysteine = −70 Cystine = −720
Determination of L-methylnicotinamide hydrochloride in standard	Standard	L-Methylni-cotinamide hydrochlo-ride	Na_2CO_3	Gc	Ag/AgCl/3M KCl	DME	DPPOL (−40 mV)	−1,300 to −1,900	Ep = −1,550
Determination of cysteine and cystine in sodium caseinate	Sodium caseinate sample containing cysteine and cystine	Cysteine and cystine	NH_4Cl buffer and CH_3COOH	pt	Ag/AgCl/3M KCl	DME	DPPOL (−50 mV)	−250 to −750 / −1,300 to −1,880	Ep = −470 Cystine = −1,650
Determination of speciation of Fe(III) and Fe(II) in standard	Standard	Fe(II) and Fe(III)	Sodium pyrophosphate	pt	Ag/AgCl/3M KCl	DME	DPPOL (−20 mV)	−50 to −1,300	Fe(II) = −320 Fe(III) = −850

Continued

Continued

Application	Samples	Elements	Electrolytes	Auxiliary electrode	Reference electrode	Working electrode /multimode electrode (MME)]	Striping method (pulse amplitude)	Scan range (mV)	Peak potential (mV)
Determination of 4-carboxybenzaldehyde (CBA) in PTA	Sample of PTA containing CBA	CBA	NH_4Cl buffer	Pt	Ag/AgCl/3M KCl	DME	DPPOL (−50 mV)	−1,050 to −1,350	Ep = −1,200
Determination of cyanide in gases resulting from the incineration of plastic insulation materials	Cable insulation	Cyanide	KOH and H_3BO_3	Pt	Ag/AgCl/3M KCl	DME	DPPOL (−50 mV)	−100 to −600	Ep = −310
Determination of free styrene in polystyrene and mixed polymers	Yoghurt beaker made of polystyrene	Styrene	$NaNO_2$ and NaAC	Pt	Ag/AgCl/3M KCl	SMDE	DPPOL (−50 mV)	0 to −400	Ep = −240
Determination of tungsten in organic phase	Olefin epoxide with tungsten as phosphorus complex	Tungsten	8-hydroxy-7-iodo-5-quinolinesulfonic acid in H_2SO_4	Pt	Ag/AgCl/3M KCl	SMDE	DPPOL (50 mV)	−680 to −1,180	Ep = −950
Determination of formaldehyde, acetaldehyde, and acetone in methanol	Methanol, puriss. p.a.	Formaldehyde, acetaldehyde, and acetone	Na_2HPO_4/citric acid buffer and hydrazine sulfate	Pt	Ag/AgCl/3M KCl	SMDE	DPPOL (−20 mV)	Formaldehyde = −850 to −1,160	Formaldehyde = −1,050
								Acetaldehyde = −1,070 to −1,320	Ep = −1,200
								Acetone = −1,250 to −1,600	Ep = −1,350

Continued

Continued

Application	Samples	Elements	Electrolytes	Auxiliary electrode	Reference electrode	Working electrode [multimode electrode (MME)]	Striping method (pulse amplitude)	Scan range (mV)	Peak potential (mV)
Determination of Cd and Pb in seawater	Seawater acidifies to pH = 2 with HCl	Cd and Pb	0.3 mol/L HCl + 10 mg/L + Hg^{2+}	GC	Ag/AgCl/3M KCl	MFE	DPASV	−900 to −300	Cd = −660 Pb = −470
Determination of Ni and Co in seawater	Seawater	Ni and Co	0.2 mol/L NH_3 + 0.1 mol/L NH_4Cl + 5.10^{-4} mol/L DMG	pt	Ag/AgCl/3M KCl	HMDE	DPAdSV	−800 to −1,300	Ni = −960 Co = −1,110
Determination of iodine in glacial CH_3COOH	CH_3COOH	I	No	pt	Ag/AgCl/3M KCl/KNO_3 salt	HMDE	DP-CSV	−300 to −600	I = −470
Determination of pt and Rg in drinking water	Drinking water	Rh	HCl + formaldehyde HCl + formaldehyde + hydrazinium sulfate	GC	Ag/AgCl/3M KCl	HMDE	DPAdSV	−1,000 to −1300	Rh = −1,180
		Pt		GC	Ag/AgCl/3M KCl	HMDE	DPAdSV	−700 to −1,000	Pt = −880
Determination of NTA and EDTA in waste water	Waste water	NTA EDTA	HNO_3 + KNO_3 + ascorbic acid	pt	Ag/AgCl/3M KCl	DME	DPAdSV	+100 to −600	NTA = −220 EDTA = −450
Determination of vitamin C in orange juice	Orange juice	Ascorbic acid	0.1 mol/L acetate buffer	pt	Ag/AgCl/3M KCl	DME	DPAdSV	−200 to +200	Ep = +110
Determination of vitamin B2 in vitamin tablets	Multivitamin tablets	Vitamin B2	0.05 mol/L KCl 0.1 mol/L K_2CO_3	pt	Ag/AgCl/3M KCl	DME	DPAdSV	−300 to −700	Ep = −550
Determination of nicotinamide (vitamin B3, vitamin PP) in vitamin tablets	Multivitamin tablets	Nicotinamide	1% tetramethylammonium hydroxide	pt	Ag/AgCl/3M KCl	DME	DPAdSV	−1,400 to −1,900	Ep = −1,700
Determination of CO in electrolytic gold baths	Gold plating bath	CO	0.1 mol/L sulfosalicylic acid + 0.1 mol/L NH_3 + 5.10^{-4} mol/L DMG	pt	Ag/AgCl/3M KCl	DME	DPAdSV	−1,000 to −1,400	Ep = −1,250

Continued

Chapter 10 — VOLTAMMETRY/POLAROGRAPHY TRACE METAL ANALYZER AND ITS APPLICATIONS

Continued

Application	Samples	Elements	Electrolytes	Auxiliary electrode	Reference electrode	Working electrode [multimode electrode (MME)]	Striping method (pulse amplitude)	Scan range (mV)	Peak potential (mV)
Determination of nickel and cobalt in zinc plant electrolytes	Concentrated zinc solution	Ni	Ammonia buffer C (HCl) = 1 mol/L + C(NH$_3$) = 3 mol/L	pt	Ag/AgCl/3M KCl	HDME	DPAdSV	−700 to −1,100	Ep = −950
		Co	Supporting electrolyte α-Benzildioxime solution	pt	Ag/AgCl/3M KCl	HMDE		−800 to −1,125	Ep = −960
Determination of antimony in Zinc electrolytes	Zinc plant electrolyte	HCl	Zinc plant electrolyte	pt	Ag/AgCl/3M KCl	HMDE	DPAdSV	Sb (total) −0.4 V to −0.1 V	Ep = −0.18 V
								Sb(III) 0.2 to −0.05	Ep = −0.13 V
Determination of GE in electroplating bath	Plating solution containing high concentrations of An, Mn, Al, and Fe	Ge	Catechol + acetate buffer	pt	Ag/AgCl/3M KCl	HMDE	DPPol	−500 to −900	Ge = −700
Determination of Ge in lead	Metallic acid	Ge	Catechol + Acetate buffer	pt	Ag/AgCl/3M KCl	HMDE	DPAdSV	−500 to −900	Ep = −700
Determination of Cu, Fe, and V in salt	Pure sample	Cu, Fe, and V	Pipes buffer with catechol	pt	Ag/AgCl/3M KCl	HMDE	DPAdSV	−340 to −600	Ep = −160
Determination of different species of Cr in seawater	Seawater	All Cr species, DTPA, and sodium nitrate, pH 6.2	Acetate buffer	pt	Ag/AgCl/3M KCl	HMDE	DPAdSV	−1,000 to −1,400	Ep = −1,200

Continued

VOLTAMMETRY/POLAROGRAPHY TRACE METAL ANALYZER AND ITS APPLICATIONS

Continued

Application	Samples	Elements	Electrolytes	Auxiliary electrode	Reference electrode	Working electrode [multimode electrode (MME)]	Striping method (pulse amplitude)	Scan range (mV)	Peak potential (mV)
Determination of zinc, cadmium, lead, and copper in wastewater after UV digestion	Wastewater	Zn, Cd, Pb, and Cu	Acetate buffer, pH 4.6 C (acetate acid) = 2 mol/L + C(NH_3) = 1 mol/L	pt	Ag/AgCl/3M KCl	HMDE	DPPol	−1,150 to +150	Zn = −980 Cd = −560 Pb = −380 Cu = +30
Determination of total Cr in wastewater after UV digestion	Wastewater	Cr	C (sodium acetate) = 0.2 mol/L + C (DTPA) = 0.05 mol/L	pt	Ag/AgCl/3M KCl	HMDE	DPASV	−1,000 to −1,450	Ep = −1,270
Determination of elemental sulfur in gasoline	Gasoline	S		pt	Ag/AgCl/3M KCl	DME	DPASV	−0.3 V to −0.6 V	Ep = −0.47 V
Determination of Cd, Pb, and Cu in drinking water	Drinking water	Cd, Pb, and Cu	Acetate buffer pH 4.6 C (Acetic acid) = 2 mol/L + C (NH_3) = 1 mol/L KCl solution C(KCl) = 3 mol/L	pt	Ag/AgCl/3M KCl	HMDE	DPASV	−900 to +100	Cd = −580 Pb = −370 Cu = −60
Determination of Ni and Co in drinking water	Drinking water	Ni and Co	Ammonia buffer	pt	Ag/AgCl/3M KCl	HMDE	DPAdSV	−850 to −1,250	Ni = −960 Co = −1,150
Determination of uranium in drinking water	Drinking water	U	Nitric acid	pt	Ag/AgCl/3M KCl	HMDE	DPAdSV	+50 to −150	Ep = −30
Determination of mercury in wastewater	Wastewater	Hg	C($HClO_4$)—0.2 mol/L C(NaCl)—3 mmol/L C(EDTA Na_2 + $2H_2O$)—1 mmol/L	GC	Ag/AgCl/3M KCl	RDE	DPCSV	+360 to +800	Ep = 550
Determination of manganese in drinking water	Drinking water	Mn	Borate buffer	pt	Ag/AgCl/3M KCl	HMDE	DPASV	−1,650 to −1,300	Ep = −1,450

Continued

VOLTAMMETRY/POLAROGRAPHY TRACE METAL ANALYZER AND ITS APPLICATIONS

Continued

Application	Samples	Elements	Electrolytes	Auxiliary electrode	Reference electrode	Working electrode [multimode electrode (MME)]	Striping method (pulse amplitude)	Scan range (mV)	Peak potential (mV)
Determination of iron in drinking water	Drinking water	Fe	Phosphate buffer	pt	Ag/AgCl/3M KCl	HMDE	DPASV	−250 to −600	Ep = −360
Determination of Ni in white wine	White wine	Ni	Ammonia buffer	pt	Ag/AgCl/3M KCl	HMDE	DPCSV	−700 to −1,250	Ep = −950
Determination of Cd, Pb, and Cu in wine	Red wine (Switzerland)	Analysis of Cd and Pb		pt	Ag/AgCl/3M KCl	HMDE	DPASV	−800 to −100	Cd = −500 Pb = −360
		Analysis of Cu	KCl electrolyte	pt	Ag/AgCl/3M KCl	HMDE	DPASV	−450 to +75	Cu = −140
Determination of platinum and rhodium in wine	Red wine	Rh	Dilute formaldehyde solution	Gc	Ag/AgCl/3M KCl	HMDE	DPCSV	−900 to −1,230	Rh = −1,170
		Pt	Hydrazine sulfate solution	Glassy carbon (GC)	Ag/AgCl/3M KCl	HMDE		−600 to −1,100	Pt = −900
Determination of quinine in bitter lemon	Bitter lemon (soft drink)	Quinine	Britton–Robinson buffer pH 7	pt	Ag/AgCl/3M KCl	DME	DPCSV	−800 to −1,250	Ep = −1,130
Determination of platinum in urine	Human urine	Pt	Hydrazine sulfate solution	Gc	Ag/AgCl/3M KCl	DME	DPASV	−700 to −1,050	Pt = −880
Determination of Chromium in sulfuric acid	Sulfuric acid	Cr	C (Sodium acetate)— 0.2 mol/L C (DTPA)—0.05 mol/L C(NaNO$_3$)—2.5 mol/L	pt	Ag/AgCl/3M KCl	HMDE	DPASV	−1,000 to −1,450	Ep = −1,230
Determination of molybdenum in sulfuric acid	Sulfuric acid	Mb	W(HNO$_3$)	pt	Ag/AgCl/3M KCl	SMDE	DPASV	+200 to −450	Mo = −150

Continued

Continued

Application	Samples	Elements	Electrolytes	Auxiliary electrode	Reference electrode	Working electrode [multimode electrode (MME)]	Stripping method (pulse amplitude)	Scan range (mV)	Peak potential (mV)
Determination of cadmium, lead, and copper in triphosphate	Pentasodium triphosphate	Cd, Pb, and Cu	Nitric acid	pt	Ag/AgCl/3M KCl	HMDE	DPASV	−750 to +150	Cd = −600 Pb = −400 Cu = +10
Determination of nickel and cobalt in triphosphate	Pentasodium triphosphate	Ni, Co	Ammonia buffer	pt	Ag/AgCl/3M KCl	HMDE	DPASV	−850 to −1,300	Ni = −990 Co = −1,150
Determination of iron in triphosphate	Pentasodium triphosphate	Fe	Catechol solution	pt	Ag/AgCl/3M KCl	SMDE	DPASV	−250 to −600	Ep = −390
Determination of manganese in triphosphate	Pentasodium triphosphate	Mn	Tartrate solution	pt	Ag/AgCl/3M KCl	HMDE	DPASV	−1,650 to −1,300	Ep = −1,530
Determination of chromium in lime (CaCO$_3$)	Lime (CaCO$_3$)	Cr		pt	Ag/AgCl/3M KCl	HMDE	DPASV	70 to −170	Ep = −30
Determination of formaldehyde in metal working lubricants	Metal working lubricant	Formaldehyde	C(LiOH)—0.1 mol/L + C(EDTA)—0.02 mol/L	pt	Ag/AgCl/3M KCl	DME	DPCSV	−1,400 to −1,850	Ep = −1,640
Determination of thallium, besides excess of Cd in Zn plant electrolytes (concentrated ZnSO$_4$ solution)	Zn plant electrolyte	Zn, Cd, and Tl	Hydrochloric acid, W(HCl)—30%, and Suprapur	pt	Ag/AgCl/3M KCl	HMDE	DPASV	Tl = −600 to −300 Cd = −450 to −750	Ep = −460 Ep = −610
Determination of nickel in wastewater	Wastewater	Ni	Ammonia buffer	pt	Ag/AgCl/3M KCl	HMDE	DPASV	−700 to −1,100	Ni = −950
Determination of Tin in wastewater	Wastewater	Tin	Supporting electrolyte	pt	Ag/AgCl/3M KCl	HMDE	DPASV	−800 to −300	Sn = −580

Continued

Chapter 10
VOLTAMMETRY/POLAROGRAPHY TRACE METAL ANALYZER AND ITS APPLICATIONS

Continued

Application	Samples	Elements	Electrolytes	Auxiliary electrode	Reference electrode	Working electrode [multimode electrode (MME)]	Striping method (pulse amplitude)	Scan range (mV)	Peak potential (mV)
Determination of thallium in wastewater	Wastewater	Tl	Acetate buffer EDTA solution	Pt	Ag/AgCl/3M KCl	HMDE	DPASV	−800 to −200	Tl = −440
Determination of selenium in wastewater	Wastewater	Se	Ammonium sulfate solution 10%	Pt	Ag/AgCl/3M KCl	HMDE	DPASV	−550 to −900	Se = −670
Determination of chromium in wasterwaste	Wastewater	Cr		Pt	Ag/AgCl/3M KCl	SMDE	DPASV	100 to −150	Cr(VI) = −20
Determination of germanium in Zn plant electrolytes (concentrated $ZNSO_4$ solution)	Zn plant electrolyte	Ge	PCV solution	Pt	Ag/AgCl/3M KCl	HMDE	DPASV	−200 to −450	Ge = −340
Determination of thiourea in nickel plating baths	Ni planting bath containing chloride	Thiourea	Acetate solution perchlorate solution Ammonia buffer	Pt	Ag/AgCl/3M KCl	HMDE	DPCSV	+100 to −800	Thiourea = −370
Determination of titanium in polyethylene terephthalate (PET)	PET pellets	Ti	C(mandelic acid) 0.4 mol/L in water	Pt	Ag/AgCl/3M KCl	HMDE	DPASV	−600 to −950	Ti = −770
Determination of cobalt in PET	PET pellets	Co	Ammonia buffer	Pt	Ag/AgCl/3M KCl	HMDE	DPASV	−900 to −1,250	Co = −1,050
Determination of antimony in PET	PET pellets	Sb	W(HCl)—30% suprapur	Pt	Ag/AgCl/3M KCl	HMDE	DPASV	−300 to −70	Sb = −200
Determination of zinc and lead in ethanol	Ethanol, food grade	Zn and Pb	Acetate buffer pH 4.6	Pt	Ag/AgCl/3M KCl	HMDE	DPASV	−1250 to −200	Zn = −980 Pb = −400
Determination of iron in ethanol	Ethanol, food grade	Iron	Pipes buffer	Pt	Ag/AgCl/3M KCl	HMDE	DPASV	−200 to −600	Fe = −390

Continued

Continued

Application	Samples	Elements	Electrolytes	Auxiliary electrode	Reference electrode	Working electrode [multimode electrode (MME)]	Striping method (pulse amplitude)	Scan range (mV)	Peak potential (mV)
Determination of gold in ammonium thiosulfate solution	Ammonium thiosulfate solution	Au	$C(KNO_3)$—0.2 mol/L + $C(Na_2EDTA)$—0.04 mol/L	Gc	Ag/AgCl/3M KCl	Ultratrace RDE	DPASV	−400 to 500	Au= +150
Determination of cyclic voltammetry with the 746 VA trace analyzer	KCl solution	Pb	$C(KCl)$—3 mol/L	pt	Ag/AgCl/3M KCl	HMDE	DPASV	−600 to −200	Pb cathodic = −420 Pb anodic = −390
Determination of total iron in wastewater after digestion (triethanolamine bromated method)	Wastewater	Total Fe	$C(triethanolamine)$ + $C(KBrO_3)$ + $C(NaOH)$	Pt 6.0343.000	Ag/AgCl/3M KCl	HMDE	DPASV	−750 to −1,200	Fe (total) = −1,010
Determination of total iron in deionized water (triethanolamine bromated method)	Deionized water	Total iron	$C(triethanolamine)$ + $C(KBrO_3)$ + $C(NaOH)$	Pt 6.0343.000	Ag/AgCl/3M KCl	HMDE	DPASV	−600 to −1,300	Fe (total) = −930
Determination of total iron in ethylene glycol (2,3-dihydroxynaphthalene method)	Monoethylene glycol	Total iron	Analysis of total Fe HEPPS buffer DHN solution bromate solution measuring solution	Pt 6.0343.000	Ag/AgCl/3M KCl	HMDE	DPASV	−0.1 to −0.8	Fe (total) = −530
Determination of traces of Fe(III) in standard solution with solochrome violet RS	Drinking water	Fe(III)	Analysis of Fe(III) Acetate buffer solution SVRS solution	Pt 6.0343.000	Ag/AgCl/3M KCl	HMDE	DPASV	−0.2 to −0.7	Fe(III) = −530
Determination of traces of iron in water (1-nitroso-2-napthal method)	Ultrapure water	Iron	Measuring solution pipes buffer pH 8.0 NN solution Measuring solution	Pt 6.0343.000	Ag/AgCl/3M KCl	HMDE	DPASV	−0.2 to −0.6	Fe = −420

Continued

VOLTAMMETRY/POLAROGRAPHY TRACE METAL ANALYZER AND ITS APPLICATIONS

Continued

Application	Samples	Elements	Electrolytes	Auxiliary electrode	Reference electrode	Working electrode [multimode electrode (MME)]	Striping method (pulse amplitude)	Scan range (mV)	Peak potential (mV)
Determination of selenium in vitamin tablets	Vitamin tablets	Se	$C[(NH_4)_2SO_4]$	pt	Ag/AgCl/3M KCl Intermediate electrolyte: C(KCl)	HMDE	DPCSV	−0.45 to −0.9	Se = −0.65
Polarographic determination of Fe^{2+} in iron sucrose injection solution according to USP26/NF21	Iron sucrose injection solution	Fe^{2+}	$\beta(CH_3COONa) = 150$ g/L	Pt 6.0343	Ag/AgCl/3M KCl	DME	DPASV	−0.1 to −1.8	Fe^{2+} = −750 −1,450
Determination of total iron in the ppm range in a chromium electroplating bath	Chromium plating bath	Fe	C(ammonium oxalate)	Pt 6.0343	Ag/AgCl/3M KCl	DME	DPASV	+0.1 to −0.5	Fe = −150
Determination of total iron in the ppm range in phosphoric acid	Phosphoric acid	Total iron	C(ammonium oxalate)	Pt 6.0343	Ag/AgCl/3M KCl	SMDE	DPASV	+0.12 to −0.3	Fe = −40
Determination of aluminum in the ppb range in aqueous elutes of filter layers. (Solochrome violet RS method)	Standard solution	Al	C(acetic acid) C(ammonia)	Pt 6.0343	Ag/AgCl/3M KCl	HMDE	DPCSV	−0.25 to −0.6	Fe = −380
Destination of nickel and cobalt in sulfuric acid	Sulfuric acid	Ni and Co	$C(NH_4Cl)$ $C(NH_3)$ DMG solution measuring solution	Pt 6.0343	Ag/AgCl/3M KCl	HMDE	DPASV	−0.8 to −1.25	Ni = −950 Co = −1,250

Continued

Continued

Application	Samples	Elements	Electrolytes	Auxiliary electrode	Reference electrode	Working electrode [multimode electrode (MME)]	Striping method (pulse amplitude)	Scan range (mV)	Peak potential (mV)
Determination of Fe in sulfuric acid	Sulfuric acid	Fe	C(pipes) C(1N2N) Measuring solution	Pt 6.0343	Ag/AgCl/3M KCl	HMDE	DPASV	−0.25 to −0.62	Fe = −410
Determination of Suppressor << Copper gleam™ 2001 Carrier >> in acid copper baths (Rohm and Haas electronic material)	Acid copper electro-plating bath	Suppressor	Virgin makeup solution	Pt 6.0343	Ag/AgCl/3M KCl KNO$_3$ saturated H$_2$O	RDE	CSV	1.575	0.2 ± 0.2
Determination of Brightener << copper gleam™ 2001 Additive >> in acid copper bath (Rohm and Haas electronic material)	Acid copper electro-plating bath	Brightener	Virgin makeup solution	Pt 6.0343	Ag/AgCl/3M KCl KNO$_3$ saturated H$_2$O	RDE	CSV	1.575	0.2 ± 0.2
Determination of Suppressor <<<Cupracid BL–CT >> in acid copper bath (Atotech)	Acid copper electro-plating bath	Suppressor	Virgin makeup solution	Pt 6.0343	Ag/AgCl/3M KCl KNO$_3$ saturated H$_2$O	RDE	CSV	1.575	0.2 ± 0.2
Determination of Brightener <<<Cupracid BL >> in acid copper baths (Atotech)	Acid copper electro-plating bath	Brightener	Virgin makeup solution	Pt 6.0343	Ag/AgCl/3M KCl KNO$_3$ saturated H$_2$O	RDE	CSV	1.575	0.2 ± 0.2
Determination of Suppressor <<Cupraspeed>> in acid copper bath (Atotech)	Acid copper electro-plating bath	Suppressor	Virgin makeup solution	Pt 6.0343	Ag/AgCl/3M KCl KNO$_3$ saturated H$_2$O	RDE	CSV	1.575	0.2 ± 0.2

Continued

Chapter 10

VOLTAMMETRY/POLAROGRAPHY TRACE METAL ANALYZER AND ITS APPLICATIONS

Continued

Application	Samples	Elements	Electrolytes	Auxiliary electrode	Reference electrode	Working electrode [multimode electrode (MME)]	Striping method (pulse amplitude)	Scan range (mV)	Peak potential (mV)
Determination of Brightener <<Cupraspeed>> in acid copper bath (Atotech)	Acid copper electro-plating bath	Brightener	Virgin makeup solution	Pt 6.0343	Ag/AgCl/3M KCl KNO$_3$ saturated H$_2$O	RDE	CSV	1.575	0.2 ± 0.2
Determination of thiourea in an acid copper bath containing chloride	Acid copper electro-plating bath	Thiourea	β(HgNO$_3$) C(HNO$_3$)	Pt 6.0343	Ag/AgCl/3M KCl KNO$_3$ saturated H$_2$O	DME	DPCSV	0.3 to 0.2	Thiourea = 0.24
Determination of total antimony in an acid copper bath	Acid Cu bath	Sb	W(HCl)	Pt 6.0343	Ag/AgCl/3M KCl KNO$_3$ saturated H$_2$O	HMDE	DPASV	-0.27 to -0.12	Sb = -0.2
Determination of Suppressor <<MACu Spec™ PPR 100 wetter>> in acid copper bath (MacDermid)	Acid-copper electro-plating bath	Suppressor	Virgin makeup solution	Pt 6.0343	Ag/AgCl/3M KCl H$_2$SO$_4$	RDE	CSV	1.575	0.25 ± 0.25
Determination of Brightener <<MACu Spec™ PPR 100 Brightener>> in acid copper baths (MacDermid)	Acid copper electro-plating bath	Brightener	Virgin makeup solution	Pt 6.0343	Ag/AgCl/3M KCl H$_2$SO$_4$	RDE	CSV	1.575	0.25 ± 0.25
Determination of Suppressor <<MultiBond™ 100 Part Azo>> in acid copper bath (MacDermid)	Acid copper electro-plating bath	Suppressor	Virgin make up solution	Pt 6.0343	Ag/AgCl/3M KCl KNO$_3$ saturated H$_2$O	RDE	CSV	1.575	0.2 + 0.2

Continued

Continued

Application	Samples	Elements	Electrolytes	Auxiliary electrode	Reference electrode	Working electrode [multimode electrode (MME)]	Striping method (pulse amplitude)	Scan range (mV)	Peak potential (mV)
Determination of Suppressor<<Ronasta-n TP additive>> in a tin-lead bath Ronasta-n TP (Rohm and Haas electronic material)	Tin-lead plating bath	Suppressor	Virgin makeup solution	Pt 6.0343	Ag/AgCl/3M KCl KNO$_3$ saturated: H$_2$O	RDE	CSV	0.475	−0.25 ± 0.1
Determination of Suppressor<<solderon ST-200 Primary>> in a tin bath	Sn plating bath	Suppressor	Virgin makeup solution	Pt 6.0343	Ag/AgCl/ 3M KCl Solderon acid HCl	RDE	CSV	0.475	0.2 ± 0.2
Determination of Suppressor<<In pulse H6>> in acid copper baths (Atotech)	Acid copper electro-plating bath	Suppressor	Virgin makeup solution	Pt 6.0343	Ag/AgCl/ 3M KCl KNO$_3$ saturated H$_2$O	RDE	CSV	1.575	0.2 ± 0.2
Determination of Brightener<<In pulse H6>> in acid copper baths (Atotech)	Acid copper electro-plating bath	Brightener	Virgin makeup solution	Pt 6.0343	Ag/AgCl/3M KCl KNO$_3$ saturated H$_2$O	RDE	CSV		
Determination of nickel in a sulfamate nickel plating bath	Sulphamate nickel bath	Ni	C(HCl) C(NH$_3$)	Pt 6.0343	Ag/AgCl/3M KCl C(KCl)	DME	DPASV	−0.7 to −1.1	Ni = −0.9
Determination of cobalt in a sulfamate nickel plating bath	Sulfamate nickel electro-plating bath	Co	C(HCl) C(NH$_3$)	Pt 6.0343	Ag/AgCl/3M KCl C(KCl)	HMDE	DPASV	−0.9 to −1.25	−1.15

Continued

Continued

Application	Samples	Elements	Electrolytes	Auxiliary electrode	Reference electrode	Working electrode (multimode electrode (MME))	Striping method (pulse amplitude)	Scan range (mV)	Peak potential (mV)
Determination of copper in a nickel plating bath	Ni electro-plating bath	CU	C(Na acetate) C(CH₃COOH)	Pt 6.0343	Ag/AgCl/3M KCl C(KCl)	DME	DPASV	0.05 to -0.2	-0.1
Determination of antimony (III) and total antimony in electroless nickel bath	Electroless Ni bath	Sb	C(HCl) = 0.6 mol/L	Pt 6.0343	Ag/AgCl/3M KCl C(KCl)	HMDE	DPASV	-0.3 to 0	-0.12
Determination of thallium in a cyanidic gold bath	Electroless cyanidic Au bath	Tl	None	Pt 6.0343	Ag/AgCl/3M KCl C(KCl)	HMDE	DPASV	-0.8 to -0.2	Ti = -0.45
Determination of gold(I) in a cyanide gold bath	Cyanidic Au bath	Au	C(KOH) C(EDTA)	Pt 6.0343	Ag/AgCl/3M KCl C(KCl)	DME	DPASV	-0.9 to -1.8	Au(I) = -1.5
Determination of Nitrilotriacetic acid (NTA) in a cyanidic gold bath	Cyanidic Au bath	NTA	β(ascorbic acid) β(Bi³⁺)	Pt 6.0343	Ag/AgCl/3M KCl C(KCl)	DME	DPCSV	0.1 to -0.4	NTA = -0.2
Determination of Suppressor <<Thrucup EVF-B>> in acid copper baths (Uyemura)	Acid copper electro-plating bath	Suppressor	Virgin makeup solution	Pt 6.0343	Ag/AgCl/3M KCl KNO₃ saturated H₂O	RDE	CSV	1.575	0.2 ± 0.2
Determination of Brightener<<Thrucup EVF-IA>> in acid copper baths (Uyemura)	Acid copper electro-plating bath	Brightener	Virgin makeup solution	Pt 6.0343	Ag/AgCl/3M KCl KNO₃ saturated H₂O	RDE	CSV	1.575	0.25 ± 0.2

Continued

VOLTAMMETRY/POLAROGRAPHY TRACE METAL ANALYZER AND ITS APPLICATIONS

Continued

Application	Samples	Elements	Electrolytes	Auxiliary electrode	Reference electrode	Working electrode [multimode electrode (MME)]	Striping method (pulse amplitude)	Scan range (mV)	Peak potential (mV)
Determination of Leveler<<Thru-cup EVF-R>> in acid copper baths (Uyemura)	Acid copper electro-plating bath	Leveler	Virgin makeup solution	Pt 6.0343	Ag/AgCl/3M KCl KNO$_3$ saturated H$_2$O	RDE	CSV	1.625	0.2 ± 0.3
Determination of indium in a tin bath	Acid Sn bath	Zn and Sn	W(HCl) C(Urotro-pin)	Pt 6.0343	Ag/AgCl/3M KCl C(KCl)	HMDE	DPASV	−0.68 to −0.53	−0.60
Determination of bismuth in a tin bath	Acid Sn bath	Bi	W(HCl) C(Urotro-pin)	Pt 6.0343	Ag/AgCl/3M KCl C(KCl)	HMDE	DPASV	−0.2 to −0.03	−0.1
Determination of palladium in an activator bath	Activator solution	Pd	C(NH$_4$Cl) C(NH$_3$) C(KCl)	Pt 6.0343	Ag/AgCl/3M KCl C(KCl)	DME	DPASV	−0.4 to −0.9	Pd = −0.71
Determination of copper in a cyanidic copper bath	Cyanidic Cu bath	Analysis of Cu	C(KCl) W(HCl)	Pt 6.0343	Ag/AgCl/3M KCl C(KCl)	DME	DPCSV	0 to −0.4	Cu = −0.17
Determination of total iron in deoxidation solution (oxalate method)	Deoxidation solution	Analysis of total Fe (total)	C(NH$_4$)$_2$C$_2$O$_4$	Pt 6.0343	Ag/AgCl/3M KCl C(KCl)	DME	DPCSV	0.2 to −0.3	Fe = 0.05
Determination of total iron in degreasing bath (triethanolamine bromated method)	Degreasing bath	Analysis of Fe(total)	C(NaOH) C(KBrO$_3$) C(Tea)	Pt 6.0343	Ag/AgCl/3M KCl C(KCl)	DME	DPCSV	−0.7 to −1.3	Fe = −1.0
Determination of titanium in a titanium pickle bath	Ti pickle bath	Analysis of Ti	C(Oxalic acid) C(H$_2$SO$_4$) C(KClO$_4$)	Pt 6.0343	Ag/AgCl/3M KCl C(KCl)	DME	DPASV	0.1 to −0.5	Ti = −0.22

Continued

VOLTAMMETRY/POLAROGRAPHY TRACE METAL ANALYZER AND ITS APPLICATIONS

Continued

Application	Samples	Elements	Electrolytes	Auxiliary electrode	Reference electrode	Working electrode [multimode electrode (MME)]	Striping method (pulse amplitude)	Scan range (mV)	Peak potential (mV)
Determination of Zinc in a phosphatation bath	Zinc phosphatation bath	Analysis of Zn	C(NH$_4$Cl) C(NH$_3$)	Pt 6.0343	Ag/AgCl/3M KCl C(KCl)	DME	DPASV	−1.05 to −1.4	Zn = −1.23
Determination of Nickel in a phophatation bath	Zinc phosphatation bath	Analysis of Ni	C(NH$_4$Cl) C(NH$_3$)	Pt 6.0343	Ag/AgCl/3M KCl C(KCl)	DME	DPASV	−0.8 to −1.15	Ni = −0.96
Determination of cadmium in a phosphatation bath	Zinc phosphatation bath	Analysis of Cd	W(HCl)	Pt 6.0343	Ag/AgCl/3M KCl C(KCl)	DME	DPASV	−0.48 to −0.7	Cd = −0.58
Determination of lead in a phosphatation bath	Zn phosphatation bath	Analysis of Pb	W(HCl)	Pt 6.0343	Ag/AgCl/3M KCl C(KCl)	HMDE	DPASV	−0.55 to −0.3	Pb = −0.43
Determination of lead in tin soldering contacts	Sn soldering contact	Analysis of Pb	C(Sodium citrate) C(Oxalic acid) C(HCl)	Pt 6.0343	Ag/AgCl/3M KCl C(KCl)	HMDE	DPASV	−0.53 to 0.25	Pb = −0.4
Determination of Selenium (IV) in zinc plant electrolyte	Zinc plant electrolyte (concentrated ZnSO$_4$ solution)	Analysis of Se(IV)	C(NH$_4$)$_2$SO$_4$) C(Na$_2$EDTA)	Pt 6.0343	Ag/AgCl/3M KCl C(KCl)	HMDE	DPASV	−0.4 to −0.95	Se = −0.73
Determination of tellurium (IV) in Zn plant electrolyte	Zinc plant electrolyte (concentrated ZnSO$_4$ solution)	Analysis of Te	C(NH$_4$)$_2$SO$_4$) C(Na$_2$EDTA)	Pt 6.0343	Ag/AgCl/3M KCl C(KCl)	HMDE	DPASV	−0.9 to −1.15	Te = −1.0
Determination of cobalt in zinc plant electrolyte with α-furildioxime as complexing agent	Neutral zinc sulfate solution	Analysis Co	C(NH$_4$Cl) C(NH$_3$)	Pt 6.0343	Ag/AgCl/3M KCl C(KCl)	HMDE	DPASV	−0.8 to −1.1	Co = −0.98

Continued

VOLTAMMETRY/POLAROGRAPHY TRACE METAL ANALYZER AND ITS APPLICATIONS

Continued

Application	Samples	Elements	Electrolytes	Auxiliary electrode	Reference electrode	Working electrode [multimode electrode (MME)]	Striping method (pulse amplitude)	Scan range (mV)	Peak potential (mV)
Determination of lead in zinc plant electrolyte	Neutral zinc sulfate solution	Analysis of Pb	W(HCl)	Pt 6.0343	Ag/AgCl/3M KCl C(KCl)	HMDE	DPASV	−0.6 to −0.2	Pb = −0.42
Determination of total arsenic in zinc plant electrolyte	Zinc plant electrolyte	Analysis of As	W(HCl)	Gc	Ag/AgCl/3M KCl C(KCl)	RDE	DPASV	−0.1 to 0.3	As = −0.13
Determination of antimony (III) in Zinc plant electrolyte with chloranilic acid as complexing agent	Zinc plant electrolyte	Analysis of Sb(III)	C(CAA)	Pt 6.0343	Ag/AgCl/3M KCl C(KCl)	HMDE	DPASV	−0.2 to −0.5	Sb(III) = −0.35
Determination of total selenium in tap water after reduction of selenium (VI) to selenium (IV) by means of 705 digester	Tap water	Analysis of Se	$(NH_4)_2SO_4$ solid	Pt 6.0343	Ag/AgCl/3M KCl C(KCl)	HMDE	DPASV	−0.45 to −0.85	Se = −0.72
Determination of total iron in a chromium bath	Cr(III/VI) electro-plating bath	Analysis of Fe (total)	C(NaOH)-0.3 mol/L	pt	Ag/AgCl/3M KCl	DME	DPASV	−0.7 to −1.3	Fe = −0.95
Determination of copper in seawater with the mercury film electrode	Seawater	Analysis of Cu	$C(CH_3COONH_4)$ −1 mol/L	Gc	Ag/AgCl/3M KCl	RDE	DPASV	−0.6 to −0.1	Cu = −0.28
Determination of iron in boiler feed water for power plants (DHN method)	Boiler feed water	Analysis of Fe (total)	C(HEPPS)-0.5 mol/L	pt	Ag/AgCl/3M KCl	HMDE	DPASV	−0.1 to −0.8	Fe = −0.55
Determination of nitrobenzene in aniline	Aniline	Analysis of nitro-benzene	$W(CH_3CH_2OH)$ −99.9%	pt	Ag/AgCl/3M KCl	DME	DPCSV	−0.25 to −0.7	−0.48
Determination of chromium in cement	Cement	Analysis of Cr(VI)	$C[(NH_4)_2C_4H_4O_6]$	pt	Ag/AgCl/3M KCl	HMDE	DPASV	0 to −0.4	Cr = −0.2

Continued

VOLTAMMETRY/POLAROGRAPHY TRACE METAL ANALYZER AND ITS APPLICATIONS

Continued

Application	Samples	Elements	Electrolytes	Auxiliary electrode	Reference electrode	Working electrode [multimode electrode (MME)]	Striping method (pulse amplitude)	Scan range (mV)	Peak potential (mV)
Determination of Suppressor in acid copper baths	Acid copper electro-plating bath	Analysis of suppressor	Virgin make up solution (VMS)	pt	Ag/AgCl/3M KCl	RDE	DPASV	1,625	0.2 ± 0.2
Determination of Brightener in acid baths	Acid copper electro-plating bath	Analysis of brightener	Virgin make up solution (VMS)	pt	Ag/AgCl/3M KCl	RDE	CSV	1,625	0.2 ± 0.2
Determination of leveler in acid copper baths by response Curve technique	Acid copper electro-plating bath	Analysis of leveler	Virgin makeup solution (VMS)	pt	Ag/AgCl/3M KCl	RDE	CSV	1,625	0.2 ± 0.2
Determination of Cadmium and lead in electronic components as part of electrochemical products	Electronic components	Analysis of Cd, Pb	Ammonium oxalate buffer pH2	pt	Ag/AgCl/3M KCl	HMDE	DPASV	−0.8 to −0.2	Cd = −0.6 Pb = −0.4
Determination of Chromium in electronic components as part of electrochemical products	Electronic components	Analysis of Cr	Ammonium buffer pH-9.6	pt	Ag/AgCl/3M KCl	DME	DPASV	−0.1 to 0.45	Cr = −0.25
Determination of Mercury in electronic components as part of electrochemical products	Electronic components	Analysis of Hg	Perchloric acid electolyte	Gc	Ag/AgCl/3M KCl	RDE	DPASV	+0.4 to +0.8	Hg = +0.64
Determination of Cadmium and lead in polymer materials as part of electro chemical products	Polymer materials	Analysis of Cd, Pb	Ammonium oxalate buffer pH-2	pt	Ag/AgCl/3M KCl	HMDE	DPASV	−0.8 to −0.2	Cd = −0.6 Pb = −0.4

Continued

Continued

Application	Samples	Elements	Electrolytes	Auxiliary electrode	Reference electrode	Working electrode [multimode electrode (MME)]	Striping method (pulse amplitude)	Scan range (mV)	Peak potential (mV)
Determination of Chromium (VI) in polymer materials as part of electro technical products	Polymer materials	Analysis of Cr(VI)	Ammonia buffer pH-9.6	pt	Ag/AgCl/3M KCl	DME	DPASV	−0.1 to −0.5	Cr = −0.25
Determination of Mercury in polymer materials as part of electrotechnical products	Polymer materials	Analysis of Hg	Perchloric acid electrolyte	Gc	Ag/AgCl/3M KCl	RDE	DPASV	+0.4 to +0.8	Hg = +0.64
Determination of Cadmium and lead in metallic materials as part of electrotechnical products	Metallic materials	Analysis Cd, Pb	Ammonium oxalate buffer pH2	pt	Ag/AgCl/3M KCl	HMDE	DPASV	−0.8 to −0.2	Cd = −0.6 Pb = −0.4
Determination of Chromium (VI) in chromate coating on metallic materials as part of electrotecnical products	Colorless and colored chromate coating on Metallic materials	Analysis of Cr(VI)	DTPA electrolyte	pt	Ag/AgCl/3M KCl	HMDE	DPASV	−1.0 to −1.5	Cr = −1.3
Determination of Mercury in metallic materials as part of electrotechnical products	Metallic materials	Analysis of Hg	Perchloric electrolyte	Gc	Ag/AgCl/3M KCl	RDE	DPASV	+0.4 to +0.8	Hg = +0.64

electrode material. We believe that each modern analytical laboratory can be equipped by voltammetric devices, which are of high quality, low cost, and the obtained results of analysis of environmental samples are fully comparable with those achieved using other techniques.

■ FURTHER READINGS

1. Al-Ghamdi AH, Al-Shadokhy MA, Al-Warthan AA. Electrochemical determination of cephalothin antibiotic by adsorptive stripping voltammetric technique. J Pharm Biomed Anal. 2004;35:1001-9.
2. Blaylock RL, Strunecka A. Immune-glutamatergic dysfunction as a central mechanism of the autism spectrum disorders. Curr Med Chem. 2009;16:157-70.
3. Delahay P. New Instrumental Methods in Electrochemistry. New York: Interscience Publishers Inc.; 1954.
4. Drago D, Cavaliere A, Mascetra N. Aluminum modulates effects of beta amyloid (1–42) on neuronal calcium homeostasis and mitochondria functioning and is altered in a triple transgenic mouse model of Alzheimer's disease. Rejuvenation Res. 2008;11(5):861-71.
5. Ferreira VS, Zanoni MVB, Fogg AG. Cathodic stripping voltammetric determination of ceftazidime with reactive accumulation at a poly-L-lysine modified hanging mercury drop electrode. Anal Chim Acta. 1999;384:159-66.
6. Filipe OMS, Brett CMA. Cathodic stripping voltammetry of trace Mn (II) at carbon film electrodes. Talanta. 2003;61:643-50.
7. Gusakova AM, Ivanovskaya EA. Determination of enalapril by stripping voltammetry at a mercury film electrode. J Anal Chem. 2005;60:436-8.
8. Fauci A, Braunwald E, Kasper D, Hauser S, Longo D, Jameson JL, et al. Harrison's Principles of Internal Medicine, 17th edition. New York: McGraw-Hill Companies Inc.; 2008.
9. Heyrovsky J, Zuman P. Practical Polarography: An Introduction for Chemistry Students. London: Academic Press; 1968.
10. Jiang HX, Chen LS, Zheng JG, Han S, Tang N, Smith BR. Aluminum-induced effects on Photosystem II photochemistry in citrus leaves assessed by the chlorophyll a fluorescence transient. Tree Physiol. 2008;28:1863-71.
11. Palacios FJJ, Machón MC, Sánchez JCJ, Carranza JH. Adsorptive stripping voltammetric determination of cefepime at the mercury electrode in human urine and cerebrospinal fluid, and differential pulse polarographic determination in serum. J Pharm Sci. 2003;92:1854-59.
12. Kissenger PT, Heineman WR. Laboratory Techniques in Electroanalytical Chemistry, 2nd edition. New York: Marcel Dekker; 1996.
13. Meites L. Polarographic Techniques, 2nd edition. New York: Interscience Publishers; 1967.
14. Merrill JC, Morton JJP, Soileau SD. Principles and Methods of Toxicology, 5th edition. United States: CRC Press; 2007.
15. Morrison GH. Trace Analysis: Physical methods, 1st edition. New York: John Wiley and Sons Inc.; 1965.

16. Ozkan SA, Uslu B, Aboul-Enein HY. Analysis of pharmaceuticals and biological fluids using modern electroanalytical techniques. Crit Rev Anal Chem. 2003;33:155-81.
17. Petersen SL, Tallman DE. Silver Composite Electrode for Voltammetry. Anal Chem. 1988;60:82-6.
18. Pravda M, Vytras K. Application of stripping voltammetry to trace lead analysis in intermediates and final products of syntheses of pharmaceuticals. J Pharm Biomed Anal. 1996;14:765-71.
19. Sabry SM. Adsorptive stripping voltammetric assay of phenazopyridine hydrochloride in biological fluids and pharmaceutical preparations. Talanta. 1999;50:133-40.

Chapter 11

Microwave Digestion System and its Applications

■ INTRODUCTION

For analysis of different elements in any material such as solid, liquid, etc., the first step is to bring the element in solution form which is achieved by acid digestion procedure. The goal of every digestion process is, therefore, the complete decomposition of the solid by avoiding loss or contamination of the analyte. The basic aims of microwave digestion are to:
- Convert the element in solution form
- Complete decomposition of the matrix
- Avoid losses and any contamination
- Reduce handling and processing time

Digestion is carried out by open acid digestion or closed digestion. There are numerous advantages of the closed procedure to open digestion such as low acid consumption, less time, good digestion quality, no loss of volatile element, and no contamination risk. Basic requirements for decomposition/digestion are:

1. Exclusion of systematic errors by preventing contamination, which can be prevented either by using pure acids or sub-boiling analytical reagent quality acids to purify them. Contamination by the vessels can be prevented by cleaning, digestion, or evaporation equipment
2. Exclusion of systematic errors by preventing contamination by the loss of analytes
3. Exclusion of systematic errors by preventing contamination by the adsorption of analytes on the vessel surface. It is prevented by using highly pure materials, which are chemically and thermally resistant, e.g., perfluoroalkoxy (PFA), polytetrafluoroethylene (PTFE), and quartz glass
4. Removal of distorting matrices and prevention of matrix extension, e.g., from the decomposition acids used
5. Simple operation with minimum required time, work, and instrument operation

All these requirements are fulfilled by microwave digestion/decomposition.

MICROWAVE DIGESTION SYSTEM AND ITS APPLICATIONS

■ PRINCIPLES OF MICROWAVE TECHNOLOGY

1. All electromagnetic waves are sky waves, which propagate at the speed of light and transport energy without loss in a vacuum and with loss in dielectric material
2. They show the same effects as light such as interference, diffraction, refraction, reflection, and polarizability
3. Microwaves are high-frequency electromagnetic waves in the same frequency band as radar waves
4. Only four microwave frequencies are permitted for industrial and scientific use. Out of these, 2.45 GHz is the most frequently used

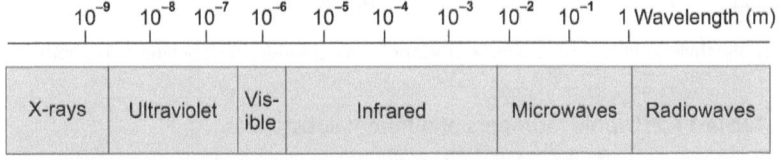

■ CHARACTERISTICS OF MICROWAVES

1. Microwaves are reflected by nonpolar materials
2. Microwaves pass through ceramic, glass, and porcelain
3. Microwaves are absorbed by food, human tissue, and polar materials
4. Microwave radiation is not an ionizing radiation and is, therefore, not hazardous for human tissue
5. Low microwave frequencies can be produced using electron tubes or transistors
6. High and very high frequencies of >100 MHz are produced by klystrons, magnetrons, or traveling wave tubes
7. In decomposition instruments, microwaves are produced using magnetrons.

■ MATERIAL BEHAVIOR OF MICROWAVE

1. The capacity of a substance to absorb microwave energy is represented by its dielectric loss factor tan δ, which is ratio of dielectric loss (ε') and' the permittivity or dielectric constant (ε'). The tan δ value of some common materials is given in **Table 11.1**

$$\tan \delta = \varepsilon'/\varepsilon'$$

2. The lower the loss factor, the lower the absorption capacity of the substance
3. Materials with a low absorption capacity can be used as neutral components, e.g., as vessel material
4. Some substances, e.g., water, have a relatively high loss factor at room temperature, but this decreases once a certain temperature has been attained

Table 11.1: Tan δ values for different materials.

Materials	Tan δ
Quartz	0.6
Borosilicate	10.6
PTFE and PFA	1.5
PE	3.1
PVC	55.0
Ceramic	5.5
Water	1570.0

(PE: polyethylene; PFA: perfluoroalkoxy; PVC: polyvinyl chloride; PTFE: polytetrafluoroethylene)

Table 11.2: Dipole moments of different substances.

Substances	Dipole moments (Debye)
Sulfuric acid (H_2SO_4)	2.964
Hydrofluoric acid (HF)	1.820
Nitric acid (HNO_3)	2.170
Hydrochloric acid (HCl)	1.030
Water (H_2O)	1.844
Ammonia (NH_3)	1.460
Carbon tetrachloride (CCl_4)	0.000
Hydrogen peroxide (H_2O_2)	2.260
Methyl chloride (CH_3Cl)	1.870

5. The dielectric loss factor is dependent on the substance, frequency, and temperature
6. To heat a substance, the material must couple to the microwaves. In other words, the substance must absorb electromagnetic energy
7. The two mechanisms for microwave are dipole rotation and ionic conductance
8. *Dipole rotation*: In a rapidly changing electric field, the molecules try to orient themselves in the direction of the field lines. This sets them in rotational vibration. The energy absorption from the microwave field is more intensive; the closer the resonance frequency of the molecule is to the frequency of the microwave. This is the case with materials, which have a pronounced dipole, e.g., water, acids, and solvents. Dipole moments of different substances are given in **Table 11.2**
9. *Ionic conductance*: Heating in the electromagnetic field also occurs when there are free ions, e.g., electrolytes, glassy materials, and ceramic materials

10. Both mechanisms, dipole rotation and ionic conductance, are influenced by various factors such as wavelength, physical properties of the solution such as permittivity dielectric constant, polarity, temperature, viscosity, thermal capacity, and ion characteristics or ionic conductor such as size, concentration, charge, and mobility.

■ ADVANTAGES OF MICROWAVE TECHNOLOGY OVER THERMAL CONVECTION

When heating material uses thermal convection, the heating occurs from the outside in. Microwave energy heats the material from the inside out. The dielectric dissipation is independent of the heat flow on the surface of the material. Major benefits are:
1. It reduces time
2. It minimizes the energy
3. When the microwave radiation is switched off, the source of heat is immediately removed from the object

Comparison of conventional method and microwave method is given in **Figures 11.1A** and **B**.

■ MICROWAVE DECOMPOSITION/DIGESTION

Microwave digestion is widely used technique for the digestion of samples for metal analysis using graphite furnace atomic absorption (GFAA), inductively coupled plasma-optical emission spectrometry (ICP-OES), inductively coupled plasma-mass spectrometry (ICP-MS), etc. Since, it operates at far higher temperature and pressure than the open digestion, it can be applied to a much wider range of samples, producing a clear digested sample from even the most refractory sample type.
1. Decomposition is the conversion of a solid sample into a homogeneous liquid

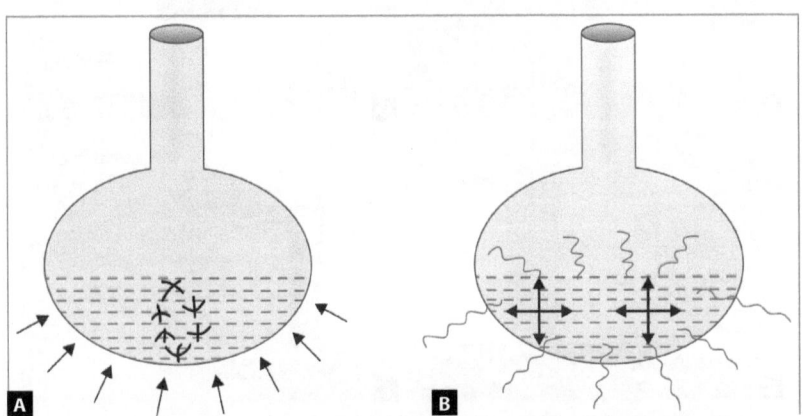

Figs. 11.1A and B: Heating a vessel. (A) Conventional method and (B) Microwave method.

MICROWAVE DIGESTION SYSTEM AND ITS APPLICATIONS

2. Digestion makes the sample easier to aliquot and has all the requirements for an interference-free qualitative and quantitative determination of the elements
3. After mechanical sample preparation, decomposition is the most time-consuming step in wet chemical procedures. It is, therefore, very useful to optimize this step and reduces the required time, while retaining or increasing the quality of the analysis

■ INSTRUMENTATION

Microwave digester is manufactured by many companies such as Aurora instruments, Lab X, Evisa, Sineo, Milestone, etc. (**Figs. 11.2A to F**). Each instrument has magnetron of different capacity and vessels of different size and volume. Solvents used for the digestion are same for all. Few important points about magnetron, vessels, and reagents are described below.

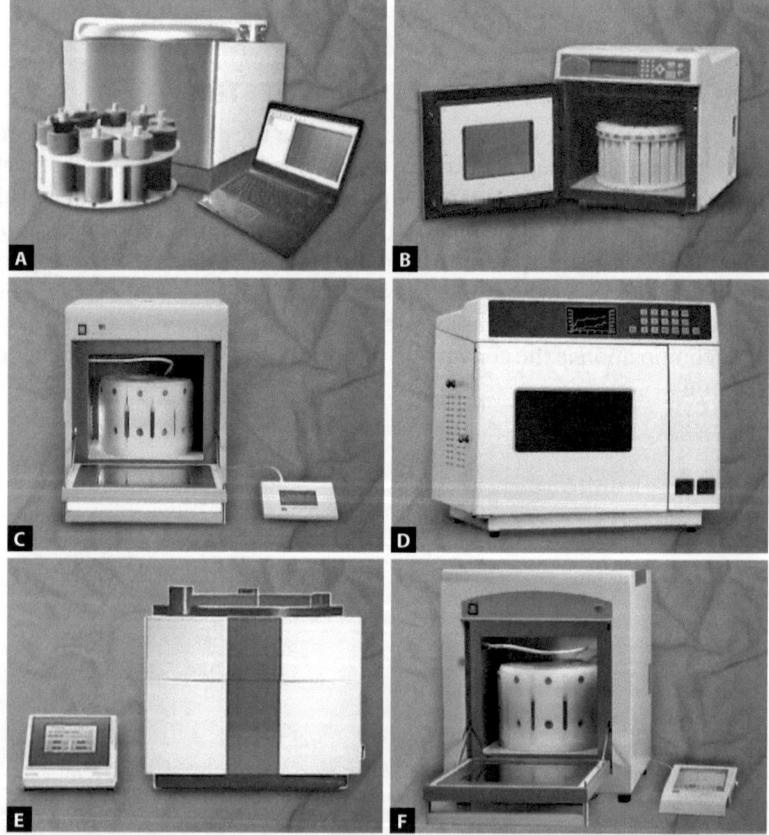

Figs. 11.2A to F: Microwave digesters from various manufacturers. (A) Aurora; (B) Lab X; (C) Evisa; (D) Sineo; (E) Analytik Jena; and (F) Milestone.

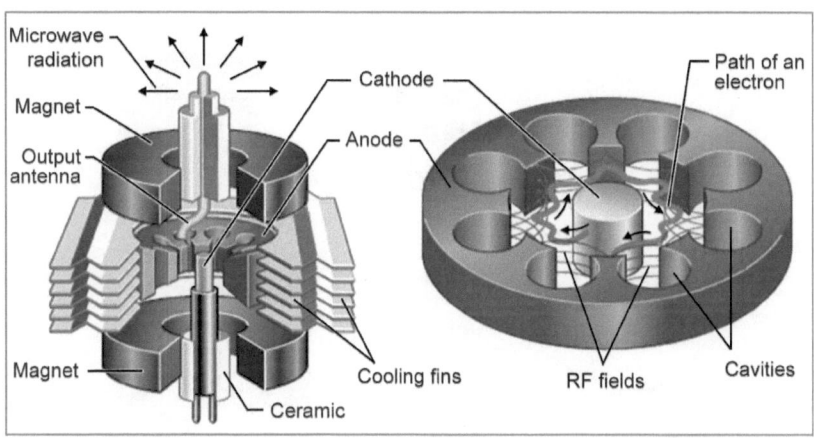

(RF: radiofrequency)

Fig. 11.3: Pictorial representation of magnetron from Encyclopedia Britannica, Inc.

Magnetron

It is the high voltage system which is the heart of the microwave digester and its purpose is to generate microwave energy. The high voltage components accomplish this by stepping up AC line voltage to high voltage, which is then changed to an even higher DC voltage. The pictorial representation of the magnetron is shown in **Figure 11.3**.

- A magnetron is a metallic vacuum tube, consisting of a cathode and an anode, which is surrounded by a permanent magnet frame
- A high voltage is applied to a heated rod (cathode) to emit electrons. These electrons are drawn into a circular path by the applied magnetic field
- These electrons hit the outer wall of the tube (anode), which is cut at regular intervals radially to the chamber (resonator)
- Within these incisions, the polarity of the electrical field reverses with the desired frequency and produces microwaves. These are emitted via an antenna, e.g., in the microwave oven

Vessels

Naturally, the employed vessels must be resistant to the acids and reagents being used. Glass, except for solution containing hydrofluoric acid (HF), polypropylene (PP), and polyethylene (PE), is all suitable for vessel in which digestion solutions are to be stored. Commonly used vessels are given in **Figure 11.4**.

Polytetrafluoroethylene -$[CF_2-CF_2]_n$-

It is perforated plastic with melting temperature of approximately 330°C; hence, it can be used at temperature up to +260°C. It is nearly universal chemical resistant and has high purity.

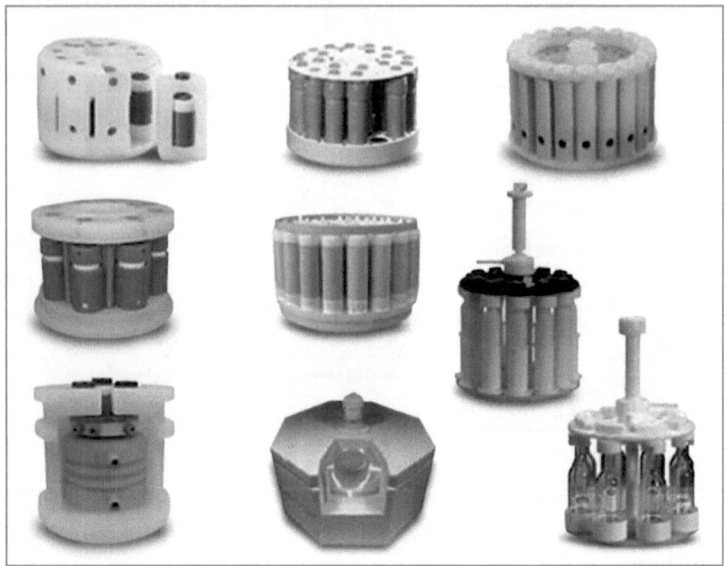

Fig. 11.4: Different types of vessels used for digestion from different manufacturers.

Thin-film Membrane-polytetrafluoroethylene

It is perforated plastic with PFA side chain (<1% by weight) with melting temperature approximately 330°C. It can be used at temperature up to +260°C. It is also nearly universal chemical resistant and has high purity. It has improved surface structure compound as compared to PTFE.

Perfluoroalkoxy -$[(CF2)_4$-$CF(-O-CF_2-CF_2-CF_3)$-$(CF_2)_5]_n$-

It is perforated plastic with PFA side chain (4–10% by weight) with melting temperature approximately 290°C. It can be used at temperature up to 220°C. It is nearly universal chemical resistant and has high purity. It has improved surface structure compared to PTFE. It is less resistant than PTFE and TFM-PTFE.

Quartz

Its melting temperature is approximately 1,100°C and can be used at temperature up to +300°C for digestion. It is attacked by HF and has high purity.

Reagents

Commonly used reagents are nitric acid (HNO_3), hydrogen peroxide (H_2O_2), hydrochloric acid (HCl), nitrohydrochloric acid, HF, and sulfuric acid (H_2SO_4). Acid digestion, whether open or closed pressure digestion, is carried out with the aid of a wide variety of reagents. Aside from the various mineral acids, other reagents, such as H_2O_2, potassium peroxide sulfate, boric acid, and many more, are also used. The selection of the reagents or the preparation of a reagent mixture depends on the sample to be digested. Organic sample materials are generally decomposed into carbon dioxide with the help of oxidizing acid, such as HNO_3 and H_2O_2. Some acids with their properties are given below.

Nitric Acid

It is frequently mixed with H_2O_2 or HCl, HF, and H_2SO_4. Boiling point of HNO_3 is 122°C (HNO_3 65%) and vapor pressure is ~25 bar (at ~225°C). It forms soluble nitrates with all elements, except Au, Pt, Al, B, Cr, Ti, and Zr. It is oxidizing acid.

$$(CH_2)n + 2HNO_3 \rightarrow CO_2 + 2NO + 2H_2O$$

Nitric Acid/Hydrogen Peroxide

It reoxidizes NO_2 into NO_3 and thus suppresses the formation of the yellow nitrous oxides typical of HNO_3. Typical HNO_3/H_2O_2 is used in 4:1 ratio. It has increased oxidation potential.

$$2H_2O_2 \rightarrow 2H_2O + O_2$$

Hydrochloric Acid

It is nonoxidizing acid with boiling point 84°C (HCl 32%) and vapor pressure ~25 bar (at ~205°C). It forms soluble chlorides with all elements, except Ag, Hg, and Ti. It dissolves the salts of weaker acids (carbonates, phosphates, borates, and iron alloys).

Nitrohydrochloric Acid

It has vapor pressure of ~25 bar (at ~200°C). It aids digestion of precious metal, sulfides. It is freshly prepared when required in the ratio 3:1. It forms nitrosyl chloride (NOCl) and releases chlorine as the active component.

$$2NOCl \rightarrow 2NO + Cl_2$$

Hydrofluoric Acid

It is nonoxidizing acid. It is used in excess otherwise, it leads to loss of BF_3, SiF_4, GeF_4, and SeF_4. It has a boiling point of 108°C (HF 40%) and its vapor pressure is ~25 bar (at ~240°C). It is usually employed in a mixture with other acids. It helps in digestion of minerals, ores, soil, stone, plants, and silicates.

$$H_3BO_3 + 4HF \rightarrow HBF_4 + 3H_2O$$
$$SiO_2 + 6HF \rightarrow H_2SiF_6 + 2H_2O$$

Sulfuric Acid

It is nonoxidizing acid. It helps in dehydration of organic materials, particularly plastics. Its boiling point is 340°C (H_2SO_4 98%). Vapor pressure is negligible. It is usually employed in a mixture with other acids. It helps in digestion of plastics, ores, and minerals. It forms insoluble sulfates with Ba, Pb, and Sr.

■ DO'S AND DON'TS FOR HANDLING MICROWAVE DIGESTOR

Do's

1. Allow the vessel temperature to come down before they can be opened. Once the temperature is observed to drop to 60°C, vessels are safe to handle
2. Clean vessel liner by 1:1 HNO_3 solution
3. Rinse with distilled water and dry well all vessel components after removal of the sample
4. Rinse the sensor vessel's thermocouple probe carefully with distilled water and leave it to dry. Care should be taken not to let water enter the sensor except on the probe
5. Any residual sample in the temperature probe or inside the vessel may bring the starting temperature/pressure up and may also result in cross-contamination of the new sample and affect the results of subsequent digestion
6. Check the ruptured disks and pressure transducer ring before starting with new digestion

Don'ts

1. Never run the sensor vessel without at least 10-15 mL volume of sample and reagent inside the vessel. Running the sensor vessel with <10-15 mL may damage the sensor vessel
2. Never heat an empty vessel, i.e., without the material
3. All vessels should be filled either with water or appropriate sample with similar volume
4. Never use >1 rupture disk in a vessel. Using >1 disk per vessel will defeat its purpose and may cause damage or failure to the vessel
5. To ensure operator safety, the rupture disk and pressure transducer ring should be checked and replaced, if needed before each run
6. Never use concentrated form of H_2SO_4 and perchloric acid because of high heat capacity and boiling point
7. It is recommended that volume in excess should not be used in the digestion vessels. The vessels should have at least 20 mL of headspace above the liquid level to avoid overpressurization

■ TECHNICAL SPECIFICATIONS FOR MICROWAVE DIGESTOR

1. Computer controlled closed vessel microwave digestion system with high pressure capabilities
2. *Number of vessels*: Five or more
3. *Operating pressure*: 400 psi and above
4. *Operating temperature*: 250°C or more

5. *Vessel volume*: Approximately 60 mL
6. *Electrical*: 220 V, 50/60 Hz, and 10 A
7. *Microwave power*: 1,200 W or more
8. *Magnetron frequency*: 2,450 Mz
9. *Weight*: Approximately 27 kg
10. Necessary accessories may be coated

Names of some manufacturers with their address, telephone number, and website are given below:

1. *Aurora Biomed*: 1001 East Pender Street Vancouver, BC, Canada, V6A 1W2. Tel: 1.604.215.8700. Fax: 1.604.215.9700. Email: info@aurorabiomed.com
2. *Milestone*: Fatebenefratelli, 1/5, 24010 Sorisole (BG) Italy. Phone: +39 035 573857. Fax: +39 035 575498/4128028. Web: www.milestonesrl.com
3. *Anton Paar USA Inc.*: 10215 Timber Ridge Drive, Ashland, VA 23005, United States. Toll Free: 800 722 7556. Fax: 804 550 1057. Email: info.us@anton-paar.com
4. *Lab X*: P.O. Box 216, 478 Bay Street, Midland, ON, Canada, L4R 1K9. Fax: 705-528-0270. Email: help@labx.com
5. *Global Spec*: Corporate Headquarters, 30 Tech Valley Dr Suite 102 East Greenbush, New York 12061. Phone: 5188800200. Fax: 5188800250
6. *Berghof Products*: Harretstr. 1, 72800 Eningen, Germany. Phone: 49 7121 894-202. Fax: 49 7121 894-300
7. *Sineo Microwave Chemistry Technology (China) Co., Ltd.*: Address: 3F, South Building, 227 Guan Sheng Yuan Road, Cao He Jing Hi-Tech Zone, Shanghai, China (200235). Tel: +86-21-54487840, 54487841. Direct Line: +86-21-64700006. Email: marketing@sineo.cn
8. *CEM*: 201, Nand Chambers, LBS Marg, Near Vandana Cinema, Thane-400 602, India. Fax: 91-22-25410420. Email: http://www.labindia.com, sales.mfd@labindia.com

■ COMPARISON OF OPEN AND CLOSED DECOMPOSITION/DIGESTION

Closed decomposition has revealed advantages over open digestion such as less acid consumption, less time taking, good digestion quality, no loss of volatile material, etc. Brief comparison between open and closed digestion/decomposition is given in **Table 11.3**.

■ BASIC PROCEDURE FOR SAMPLE DIGESTION IN THE MICROWAVE DIGESTOR

Digestion of sample in microwave is very easy and various steps in this process are:

Step 1: Vessels are cleaned with HNO_3 water mixture (1:1) followed by water and dried

Table 11.3: Comparison of the open and closed digestors.

Properties	Open decomposition	Closed decomposition
General	1. Samples and reagents are heated on a hot plate or in a sand bath, etc. 2. The sample and reagents are heated in open vessels made of glass, quartz, glassy carbon, or PTFE 3. The gas vapors, which are produced, are either extracted or caught by a reflux condenser and returned to the reaction mixture 4. Maximum temperature is limited by the solution's boiling point 5. It is employed in homogeneous samples 6. Sample amount is approximately 0.5–10 g 7. Acid used is approximately 10–100 mL 8. Decomposition time is approximately 2–10 hours 9. There is loss of volatile elements, e.g., Hg, Pb, and As 10. There is contamination risk	1. The pressure vessels can be heated conventionally 2. Sample and reagents are heated in closed pressure vessels made of fluoroplastics, such as PFA, PTFE, PTFE-TFM, or quartz 3. The reaction is controlled via temperature and pressure sensors 4. Maximum temperature is up to 300°C 5. It is employed for any type of sample 6. Sample amount is approximately 0.1–1 g 7. Acid used is approximately 2–15 mL 8. Decomposition time is approximately 0.5–2 hours 9. There is no loss of volatile material 10. There is no contamination risk
Use	1. Easy to dissolve limited samples 2. High analyte concentration	1. Easy to dissolve all samples 2. Matrices which are difficult to dissolve
Benefits	1. Simple and reasonably priced equipment 2. It is easy to use 3. Very good for homogeneous samples	1. High temperatures up to 350°C depending on the instrument and vessel 2. High pressures up to 400 bar depending on the instrument and vessel. 3. Complete decomposition results due to the high temperatures and pressures 4. Only HNO_3 is sufficient for organic samples 5. H_2SO_4 or $HClO_4$ is not required 6. Short reaction time 7. It does not lead to corrosive air in the laboratory

Continued

Continued

Disadvantages	1. Maximum temperature is limited to the boiling point of the reagent mixture 2. Poor decomposition quality 3. Long decomposition time 4. There is loss of volatile elements 5. It leads to corrosive air in the laboratory 6. Use of H_2SO_4 or $HClO_4$ is required to increase the decomposition rate	1. Higher purchase cost 2. Limited sample weight 3. Higher weights produce larger amounts of reaction gases which remain in the vessels and lead to pressure which must be controlled
Pictorial diagram	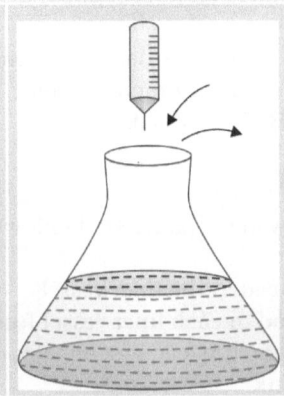	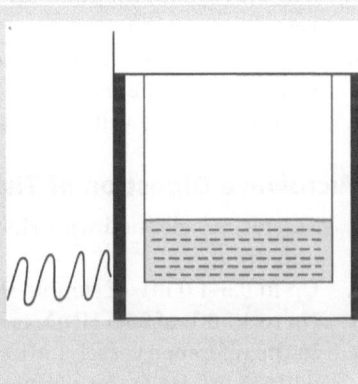

($HClO_4$: perchloric acid; HNO_3: nitric oxide; H_2SO_4: sulfuric acid; PFA: perfluoroalkoxy; PTFE: polytetrafluoroethylene)

Step 2: The weighed sample is taken into the liner vessel

Step 3: 15 mL HNO_3 (concentration depending on the sample) is added to each vessel inside the fume hood to allow the sample to outgas and then the vessels are sealed

Step 4: In the reference vessel, 1 mL of water (instead of sample) is added along with 15 mL HNO_3 for sample blank

Step 5: Vessel carrousels are loaded in the microwave digestion oven and the microwave is run with various programs specific for different substances

Step 6: After digestion, the samples are allowed to cool down and then each vessel is opened in the fume hood

Step 7: Digested sample is transferred to suitable volumetric flask and then the volume is made up to the mark with the help of ultrapure water

FORENSIC APPLICATIONS OF MICROWAVE DIGESTOR

Microwave Digestion of Blood

1. Vessels are cleaned with HNO_3 water mixture (1:1) followed by water and dried
2. Up to 1.0 mL of blood sample is placed in the liner vessel
3. Up to 15 mL of 35% HNO_3 is added in each liner vessel fume hood
4. In the reference vessel, 1 mL of water (instead of sample) is added along with 15 mL HNO_3 for sample blank
5. Vessel carrousels are loaded in the microwave digestion oven and the microwave is run with the program given in **Table 11.4**.
6. After digestion, the samples are allowed to cool down and then each vessel is opened in the fume hood
7. Digested sample is transferred to volumetric flask and then the volume is made up to the mark with the help of ultrapure water
8. If sample is pale yellow, 1–2 mL H_2O_2 is added.

Microwave Digestion of Tissue

1. Vessels are cleaned with HNO_3 water mixture (1:1) followed by water and dried
2. Up to 0.5–1.0 mL of sample is placed in the liner vessel
3. Up to 15 mL of 35% HNO_3 is added in each liner vessel fume hood
4. In the reference vessel, 1 mL of water (instead of sample) is added along with 15 mL HNO_3 for sample blank
5. Vessel carrousels are loaded in the microwave digestion oven and the microwave is run with the program given in **Table 11.5**.
6. After digestion, the samples are allowed to cool down and then each vessel is opened in the fume hood
7. Digested sample is transferred to volumetric flask and then the volume is made up to the mark with the help of ultrapure water.

Table 11.4: Program for microwave digestion of blood.

Step	Time (seconds)	Starting temperature (°C)	Ending temperature (°C)
1	210	28	100
2	600	100	160
3	600	160	170

Table 11.5: Program for microwave digestion of tissue.

Step	Time (seconds)	Starting temperature (°C)	Ending temperature (°C)
1	210	28	120
2	600	120	180
3	600	180	200

Table 11.6: Program for microwave digestion of nails/hair.

Step	Time (seconds)	Starting temperature (°C)	Ending temperature (°C)
1	300	28	100
2	700	100	160
3	700	160	170

Table 11.7: Program for microwave digestion of urine.

Step	Time (seconds)	Starting temperature (°C)	Ending temperature (°C)
1	200	28	100
2	400	100	160
3	400	160	170

Microwave Digestion of Nails/Hair

1. Vessels are cleaned with HNO_3 water mixture (1:1) followed by water and dried
2. Up to 0.10-1.00 g sample of hair/nail is placed in the liner vessel
3. 15 mL of HNO_3 is added in each liner vessel fume hood
4. In the reference vessel, 1 mL of water (instead of sample) is added along with 15 mL HNO_3 for sample blank
5. Vessel carrousels are loaded in the microwave digestion oven and the microwave is run with the program given in **Table 11.6**
6. After digestion, the samples are allowed to cool down and then each vessel is opened in the fume hood
7. Digested sample is transferred to volumetric flask and then the volume is made up to the mark with the help of ultrapure water

Microwave Digestion of Urine

1. Vessels are cleaned with HNO_3 water mixture (1:1) followed by water and dried
2. Up to 5-10 mL of urine sample is placed in the liner vessel
3. Up to 15 mL of 35% HNO_3 is added in each liner vessel fume hood
4. In the reference vessel, 1 mL of water (instead of sample) is added along with 15 mL HNO_3 for sample blank
5. Vessel carrousels are loaded in the microwave digestion oven and the microwave is run with the program given in **Table 11.7**
6. After digestion, the samples are allowed to cool down and then each vessel is opened in the fume hood
7. Digested sample is transferred to volumetric flask and then the volume is made up to the mark with the help of ultrapure water

Microwave Digestion of Leaves (Dried), e.g., Tea, Mint

1. Vessels are cleaned with HNO_3 water mixture (1:1) followed by water and dried

Table 11.8: Program for microwave digestion of dried leaves.

Step	Time (seconds)	Starting temperature (°C)	Ending temperature (°C)
1	250	28	100
2	310	100	160
3	410	160	170

Table 11.9: Program for microwave digestion of milk powder

Step	Time (seconds)	Starting temperature (°C)	Ending temperature (°C)
1	300	28	100
2	350	100	160
3	400	160	170

2. Up to 0.2 g of leaves is placed in the liner vessel
3. Up to 15 mL of 50% HNO_3 is added in each liner vessel fume hood
4. In the reference vessel, 1 mL of water (instead of sample) is added along with 15 mL HNO_3 for sample blank
5. Vessel carrousels are loaded in the microwave digestion oven and the microwave is run with the program given in **Table 11.8**
6. After digestion, the samples are allowed to cool down and then each vessel is opened in the fume hood
7. Digested sample is transferred to volumetric flask and then the volume is made up to the mark with the help of ultrapure water

Microwave Digestion of Milk Powder

1. Vessels are cleaned with HNO_3 water mixture (1:1) followed by water and dried
2. Up to 1.0 g of milk powder is placed in the liner vessel
3. Up to 15 mL of 50% HNO_3 is added in each liner vessel fume hood
4. In the reference vessel, 1 mL of water (instead of sample) is added along with 15 mL HNO_3 for sample blank
5. Vessel carrousels are loaded in the microwave digestion oven and the microwave is run with the program given in **Table 11.9**.
6. After digestion, the samples are allowed to cool down and then each vessel is opened in the fume hood
7. Digested sample is transferred to volumetric flask and then the volume is made up to the mark with the help of ultrapure water

Microwave Digestion of Fertilizer

1. Vessels are cleaned with HNO_3 water mixture (1:1) followed by water and dried
2. Up to 0.5 g of fertilizer is placed in liner vessel
3. Up to 15 mL of 50% HNO_3 is added in each liner vessel fume hood

Table 11.10: Program for microwave digestion of fertilizer.

Step	Time (seconds)	Starting temperature (°C)	Ending temperature (°C)
1	300	28	100
2	350	100	160
3	450	160	170

Table 11.11: Program for microwave digestion of soil

Step	Time (seconds)	Starting temperature (°C)	Ending temperature (°C)
1	300	28	100
2	350	100	160
3	400	160	170

4. In the reference vessel, 1 mL of water (instead of sample) is added along with 15 mL HNO_3 for sample blank
5. Vessel carrousels are loaded in the microwave digestion oven and the microwave is run with the program given in **Table 11.10**
6. After digestion, the samples are allowed to cool down and then each vessel is opened in the fume hood
7. Digested sample is transferred to volumetric flask and then the volume is made up to the mark with the help of ultrapure water

Microwave Digestion of Soil

1. Vessels are cleaned with HNO_3 water mixture (1:1) followed by water and dried
2. Up to 0.50–1.00 g of soil is placed in the liner vessel
3. Up to 15 mL of 50% HNO_3 is added in each liner vessel fume hood
4. In the reference vessel, 1 mL of water (instead of sample) is added along with 15 mL HNO_3 for sample blank
5. Vessel carrousels are loaded in the microwave digestion oven and the microwave is run with the program given in **Table 11.11**
6. After digestion, the samples are allowed to cool down and then each vessel is opened in the fume hood
7. Digested sample is transferred to volumetric flask and then the volume is made up to the mark with the help of ultrapure water.

Microwave Digestion of Sauce/Jam

1. Vessels are cleaned with HNO_3 water mixture (1:1) followed by water and dried
2. Up to 1.0 g of sauce/jam is placed in the liner vessel
3. Up to 15 mL of 50% HNO_3 is added in each liner vessel fume hood
4. In the reference vessel, 1 mL of water (instead of sample) is added along with 15 mL 50% HNO_3 for sample blank

Table 11.12: Program for microwave digestion of sauce/jam.

Step	Time (seconds)	Starting temperature (°C)	Ending temperature (°C)
1	310	28	100
2	320	100	160
3	400	160	170

5. Vessel carrousels are loaded in the microwave digestion oven and the microwave is run with the program given in **Table 11.12**.
6. After digestion, the samples are allowed to cool down and then each vessel is opened in the fume hood
7. Digested sample is transferred to volumetric flask and then the volume is made up to the mark with the help of ultrapure water

CONCLUSION

If there is no confidence in initial sample preparation stage, then there can be no confidence in the results from subsequent analyses. Complete and proper digestion is therefore essential for achieving accurate and precise results in metal analysis. Microwave digestion is a very common technique used by scientists/chemist/toxicologist to dissolve heavy metals in the presence of organic molecules prior to analysis using common analytical techniques such as AAS, ICP-OES, ICP-MS, TMA, etc. Microwave digestion method in a closed vessel has been developed for the simultaneous determination of trace and major elements, with the highest recoveries.

FURTHER READINGS

1. Abu-Samra A, Morris JS, Koirtyohann SR. Wet ashing of some biological samples in a microwave oven. Anal Chem. 1975;47:1475-7.
2. Agazzi A, Pirola C. Fundamentals, methods and future trends of environmental microwave sample preparation. Microchem J. 2000;67:337-41.
3. Agazzi A, Pirola. Fundamentals, methods and future trends of environmental microwave sample preparation. Anal Chem. 2001;73:4711-6.
4. Chakraborty R, Das AK, Cervera ML, de la Guardia M. Determination of cadmium by electrothermal atomic absorption spectrometry after microwave-assisted digestion of animal tissues and sewage sludges. Anal Bioanal Chem. 1996;355:43-7.
5. Dharmadhikari DM, Vanerkar AP, Barhate NM. Chemical oxygen demand using closed microwave digestion system. Environ Sci Technol. 2005;39:6198-201.
6. de la Guardia M, Morales-Rubio A. Modern strategies for the rapid determination of metals in sewage sludges. Trends Anal Chem. 1996;15:311-8.
7. de la Guardia M, Salvador A, Burguera JL, Burguera MJ. Flow Injection Anal. J Anal Atomic Spectr. 1988;5:121.
8. Ko FH, Chen HL. Study of microwave digestion kinetics and establishment of a model for digestion efficiency prediction. J Anal Atomic Spectr. 2001;16:1337-40.

9. Evisa. (2003). Instrument Database: Milestone S.r.l.—START D—Microwave Digestion System. [online] Available from http://www.speciation.net/Database/Instruments/Milestone-Srl/START-D—Microwave-Digestion-System-;i2571. [Last accessed March, 2021].
10. Kingston HM, Jassie LB. Introduction to Microwave Sample Preparation: Theory and Practice. Washington: American Chemical Society; 1988.
11. Kotz L, Kaiser, Tschopel T, Tolg GZ. Aufschluss biologischer Matrices fur die Bestimmung sehrniedriger Spurenelementgehalte bei begrenzter Einwaage mit Salpetersaure unter Druck ineinem Teflongethss. Anal Chem. 1972;260:207-9.
12. Kuss HM. Applications of microwave digestion technique for elemental analyses. Fresenius J Anal Chem. 1992;343:788-93.
13. Matusiewicz H, Sturgeon RE. Applications of microwave technique to sample dissolution in analytical chemistry. Prog Anal Spectrosc. 1989;12:21-9.
14. Meeravali NN, Kumar SJ. Comparison of open microwave digestion and digestion by conventional heating for the determination of Cd, Cr, Cu and Pb in algae using transverse heated electrothermal atomic absorption spectrometry. Fresenius J Anal Chem. 2000;366:313-5.
15. Rechcigi JE, Payne GG. (1990). Comparison of a microwave digestion system to other digestion methods for plant tissue analysis. [online] Available from https://www.researchgate.net/publication/232935046_Comparison_Of_a_Microwave_Digestion_System_to_Other_Digestion_Methods_for_Plant_Tissue_Analysis. [Last accessed March, 2021].
16. Schnitzer G, Soubelet A, Testu C, Mikrochim CC. Comparison of open and closed focused microwave digestions in view of total mercury determination by cold vapor atomic absorption spectrometry. Acta Chem. 1995;119:199-209.
17. Sedo G, Curtis J, Leopold KR. (2010). Dipole moment of the sulfuric acid monomer. [online] Available from https://www.asc.ohio-state.edu/miller.104/molspect/symposium_62/symposium/Abstracts/p035.pdf. [Last accessed March, 2021].
18. Smith FE, Arsenault EA. Microwave-assisted sample preparation in analytical chemistry. Talanta. 1996;43:1207-68.
19. Anton Paar. (2021). Introduction. [online] Available from www.anton-paar.com. [Last accessed March, 2021].
20. Zlotorzynski A. The Application of Microwave Radiation to Analytical and Environmental Chemistry. Crit Rev Anal Chem. 1995;25:43-76.

Chapter 12

Breath Alcohol Analyzer and its Applications

■ INTRODUCTION

Alcohol is the most common drug of abuse all over the world and it is related to various kinds of crimes such as drunken driving causing accidents, suicides, homicides, etc. Carefully performed experiments have tended to show that the consumption of alcohol increases neither our mental nor physical abilities. Shakespeare points concerning alcohol and sexual activity: "it provokes the desire but it takes away the performance" (Macbeth). It is important to check the misuse of alcohol. The breathalyzer plays an important role in its detection and legal action.

The breathalyzer is used by traffic police all over the world. Numerous studies have been done, which show that breathalyzer is a useful and reliable instrument. Gas-liquid chromatography (GLC) has been used to measure the blood alcohol level. It provides accurate results due to its sensitivity. But it has the disadvantage that it is a costly instrument, heavy, and takes more time for the report; on the other hand, breathalyzer is cheaper, portable, reliable, reproducible, and easy to handle by the police.

The modern type of breathalyzer was introduced by Dr Robert Borkenstein in 1954 and became the most widely used breath alcohol testing device. Since then, the breathalyzer has been improvised to great extent due to extensive research and latest microcomputer technology. There are numerous patented alcometer manufactured all over the world. This is an instrument, which is portable (**Figs. 12.1A** and **B**) and convenient to use. In most of the Western countries, traffic police use portable breath alcohol analyzer to detect alcohol in the breath of a suspected driver. It serves as an "on-the-spot" test. If this is positive, then the individual is taken into custody and a detailed analysis of his blood or urine is done.

■ TYPES OF BREATHALYZERS

1. *Based on type of use*:
   a. Active
   b. Passive

BREATH ALCOHOL ANALYZER AND ITS APPLICATIONS

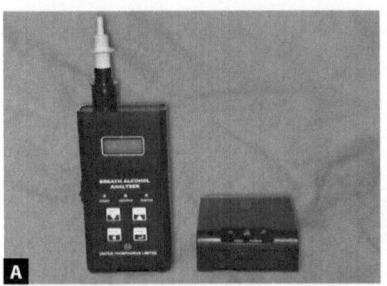 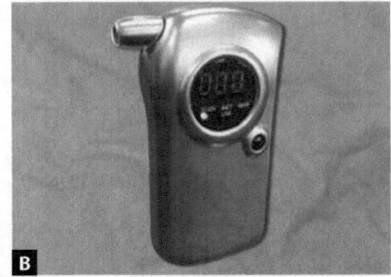

Figs. 12.1A and B: Portable breath analyzer of different companies. (A) Alcometer with printer, Uniphos (India) and (B) Alcometer (USA).

2. *Based on detectors*:
   a. Electrochemical detectors
   b. Infrared detectors
   c. Photocell detectors

The active breathalyzer needs the subject to blow deep lung air moderately and continuously until instructed to stop. The passive breathalyzer is used in case of unconscious or weak person unable to provide active breath sample. The operator focuses the sampling unit toward the person's mouth while observing the correct distance. It gives the alcohol reading from the passive breath. There is also small handset breathalyzer available for personal use. In many European countries, there is also fixed breathalyzer for public use to know your blood alcohol level.

■ PRINCIPLE OF BREATH ALCOHOL TESTING

In the simplest type, the first practical device for breath alcohol analysis was introduced in 1930. The early screening instruments were based on chemical principles for the determination of ethanol using potassium dichromate or potassium permanganate. The individual concerned is asked to blow into a plastic balloon containing a crystalline dichromate sulfuric acid mixture. If the blood alcohol is above a certain prescribed limit, the crystals turn green to a predetermined distance. But it was Dr Robert Borkenstein who first introduced the modern breath analyzer in 1954, which became the most widely used breath alcohol testing device. Currently, the methodology for breath alcohol analysis has mainly been concerned with physical-chemical principle for the assay of ethanol which has minimized erroneous results. The latest breathalyzer uses microcomputer technology and sensitive-specific detectors to detect alcohol. In the breathalyzer using electrochemical oxidation system, the alcohol present in a measured volume of breath from the individual is oxidized at a platinum electrode surface to generate an electric potential proportionate to the concentration of the ethanol in the sample, which can be registered and displayed in the screen. This oxidation reaction on the sensor is specific to ethanol and is not influenced by contaminants, such as ketones or hydrocarbons. The

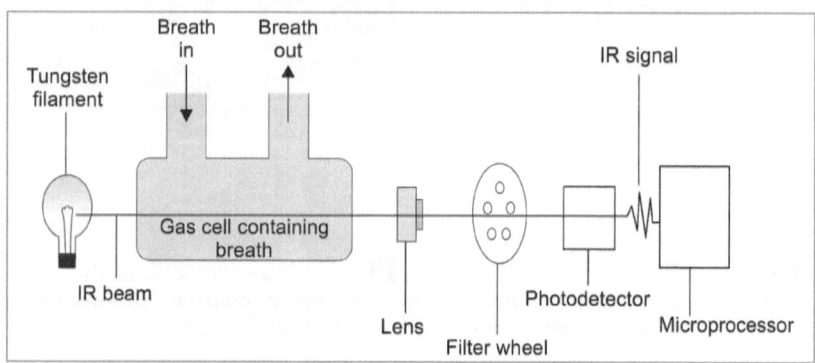

Fig. 12.2: Infrared (IR) photometric system of breath analyzer.

instrument is calibrated periodically with alcohol in air standard vapor mixture at a blood alcohol equivalent concentration of 50 mg/100 mL or 100 mg/100 mL. The calibration of breathalyzer is done using the standard 2,100:1 blood-to-breath ethanol ratio at the mean temperature of end-expired breath of 34°C.

The alcohol in alveolar air is in equilibrium with that in pulmonary capillary blood; hence, the result of the breath analysis is an indicator of the blood alcohol level. This breath alcohol concentration is multiplied by a factor called the partition ratio (i.e.) 2,100:1 to convert the concentration in blood. The direct correlation assumed between the concentration of alcohol in the alveolar air and in pulmonary capillary blood is based on Henry's law, which states that at constant temperature, the concentration of gas dissolved in a liquid is proportional to its concentration in the air directly above the liquid.

The infrared photometric system (**Fig. 12.2**) of the breathalyzer was introduced in UK in 1983. It uses detectors which are based on the absorption of infrared radiation at a wavelength around 3.4 μ corresponding to the carbon-hydrogen stretch of ethanol. It also incorporates a second (semiconductor) detector to detect abnormal levels of acetone in a breath sample and in such circumstances corrects the alcohol reading given by the infrared detector. There is also a type of breathalyzer using photocell mechanism as shown in **Figure 12.3**.

■ PRECAUTIONS

The following precautions have to be observed while conducting alcometer testing:
1. If a subject has been smoking, wait 3 minutes before conducting a test
2. Insure that a test subject has taken nothing by mouth for at last 15 minutes or rinses the mouth cavity with water prior to a breath test
3. Instruct the subject to blow moderately hard and continuously until a read out appears. Thereby, a proper sample of deep lung air will be automatically collected and analyzed

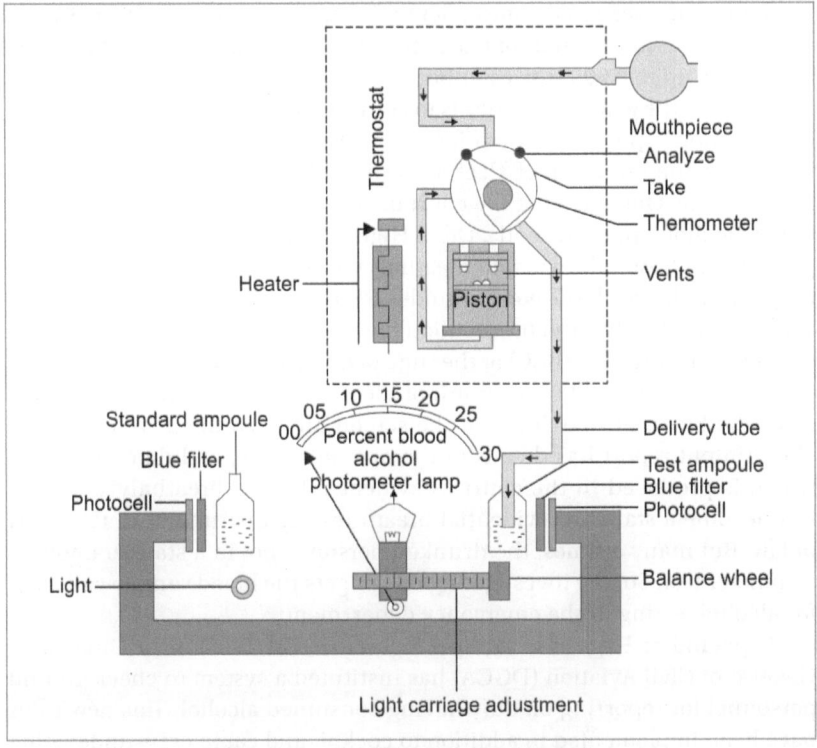

Fig. 12.3: Breathalyzer using photocell.

4. The breathalyzer operators must be trained to follow the standard protocol that includes sequential analysis of a room air blank, the subject's breath, and sample from a breath-alcohol simulator
5. He must hold a current breath testing permit issued, only after the operator has successfully completed a 40-hour basic training course in the theory and operation. Recertification is required every 2 years and is contingent upon satisfactory demonstration of continued proficiency
6. The breathalyzer should be calibrated regularly as per the specifications

LEGAL STATUS

Section 185 of the Indian Motor Vehicle Act, 1988 says that whoever person under the influence of drugs, while driving, or attempting to drive a motor vehicle:
1. Has, in his blood, alcohol exceeding 30 mg% of blood detected by a breath analyzer
2. Under the influence of a drug to such an extent as to be incapable of exercising proper control over the vehicle shall be punishable for the first offence with imprisonment up to 6 months or fine up to 2,000 rupees or

both and a second or subsequent offence, if committed within 3 years of the previous similar offence, the imprisonment may go up to 2 years or fine up to 3,000 rupees or both.

In India, the general practice is to convict only on the basis of a medical examination report, i.e., when it is proved that the driver of the vehicle was under the influence of alcohol, certified by a qualified doctor. But, it is liable to be challenged in the court of law without an alcometer test and blood alcohol report. Recently, Delhi High Court had issued an order to all government hospitals to install breathalyzer in the emergency department to test the alcohol level booked under Section 185 of Motor Vehicle Act, 1988. Under this Act, the prosecution has to prove that the accused blood alcohol concentration (BAC) at the time of offence is at or above a statutory concentration, i.e., 30 mg/100 mL of alcohol in blood. The breathalyzer gives the blood alcohol level on the screen and also the printout report. The printout report has details of the operator, time, and date of testing, which is produced in the court as evidence. Hence, breathalyzer report has become a standard evidential breath testing instrument in the court of law. But many a times, the drunken person is not in a state to undergo alcometer test. So, the investigating officer gets the blood sample collected for alcohol testing in the emergency department.

As per Indian Express newspaper report dated 21/10/2019, the Directorate General of Civil Aviation (DGCA) has instituted a system to check ground personnel for reporting on duty having consumed alcohol. This new rules have been implemented in addition to cockpit and cabin crew undergoing breath analyzer tests to check the level of alcohol in their blood; airside ground personnel and air traffic controller have also been undergoing the test. The DGCAs plan to cover ground personnel under breathalyzer examination was kicked off at over 17 airports on October 2, with more airports starting the process later. The rules say that the organizations engaged in the provision of air navigation services, aerodrome management, and aircraft maintenance and repair shall ensure that at least 10% individuals employed in their respective organizations engaged in such functions are randomly subjected to breathalyzer examination on daily basis. First-time violation—3 months suspension, second-time violation—1 year suspension, third-time violation—3 years suspension, and fourth-time violation—license should be suspended. This test ensures passenger safety.

■ LEGAL DEFENSE CHALLENGES IN DRUNKEN DRIVING

There are numerous court room challenges to the breath test resulting from several issues such as the operator falsified breath results, substances other than alcohol appeared on the subject's breath and increased the reading, the 2,100:1 blood-to-breath ratio employed in the breathalyzer was not valid for the subject tested, and random error such as radiofrequency interference falsely elevated the result. In a study done at Sweden, they encountered the following defense challenges according to priority order.

Drinking after the Offence
This is one of the most common defense tactic (90%) called hip-flask ploy. The suspect alleges consumption of alcohol after driving but before the blood specimen was obtained for forensic analysis.

Laced Drinks
The suspect claims that he or she unwittingly consumed alcohol, raising the BAC above the legal limit.

Inhalation of Ethanol Vapors from the Work Environment
Alleged inhalation of ethanol vapors from the work environment is a recurring defense challenge in drunken driving litigation.

Pathological Condition and Trauma
Various medical conditions and pathological states are sometimes suggested to account for a suspect's BAC being above the legal limit.

Use of Alcohol for Skin Disinfection when Drawing Blood
If the swabs used contain ethanol, then there is a potential risk that the blood specimen will become contaminated during the collection procedure.

Alleged Mix-up of Specimen
Very often, the reported BAC and the drinking history given to the court are grossly inconsistent. A persuasive defense counsel might manage to convince the court that a mix-up of blood specimen has occurred either at the police station or at the forensic laboratory. The chain of evidence has to be maintained and proved beyond doubt.

Postsampling Formation of Alcohols
The possibility of various alcohols being produced in the blood specimen after sampling is sometimes put forward to account for the BAC being above the legal limit.

Drug-alcohol Interactions
Drugs that interact with the pharmacokinetics of ethanol have social and medicolegal implications. Defense lawyers are always eager to learn about new drugs that might interact with pharmacokinetics of ethanol.

Intake of Alcohol from Tonics, Elixir, and Cough Syrups
Unintentional intake of alcohol from the regular use of elixirs and health tonics occurs as a defense challenges from time to time.

Dilution of Blood during Collection

People involved in traffic accidents sometimes require emergency hospital treatment. This might entail infusion of various solutions to counteract shock or a blood transfusion might be necessary. All infusion solutions should obviously be free of alcohol.

In Indian scenario, the court has not yet experienced strong trial and defense in drunken driving cases. Most of the accused accept their guilt to the police or the court and get away by paying fine and also the court is very lenient in such cases, especially when youth is involved. But with increasing awareness, prosecution challenges are likely to increase.

Evidential breath alcohol testing was introduced into Great Britain on 6th May, 1983 as part of the Transport Act, 1981. A prescribed legal limit of 35 μg/100 mL of alcohol in breath was set but police forces adopted procedures whereby no prosecutions below 40 μg/100 mL are instigated to allow for intrinsic measurement variations. A further safeguard was introduced to allow a driver to elect to give a sample of blood or urine if the breath alcohol concentration was in the range of 40–50 μg/100 mL. Two types of instrument were approved by home secretary for evidential breath testing: (1) The Lion Intoximeter 3000 and (2) the Camic Breath Analyzer. But since the breathalyzer was introduced in 1983 in UK, there have been many discussions about its accuracy and specificity.

In UK, Mr Stephen Gumbley was convicted for drunken driving. He was a motorist who provided a sample of blood 4 hours after he had been involved in a road accident. The resulting blood analysis was below the limit. However, the prosecution, relying on the fact that the blood alcohol is eliminated from everybody at a constant rate of 13–19 mg/100 mL/h, charged Mr Gumbley, claiming that he must have over the limit at the time of driving. The conviction at the magistrate court was later upheld by the high court. Such back calculations have been used in Germany, Finland, and Australia. In India also, such situation may be encountered in coming years.

There is strong evidence to suggest that a 2,300:1 ratio is physiologically more appropriate. If the breath instrument is recalibrated, so that the expired air concentration of alcohol is multiplied by 2,300 rather than 2,100, the estimated blood levels will be correspondingly higher. But calibration of breath alcohol instruments with 2,100:1 blood-to-breath ratio means that the lower estimates of the actual blood level given an advantage to the person tested.

This may be more acceptable from a medicolegal standpoint. Moreover, because of the time interval between roadside breath test and blood sampling, the alcohol concentration in blood will decrease. This means that in borderline cases, where a breath screening test might indicate above the legal limit, it will, in fact, turn out below the limit at the time of blood sampling. This so-called false-positive breath screening results can be minimized if the 2,100:1 blood-to-breadth ratio is used for calibration.

This is because an underestimation of the actual BAC in the roadside breath test will compensate for the metabolism of alcohol over the time interval between roadside test and blood sampling.

Study by R Gill et al. showed that there was no interference with the breath alcohol instruments when the subjects were exposed to toluene and 1,1,1-trichloroethane. A short-term response immediately after exposure was observed for subjects exposed to butane. Experimental study by TB Begg et al. showed that the effect of any "mouth alcohol" becomes negligible 15 minutes after ingestion and that the results of the breath analysis are unaffected by the wearing of dentures or by rinsing the mouth with water. The study done by PJ Gomm et al. showed that the use of salbutamol by asthmatics does not affect the reliability of measurements made by evidential breath alcohol testing device. Patrick H et al. in their study found that breathalyzer and blood-alcohol results correlated well and the BACs tended to be underestimated by the breathalyzer. He also found no evidence of operators altering breathalyzer results, radiofrequency interference causing elevated breathalyzer reading, or volatile substances other than ethanol causing elevated breathalyzer readings.

■ CONCLUSION

Breathalyzer has become a very useful instrument for screening for alcohol by noninvasive method. But its authenticity depends on various factors.

The performance evaluation of the breathalyzer should emphasis on: (1) Reproducibility and precision under various conditions, (2) accuracy of breath alcohol determinations in relation to blood alcohol levels, (3) variability between instruments as well as between test subjects, and (4) precision of estimating blood ethanol from analysis of breath.

Various studies have shown that there is variability in breathalyzer reports also. But these can be avoided by taking various precautions:
1. Breathalyzer should be calibrated regularly and properly every week or as per the specification. The calibration procedure requires that the instrument response is adjusted if it deviates from the expected value determined from the analysis of an ethanol-standard gas mixture
2. The operator should be trained properly and certified every 2 years or as per standard protocol
3. The breathalyzer report becomes an exhibit in the court of law. On such cases, the doctor may have to appear in the court of law. He should be aware of the defense techniques of the defense lawyer and be a good scientific witness
4. More studies should be done to study the accuracy of breathalyzer and compared with GLC report before approving the instrument for use by traffic police.
5. There is a need to study the alcohol metabolism pattern in Indian population to correlate the report reasonably.

BREATH ALCOHOL ANALYZER AND ITS APPLICATIONS

■ FURTHER READINGS

1. Begg TB, Hill ID, Nickolls LC. Breathalyzer and kitagawa-Wright methods of measuring breath alcohol. BMJ. 1964;1:9-15.
2. Gill R, Warner HE, Broster CG, Ramsey JD, Wilson HK, Wilcox AH. The response of evidential breath alcohol testing instruments with subjects exposed to organic solvents and gases-white spirit and Nonane. Med Sci Law. 1991;31(2):201-13.
3. Gill R, Hatchett SE, Broster CG, Ramsey JD, Wilson HK, Wilcox AH. The response of evidential breath alcohol testing instruments with subjects exposed to organic solvents and gases-toluene, 1,1,1-trichloroethane and butane. Med Sci Law. 1991;31(3):187-200.
4. Gomm PJ, Osselton MD, Broster CG, Johnson MN, Upton K. The effects of salbutamol on breath alcohol testing inasmathics. Med Sci Law. 1991;31(3):226-8.
5. Harding P, Patricia HF. Breathalyzer accuracy in law enforcement practice: A comparison of blood and breath-alcohol results in Wisconsin drivers. JFSCA. 1987;32(5):1235-40.
6. Jones AW. Evaluation of breath-alcohol instruments IV. Roadside tests with alcometer pocket model. For Sci Int. 1985;28:157-65.
7. Jones AW. Top ten defense challenges among drinking drivers in Sweden. Med Sci Law. 1991;31(3):229-38.
8. Raina A, Shrivastava HC, Dogra TD. Reliability factor of different breathalyzer and its co-relation with blood concentration by GLC-A pilot study. Ind Int J For Med Tox. 2003;1(1):1-5.
9. Rod G Gullberg, Barry KL. Reproducibility of within-subject breath alcohol analysis. Med Sci Law. 1998;38(2):157-62.
10. Technical manual of alcometer model datatest JE-1100 and PBA 3000. Canada: Alcohol Countermeasure Systems Corporation, 2018.
11. Government of India. (1988). The Indian Motor Vehicle Act.
12. Toseland PA. Editorial—alcohol and driving. Med Sci Law. 1991;31(3):185-6.

Chapter 13

Laboratory Accreditation: A Tool for Quality Management System

■ HISTORY OF ACCREDITATION

During World War I (1914–1918), munitions of war provided by Australia to United Kingdom were an acute embarrassment. It was a shock to the Australian's industry leaders. Later on, it was realized by the Australian that it happens due to the following:
- Lack of national standards of measurement
- Lack of national standardizing body

In June 1916, the Commonwealth Government established the Commonwealth Advisory Council of Science and Industry. In its 1916–1917 report, the Council recommended that arrangements be made for:
- The standardization of scientific apparatus and instruments
- The testing of electric lamps, apparatus, and machinery
- The testing of instruments of precision used in industry
- The physical testing and standardization of materials used by industry and by the Commonwealth Government

In September 1920, the Commonwealth Government assented to the Institute of Science and Industry Act, No. 22 of 1920, which established a permanent institute in place of the temporary Advisory Council. This act stated the powers and functions of the new institute including: "The testing and standardization of scientific apparatus and instruments and of apparatus, machinery, materials, and instruments used in industry".

This was the initial thought, which finally led to the concept of laboratory accreditation.

■ TERMS AND DEFINITIONS

Management System
Set of interrelated or interacting elements of an organization to establish policies and objectives and processes to achieve those objectives.

Accreditation

Third-party attestation related to a conformity assessment body conveying formal demonstration of its competence to carry out specific conformity assessment tasks.

Quality

The standard of something as measured against other things of a similar kind; the degree of excellence of something.

Quality Manual

A quality manual is a document that states the company's intentions for operating the processes within the quality management system (QMS). It can include policies for all areas of the business that affect ability to make high quality products and meet the customers' and standards requirements.

Quality Manager

The person nominated by the organization, who is responsible for overall management of quality systems within the organization.

Total Quality

Total quality management (TQM) describes a management approach to long-term success through customer satisfaction. In a TQM effort, all members of an organization participate in improving processes, products, services, and the culture in which they work.

Quality Assurance

The maintenance of a desired level of quality in a service or product, especially by means of attention to every stage of the process of delivery or production.

Quality Control

- A system of maintaining standards in manufactured products by testing a sample of the output against the specification
- The International Organization for Standardization (ISO) 9000 defines quality control as "a part of quality management focused on fulfilling quality requirements"

Quality Planning

A quality plan is a document, or several documents, that together specify quality standards, practices, resources, specifications, and the sequence of activities relevant to a particular product, service, project, or contract.

Quality plans should define a method for measuring the achievement of the quality objectives.

Competence
Demonstrated ability to apply knowledge and skills or ability to apply knowledge and skills to achieve intended results.

Audit
Systematic, independent, and documented process for obtaining objective evidence and evaluating it objectively to determine the extent to which the audit criteria are fulfilled.

Audit Program
Arrangements for a set of one or more audits planned for a specific time frame and directed toward a specific purpose.

Objective Evidence
Data supporting the existence or verity of something.

Audit Criteria
Set of requirements used as a reference against which objective evidence is compared.

Audit Evidence
Records, statements of fact, or other information, which are relevant to the audit criteria and verifiable.

Audit Findings
Results of the evaluation of the collected audit evidence against audit criteria and audit conclusion.

Conformity
Fulfillment of a requirement.

Nonconformity
Nonfulfillment of a requirement.

Validation
Confirmation, through the provision of objective evidence, that the requirements for a specific intended use or application have been fulfilled.

Verification
Confirmation, through the provision of objective evidence, that specified requirements have been fulfilled.

QUALITY MANAGEMENT SYSTEM

A QMS is a system of documented processes, procedures, and responsibilities for achieving quality policies and objectives.

Quality management system supports in coordination and direct organization's activities to meet customer and regulatory requirements and improve its effectiveness and efficiency on a constant basis. QMS serves many purposes including:
- Improving processes
- Reducing waste
- Lowering costs
- Facilitating and identifying training opportunities
- Engaging staff
- Setting organization-wide direction

INTERNATIONAL ORGANIZATION FOR STANDARDIZATION QUALITY MANAGEMENT PRINCIPLES

Quality management principles (QMPs) are a set of fundamental beliefs, norms, rules, and values that are accepted as true and can be used as a basis for quality management. The QMPs can be used as a foundation to guide an organization's performance improvement. They were developed and updated by international experts of ISO/TC 176, which is responsible for developing and maintaining ISOs quality management standards.

The seven quality management principles are:
1. QMP 1—customer focus
2. QMP 2—leadership
3. QMP 3—engagement of people
4. QMP 4—process approach
5. QMP 5—improvement
6. QMP 6—evidence-based decision-making
7. QMP 7—relationship management

These principles are not listed in priority order. The relative importance of each principle will vary from organization to organization and can be expected to change over time.

QMP 1—Customer Focus

The primary focus of quality management is to meet customer requirements and to strive to exceed customer expectations. Sustained success is achieved when an organization attracts and retains the confidence of customers and other interested parties. Every aspect of customer interaction provides an opportunity to create more value for the customer. Understanding current and future needs of customers and other interested parties contributes to sustained success of the organization. Key benefits are:
1. Increased customer value
2. Increased customer satisfaction
3. Improved customer loyalty

4. Enhanced repeat business
5. Enhanced reputation of the organization
6. Expanded customer base
7. Increased revenue and market share

QMP 2—Leadership

Leaders at all levels establish unity of purpose and direction and create conditions in which people are engaged in achieving the organization's quality objectives. Creation of unity of purpose and direction and engagement of people enable an organization to align its strategies, policies, processes, and resources to achieve its objectives. Key benefits are:

1. Increased effectiveness and efficiency in meeting the organization's quality objectives
2. Better coordination of the organization's processes
3. Improved communication between levels and functions of the organization
4. Development and improvement of the capability of the organization and its people to deliver desired results

QMP 3—Engagement of People

Competent, empowered, and engaged people at all levels throughout the organization are essential to enhance its capability to create and deliver value. To manage an organization effectively and efficiently, it is important to involve all people at all levels and to respect them as individuals. Recognition, empowerment, and enhancement of competence facilitate the engagement of people in achieving the organization's quality objectives. Key benefits are:

1. Improved understanding of the organization's quality objectives by people in the organization and increased motivation to achieve them
2. Enhanced involvement of people in improvement activities
3. Enhanced personal development, initiatives, and creativity
4. Enhanced people satisfaction
5. Enhanced trust and collaboration throughout the organization
6. Increased attention to shared values and culture throughout the organization

QMP 4—Process Approach

Consistent and predictable results are achieved more effectively and efficiently when activities are understood and managed as interrelated processes that function as a coherent system. The QMS consists of interrelated processes. Understanding how results are produced by this system enables an organization to optimize the system and its performance. Key benefits are:

1. Enhanced ability to focus effort on key processes and opportunities for improvement

2. Consistent and predictable outcomes through a system of aligned processes
3. Optimized performance through effective process management, efficient use of resources, and reduced cross-functional barriers
4. Enabling the organization to provide confidence to interested parties as to its consistency, effectiveness, and efficiency

QMP 5—Improvement

Successful organizations have an ongoing focus on improvement. Improvement is essential for an organization to maintain current levels of performance, to react to changes in its internal and external conditions, and to create new opportunities. Key benefits are:
1. Improved process performance, organizational capabilities, and customer satisfaction
2. Enhanced focus on root-cause investigation and determination, followed by prevention and corrective actions
3. Enhanced ability to anticipate and react to internal and external risks and opportunities
4. Enhanced consideration of both incremental and breakthrough improvement
5. Improved use of learning for improvement
6. Enhanced drive for innovation

QMP 6—Evidence-based Decision-making

Decisions based on the analysis and evaluation of data and information are more likely to produce desired results. Decision-making can be a complex process and it always involves some uncertainty. It often involves multiple types and sources of inputs as well as their interpretation, which can be subjective. It is important to understand cause-and-effect relationships and potential unintended consequences. Facts, evidence, and data analysis lead to greater objectivity and confidence in decision-making. Key benefits are:
1. Improved decision-making processes
2. Improved assessment of process performance and ability to achieve objectives
3. Improved operational effectiveness and efficiency
4. Increased ability to review, challenge, and change opinions and decisions
5. Increased ability to demonstrate the effectiveness of past decisions

QMP 7—Relationship Management

For sustained success, an organization manages its relationships with interested parties, such as suppliers. Interested parties influence the performance of an organization. Sustained success is more likely to be achieved when the organization manages relationships with all of its interested parties to optimize their impact on its performance. Relationship

management with its supplier and partner networks is of particular importance. Key benefits are:
1. Enhanced performance of the organization and its interested parties through responding to the opportunities and constraints related to each interested party
2. Common understanding of goals and values among interested parties
3. Increased capability to create value for interested parties by sharing resources and competence and managing quality-related risks
4. A well-managed supply chain that provides a stable flow of goods and services

QUALITY AUDIT

Audit results can provide input to the analysis aspect of business planning and can contribute to the identification of improvement needs and activities. An audit can be conducted against a range of audit criteria, separately or in combination, including but not limited to:
1. Requirements defined in one or more management system standards
2. Policies and requirements specified by relevant interested parties
3. Statutory and regulatory requirements
4. One or more management system processes defined by the organization or other parties
5. Management system plan(s) relating to the provision of specific outputs of a management system (e.g., quality plan, project plan)

Audit Types

- *First-party audit*: Internal audit
- *Second-party audit*: External provider audit and other external interested party audit
- *Third-party audit*: Certification and/or accreditation audit and statutory, regulatory, and similar audit

Principles of Auditing

Basic principles of auditing are:
1. *Integrity*: Integrity is the foundation of professionalism. Auditors and the individual(s) managing an audit program should:
   - Perform their work ethically with honesty and responsibility
   - Only undertake audit activities, if competent to do so
   - Perform their work in an impartial manner, i.e., remain fair and unbiased in all their dealings
   - Be sensitive to any influences that may be exerted on their judgment while carrying out an audit
2. *Fair presentation*: It is the obligation to report truthfully and accurately. Audit findings, audit conclusions, and audit reports should reflect truthfully and accurately the audit activities. Significant obstacles

encountered during the audit and unresolved diverging opinions between the audit team and the auditee should be reported. The communication should be truthful, accurate, objective, timely, clear, and complete.
3. *Due professional care*: It is the application of diligence and judgment in auditing. Auditors should exercise due care in accordance with the importance of the task they perform and the confidence placed in them by the audit client and other interested parties. An important factor in carrying out their work with due professional care is having the ability to make reasoned judgments in all audit situations.
4. *Confidentiality*: It is the security of information. Auditors should exercise discretion in the use and protection of information acquired in the course of their duties. Audit information should not be used inappropriately for personal gain by the auditor or the audit client or in a manner detrimental to the legitimate interests of the auditee. This concept includes the proper handling of sensitive or confidential information.
5. *Independence*: It is the basis for the impartiality of the audit and objectivity of the audit conclusions. Auditors should be independent of the activity being audited wherever, practicable and should in all cases act in a manner that is free from bias and conflict of interest. For internal audits, auditors should be independent from the function being audited, if practicable. Auditors should maintain objectivity throughout the audit process to ensure that the audit findings and conclusions are based only on the audit evidence.

   For small organizations, it may not be possible for internal auditors to be fully independent of the activity being audited, but every effort should be made to remove bias and encourage objectivity.
6. *Evidence-based approach*: It is the rational method for reaching reliable and reproducible audit conclusions in a systematic audit process. Audit evidence should be verifiable. It should, in general, be based on samples of the information available, since an audit is conducted during a finite period of time and with finite resources. An appropriate use of sampling should be applied, since this is closely related to the confidence that can be placed in the audit conclusions.
7. *Risk-based approach*: It is an audit approach that considers risks and opportunities. The risk-based approach should substantively influence the planning, conducting, and reporting of audits in order to ensure that audits are focused on matters that are significant for the audit client and for achieving the audit program objectives.

■ MANAGING AN AUDIT PROGRAM

An audit program should be established, which can include audits addressing one or more management system standards or other requirements, conducted either separately or in combination (combined audit).

The extent of an audit program should be based on the size and nature of the auditee as well as on the nature, functionality, complexity, the type of risks and opportunities, and the level of maturity of the management system(s) to be audited.

The functionality of the management system can be even more complex when most of the important functions are outsourced and managed under the leadership of other organizations. Particular attention needs to be paid to where the most important decisions are made and what constitutes the top management of the management system.

In order to understand the context of the auditee, the audit program should take into account the auditee's:
- Organizational objectives
- Relevant external and internal issues
- The needs and expectations of relevant interested parties
- Information security and confidentiality requirements

The audit program should include information and identify resources to enable the audits to be conducted effectively and efficiently within the specified time frames. The information should include:
1. Objectives for the audit program
2. Risks and opportunities associated with the audit program and the actions to address them
3. Scope (extent, boundaries, and locations) of each audit within the audit program
4. Schedule (number/duration/frequency) of the audits
5. Audit types such as internal or external
6. Audit criteria
7. Audit methods to be employed
8. Criteria for selecting audit team members
9. Relevant documented information

The implementation of the audit program should be monitored and measured on an ongoing basis to ensure its objectives have been achieved.

The audit program should be reviewed in order to identify needs for changes and possible opportunities for improvements.

■ ESTABLISHING AUDIT PROGRAM OBJECTIVES

The audit client should ensure that the audit program objectives are established to direct the planning and conducting of audits and should ensure the audit program is implemented effectively. Audit program objectives should be consistent with the audit client's strategic direction and support management system policy and objectives. These objectives can be based on consideration of the following:
1. Needs and expectations of relevant interested parties, both external and internal
2. Characteristics and requirements for processes, products, services and projects, and any changes to them
3. Management system requirements

4. Need for evaluation of external providers
5. Auditee's level of performance and level of maturity of the management system(s), as reflected in relevant performance indicators and the occurrence of nonconformities (NCs) or incidents or complaints from interested parties
6. Identified risks and opportunities to the auditee
7. Results of previous audits

Examples of audit program objectives can include the following:
1. Identify opportunities for the improvement of a management system and its performance
2. Evaluate the capability of the auditee to determine its context
3. Evaluate the capability of the auditee to determine risks and opportunities and to identify and implement effective actions to address them
4. Conform to all relevant requirements, e.g., statutory and regulatory requirements, compliance commitments, and requirements for certification to a management system standard
5. Obtain and maintain confidence in the capability of an external provider
6. Determine the continuing suitability, adequacy, and effectiveness of the auditee's management system
7. Evaluate the compatibility and alignment of the management system objectives with the strategic direction of the organization

■ IMPLEMENTING AUDIT PROGRAM

Once the audit program has been established and related resources have been determined, it is necessary to implement the operational planning and the coordination of all the activities within the program. The individual(s) managing the audit program should:
1. Communicate the relevant parts of the audit program, including the risks and opportunities involved, to relevant interested parties and inform them periodically of its progress, using established external and internal communication channels
2. Define objectives, scope, and criteria for each individual audit
3. Select audit methods
4. Coordinate and schedule audits and other activities relevant to the audit program
5. Ensure the audit teams have the necessary competence
6. Provide necessary individual and overall resources to the audit teams
7. Ensure the conduct of audits in accordance with the audit program, managing all operational risks, opportunities, and issues (i.e., unexpected events), as they arise during the deployment of the program
8. Ensure relevant documented information regarding the auditing activities is properly managed and maintained
9. Define and implement the operational controls necessary for audit program monitoring
10. Review the audit program in order to identify opportunities for its improvement

MANAGING AUDIT PROGRAM RESULTS

The individual(s) managing the audit program should ensure that the following activities are performed:
1. Evaluation of the achievement of the objectives for each audit within the audit program
2. Review and approval of audit reports regarding the fulfillment of the audit scope and objectives
3. Review of the effectiveness of actions taken to address audit findings
4. Distribution of audit reports to relevant interested parties
5. Determination of the necessity for any follow-up audit

MANAGING AND MAINTAINING AUDIT PROGRAM RECORDS

The individual(s) managing the audit program should ensure that audit records are generated, managed, and maintained to demonstrate the implementation of the audit program. Processes should be established to ensure that any information security and confidentiality needs associated with the audit records are addressed. Records can include the following:
- Records related to the audit program such as:
  - Schedule of audits
  - Audit program objectives and extent
  - Those addressing audit program risks and opportunities and relevant external and internal issues
  - Reviews of the audit program effectiveness
- Records related to each audit such as:
  - Audit plans and audit reports
  - Objective audit evidence and findings
  - Nonconformity (NC) reports
  - Corrections and corrective action reports
  - Audit follow-up reports
- Records related to the audit team covering topics such as:
  - Competence and performance evaluation of the audit team members
  - Criteria for the selection of audit teams and team members and formation of audit teams
  - Maintenance and improvement of competence

MONITORING AUDIT PROGRAM

The individual(s) managing the audit program should ensure the evaluation of:
1. Whether schedules are being met and audit program objectives are being achieved
2. The performance of the audit team members including the audit team leader and the technical experts
3. The ability of the audit teams to implement the audit plan

4. Feedback from audit clients, auditees, auditors, technical experts, and other relevant parties
5. Sufficiency and adequacy of documented information in the whole audit process

■ REVIEWING AND IMPROVING AUDIT PROGRAM

The individual(s) managing the audit program and the audit client should review the audit program to assess whether, its objectives have been achieved. Lessons learned from the audit program review should be used as inputs for the improvement of the program.

The individual(s) managing the audit program should ensure the following:
1. Review of the overall implementation of the audit program
2. Identification of areas and opportunities for improvement
3. Application of changes to the audit program, if necessary
4. Review of the continual professional development of auditors
5. Reporting of the results of the audit program and review with the audit client and relevant interested parties, as appropriate

■ ACCREDITATION

Accreditation is the third-party attestation related to a conformity assessment body conveying the formal demonstration of its competence to carry out specific conformity assessment task. A Conformity Assessment Body (laboratory) is a body, which includes testing including medical laboratory, calibration laboratory, proficiency testing provider, and reference material producers.

Laboratory accreditation is a procedure by which an authoritative body gives formal recognition of technical competence for specific tests/measurements based on third-party assessment and following international standards.

In India, the National Accreditation Board for Testing and Calibration Laboratories (NABL) has been established with the objective of providing accreditation scheme for Conformity Assessment Bodies, which involves third-party assessment of the technical competence of testing including medical and calibration laboratories, proficiency testing providers, and reference material producers.

The laboratory accreditation services to testing and calibration laboratories are provided in accordance with:
- ISO/IEC 17025 "General Requirements for the Competence of Testing and Calibration Laboratories"
- ISO 15189 "Medical Laboratories—Requirements for Quality and Competence"

The accreditation to proficiency testing providers is based on ISO/IEC 17043 "Conformity Assessment—General Requirements for Proficiency Testing" and to reference material producers based on ISO 17034 "General Requirements for the Competence of Reference Material Producers".

Accreditation body (AB) (e.g., NABL) has established its accreditation system in accordance with ISO/IEC 17011 "Conformity assessment—requirements for accreditation bodies accrediting conformity assessment bodies".

Accreditation body's (such as NABL) accreditation system also needs to fulfill the requirements of Mutual Recognition Arrangements (MRAs) as defined by the Asia Pacific Accreditation Cooperation (APAC) and the International Laboratory Accreditation Cooperation (ILAC).

In the current global scenario, an essential prerequisite of trade is that any product or service accepted formally in one economy must also be free to circulate in other economies without having to undergo extensive retesting. The World Trade Organization (WTO) recognizes that nonacceptance of test results and measurement data is a technical barrier to trade. Global sourcing of components calls for equivalence of measurement, which can be facilitated by a chain of accredited laboratories. Accreditation is considered as the first essential step for facilitating mutual acceptance of test results and measurement data.

The NABL is a AB in India, which provides accreditation in all major fields of Science and Engineering such as Biological, Chemical, Electrical, Electronics, Mechanical, Fluid Flow, Nondestructive, Photometry, Radiological, Thermal, and Forensics under testing facilities and Electrotechnical, Mechanical, Fluid Flow, Thermal, Optical, Medical Devices, and Radiological under calibration facilities. The NABL also provides accreditation for medical testing laboratories. In addition, the NABL also offers accreditation for proficiency testing providers and reference material producers.

Accreditation—Need

1. To ensure accurate, reliable, and reproducible test results and measurement data
2. To achieve consistency and uniformity in test results and measurement data
3. To have confidence in the quality of goods and services we use
4. To meet customer's requirement who specify testing or calibration by accredited laboratories
5. To meet requirements of regulatory and government agencies who sometimes require testing by accredited laboratories
6. To ensure equivalence of results produced by different laboratories

Benefits of Accreditation

Formal recognition of competence of a laboratory by an AB in accordance with international criteria has many advantages:
1. *Global acceptance of reports*: Test reports issued by an Indian accredited laboratory are acceptable among all the ILAC MRA partners and considered equivalent to those issued by the ILAC/APLAC MRA partners

2. Better control of laboratory operations
3. Improves staff confidence and enhances business
4. Enhanced customer confidence and satisfaction
5. Reliability of data for research and development (R&D)
6. Insurance companies can rely on test results
7. Ensures better support in the event of legal cases
8. Provides traceability in measurements to national standards
9. Provides global equivalence
10. Saving of time and money due to retesting

How to prepare for accreditation?
1. Once the laboratory decides to take accreditation, it should make a detailed plan of action for obtaining accreditation
2. Person responsible for QMS has to be identified who will coordinate all accreditation-related activities during accreditation process. This person should be aware about the standard
3. The laboratory has to make its quality documentation as per applicable standard ISO/IEC 17025 (Testing and Calibration Laboratories) or ISO 15189 (Medical Laboratory)
4. Once documentation is ready, the laboratory has to ensure that same is implemented effectively
5. To verify the effectiveness of management system, the laboratory has to conduct internal audit. This internal audit should be conducted as per the requirements stated in relevant standard
6. Management review meeting should also be conducted by the laboratory as per applicable standard
7. The laboratory should also participate in proficiency testing programs, so that confidence can be achieved on technical competence
8. The laboratory should understand the AB requirements such as application process, specific criteria, and any other requirements
9. The laboratory should also understand the accreditation process followed by AB

Accreditation Process

1. The laboratory is required to apply in the prescribed application form to AB along with required documents (e.g., quality manual and fee)
2. The laboratory will receive acknowledgement on receipt of application form from AB
3. The laboratory will also receive scrutiny report. If any additional information/documents are required by AB, the laboratory has to submit these information/documents to AB. For clarifications, laboratory has to submit response
4. If there are no inadequacies in the documents or after satisfactory corrective action by the laboratory, a preassessment is conducted by AB by sending lead assessor

5. This preassessment is conducted:
    - To evaluate the implementation of quality system in the laboratory
    - To assess the preparedness of the laboratory for final assessment
    - To determine the number of days and technical assessors for conducting complete assessment as per applied scope
6. Assessment team submits preassessment report to AB and provides copy to laboratory
7. The laboratory should take corrective actions against the NCs raised and documentary evidences are to be submitted to AB
8. After the laboratory has taken satisfactory corrective actions, AB schedule the final assessment for the laboratory
9. The final assessment team consisting of lead assessor and technical assessors
10. The assessment team reviews the laboratory's documented management system and verifies its compliance with the requirements of applicable standard (ISO/IEC 17025 or ISO 15189)
11. The assessment team also verifies the requirements as per specific criteria and AB policies
12. Through test witnessing, the laboratory's technical competence to perform specific tasks is also evaluated
13. The NCs, if observed and identified, are reported in the assessment report
14. The assessment team also provides recommendation toward grant of accreditation or otherwise
15. The assessment report prepared by the assessment team is submitted to AB
16. The assessment team also provides copy of assessment report to the laboratory
17. Laboratory is required to submit the corrective actions against each NC to the assessment team and AB. Laboratory to ensure that the corrective actions are based on root cause analysis
18. The assessment report along with corrective action (including root cause analysis) will be reviewed by AB and laboratory has to submit response against the observations, if any made by AB
19. Once satisfactory corrective actions are taken by the laboratory against the NCs and observation by AB, AB will take the decision on accreditation and same will be communicated to the laboratory
20. After receiving the decision on grant of accreditation, the laboratory can claim its accreditation status
21. It is necessary that the accredited laboratory shall conform to the requirements of relevant standard (ISO/IEC 17025 or ISO 15189) specific criteria, if applicable and AB policies at all times
22. As the AB grants accreditation for certain period, the laboratory has to reapply for accreditation as per AB policy to maintain continuity in accreditation

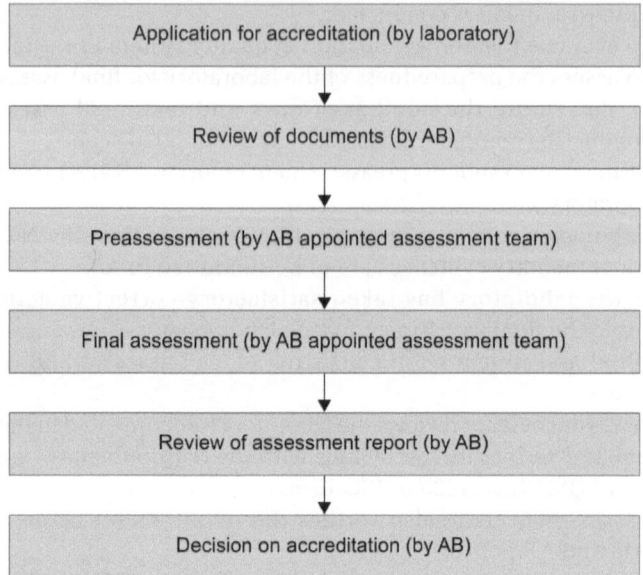

During each step, AB can ask clarification from laboratory and laboratory has to take appropriate corrective actions and documentary evidences to be submitted to AB.

Assessor Role

The objective of any on-site assessment is to obtain evidence on compliance with respect to the relevant standard. Basically, the assessor's role is to conduct on-site assessment of laboratory to adjudge the compliance.

The assessor shall also check that the laboratory meets other requirements of AB including specific criteria and has competence to perform the specific test.

Assessor shall ensure that latest documents have been used during assessment. The assessor shall also aware about the changes announced by the AB.

Since laboratory accreditation requires formal recognition of competence to carry out specific test by a laboratory, an assessor has also to consider conformities against these aspects in the assessment. Thus, an assessor would be required to exercise his scientific and technical judgment and form his opinion regarding extent of conformity with respect to accreditation criteria. Assessors are required to maintain the confidentiality on the matters/subjects related to laboratory.

The success of the accreditation scheme depends on the assessors who perform on-site assessment. Thus, the assessors play a vital role in determining the credibility and value of the accreditation.

Role of Lead Assessor

Before the start of assessment, the lead assessor should prepare an assessment schedule which should include the laboratory locations/departments/sections/areas/activities to be assessed and assignment to various assessors based on their expertise.

The lead assessor must review the laboratory's documented management system to verify compliance with the requirements of relevant standard (ISO/IEC 17025 or ISO 15189). Lead assessor should assess that the documented management system is indeed implemented and effective as described and record observations. Lead assessor should also complete checklist and record conclusion/comments related to the requirements of respective clause number. All NCs must be identified and reported separately on each sheet. No NC shall be closed during the assessment. Laboratory shall evaluate the root cause of the NC and propose correction and corrective action.

As a leader of the assessment team, lead assessor would collect the reports and documents from all technical assessors including his/her own report and compile it. A consolidated statement of NCs raised during the assessment shall be listed. If, during assessment, a case of critical system failure and gross negligence in technical aspects is noticed, the lead assessor will at the earliest inform AB and elaborately bring it out in the assessment summary of assessment report. Lead assessor should finally summarize the conduct of assessment and record the recommendations. The lead assessor is also required to monitor the performance of technical assessor.

Role of Technical Assessor

The technical assessor should clearly understand the areas/activities to be assessed by him. He must review the laboratory's documented system to verify compliance with the requirements of relevant standard (ISO/IEC 17025 or ISO 15189), specific criteria, and other policies of AB. He should assess to verify that the documented standard operating procedures (SOPs), test methods, and records are indeed implemented and effective and record observations. He should also complete checklist related to the requirements of respective clauses for the calibration(s) and test(s)/retesting witnessed by him. The technical assessor must review and endorse the uncertainty calculations for each test/calibration witnessed. For testing the datasheet for the test(s), witnessed should be prepared.

All NCs must be identified and reported separately on each sheet. The scope of accreditation to be granted to the laboratory must be checked thoroughly with necessary recommendations for testing laboratories or calibration laboratories. Any deletions or alterations in the scope must be clearly brought out and signed by both the laboratory representative and the assessor.

IDENTIFICATION, CLASSIFICATION, AND EXPRESSION OF NONCONFORMITY

The identification, classification, and expression of NC are given below:
- A NC can be identified and can be one or more of the following:
  - Related to the management system
  - Related to technical activities
  - Failure to fulfill the required objectives
  - Difference between work practices and documented instructions
- A NC can be classified as major or minor
- A major NCs are:
  - Absence of a procedure required by standard
  - Significant failure to implement a procedure
  - Direct effect on quality of results
- All other NCs are minor
- The statement of NC must be expressed as at least one of the following:
  - Nonblaming statements of fact
  - Based on recorded objective evidence
  - Directly related to specific documented requirement

PREASSESSMENT VISIT

During the preassessment visit made by the lead assessor, the following actions should be carried out in every case:
1. Explaining the purpose of the assessment, the tasks of assessors, and making clear to the laboratory the methodology to be adopted
2. Explaining the obligations on the part of the laboratory to confirm by demonstration that the management of the laboratory understands the procedures
3. Reviewing the management system documents including the availability of SOPs to cover the tests/measurements that it is carrying out internal audit and management review reports
4. Reviewing the scope of the accreditation
5. Giving an overview of the accreditation process

The objectives of a preassessment visit are:
1. To have a better understanding of the documentation
2. To familiarize with the facilities, sites/location, circumstances, and to have better knowledge of operations
3. To make the methodology to be adopted for the assessment
4. To check the preparedness of the laboratory to undergo assessment
5. To review the scope of accreditation and to ascertain the requirement of the number of assessors and the duration of assessment

ON-SITE ASSESSMENT

Before assessment, the assessment team shall plan assessment program.

Opening Meeting

1. Lead assessor and the team shall have an opening meeting with laboratory representatives where the team and the laboratory personnel will introduce each other
2. The assessment team should get acquainted with the laboratory, the departments/sections, and their locations
3. The lead assessor should make it clear in his opening remarks that the object of the assessment is to assess the work of laboratory according to ISO/IEC 17025 "General Requirements for the Competence of Testing and Calibration Laboratories" or ISO 15189 "Medical Laboratories—Requirements for Quality", whichever is applicable
4. The lead assessor shall ensure that he/she explains the objective and scope of assessment and what is expected from the laboratory during the assessment
5. The lead assessor shall confirm the scope of accreditation, etc.
6. The lead assessor shall present the assessment plan to laboratory representatives. The laboratory will be requested to assign guide/co-coordinator to accompany each assessor
7. The lead assessor shall assure the laboratory that all findings will be treated in strict confidence
8. The lead assessor shall inform the laboratory that the team members shall not be approached by the laboratory for closure of NCs during the assessment and the response to the closure of NCs has to be sent by laboratory after conducting root cause analysis
9. Lead assessor shall have record of all participants of opening meeting

On-site Assessment Procedure

1. The assessment team shall proceed to various sections of the laboratory as planned earlier. Assessors must be objective and should not convey the impression of having superior knowledge and judgment
2. Assessor(s) should thoroughly examine the technical competence of the laboratory in terms of manpower, qualification, experience, up-to-date knowledge, equipment, and other related elements. Assessor(s) shall also verify the confidentiality by laboratory personnel including those on contract/outsourced
3. While interviewing the laboratory personnel, the assessors should create a comfortable environment to gather all information needed to accurately evaluate the competence of the laboratory
4. The technical competence of the laboratory personnel could be verified by examining their qualification, experience, training relevant to the job/responsibilities assigned, and observations during the activities related to the scope of accreditation
5. Assessors shall track the status of the laboratory's authorized signatories, which are detailed in the laboratory's application form. Assessors shall also check that the authorized signatories of the laboratory are meeting the criteria set by AB

6. Knowledge of the procedures for recording, reporting, and checking results should also be verified by the assessment team
7. If the laboratory is functioning in shifts, the assessor shall ensure the competence of staff working in shift operations and report the details
8. The assessment team should show a positive attitude during the process of assessment. The objective of assessment is to ascertain by observations of the activities whether, the work of the laboratory is being carried out in accordance with ISO/IEC 17025 "General Requirements for the Competence of Testing and Calibration Laboratories" or ISO 15189 "Medical Laboratories—Requirements for Quality and Competence".
9. Favorable and adverse noting must be based on objective evidence and be recorded and verified before leaving the area under assessment. To secure agreement on the facts and to avoid subsequent disputes, assessors shall record detailed NCs as they occur. Each NC shall be accepted by the laboratory representative.
10. At the time of assessment of the laboratory, assessors will discuss with the quality manager of the laboratory whether the laboratory is participating in any national/international proficiency testing/interlaboratory comparison program (wherever applicable), their performance, and the action taken by the laboratory, if the performance was unsatisfactory
11. Lead assessor shall, during the course of on-the-spot assessment, verify the effectiveness of management system and related documents using the audit techniques and shall raise the relevant NC. The lead assessor shall record the findings
12. Since it is not possible to assess every procedure in operation, assessors should use his own judgment to select one or more calibration/test for their demonstration. The selection of the calibration/test would have to be such that it can help assess the laboratory's competence in terms of equipment and capabilities of experts
13. The assessors are required to witness the conduct of some replicate tests using old samples whose reported results are available to study repeatability and reproducibility of measurements
14. In some cases, assessors may trace back results from previously issued certificates or reports to the original entries in the laboratory's registers/notebooks/worksheets. Aspects, which require evidence from some other area of laboratory before they can be settled, may be perused for further investigation. The assessors shall record the findings
15. Using the checklist, the assessors shall conduct the technical assessment and examine the management system. They shall raise the NC as may be relevant. The assessors shall record the findings
16. At the end of each assessment day, the lead assessor shall consolidate their findings. The lead assessor shall brief the laboratory about the NCs noticed by the team. The above would facilitate laboratory to take corrective actions on the NC observed
17. The lead assessor and assessors shall individually complete assessment report, which shall be accepted by the laboratory representative

18. After the assessors have completed their individual assessment, a preliminary meeting of assessment team is held to summaries their conclusions

Compilation Report
1. Each assessor, based on his verification, shall prepare as part of his recommendations the details of calibration/test of the laboratory is to be accredited
2. The lead assessor shall consolidate the findings based on individual assessor's report(s)

Closing Meeting
1. The lead assessor shall summarize the findings of the assessment team and present it to the laboratory representatives. The lead assessor shall invite each assessor to summarize his/her findings
2. During the closing meeting, the management representative present shall be asked to suggest a date for completion of corrective action of all NC and to acknowledge this by signing. A copy of this form along with NC, scope, and authorized signatories is to be shared with the laboratory representative
3. The closing meeting is to end with thanks giving for the cooperation and assistance given by laboratory

Procedure for Conducting Closing Meeting
The purpose of the closing meeting is to enable the team to present the laboratory management with a summary of the findings of the assessment and to inform the management of the recommendations that the team will make to the AB. The concluding report shall be based on the summary report prepared by assessment team.
1. Final meeting shall be chaired by the lead assessor, who should:
   - Thank the laboratory for its assistance and cooperation. He shall also refer to individuals as may be appropriate
   - Explain the significance of the type of NCs
   - Ask for questions to be deferred until the findings have been presented, although points of clarification should not be refused
   - Invite each assessor to summarize his or her findings based on the report, but it should not be discussed in detail. He should present his/her findings as individual assessor
   - Invite the laboratory to specify the date by which any required corrective actions will be implemented. It should be in line with the NABL norms
   - Provide the laboratory with an opportunity to discuss the assessment and answer any questions
   - Apprise laboratory with the specific requirements of AB

LABORATORY ACCREDITATION: A TOOL FOR QUALITY MANAGEMENT SYSTEM

2. During the closing meeting, the assessment team should not enter into debating the validity of their conclusions or recommendations. If these are questioned, the assessor may, however, enumerate individual NCs, which justify the recommendations in question and point out the combined effect of the observations of the assessment. If the laboratory is still unwilling to implement the recommendations, the lead assessor should advise them to take up the matter with AB
3. Lead assessor should also have record of personnel who has attended the closing meeting

■ ISO/IEC 17025: 2017: SUMMARY AT A GLANCE

Laboratory (Testing and Calibration) Accreditation is based on the ISO/International Electrotechnical Commission (IEC) 17025.

The structure of standard is as follows:
1. Scope
2. Normative references
3. Terms and definitions
4. General requirements
5. Structural requirements
6. Resource requirements
7. Process requirements
8. Management requirements:
   - Annexure A—metrological traceability (informative)
   - Annexure B—management system (informative)
   - Bibliography

The ISO/IEC 17025: 2017 standard was developed with the objective of promoting confidence in the operation of laboratories (testing and calibration) and contains requirements for laboratories (testing and calibration) to enable them to demonstrate that they operate in a competent and impartial way and that they are able to provide valid results consistently.

The ISO/IEC 17025 consisting principles of ISO 9001. This standard can be used for accreditation purposes, self-assessment by the laboratories, and it can also be used for second-party assessments by the laboratory customers, regulators, etc.

Its requirements are applicable to all organization, which are involved in the activities of testing and/or calibration and/or sampling associated with subsequent testing or calibration. Therefore, accreditation can be also achieved by organizations which are involved in sampling associated with subsequent testing or calibration as per this standard.

When the standard uses the term "laboratory", then it is referring to any of the three options mentioned below:
1. Testing
2. Calibration
3. Sampling

Accreditation to sampling activities is a new component in this standard.

Examples:
- *Organization involved in sampling activity*: If there is an organization which is doing sampling and forwarding these samples to a testing or calibration laboratory, then such type of organization should meet the requirements of this standard with respect to sampling and management system comply with the requirements related to competence of the personnel
- *Organization performing sampling and testing/calibration*: If the testing/calibration laboratory is taking samples by its own, then it should comply with all requirements of this standard which are related to sampling and testing/calibration

ISO/IEC 17025 Main Requirements

The standard mentions its requirements in the clauses from 4 to 8.

Clause 4—General Requirements

4.1 Impartiality: Clause 4.1 states the impartiality requirements. Commitment to impartiality by laboratory management can be evident from the structure of the organization. This standard addresses the importance of management of laboratory and other activities, which may affect impartiality. Introduction to risk-based approach in this standard is the new concept, which has to be used to identify risk to its impartiality on an ongoing basis. This standard also requires that the identified risk should be eliminated or minimized.

4.2 Confidentiality: The laboratory is responsible for maintaining the confidential information about the sample, organization, etc. It is the responsibility of the laboratory to inform its customer in advance about the information to be put in public domain. It is also required that how the confidential information is to be released if required by laboratory or authorized by contractual arrangements. Mechanism to maintain confidentiality of the information received from complainant, regulators, etc., should be ensured by the laboratory. The laboratory personnel (including committee members, contractors, personal of external bodies, or individuals acting on the laboratory behalf) is also required to comply with confidentiality requirements.

Clause 5—Structural Requirements

Structural requirements are defined, which require: Legal status of the laboratory, identification of laboratory management, range of laboratory activities, organization and management structure, documenting its procedures, availability of personnel responsible for the implementation, maintenance and improvement of the management system, and communication mechanism to ensure integrity of the management system.

Clause 6—Resource Requirements

Resource requirements are addressed in clause 6, which include personnel, facilities and environmental conditions, equipment, metrological traceability, and externally provided products and services.

6.1 General: To manage laboratory activities, it is essential to have competent personnel, suitable facilities, calibrated equipment, and other required services.

6.2 Personnel: The laboratory is required to ensure availability of the competent personnel (internal or external) and they act impartially. It is expected from the laboratory that it should have procedure and records related to competence requirements, selection, training, and supervision of personnel. Laboratory to ensure proper authorization of personnel and competence of personnel is monitored.

6.3 Facilities and environmental conditions: To ensure that the validity of the results is not adversely affected due to facilities and environmental conditions, it is expected from the laboratory to maintain suitable environmental conditions according to the laboratory activities. It is also expected from the laboratory that the environmental conditions are monitor, control, and recorded as per the requirements mentioned in specification, methods, procedure, etc. Measures to control facilities should include access to and use of areas affecting laboratory activities, prevention of contamination, interference or adverse influences on laboratory activities, and effective separation of areas.

6.4 Equipment: The laboratory should have required equipment that is required for the correct performance including procedure for handling, transport, storage, and use and planned maintenance of equipment is required. Equipment requirements are applicable to hardware, software, measurement standards, reference materials, reference data, reagents, consumables, or auxiliary apparatus—whatever is required for achieving correct results during laboratory activities. The laboratory should ensure that the equipment is capable of achieving the measurement accuracy and calibration program is established and followed.

6.5 Metrological traceability: The laboratory is required to maintain metrological traceability of its measurement results. This traceability can be achieved through unbroken chain of calibrations to SI units.

6.6 Externally provided products and services: The laboratory is required to ensure the quality of products and services, which are used during laboratory activities. Procedure is to be made to define, review, and approve the laboratory's requirements for externally provided products and services, defining the criteria for evaluation, selection, monitoring of performance, and re-evaluation of the external providers, ensuring that they conform to requirements provided by laboratory and taking suitable actions, if quality is not as per the specifications.

Clause 7—Process Requirements

7.1 Review of requests, tenders, and contracts: A procedure is required to address the understanding of requirements, which include laboratory's capability and resources, prior approval from customer for the specific laboratory activities performed by the external providers, and selection of appropriate methods which should meet the customers' requirements. When the method requested by customer is considered to be inappropriate or out of date, then the laboratory is required to inform the same to the customer. It is expected that the laboratory shall have decision rule in case when the customer requests a statement of conformity to a specification or standard for the test or calibration (e.g., pass or fail). It is also required that the deviation from the contract should be bring into the notice of customer and if contract is amended after work has been started then due process is to be repeated. In all cases, the laboratory should cooperate with customer.

7.2 Selection, verification, and validation of methods: The laboratory should use suitable method for all its measurement and all these methods should be kept up to date (latest version of standard to be followed). In case when customer has not specified the method, then laboratory has to use appropriate method which includes methods published in international, regional or national standards, or by reputable technical organizations, or in relevant scientific texts or journals, or as specified by the manufacturer of the equipment, or laboratory-developed or laboratory-modified methods. The laboratory should verify that they can properly perform selected methods. Deviations from methods should be accepted only if the deviation has been documented, technically justified, authorized, and accepted by the customer. Nonstandard methods, laboratory-developed methods, and modified standard methods are to be used, if these methods are validated.

7.3 Sampling: This clause is applicable for those laboratories, which are involved exclusively in sampling activities and the laboratory which are taking samples by its own and subsequently doing testing or calibration. In both of the cases, the laboratory should have sampling plan and method which should be available and implemented when the laboratory carries out sampling of substances, materials, or products.

7.4 Handling of test or calibration items: The laboratory should have a procedure for the transportation, receipt, handling, protection, storage, retention and disposal, or return of test or calibration items to protect integrity of the sample. Necessary precautionary measures should be taken to avoid deterioration, contamination, loss, or damage to the sample in any of the activities carried out by the laboratory. Specified conditions are expected to be recorded and the customer to be consulted for next steps. The laboratory has to be maintained and monitored the environmental conditions, whenever specific storage conditions are specified.

7.5 Technical records: The laboratory should address the requirements to retain technical records to ensure the traceability of laboratory activities and provide the exact information in which laboratory activities are performed. The technical records should contain the results, report and sufficient information to facilitate, if possible, identification of factors affecting the measurement result, and its associated measurement uncertainty and enable the repetition of the laboratory activity.

7.6 Evaluation of measurement uncertainty: Testing laboratories are required to evaluate measurement uncertainty considering all significant contributions, including those arising from sampling. In a note, it has been clarified that if laboratory is using well-recognized test method which specifies limits to the values of the major sources of measurement uncertainty and specifies the form of presentation of the calculated results, then laboratory is meeting the standard requirements.

Calibration laboratories are required to evaluate the measurement uncertainty for all calibrations considering all significant contributions, including those arising from sampling.

7.7 Ensuring the validity of results: The laboratory should have a procedure for monitoring the validity of results and the trends are visible. This monitoring should include, but not limited to, use of reference materials or quality control materials, use of alternative instrument, functional checks, use of reference standards with control charts, intermediate checks, replicate tests or calibrations, retesting or recalibration, correlation of results, review of reported results, intralaboratory comparisons, and testing of blind samples.

Wherever available and appropriate, the laboratory should participate in proficiency testing programs. It is expected from the laboratory that if the results of analysis of monitoring data are outside the predefined criteria, then suitable actions to prevent incorrect results should be taken.

7.8 Reporting of results: The laboratory has to be reviewed the results before release. The report should have all information as agreed with the customer and results are provided accurately, clearly, unambiguously, and objectively. Common and specific requirements for reports are stated in the standard. When the laboratory is reporting statements of conformity, then laboratory should apply a decision rule which has to be formulated by using risk-based approach. The laboratory is also required to document on which opinions and interpretations are made. Traceability is to be maintained for all the changes made in the report.

7.9 Complaints: The laboratory should have a documented process for receiving, evaluating, and making decisions on complaints. This process is to be available to any interested party. This process should include the description of complaint receiving process, validity of complaint, investigation of complaint, and actions to be taken. Each complaint has to be tracked and suitable actions should be taken by the laboratory. The outcomes should be communicated to the complainant, which should be made by, or reviewed and approved by, individual(s) not involved in the original laboratory activities in question.

7.10 Nonconforming work: To deal with the nonconforming work, the laboratory should have a procedure in place which includes the responsibilities and authorities for the management of nonconforming work, subsequent actions which are based upon the risk levels, evaluation of the significance of the nonconforming work, decision process for the acceptability of the nonconforming work, process to notify the customer, if necessary, and the responsibility for authorizing the resumption of work.

7.11 Control of data and information management: This clause specifies the requirements for the laboratory information management system(s) used for the collection, processing, recording, reporting, storage, or retrieval of data. It is expected from the laboratory that the laboratory information management system should be protected from unauthorized access, tampering, loss, and maintained to ensure integrity of the data and information.

Clause 8—Management System Requirements

8.1 Options: The laboratory can choose either option A or option B for implementation of management system.

Option A lists the minimum requirements for implementation of a management system in a laboratory, which includes management system documentation, control of management system documents, control of records, actions to address risk and opportunities, improvement, corrective actions, internal audits, and management reviews.

Option B is applicable for those laboratories, which has established and maintained a management system in accordance with the requirements of ISO 9001. Such laboratories are required to demonstrate the consistent fulfillment of the requirements of clauses 4–7 of this standard and also fulfill the intent of the management system as specified in clauses 8.2–8.9 of this standard.

8.2 Management system documentation: The laboratory has to establish and document the management system for maintaining the policies and objectives, which should address the competence, impartiality, and consistent operation of the laboratory. The laboratory should be committed for development and implementation of management system and its effectiveness should be continuously improved.

8.3 Control of management system documents: It is expected from the laboratory that all documents (internal or external) are reviewed and updated periodically, identified changes and the latest standard is available at the points of use; unique identification for all documents and obsolete documents should not be used.

8.4 Control of records: The laboratory should ensure that all records are retained for a period to meet its contractual obligations. Necessary controls are to be implemented for its identification, storage, protection, backup, achieve, retrieval, retention time, and disposal.

8.5 Actions to address risk and opportunities: The laboratory should have an action plan to address risks and opportunities for its management system. By considering risks and opportunities associated with laboratory activities, the laboratory can give assurance to achieve its expected results, enhance opportunities, prevent or reduce undesired impacts, and potential failures in the laboratory activities.

8.6 Improvement: Through strong feedback mechanism, the laboratory has to improve its services on a continuous basis.

8.7 Corrective actions: It is expected from the laboratory that whenever NC is observed, its consequences are to be addressed and immediate actions are to be taken to control and correct it. Measure should be taken to identify cause of NC and eliminate it.

8.8 Internal audits: Laboratory has to conduct internal audit on frequent basis to ensure that the laboratory management system conforms to the standard requirements, its own requirements, and its effective implementation. The laboratory has to plan, establish, implement, and maintain an audit program.

8.9 Management reviews: The laboratory management has to review its management system at planned interval to ensure its continuing suitability, adequacy, and effectiveness. The management review should include changes in internal and external issues that are relevant to the laboratory, fulfillment of objectives, suitability of policies and procedures, status of actions from previous management reviews, outcome of internal audits, corrective actions, assessments by external bodies, changes in the volume and type of the work or in the range of laboratory activities, customer and personnel feedback, complaints, effectiveness of any implemented improvements, adequacy of resources, results of risk identification, outcomes of the assurance of the validity of results, and other relevant factors, such as monitoring activities and training.

■ CONCLUSION

It is essential for any laboratory to have QMS to produce reliable and accurate results. Further to ensure the consistency in the laboratory operation, it is most important that laboratory is having confidence in its management system. This confidence can be achieved through accreditation.

The concept of laboratory accreditation was not in much use before 1970, but now laboratory accreditation is household name in laboratory community. Laboratory accreditation is internationally recognized concept. The ILAC and the APAC are playing pivotal role in international recognition of laboratory accreditation.

LABORATORY ACCREDITATION: A TOOL FOR QUALITY MANAGEMENT SYSTEM

■ DISCLAIMER

Contents of this chapter have been taken from the reference mentioned in further readings. The objective of writing this chapter is to spread awareness about accreditation. Students can be benefitted by this chapter to understand the concept of accreditation, its need, and benefits. In India, the NABL is the AB; hence, accreditation process followed by the NABL (as available on NABL website and its documentation) is taken for reference. The NABL 201 is referred for assessor roles, responsibility, and steps to be followed by assessors and the NABL.

■ FURTHER READINGS

1. Stanton K. Laboratory Accreditation: Origins of a Concept. Australia: National Association of Testing Authorities; 1998. p. 55.
2. ISO Quality management principles.
3. International Organization for Standardization (ISO). (2018). ISO 19011: 2018: Guidelines for auditing management systems. [online] Available from https://www.iso.org/obp/ui/#iso:std:iso:19011:ed-3:v1:en. [Last accessed March, 2021].
4. International Organization for Standardization (ISO). (2017). ISO/IEC 17025: 2017: General requirements for the competence of testing and calibration laboratories. [online] Available from https://www.iso.org/standard/66912.html. [Last accessed March, 2021].
5. National Accreditation Board for Testing and Calibration Laboratories (NABL). (2018). Accreditation process is based on the process defined by NABL on NABL website and corresponding documents.
6. National Accreditation Board for Testing and Calibration Laboratories (NABL). (2016). NABL 210: Assessor Guide. [online] Available from https://nabl-india.org/nabl/file_download.php?filename=201707100431-NABL-210-doc.pdf. [Last accessed March, 2021].
7. Kanipayor R, Bax C, Anastasopoulos G. (2019). The new ISO/IEC 17025:2017: The Updated Standard. [online] Available from https://cannabisindustryjournal.com/feature_article/the-new-iso-iec-170252017-the-updated-standard/. [Last accessed March, 2021].

Chapter 14

Forensic Toxicology Reporting and Interpretation

■ INTRODUCTION

The forensic toxicologist has an important role in analysis and identification of drug and poison in the suspect samples to help in ruling out or confirming the presence of the poison in the sample. The poisoning deaths may be accidental, suicidal, or rarely homicidal. In India, the viscera exhibits in poisoning deaths or suspected cases are preserved by the forensic medicine doctors who conduct the postmortem on the case which is mandatory as per the law. These samples are then forwarded through the investigating officer to the state forensic science laboratories located in the respective state. The toxicology report is collected by the investigating officer and submitted to the forensic medicine doctor for the final opinion on the cause of death. In India, it takes about 3–6 months for the toxicology report due to the heavy load of cases and lack of sufficient forensic science laboratories and manpower.

■ CLASSIFICATION OF POISONS

Drugs and poisons can be classified in many ways. It can be classified alphabetically, pharmacologically, or by chemical structure. However, for analytical purposes, it is more useful and practical to classify poisons according to the method used for extraction. Seven major groups are usually considered:
1. *Gases*: Carbon monoxide (CO), phosphine, cyanide, etc.
2. *Volatile substances*: Ethanol, methanol, ethylene dibromide, chloral hydrate, ethylene glycol, etc.
3. *Drugs*: Barbiturates, benzodiazepines, phenothiazine, salicylates, amitriptyline, opiates and narcotics, amphetamines, etc.
4. *Metals*: Thallium, selenium, lead, mercury, arsenic, antimony, etc.
5. *Pesticides*: Organochlorine and organophosphorus, carbonates, allenthrone, pyrethroids, etc.
6. *Anions*: Bromides, chlorates, fluorides, nitrates, etc.
7. *Miscellaneous substances*: Kaner, Datura, fertilizer, insulin, digitalis, etc.

Gases and volatile are isolated by distillation or by sampling the headspace above the sample held in a closed container. The drugs and pesticides are organic nonvolatile substances isolated by solvent extraction method. Metallic poisons are isolated by ashing, by wet oxidation of the organic matter, or by enzymatic hydrolysis of the tissue. The ions are isolated by dialysis. The miscellaneous poisons will require immunoassay or special extraction techniques such as ion exchange columns, formation of derivatives or ion pairs, freeze drying, and continuous extraction with a polar solvent.

■ GENERAL STEPS IN TOXICOLOGICAL EXAMINATION
1. *Detection*: To detect drugs or poisons in the samples submitted by screening methods
2. *Identification*: To identify conclusively any drugs, metabolites, or poisons present by specific relevant physiochemical confirmatory test
3. *Quantification*: To quantify accurately those drugs, metabolites, or poisons present
4. *Interpretation*: To interpret the analytical findings in (2) and (3) in the context of the case, the information given, and the question asked by the investigating officer

■ OBJECTIVES OF TOXICOLOGY REPORTING
In cases of death due to suspected poisoning, relevant biological samples are preserved by forensic pathologist for toxicological analysis. In some case, the evidence of particular poison may be present at the scene or at the autopsy which can give a hint to the toxicologist to directly test for that substance. However, in many cases, the forensic expert and the investigating officer may not get any specific hint or clue to guide the toxicologist and the toxicologist cannot practically screen for all poisons. In such cases, the forensic toxicologist can screen for the common poisons or general drug screening (GDS). This list of common poisons may vary from region to region.

After analyzing the sample, the forensic toxicologist has to answer the following questions:
1. Whether any poison was detected?
2. If the poison was detected, what was the level of the poison?

Even when the cause of death is clear, a GDS may be required in case of suspected intoxication. GDS is a broad-spectrum analysis for many drugs. The GDS usually involves methods such as thin-layer chromatography (TLC), gas-liquid chromatography (GLC), high-performance liquid chromatography (HPLC), and gas chromatography (GC) mass and is applicable to many different specimens, including urine, blood, gastric lavage, and tissue homogenates.

■ WAYS OF EXPRESSING REPORT
Forensic toxicology reports are usually expressed in different ways by different laboratories. Here are some patters of reporting:
1. Common poison could not be detected in the exhibit.

It indicates that the viscera have been examined for all the common poisons and none of these was found positive.
2. On chemical, microscopic, TLC and GC-HS examination, metallic poisons, ethyl and methyl alcohol, cyanide, phosphide, alkaloids, barbiturates, tranquilizers, and pesticides could not be detected in the exhibits.
3. Sample is not fit for analysis or sample is insufficient for analysis.

Sometime, sample received for analysis is in decomposed or dried form. Moreover, quantity may be very less to carry out all the possible analysis. In such condition, it is reported in this way.

Example: In burn cases, if the blood is completely charred and dried, in the case of alcohol, if the sample is not preserved properly in sodium fluoride and analyzed within few days, it gets decomposed and results are not dependable.
4. Various laboratory tests such as color tests, chromatographic analysis and Kozelka–Hine Method were carried out with the exhibits-1, 2, 3 and 4 for the detection of common insecticide, volatile, metallic/inorganic, gaseous and sedative poisons in them. The results thus obtained have been analyzed as given below:
   i. Ethyl alcohol has been detected in exhibits-1, 2 and 3
   ii. The percentage of ethyl alcohol in exhibit-3 was found to be 165.08 mg%

None of the above said common poisons was detected in exhibit 4.

It is a good practice to specify the group or specific poison screened, instrument used and its limitations. It will assist in the better interpretation of the results. The toxicologists are discouraged from including interpretive comments on the toxicology report. The sample of forensic toxicology reporting form of the Forensic Science Laboratory (FSL), Delhi and the Central Forensic Science Laboratory (CFSL), Hyderabad is shown in **Annexures I** and **II**, respectively.

As per our observation, the forensic toxicological laboratories in India usually give the qualitative report only except for the alcohol. Probably there is limitation of sophisticated instruments or trained scientists. But it affects the interpretation of the results. Therefore, the quantitative report should be given wherever possible. The FSLs in India generally maintain a list of common poisons screened in their laboratories. The names of the common poisons screened should be mentioned in the report as the list of common poisons screened may vary for different laboratories.

The following are the list of common poisons generally tested in India in the FSLs:
1. Cyanide
2. Ethyl alcohol
3. Methyl alcohol
4. Phosphide
5. Metallic poisons such as Pb, As, Sb, Hg, Bi, etc.
6. Acidic extracts for barbiturates, etc.
7. Basic extract for alkaloids and its derivatives

8. Neutral hexane extract
9. Organochlorine compounds
10. Organophosphorus compounds
11. Carbamates
12. Pyrethroids
13. Miscellaneous such as Datura particles, kaner, bhang, etc.

■ LEGAL STANDING OF THE TOXICOLOGY REPORT

As per Section 293 in the Code of Criminal Procedure (CrPC), 1973, the report signed by any chemical examiner or assistant chemical examiner as a scientific expert of the government upon any matter or thing duly submitted to him for examination or analysis, report may be admitted as evidence without requiring the officer concerned to be examined in court to prove the report. The court may, if it thinks fit, summon and examine any such expert as to the subject matter of his report. Wherever, any such expert is summoned by a court and he is unable to attend personally, he may, unless the court has expressly directed him to appear personally, depute any responsible officer working with him to attend the court, if such officer is conversant with the facts of the case and can satisfactorily depose in court on his behalf. No hard and fast rule can be laid down regarding the value attached to the report. Chemical examiner does not give opinion as to cause of death. He merely gives report of chemical examination of samples sent to him. Report is a piece of scientific evidence and does not require any formal proof. The report is forwarded to the forensic pathologist who conducted the autopsy. The forensic pathologist in the light of the autopsy findings, toxicology report and circumstantial findings gives the opinion about the final cause of death.

■ INTERPRETATION OF RESULTS

In India, the toxicology report from the FSL is sent to the investigating officer of the case. The report is then submitted to the forensic expert who conducted the autopsy on the deceased for finalizing the opinion on the cause of death. The forensic expert has to interpret the report as to the physiological effects of the analytes in respect to their concentration and the postmortem findings. Interpretation generally requires a holistic approach, considering all relevant information in formulating an opinion. The forensic toxicologists are discouraged from including interpretive comments on toxicology reports. It must be remembered that forensic experts must be aware that it is mandatory the collaboration of a forensic toxicologist in the interpretation of toxicology results. Although there is no universally accepted standard education, the forensic toxicologist should be endowed with adequate training in analytical chemistry, but especially in depth knowledge of the toxicokinetic of poisons and be attentive for variables that can influence them. It would be advisable that the collection procedure of forensic expert can be audited by toxicologists to avoid errors. Absolute rules for the interpretation of toxicological results are absent, since each case is unique. It is almost impossible to know the true concentration of a poison in a sample. Attempts to interpret toxicology findings exclusively based on the therapeutic, toxic, and fatal ranges are irreversible, especially in postmortem toxicology. These intervals frequently overlap.

The specific questions that must be answered are whether the concentration of any analyte or combination of analytes were:
1. Sufficient to cause death or is this a fatal level
2. Sufficient to have affected the actions of the deceased so as to cause the death
3. Insufficient to have any involvement in the cause of death
4. Insufficient to protect the individual from an underlying mechanism of death such as an epileptic seizure (therapeutic drugs)

It is the prerogative of the investigating officer or the judge to decide the manner of death, whether the poisoning was suicidal, accidental, or homicidal, but the forensic expert can assist them to come to a logical conclusion on the basis of toxicological report and postmortem findings and other circumstantial evidences.

The forensic expert must take into account many factors, while interpreting the toxicology report.
1. *Route of administration*: The route of administration, together with the nature of the dosage form, determines the rate and extent of absorption. Administration by inhalation, intravenous, or intramuscular injection leads to a high bioavailability and quick and often intense response, while oral administration produces lower concentration of longer duration. Thus, a fatal drug dose given intravenously is often much smaller than a fatal dose given by mouth because the injected drug is able to reach the site of action very rapidly. The most common methods of administration of poisons are oral, intravenous, and inhalation. In poisoning cases, the route may not be always known unless the evidence is found at the scene such as syringe and the deceased has very recent injection marks. There may also be tablets found in the stomach on autopsy indicating an oral route of administration. The other findings, such as extremely high lung concentrations of drug or chemical, are suggestive of an inhalation route. It must be remembered that drug administered intravenously can cause death in a lower dose than those found in oral overdoses. It also should be noted that some drugs are absorbed very rapidly such as tricyclic antidepressant and even when massive overdoses are ingested, only traces may be found in the gastric content.
2. *Synergistic effect of drugs*: It is important to know that drugs taken in combination can be more toxic than if considered separately. Knowledge of the interaction of toxicant is important for proper interpretation of the toxicity of the analyte. Most analytes are more toxic in the presence of alcohol, especially the barbiturates. The use of cocaine or amphetamine in combination with diamorphine (heroin) is more toxic than one drug alone.

3. Age, sex, body weight, genetic factors, tolerance, environmental exposure, and general health states of the individual. All these factors can influence the response of a given concentration of an analyte or combination of analytes. For example, a patient of liver diseases may prevent the metabolism of analytes, resulting in the accumulation of the drug to toxic concentration.
4. Whether drug/poison is therapeutic, chronic high level, or acute overdose. It is common to find blood levels in case of acute poisoning that fall within therapeutic range either because death has occurred rapidly or has occurred in a considerable time after ingestion or metabolism has destroyed the bulk of poison.
5. When the presence of even trace amount of highly toxic substance is established, the cause of death may be justified as poisoning.
6. In case of poisoning by ingestion, the amount remaining in the stomach at death is what remains after vomiting and absorption. When a small amount is found in the alimentary canal, then the question arises whether it is the residue of toxic dose or therapeutic dose. An important source of variable absorption is through oral dosing, since this route is probably the most common. Most of the variable is related to any first-pass metabolism that occurs for drugs with low bioavailability. A number of factors can influence bioavailability. These include the motility of the stomach and bowel, pH, and (for a small number of drugs) activity of gut enzymes that metabolize the drug before it is even absorbed.
7. In case of poisoning by CO, total hemoglobin also has to be taken into consideration, because at a particular carboxyhemoglobin (COHb) level, it will indicate different pictures in two people having different Hb level. Secondly, in the fire deaths, it is always advisable to analyze the blood for cyanide along with CO because in these cases, person may die due to low CO levels but as a cumulative effect of cyanide and CO produced in fire due to burning of plastic. Otherwise, low levels of CO may indicate early death due to shock, coexistence of any respiratory or circulatory deficiency, anemia, or drugs such as barbiturates.
8. It has been observed that values vary between blood samples taken from different sites on the same body. These anatomical site concentration differences have shown that in most cases, femoral blood is more likely to be a better indicator of the postmortem concentration of the analyte.
9. *Postmortem drug redistribution*: Blood drug concentrations change significantly with increasing postmortem period. The concentrations tend to increase with increasing postmortem interval. The drugs, such as tricyclic antidepressant, have shown to be higher in the postmortem period than in the premortem period.

Hence, the case should be interpreted taking into account antemortem or postmortem toxicology results, circumstances of the death and scene, medical history, autopsy findings, influence of postmortem redistribution, tolerance, application of common sense, etc.

FORENSIC TOXICOLOGY REPORTING AND INTERPRETATION

■ CAUSES OF FALSE-NEGATIVE REPORT

In some cases, the history, circumstances, and the postmortem findings may clearly suggest that poisoning is the most likely cause of death but the toxicology report may be still negative.

The possible explanations of false-negative reports are:

1. As stated earlier, in the case where the victim/deceased was admitted in the hospital for a considerable time, the possibility of detecting poison in the viscera gets lesser. In such conditions, often viscera report may be negative in real poisoning cases and some other substances other than the poison may come positive which was taken in the hospital for therapeutic reason such as promethazine, etc. The medication itself may alter the poisonous substance and make its detection difficult or even impossible. Hence, it is important to know about the treatment records.
2. Insufficient biological material, such as tissue, blood, urine, etc., for analysis.
3. In postmortem decomposition, many poisons present in the tissue undergo chemical changes which cannot be detected. Putrefaction of normal tissue may produce substances, which may give chemical reactions similar to those obtained from toxic compounds. Most volatile compounds are lost due to putrefaction.
4. The whole poison may disappear from the lungs in case of volatile poison by evaporation or oxidation due to faulty preservation such as dried up blood sample. Organic solvent poison gets evaporated during extraction and concentration.
5. The poison might have been vomited out, excreted, neutralized, metabolized, and detoxified to such a quality that it cannot be detected by general scheme of chemical analysis and by available methods of chemical analysis. The poison after absorption may be detoxified and eliminated.
6. Some vegetable alkaloids cannot be detected by chemical analysis.
7. It is well known that usual routine toxicological screening procedures may not detect hemoglobin such as COHb, sulfmethemoglobin and methemoglobin, diuretics, solvents, radioactive compounds, antibiotics, nonsteroidal anti-inflammatory substances, except aspirin and paracetamol, calcium channel blockers, and beta-blockers.
8. Some drugs are rapidly metabolized and there may be complete metabolism of the poison in the body. Drugs, such as haloperidol and oxycodone, are rapidly metabolized and only metabolite can be detected. Early disintegration of poison, like IV narcotism, the substances are rapidly metabolized and create difficulty in analysis. Some drugs have short half-life and are rapidly metabolized. In delayed death cases, poison may be excreted or detoxified completely.
9. Biological toxins and snake venom are protein and cannot be separated from the body tissues. Immunoassay method may detect these poisons, but this facility is not easily available in all laboratories.

10. Some organic poisons decompose due to improper preservation. Drugs, which have been found to decompose during the storage at 40°C, are clonazepam, cocaine, isoniazid (INH), methadone, morphine, and nitrazepam. Cocaine gets hydrolyzed in alkaline medium. Alkaloids and phenothiazines, such as lysergic acid diethylamide (LSD) and psilocybin, are photolabile. Catecholamines are easily oxidized, if container is not airtight.
11. Some drugs are in very small amount and need considerable amount of viscera and sensitive analysis procedures. For example, amphetamine may be undetected in the blood owing to very low concentration present, even after fatal dose. Many potent drugs, such as clonidine, ergot alkaloids, dioxin, digoxin, and tetrahydrocannabinol (THC), pose such problems.
12. Diamorphine (heroin) is rarely detected as it gets rapidly hydrolyzed to 6-monoacetylmorphine, which is present in urine in small concentration.
13. Some inorganics are too polar, e.g., Hg, phosphorus.
14. Anesthetics are mostly esters and get hydrolyzed at room temperature. Many highly volatile substances, such as aromatic and halogenated hydrocarbons, solvents, anesthetic agents, noxious gases such as hydrogen sulfide (H_2S), CO, and nitric oxide (NO_2), behave in this manner.
15. Some substances, such as fentanyl, may have structural dissimilarity from their drug class prototype and give negative results for that particular group.
16. Tampering of viscera during preservation and in preserved bottles with vested interests or wrong motive. Addition of strong chemicals, such as soap, bleach powder, or glutaraldehyde, alters the results in immunoassay.
17. Use of wrong analytical techniques.
18. Some laboratories do not test for drugs, enzymes, and toxins.
19. Poor laboratory quality assurance and defective analysis, as many laboratories are not accredited and upgraded with modern facilities.
20. As a protocol, substances detected may not be reported as these are naturally occurring substances or are constituents of the body such as phosphates.
21. Nonavailability of sophisticated instrument such as GC mass, LC mass, etc.
22. Lack of expertise, qualified, and experienced toxicologists.

It has been observed by many researchers in routine practice that too polar such as INH, iron, lead and ethyl glycol, volatile-like solvents, and aromatic or halogenated hydrocarbons gases; nonvolatile such as plant or fungal alkaloids; low concentration such as very potent drugs and substances; toxic anions such as thiocyanate, cyanide, fluoride, and nitrites; and new substances such as buspirone are not detected by conventional toxicological screening.

A negative screen does not necessarily mean that a toxin is not present. It says only that none on the list of those that were screened has been found.

FORENSIC TOXICOLOGY REPORTING AND INTERPRETATION

■ CAUSES OF FALSE-POSITIVE REPORT

1. *Decomposition*: When the sample is not properly preserved and sent for analysis after a lapse of time, there is every possibility of postmortem production of ethyl alcohol, cyanide, CO, ketones, sulfides, etc., which can give false-positive result. Therefore, it should always be taken into consideration before finalizing the report. In such cases, interpretation needs extra attention. It is observed that the autogenous production of alcohol in tissues of decomposed body may occur due to the action of certain microorganism. This may result in a blood alcohol concentration (BAC) up to 30 mg/100 mL even in a person who has not consumed alcohol prior to his death. In general, in the absence of other information or available specimens, one can estimate that a BAC of 30 mg% or higher was the result of antemortem ingestion. Although this criterion cannot absolutely distinguish between antemortem ingestion and postmortem synthesis of ethanol, it presents a valuable initial guide for postmortem interpretation. There is no known correlation between the degree of putrefaction of a specimen and the production of ethanol. It is advised to analyze multiple samples from different anatomical sites such as vitreous humor and urine. If ethanol is detected in blood, but is not detected in vitreous humor and urine, it can be assumed that postmortem alcohol production has occurred. It is also known that there is sporadic production of small amount of CO (10%) in stored blood. Amines are also produced in putrefaction, which may interfere with drug analysis. In general, putrefactive bases tend to give reactions expected of simple primary and secondary aliphatic amines and also complex tertiary amine structures found in alkaloid drugs and thus, these substances can create considerable interference problems. The presence of interfering phenolic substances can also be expected. In the putrefied tissue, there is also possibility of phosphine production from bacterial reduction of phosphate. This may cause difficulty in the interpretation of the result in the suspected case of zinc or aluminum phosphide poisoning because phosphine is the major metabolite of these poisons. Therefore, it is important to absorb the H_2S gas in the putrefied sample before testing for phosphide to avoid false-positive result. Fatty liver and intestine walls not containing poison may produce a yellow stain on the silver nitrate paper, which is of no significance. However, insecticide such as parathion is relatively stable compound and even in exhumed body, it is worth trying if parathion poisoning is suspected.
2. *Using wrong preservative*: If viscera is preserved in formalin or denatured spirit, it may give false-positive test as these are contaminated with methanol, butanol, and copper sulfate.
3. False-positive results in immunoassays are mainly due to cross-reactivity and structural similarity. For example, false-positive reaction for opiate group can be seen on consumption of poppy seeds, chlorpromazine, dextromethorphan, and diphenyl oxalate tablets. There may be false-positive reaction for amphetamine due to cross-reactivity on account of consumption of ephedrine nasal drops, pseudoephedrine in cough

syrups, chloroquine, and procainamide. Phencyclidine is falsely represented by dextromethorphan, diphenhydramine, doxylamine, and thioridazine.
4. Faulty instrument and lack of standardization may lead to false-positive or false-negative results.
5. Faulty figures of substances in reporting due to human error on viscera examination from laboratories. It is suggested that chemical examination report should not be taken as a gospel truth in each and every case.
6. Tampering of viscera during preservation and in preserved bottles with vested interests or wrong motive.

CONCLUSION

Orfila is considered as the father of toxicology. He established many of the guiding principles of toxicology, which still holds true today. They are as follows:
1. Experience is paramount for credibility and reliability.
2. All facts surrounding the case must be given to the analysts.
3. All the evidences must be submitted properly, identified and labeled, and sealed.
4. All tests should be run and properly recorded.
5. Reagents must be pure and control samples free of the analytes of interest must be tested.
6. All tests must be repeated and compared with specimens to whom known amounts of the analytes of interest have been added.

It is mandatory that positive test using one methodology preferably should be confirmed with another technique, whenever major decisions are based on the results. A combination of the clinical examination findings of the patient, treatment records, autopsy appearances, and spot tests with toxicological laboratory report play a major role in concluding the final opinion. We have seen many cases of clear poisoning, such as celphos and baygon, brought to the emergency, diagnosed and treated, admitted in the ward, and expired after few days. However, the viscera analysis report has come negative for the poison consumed. Therefore, the toxicological report should not be treated as the gospel truth. In such cases, the doctor may conclude the case based on the findings of treatment records and autopsy findings. In this case, the treatment records prepared by the first hand treating physician play a vital role along with the supporting autopsy findings. The court has not objected to such opinion as long as it is scientific and authentic. Above all, it is important for the forensic toxicologist to apply the best possible way of analyzing the biological sample, reporting and interpreting the report in the context of the case, and help the investigating officer to come to a logical conclusion. In any laboratory, experience, availability of facts, proper chain of custody, pure reagents, double confirmation, and repetition of tests still hold the key of success for good laboratory report. The doctor who conducts the autopsy has to interpret the toxicology report in the light of his knowledge of the history, clinical features, treatment records, and autopsy findings.

FORENSIC TOXICOLOGY REPORTING AND INTERPRETATION

■ FURTHER READINGS

1. Bailey DN, Dyke CV, Langou RA, Jatlow Pl. Tricyclic antidepressants: plasma levels and clinical findings in overdose. Am J Psychiatry. 1978;135:1325-8.
2. Ballantyne B, Marrs T, Syversen T. General and Applied Toxicology, 2nd edition. London: Macmillan Publishers Ltd.; 2000.
3. Negrusz A, Cooper G. Clarke's Analytical Forensic Toxicology, 2nd edition. London: Pharmaceutical Press; 2013.
4. ÓNeal CL, Poklis A. Postmortem production of ethanol and factors that influence interpretation: a critical review. Am J Forensic Med Pathol. 1996;17:8-20.
5. Clark MA, Jones JW. Studies on putrefactive ethanol production. J Forensic Sci. 1982;2:366-71.
6. Nelson LS, Howland MA, Lewin NA, Smith SW, Goldfrank LR, Hoffman RS. Goldfrank's Toxicologic Emergencies, 11th edition. California: Tata McGraw Hill; 1990.
7. Jickells S, Negrusz A. Clarke's Analytical Forensic Toxicology, 1st edition. London: Pharmaceutical Press; 2008.
8. Levine B, Smith ML, Smialek JE, Caplan YH. Interpretation of low postmortem concentrations of ethanol. J Forensic Sci. 1993;38:663-7.
9. Murty OP. Postmortem production of alcohol in viscera. Int J Med Tox Leg Med. 2002;4:34-5.
10. Osterloh JD. Laboratory diagnosis and drug screening. In: Osterloh JD (Ed). Clinical Management of Poisoning and Drug Overdose, 3rd edition. Philadelphia: WB Saunders Company; 1998.
11. Prouty R, Anderson W. The forensic science implication of site and temporal influences on postmortem blood drug concentrations. J Forensic Sci. 1990;35:243-70.
12. Sarkar PC. Criminal Major Acts: A Complete Handbook, 6th edition, New Delhi: Orient Law Book House; 2015.
13. Sharma VK, Badkur DS, Satpathy DK. Artefacts in the estimation of carboxyhaemoglobin in burn deaths. Int J Med Tox Leg Med. 1999;2:21-3.
14. Sharma VK. Poisons, viscera analysis, report and its interpretation. Int J Med Tox Leg Med. 1999;6:49-54.
15. Singh RK, Chandra H. Estimation of postmortem production and loss of ethanol in blood with respect to duration of storage at room temperature. Int J Med Tox Leg Med. 1999;2:21-3.
16. Society of Forensic Toxicologists (SOFT)/American Academy of Forensic Sciences (AAFS). (2006). Forensic Toxicology Laboratory Guidelines: 2006 Version. [online] Available from http://www.soft-tox.org/files/Guidelines_2006_Final.pdf. [Last accessed March, 2021].
17. Tabin M, Jaiswal AK, Jhamad AR, Murty OP. Forensic toxicology: reporting and interpretation. Indian J Criminol Criminal. 2010;31:76-85.
18. Winek DL. Reliability of 22 hours postmortem blood and gastric alcohol samples. JAMA. 1975;233:912.
19. Mortuary manual. Department of Forensic Medicine and Toxicology. New Delhi: AIIMS; 2018.

FORENSIC TOXICOLOGY REPORTING AND INTERPRETATION

Annexure I: Forensic toxicology reporting form—Forensic Science Laboratory (FSL), Government of NCT of Sector 14, Rohini, Delhi-110085.

REPORT No. FSL: Dated:

1. Please quote the report (opinion) no. and date in all future correspondence and summons.
2. This report is per se admission U/S. 293 CrPC.

To

The Station House Officer

PS:

New Delhi

Your letter No. _____ dated _____ regarding one parcel in connection with case DD No. _____ dated _____ U/S _____ PS duly received in this office on _____ through constable _____ No. _____.

DESCRIPTION OF PARCEL(S)

Sealed corrugated box: 1 (one)

One sealed parcel marked as "1". Seals were intact and tallied with the specimen seal as per forwarding letter (FSL Form).

DESCRIPTION OF ARTICLES CONTAINED IN THE PARCEL(S)/EXHIBIT(S)

Parcel-"1":

Exhibit-"1A":

Exhibit-"1B":

Exhibit-"1C":

Exhibit-"1D":

RESULTS OF EXAMINATION

On chemical and TLC examination, metallic poisons, ethyl and methyl alcohol, cyanide, phosphide, alkaloids, barbiturates, tranquilizers and pesticides _____ in exhibits _____.

Note: Case exhibits/remnants of exhibits sent to this laboratory for examination have been sealed with the seal of "AR FSL Delhi".

(Authorized Signatory)

FORENSIC TOXICOLOGY REPORTING AND INTERPRETATION

Annexure II: Forensic toxicology reporting form—Central Forensic Science Laboratory (CFSL), MoH, Govt of India Hyderabad, Andhra Pradesh-500013.

EXAMINATION REPORT
[Admissible under Section 293 Code of Criminal Procedure (CrPC) of India]

1. Report No.:_____ Dt. __ /__ /__
2. No. of pages of Report
3. Ref. No.: Dt. __ /__ /__ From:
4. Case/FIR/DD/RC No.: Dt. __ /__ /__ U/S: _____ PS
5. Mode of receipt:
6. Date of receipt:
7. Article(s) received:
8. Details of the parcels/exhibits received:

Parcel No.	No. of seals and impression	Description of exhibits
		One sealed cardboard box containing four sealed glass jars, marked as exhibits 1, 2, 3, and 4, respectively, relating to the deceased .... Age/Sex .... (PM No .... Dt. __ /__ /__)
		Exhibit-1:
		Exhibit-2:
		Exhibit-3:
		Exhibit-4:

9. Condition of the seal(s)/parcel(s):
10. Purpose of reference:
11. Dates of examination:

RESULTS OF EXAMINATION REPORT
(Use separate sheets, if necessary)

The exhibits were analyzed by color tests, chemical tests, and chromatographic techniques.

FORENSIC TOXICOLOGY REPORTING AND INTERPRETATION

The result of examination, thus, obtained was as follows:

Ref: Working Procedure Manual of Toxicology, DFS, MHA, New Delhi.

Note:
1. Results related only to the exhibits tested.
2. Reports shall not be reproduced except in full, without the written approval of the Director.
3. After the examination, the remnants of the exhibits have been sealed with the seal of CFSL, Toxicology, Hyderabad.

Specimen Seal   Examined by:

                                  Name:

                                  Designation:

(*Note*: If evidence is required, correspondence may be made with examining officer)

I caused it examined and forwarded to _____.

Director

CFSL, Hyderabad

Endst. No. _____   Dated_____

The sealed case report along with/without case property in _____ handed over to Const. _____ No. _____ of P.S. _____ or sent by post on _____.

Director

CFSL Hyderabad

FORENSIC TOXICOLOGY REPORTING AND INTERPRETATION

Annexure III: Viscera Forwarding Letter

All India Institute of Medical Sciences
Department of Forensic Medicine and Toxicology
New Delhi India
Ph. No. 91-11-26593202 Fax No. 91-11-26588663

PM No.:   Dated:

The Director

CFSL/SFSL/RFSL

Through DCP, South/South East Delhi

Dear Sir,

I am sending herewith a sealed box containing the viscera of deceased.

Mr./Ms.: ....

S/D/W of .... Age .... Sex ....

PM No. .... dated ....

R/o ....

for chemical analysis to determine intoxication/poisoning. Details of viscera are as follows:

Jar No. 1:   A. Stomach with contents.   B. Segment of small intestine with contents

Jar No. 2:   A. Liver section   B. Spleen full   C. Kidney (half of each). D. Other viscera

Bottle No. 3: Sample of preservative used: saturated solution of common salt.

Bottle No. 4: Blood of the deceased.

Also find enclosed a sample of seal. The IO has to submit the copy of postmortem report and details of investigative findings which can be of help in chemical analysis of viscera.

Thanking you,

Yours Faithfully

Signature..

Name of the Doctor...........................

Designation..

Department of Forensic Medicine and Toxicology

All the above necessary papers, wooden box containing the viscera and blood under six seals, handed over to PC ....

No. .... PS ....

New Delhi on ....

Chapter 15

Do's and Don'ts for Different Personnel Involved in Crime Investigation of Poisoning Deaths

■ INTRODUCTION

The investigation of poisoning deaths is a common challenge faced by the forensic pathologists, forensic toxicologists, and the police investigating officer. The manner of death may be accidental, suicidal, or homicidal. The homicidal poisoning deaths are the most difficult case to handle. The investigation commences from the visit of the scene of death, followed by collection of relevant evidences, statements of the eye witnesses, deceased's hospital medical history, and treatment documents. The autopsy and toxicological report forms vital positive evidence in proving the case of homicidal poisoning deaths. In homicidal poisoning, the investigation officer has to prove that the death has taken place by poisoning, the accused had the poison in his possession, and the accused had the opportunity to administer poison to the deceased. The circumstantial evidence can play an important role. This article deals with detailed guideline of do's and don'ts for the personnel involved in the investigation of deaths due to poisoning such as police officers, forensic toxicologists, and the medical officers. It can be a useful checklist when dealing with such cases.

■ GENERAL INSTRUCTIONS FOR EXAMINING SCENE OF CRIME

Usually, the police officer and the crime scene investigation team are the first to reach the scene of incidence. The place of incident may be the home, hotel room, park area, secluded jungle area, etc.

Do's

1. Immediately secure the scene of incident to prevent any interference and loss of trace evidence, till all details are recorded, samples collected, and photographed.
2. Search for the cause and source of poison or agent administered such as medicinal drugs, domestic or industrial compounds, insecticide/rodenticide, gas, etc.

3. If some medicinal drugs have been consumed, then find out the name of the drug, amount, quantity found unused, amount prescribed, date of prescription, date of dispensation, name of the doctor, and pharmacy.
4. Search for the motive behind the poisoning.
5. Look for the method of administration of poison.
6. Find out from whom poison was obtained or from where it was brought or bought?
7. For which/what purpose was it brought?
8. Is there any remnant portion of the poison? Where it was found and in which form? Search for it.
9. Is it accidental, suicidal, or homicidal poisoning? Look for clues from the scene of occurrence.
10. Is there any suicidal note? Was there any history of prior attempts or threats of suicide?
11. Ask about the last meal taken, its constituents, and time of intake.
12. What was the interval between last meal and commencement of symptoms?
13. Was any medical assistance given before death? Get the medical records.
14. Where was the dead body found?
15. What things were found near the body?
16. How was the clothing? Was it soiled or stained?
17. Was there any struggle mark or sign on the scene? (If yes, it could be a homicidal poisoning).
18. Was the body displaced from original scene? Why it was displaced? Examine the primary place.
19. Give every minute detail of the body appearance in *panchnama*.
20. Look for any unusual mark on the body (any injury or injection mark, bite mark, etc.).
21. Take color photographs of the scene and the seized items.
22. Send the body for postmortem (PM) as early as possible.
23. Ask the autopsy doctor regarding type of poison, effect on the body, internal findings and to preserve the relevant parts (viscera) for chemical analysis, and confirmation of poison.

When investigating a case of suspicious death due to poisoning, take particular care to see that the investigation is meticulous and obtain the following detailed information:
1. Was the deceased in good health before the incident?
2. If he was not in good health, what was he suffering from?
3. What medicine was he taking?
4. What were the first symptoms and signs?
   - Was he thirsty?
   - Did he faint?
   - Did he complain of headache or giddiness?
   - Did he appear to have lost the use of his limbs?
   - Did he sleep heavily?
   - Was he at any time insensible?
   - Did convulsions occur?

- Did he complain of any particular taste in his mouth?
- Did he notice any peculiar taste in his food or drink?
- Was he sensible in the intervals between the convulsions?
- Did he complain of burning or tingling in the mouth and throat or of numbness and tingling in the limbs?
- Was there any vomiting?
- Was there purging?
- Was there any pain in the stomach?
- Mention any other symptoms and signs?
- Had he ever suffered previously from a similar attack?
5. How many other persons took the meal or food or drink by which the deceased is supposed to have been poisoned?
6. How many were affected and in which way?
7. Did the deceased move from the place where the first symptom was noticed, if so, how far?
8. If the deceased vomited before death, secure the vomited matter in a clean glass container, seal it, label it along with your signature, and hand it over to the police for toxicological analysis.

Don'ts
1. Do not test or smell the poisons found on the spot of scene or nearby.
2. Do not leave any related physical evidence on the scene.
3. Do not leave any poisonous remain on the scene.
4. Do not overcrowd the scene of incident to avoid contamination and interference.

■ DO'S AND DON'TS FOR COLLECTION AND PRESERVATION OF SAMPLES

Do's
1. Collect the poison remains from the scene or near the body.
   - If solid, pack it in airtight polythene bag.
   - If liquid, pack it in airtight nonleaking plastic or glass container with screw cap and then in airtight polythene bag.
   - If gas, by suction in airtight tube.
2. Poison remains should be collected and packed in original form.
3. Collect vomiting or stomach wash from home or hospital and it should be collected in transparent glass or plastic jar with screw cap which must be nonleaking and airtight.
4. Sample of food consumed should be preserved.
5. Vomiting, if on cloths, cloths should be shade dried and then packed in airtight polythene bags.
6. Empty wrappers, medicine bottles, utensils, glasses, cups, etc., related to poisoning must be collected, packed properly, and sent with viscera for analysis.

7. Vomitus-stained soil should be collected with control sample in plastic jar.
8. Any syringe, needle, or such type of things found nearby body or in suspicious state should be collected and packed in clean polythene bag and sent for analysis.
9. The autopsy doctor should be asked to collect blood and urine sample with viscera for chemical analysis.
10. If there is any bite mark or injection mark found on the body, ask the autopsy doctor to preserve the skin and subcutaneous tissue for analysis.
11. Viscera should be collected in wide mouth bottle of glass or plastic jar (airtight and leak proof) with screw cap. The best preservative is alcohol (rectified spirit) and after that is saturated saline solution. But saturated solution of common salt is the most commonly used preservative as it is easily available and cheap.
12. Viscera should be collected in two separate glass jars. First jar should contain stomach and small and large intestine. Second jar should contain liver, lung, kidney, heart, brain, and relevant organs.
13. Blood and urine should also be collected in separate glass jars.
14. Sample of preservative must be sent in small bottle with viscera.
15. Amount of preservative in jar must be more than the viscera, so that the viscera are completely immersed in preservative.
16. Proper preservative should be used by doctor according to the nature of poison.

Don'ts

1. Do not send cloths (with vomit) in wet condition for analysis (fungus growth and decomposition will take place).
2. Do not contaminate the sample by careless handling or using unclean containers.
3. Do not add any chemical compound except the preservative.
4. Do not use spirit as preservative in case of alcohol poisoning.
5. Do not completely fill the viscera container and keep some free space to accommodate the gas formation.

■ DO'S AND DON'TS FOR PACKING/LABELING THE SAMPLES

Do's

1. All viscera samples should be preserved in wide mouth jar of plastic or glass.
2. Packing must be leak proof and airtight.
3. All articles should be packed separately to avoid the contamination.
4. All articles should be packed properly and sealed.
5. The seal must be on the knot of the thread or bandage strip so that the article will be intact.
6. Every article must be labeled and marked properly in sequential order of seizure.

7. Label of each article must contain the following information: (1) police station, (2) district, (3) crime or first information report (FIR) no./Indian Penal Code (IPC) section, (4) name of deceased, s/o, d/o, w/o, (5) age, (6) sex, (7) date of PM (in viscera), (8) article label must be on the top of the article in capital letters, and (9) signature of IO and date.
8. Articles sealed in acrolite (transparent) box are better than in wooden box.
9. Seal on the article must be authentic, proper, full, and legible.
10. Sample of seal must be sent with the memo (doctor's medicolegal seal and IO personal or PS seal).
11. Packing and sealing of the article should be done properly, so that inside material cannot be tampered without breaking of seal.
12. A designated staff should be assigned for sealing the samples under the supervision of the autopsy doctor.
13. Doctor and IO should attest sample of seal accordingly.

Don'ts
1. Do not forget to countercheck the label, when it is done by staff under you, before signing.
2. Do not use low quality containers or sealing material or label.

DO'S AND DON'TS FOR DISPATCH AND FORWARDING THE SAMPLES
Do's
1. Article should be sent to laboratory for analysis as early as possible (time lapse destroys the evidences).
2. Draft form (memo) must contain the brief history of case.
3. With the memo, the following documents must be sent (attested photocopies):
   - FIR or first information report
   - Panchnama
   - Postmortem report
   - Medical treatment papers
   - Dying declaration, if any
   - Sample of seal
4. Memo should be addressed to the director/chemical examiner and forwarded by the SP or DCP or by the authorized person with proper seal and sign with date.
5. In memo, the details of the articles must be very clear and described properly.
6. Memo should include the name and identification of the person who is coming to deposit the article in laboratory for analysis, so that the legal continuity of chain of evidence is maintained.
   - If forensic scientist has visited the scene, his report regarding scene of crime (SOC) visits must be included and sent with memo to the

laboratory, which will enlighten the case and will be very much helpful in the analysis.
- All documents with memo should be packed in large envelope, which must be closed and sealed accordingly.
- Sample of seal must be very legible on the wax, on the sealed items, which must be attested and signed by proper authority.

Don'ts
1. Never use button or coin-like seals on articles.
2. Do not keep the packed sample in unsafe custody.
3. Do not delay in forwarding the sample for chemical analysis.

■ DO'S AND DON'TS FOR POLICE INVESTIGATING OFFICERS

Do's
1. Statement of witnesses (relatives, neighbors, and friends) must be taken.
2. Clinical history of the case of deceased admitted in the hospital should be collected.
3. They must collect the visceral material immediately after PM, i.e., on the same day.
4. They must send the viscera to concerning forensic science laboratory (FSL) as early as possible.
5. They should collect the following articles from the SOC, preserve and pack them separately:
   - Poison container, e.g., pesticide
   - Vomitus-mixed soil along with the control sample
   - Vomited matter
   - Glass vessel or container used
   - Clothing's, etc.
   - The above article must be sent for analysis along with the viscera
6. They should request the autopsy surgeon to preserve viscera only in the case of suspected poisoning.
7. They must make sure that the articles are properly marked according to the requisition letter (memo).
8. The copy of PM report, *Panchnama*, FSL form duly filled, sample of seal of PM center and police station, and seizure memo must be sent with the case.

Don'ts
1. There should be no delay in reaching the scene of event, otherwise crucial evidence will be lost.
2. The scene of event should not be allowed to be tempered by anyone.
3. The IO should not leave any work pending, e.g., collection of samples, statement of witness, relatives, etc., in the first visit as the first visit is the most reliable and important visit.

■ DO'S AND DON'TS FOR MEDICAL OFFICERS

Do's

1. Collect all information from the inquest report and from the IO, witnesses, and relatives.
2. A complete autopsy must be done. All the body cavities should be opened and every organ must be examined.
3. The PM should be conducted in the mortuary, except in some exceptional cases, where the body is in an advanced stage of putrefaction and its transportation will be difficult and material of evidential value may be lost during the transport.
4. It should be conducted only when there is an official order authorizing the autopsy from the police or magistrate.
5. It should be performed as early as possible after receiving the requisition.
6. The medical officer should first read the inquest paper carefully and find out the apparent cause of death and obtain all the available details of the case from case sheets, accident register, etc., so that attention may be diverted to the significant points, while doing the PM examination and to carry out appropriate investigations.
7. The autopsy should be conducted generally in daylight as far as possible because color changes cannot be appreciated well in the artificial light. However, in some states such as Maharashtra, it is done 24 hours with good lightning facility.
8. The police constable, who accompanies it, must identify the body of the deceased and the names of the relatives who identify the body should be recorded.
9. In case of unknown bodies, the marks of identification, photographs, and fingerprints should be recorded.
10. As the autopsy is conducted, details of examination should be noted verbatim by an assistant and sketches made of all the important injuries.
11. Even if the body is decomposed, autopsy should be conducted.
12. Color photographs should be taken with proper label for record and evidence.
13. The PM should be detailed, honest, objective, and scientific.
14. Maintain aseptic measures while conducting autopsy.
15. The medical officer must preserve the following viscera for chemical analysis: (1) stomach and its content (up to 300 mL), (2) small intestine and its contents (about 30 cm, up to 100 mL), (3) liver (about 500 g), (4) kidney (one half of each kidney), (5) blood (10–20 mL), (6) urine (up to 200 mL), and (7) special viscera as per indication.
16. The right preservative and amount should be used according to the nature of poison.
17. The label of the viscera must contain the following information: Name of the deceased, age, sex, PM no., date of PM, police station, name of viscera items, and signature of medical officer.

18. For viscera, wide mouth airtight container of glass or plastic with screw cap must be used. For blood and other body fluid, small glass/plastic vial can be used.
19. The sample of preservative must be sent with the viscera. The amount of preservative added must be recorded.
20. The chain of custody of the viscera must be maintained.
21. The seal of the PM center must be on the knot of the thread or bandage strip.
22. In special case such as snakebite or drug reaction after injection, the skin with the underneath muscle tissue from the bite mark or injection site should be preserved.
23. In decomposed body, vitreous humor from eye should be preserved for analysis.

Don'ts

1. The autopsy must never be conducted in a private room or unauthorized venue.
2. Preferably, autopsy should not be conducted in the night.
3. No unauthorized person should be present at the autopsy. The investigating officer may be allowed with permission.
4. Nothing should be erased in the PM report and all alterations should be initialed in the report.
5. Precautions should be taken not to mix-up the sample.

■ DO'S AND DON'TS FOR FORENSIC TOXICOLOGISTS/SCIENTISTS

Do's

1. Forensic scientist/toxicologist may be asked to visit the SOC and he must be well equipped to collect all the necessary samples in a proper scientific way.
2. It must be made sure that the chain of custody of evidence is maintained.
3. In the laboratory, before receiving the viscera box, the intact seal should be checked properly and the name of the person who delivered should be mentioned.
4. The viscera analysis should be done by standard scientific methods.
5. The test should be reproducible.
6. The background information concerning the case must be made available, e.g., autopsy report, the police report, and the medical history.
7. The forensic toxicologist must keep in touch with the forensic pathologist whenever necessary to make the appropriate analysis.
8. To make the results reliable beyond reasonable doubt, the samples must be analyzed by a screening test and then by a confirmatory test.
9. A qualified analyst must only issue toxicology report.
10. The analytical work should be carried out entirely by the reporting scientist or under the direct supervision of the scientist with assistance from the technician.

11. To safeguard the reliability of the results, the laboratory must have a strict quality control system.
12. A toxicology report must have the following information:
    - Date and reference number of the report
    - The case name (the deceased or specimen donor)
    - The instructing authority, e.g., the police officer or magistrate
    - The name of the medical officer or police officer from whom the specimen was received
    - The date on which the specimen was received
    - The test that was carried out
    - The result of the test
    - Limitations in the test
    - The signature of the analyst

Don'ts

1. Do not discard the sample immediately. It may be needed for repeat test. Preserve it safely for specific period as per the laboratory protocol. It can be returned to the IO along with the report.
2. Avoid contamination of samples during analysis to prevent false-positive results.
3. Do not give report or opinion carelessly. Care must be taken in the interpretation of some results, since there could be alternative explanations.
4. Do not use methods, which are still under research and not well authenticated.

■ CONCLUSION

Poisoning is a common cause of death in India and other countries. The manner of death may be accidental, suicidal or homicidal in nature. It is a medicolegal case and needs proper investigation by the police. These ready made checklist of do's and don'ts will help all the professionals involved in investigation of poisoning deaths to do the right thing and not miss any crucial evidence.

■ FURTHER READINGS

1. Goel MR. Manual of Medicolegal Practice, 1st edition. Ajmer: Unique Books; 1996.
2. Jaiswal AK, Millo T. Do's and Don'ts for sophisticated analytic instruments. Int J Med Tox Leg Med. 2006;9(1):6-8.
3. Murty OP. Crime Investigation, 1st edition. New Delhi: National Academy of Medical Sciences; 1999.
4. Vanezis P, Busuttil A. Suspicious Death Scene Investigation, 1st edition. London: Arnold; 1996.
5. White P. Crime Scene to Court—The Essentials of Forensic Science, 1st edition. London: Royal Society of Chemistry; 1998.

Chapter 16

Safety Measures in the Laboratory

■ INTRODUCTION

There are always chances of chemical, physical, and biological hazards during various phases of analysis, operation, instrumentation, handling, and ultimate disposal of hazardous wastes. The laboratory should have a clear safety policy in the form of manual to insure the health and safety of the personnel working in various areas of the laboratory. It should address a minimum of the following issues:
1. Specimen handling including the handling of infectious material and the disposal of specimens.
2. Handling and disposal of solvents, reagents, and other chemicals in the laboratory.
3. Handling and disposal of any reactive materials used in the laboratory.
4. Handling and disposal of laboratory glassware.
5. Responses to personal injuries and spillage of biological specimens, chemicals, solvents, reagents, or radioactive materials.
6. Regulation governing dress (e.g., laboratory coats and safety glasses), eating, drinking, or smoking in the laboratory.
7. The management policy of a chemical control program.
8. Basic principles of prevention.
9. Health risks resulting from exposure to chemical hazards during work.
10. Specific procedures for safety and health in various areas in laboratory.

Each laboratory must be aware of the respective state law or regulations in relation to the laboratory standard requirements.

■ COMMON SAFETY AND HEALTH MEASUREMENTS IN THE LABORATORY

The following are some useful guidelines for the safety of the personnel working in the laboratory.
1. Always wear an apron (laboratory coat) (**Figs. 16.1A** to **C**).
2. Keep your seat and the working place clean.
3. Do not touch a chemical with hand. Use a spatula.

SAFETY MEASURES IN THE LABORATORY

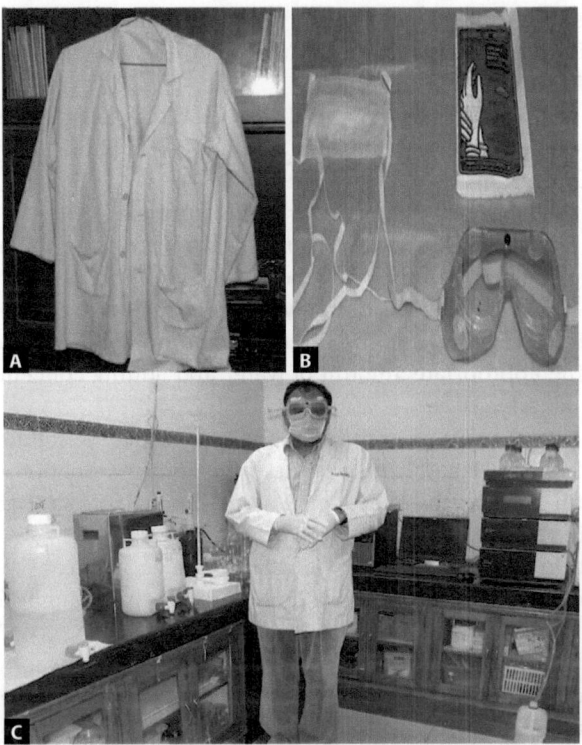

Figs. 16.1A to C: (A) Apron; (B) Mask, surgical gloves, and safety goggles; and (C) Working person wearing all safety articles.

4. Never taste a chemical.
5. Do not keep the reagent bottle open.
6. Place the reagent bottle in the shelf at the appropriate place.
7. Do not keep the water tap running when not required.
8. Do not keep the burner on if you have finished your work.
9. Do not throw solid waste materials such as filter paper pieces, etc., in the sink. Throw them in the waste box only.
10. Do not throw very hot solutions in the sink.
11. Do not heat beakers and China dishes directly on the flame. Use wire gauge or water bath.
12. Do not use filter paper for taking solid substances on it. Use ordinary piece of paper for this work.
13. Do not waste any chemical. Use the minimum quantity required.
14. Before leaving the laboratory, wash your hands with soap and dry them with a clean towel.
15. Avoid wearing loose dresses such as kurta, pajama, or sari, etc.
16. Long hair should be tied back out of the way of flames. Avoid long beard or moustache.

SAFETY MEASURES IN THE LABORATORY

17. Wear safety glasses but do not use contact lens as some corrosive material may be entrapped between the lens and the cornea of the eye (**Fig. 16.1B**).
18. Never smell the vapors or gases directly. Do it by keeping the test tube at least 6 inches away from your nose and with hands fan the vapors toward your nose.
19. Never use laboratory water for drinking purpose.
20. Never point test tube toward yourself or toward your neighbor, while heating any liquid in the test tube.
21. Never dilute an acid by adding water to concentrated acid, as it is an exothermic reaction and the liquid may bump out. Always dilute acid by taking appropriate amount of water and adding concentrated acid to it gradually.
22. Never heat the bottom of the test tube containing the solution to avoid splashing out. Heat it from a point at the highest level of the solution.
23. Never fill the test tube or beaker to more than half of its capacity during a heating operation.
24. Do not throw a burning matchstick into the waste box.
25. Sufficient space should be available for each instrument for smooth operation.
26. Safety equipment such as fire extinguishers, eyewash facilities, emergency showers, and spill kits should be identified by proper sign boards.
27. Equipment and materials should be made available for handling of carcinogenic, toxic, biological, and other dangerous materials.
28. Appropriate disinfectants must be regularly used in the laboratory. First aid kit should be present in laboratory.
29. Sufficient space must be there for storage of supplies, equipment, and tools.
30. Laboratory design must be in such a way that it permits the effective circulation of evidence/sample from the time of its acceptance to its proper disposal.
31. Proper lighting should be there for the personnel to carry out the assigned task.
32. Proper temperature and humidity control measures should be taken.
33. Flammable liquid should be stored separately in a proper storage cabinet and at low temperature; acid and solvents should be stored separately.
34. Emergency exit from the laboratory is essential for the safe exit in an emergency.
35. A register should be maintained to record the laboratory accidents, injuries, and the follow-up action taken. Immunization facility should be available for laboratory staff.
36. Cleaning agents and handwashing facility should be available.
37. Laboratory should not accept any radioactive material for examination.
38. Smoking should be strictly prohibited in the laboratory premises.

39. Safety audits should be conducted in the laboratory once in every 6 months and the records of the safety audits should be maintained properly.
40. Air purifier equipment must be in extraction and isolation unit area.
41. Electric equipment should be free from recognized hazard.
42. The safety manual should be easily available to all staffs.

■ SAFETY MEASUREMENTS TO CHEMICAL EXPOSURE

1. The list of common chemical substances used in the laboratory and precautionary measures must be prominently displayed at working area.
2. Food and cosmetic application must be strictly prohibited in working area.
3. List of common chemical showing flammability must be displayed in each working area.
4. To prevent chemical hazards, the storage of chemicals should be by the hazard class of chemical.
5. Refrigerator or freezer should be used for storing flammable chemicals.
6. Ignition source should be kept out of the immediate area during flammable liquids use.
7. Flames and liquefied petroleum gas (LPG) cylinders should be kept away from solvents.
8. Not more than 2.5 L of particular solvent should be allowed to the working area at a time. The excess stock must be kept in storeroom.
9. The chemicals and other reference materials should be stored in isolated place to avoid contamination and chemical hazard.
10. Good ventilation is must in the laboratory to prevent the accumulation of the vapor of hazardous chemicals.
11. The senior scientist should insure that the chemicals having proper label are used in the laboratory. The unlabeled chemicals must be disposed off.
12. Chemical reaction using mineral acids should be done in fume hoods.
13. List of common chemicals and procedures to deal with spillage or leakage must be displayed in working place.
14. Cryogenic liquid (boiling point < −90°C) (liquid nitrogen, liquid oxygen, liquid helium, liquid argon, etc.) should be typically stored in low pressure, multiwalled containers with vacuum insulated walls in order to keep them in liquid form.
15. In compressed gas cylinders, typical pressure relief devices should be included such as spring-loaded safety valves. Hydrogen should be stored according to the local fire and health and safety regulation.
16. Appropriate and adequate ventilation in toxicology laboratory should have extreme importance. Commonly used modes are exhaust ventilation and chemical fume hoods, biological safety cabinets, and other type of local exhaust.
17. Use acid-resistant gloves and masks while working.

■ WASTE DISPOSAL PROCEDURES FOR BIOLOGICAL MATERIAL

The laboratory should have documented waste management policy. There must be a clear policy in place for the disposal of materials on completion of examination. After examination of the samples, the reporting officer should insure that the waste materials are collected in the designated container with proper lids and these waste materials should be destroyed properly under the supervision of senior officer. An incinerator of suitable capacity should be installed to destroy the biological waste material. In some instances, this involves returning what remains of the sample to the customer, subject, or legal custodian. In other cases, the sample needs to be destroyed safely and statutory requirements may have to be observed in doing this. However, in no circumstances should anything be disposed off without the consent of the customer or other relevant authority and records should be maintained of what has been disposed off and what has been retained.

There is no separate act or rule for the forensic laboratory biological waste management, but the Biological Waste Management Rules, 2016 applied for the hospitals will also apply to the forensic science laboratories.

■ BIOMEDICAL WASTE MANAGEMENT RULES, 2016

Biomedical waste is defined as "any solid, fluid, and liquid or liquid waste, including its container and any intermediate products, which is generated during the diagnosis, treatment, or immunization of human being or animals, in research pertaining thereto or in the production or testing of biologicals and the animal waste from slaughter houses or any other similar establishments". All biological wastes are hazardous. The following are the brief contents of the Biological Waste Management Rules, 2016.

Steps in the management of biomedical waste include:
- Generation
- Segregation
- Collection
- Storage
- Treatment
- Transport
- Disposal

Thus, the Biomedical Waste Management Rules are applicable to all persons who generate, segregate, collect, receive, store, treat, transport, dispose, or handle biomedical waste in any form.

In addition to Biomedical Waste Management Rules, 2016, the following types of wastes are also covered under different other acts:
1. Radioactive wastes (Atomic Energy Act, 1962)
2. Hazardous chemical (Manufacture, Storage and Import of Hazardous Chemical Rules, 1989)

3. Lead acid batteries [Batteries (Management and Handling) Rules, 2001]
4. Hazardous wastes [Hazardous and Other Wastes (Management and Transboundary Movement) Rules, 2016]
5. E-waste [E-Waste (Management) Rules, 2016]
6. Municipal solid wastes (Solid Waste Management Rules, 2016)
7. Hazardous microorganisms, genetically engineered microorganisms, and cells (Manufacture, Use, Import, Export, and Storage of Hazardous Microorganisms, Genetically Engineered Microorganisms or Cells Rules, 1989)

Salient features of Biomedical Waste Management Rules, 2016 along with Biomedical Waste Management (Amendment) Rules, 2018 are:

1. The scope of the rules has been expanded to include vaccination camps, blood donation camps, surgical camps, or any other healthcare activity.
2. Phaseout the use of chlorinated plastic bags, gloves, and bags within 2 years of notification of Biomedical Waste Management Rules, 2016, i.e., by 27th March, 2018. But as per the Biomedical Waste Management (Amendment) Rules, 2018, use of chlorinated plastic bags (excluding blood bags) and gloves has to be phased out by the 27th March, 2019.
3. Pretreatment of the laboratory waste, microbiological waste, blood samples, and blood bags through disinfection sterilization on-site in the manner as prescribed by the World Health Organization (WHO) or the National AIDS Control Organization (NACO).
4. Provide training to all its healthcare workers and immunize all health workers regularly against diseases such as tetanus and hepatitis B.
5. Establish a barcode system for bags or containers containing biomedical waste for disposal within 1 year of notification of rules, i.e., 27th March, 2017. But as per the Biomedical Waste Management (Amendment) Rules, 2018, barcode system has to be established in accordance with the guidelines issued by the Central Pollution Control Board by 27th March, 2019.
6. Report major accidents such as needlestick injuries, broken mercury thermometer, accidents caused by fire, and blasts during handling of biomedical waste and the remedial action taken and record the same in prescribed form.
7. Procedure to get authorization is simplified.
8. The new rules prescribe more stringent standards for incinerator to reduce the emission of pollutants in environment.
9. No hospital/healthcare facility (occupier) shall establish on-site treatment and disposal facility, if a service of "Common Biomedical Waste Treatment Facility (CBMWTF)" is available at 75 km.
10. Operator of a common biomedical waste treatment and disposal facility to ensure the timely collection of biomedical waste from the healthcare facility and assist the healthcare in conducting training.
11. Biomedical waste has been classified into four categories instead of 10 categories as per Biomedical Waste (Management and Handling) Rules, 1998 to improve the segregation of waste at source (**Table 16.1**).

SAFETY MEASURES IN THE LABORATORY

Table 16.1: Classification of biomedical waste (BMW) based on treatment.

Categories	Type of bag/ container used	Types of waste	Treatment/ Disposal options
Yellow	• Nonchlorinated plastic bags • Separate collection system leading to effluent treatment system	• Human anatomical waste • Animal anatomical waste • Soiled waste • Expired or discarded medicines and cytotoxic drugs along with glass or plastic ampoules, vials, etc. • Chemical waste • Microbiology, biotechnology, and other clinical laboratory waste • Chemical liquid waste • Discarded linen, mattresses, and beddings contaminated with blood or body fluids. Also, routine mask and gown as per BMW rules, 2018	Incineration or plasma pyrolysis or deep burial
Red	Nonchlorinated plastic bags or containers	• Contaminated waste (recyclable) • Vacutainers, tubing, bottles, intravenous tubes and sets, catheters, urine bags, and syringes (without needles and gloves)	Autoclaving/ microwaving/ hydroclaving and then sent for recycling, not sent to landfill
White (translucent)	Translucent puncture, leak, and tamper proof containers	Waste sharps including metal sharps: Needles, syringes with fixed needles from needle tip cutter/burner, scalpels, and blades	Auto or dry heat sterilization followed by shredding or mutilation or encapsulation
Blue	Cardboard boxes with blue-colored marking. Puncture proof and leak proof boxes or containers with blue-colored marking as per BMW rules, 2018	Broken/discarded glass medicine vials, ampoules, except those contaminated with cytotoxic wastes, and metallic body implants	Disinfection or autoclaving, microwaving, hydroclaving, and then sent for recycling

FIRST AID EMERGENCY TREATMENT IN THE LABORATORY ACCIDENTS

Accidents in the laboratory usually occur due to carelessness. However, accident may occur by chance also. In case, if it occurs, do not be confused. Take the necessary steps immediately as your laboratory has a first aid box (**Figs. 16.2** and **16.3**). The management protocol is shown in **Table 16.2**. The

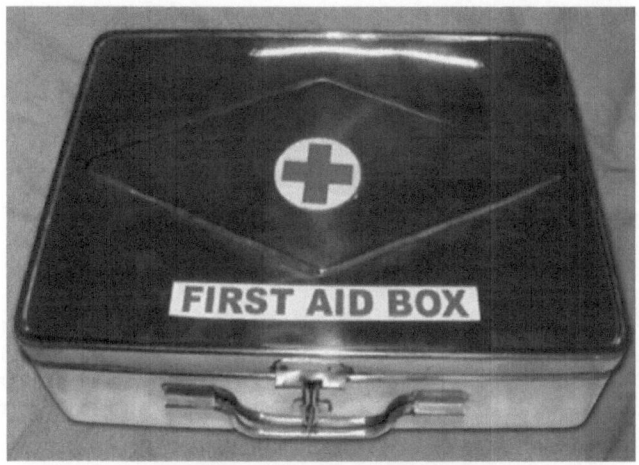

Fig. 16.2: First aid box for laboratory.

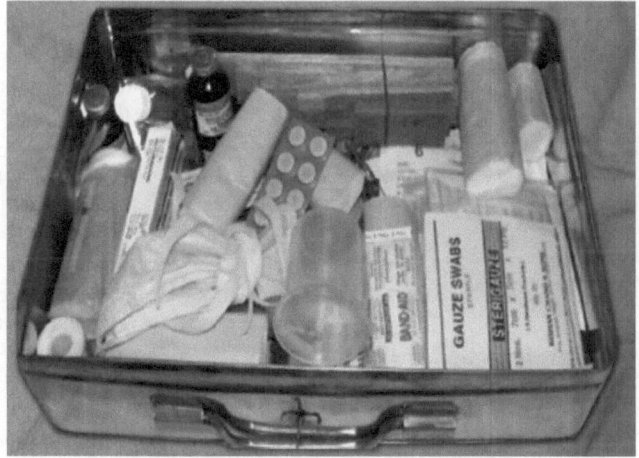

Fig. 16.3: Contents of the first aid box.

probable accidents and their first aid emergency treatments are given in **Table 16.2**. The first aid box consists of the following items:
- Bandage
- Cotton
- Surgical gloves
- Distilled water
- Methylated spirit
- Handyplast
- Paracetamol
- Cetirizine
- Flexon tablets
- Betadine ointment
- Silver sulfadiazine cream

The medicine should be regularly replaced with new one on expiry.

SAFETY MEASURES IN THE LABORATORY

Table 16.2: Emergency management of laboratory accidents.

Types of accident		First aid emergency treatment
Burns	Burn by dry heat (i.e., flame, hot objects, etc.). Burns causing blisters. *Caution*: Dry heat burns should never be washed	Apply 1% silver sulfadiazine cream
	Acid burns	Wash freely with water for about 15 minutes. No attempt must be made at neutralization with alkalis, since the resulting exothermic reaction can cause more harm than benefit. Take him to the doctor
	Bromine burns	Wash liberally for about 15 minutes with water
Cuts	Minor cuts	• Allow to bleed for a few seconds • Remove the glass piece, if any. Apply a little methylated spirit and cover with a piece of sterile cotton pad. Take him to the doctor
	Serious cuts	Apply pressure over the cut with sterile cotton pad to stop bleeding. Take him to the doctor
Eye accident	Acid in eye	Rinse the eye copiously with distilled water or clean water for about 15 minutes. No attempt must be made at neutralization with alkalis, since the resulting exothermic reaction can cause more harm than benefit. Take him to doctor
	Alkali in eye	Rinse the eye copiously with distilled water or clean water for about 15 minutes. No attempt must be made at neutralization with acid solutions, since the resulting exothermic reaction can cause more harm than benefit
Poisons	Poisons not swallowed	Spit out immediately. Rinse the mouth copiously with water
	Acid swallowed	Diluent such as cold water can be given (not more than one or two glass in adult) followed by cold milk or egg emulsion, if available. No emetic should be taken
	Caustic alkali swallowed	
	Inhalation of gases such as Cl_2, SO_2, Br_2, etc., causing suffocation	Loosen the clothes at the neck. Go in the open air and breath
Fire	Clothes catch fire	Do not run. Wrap with a blanket. Lie down on the floor and roll
	Beaker containing inflammable liquid catches fire	Cover the beaker with duster or damp cloth

FURTHER READINGS

1. Crees Z, Fritz C, Huedebert A, Noe J, Rengarajan A, Wang X. The Washington Manual of Medical Therapeutics, 36th edition. New Delhi: Wolters Kluwer (India) Pvt. Ltd.; 2019.
2. Sharma S, Sethi GR, Gulati RK. Standard Treatment Guidelines: A Manual for Medical Therapeutics. New Delhi: Wolters Kluwer (India) Pvt. Ltd.; 2002.
3. Jaiswal AK, Millo T, Mishra S, Rai A, Murthy OP. Planning and designing of modern forensic toxicology laboratory. J Forensic Med Toxicol. 2007;2:43-60.
4. Pillay VV. Comprehensive Medical Toxicology, 3rd edition. Hyderabad: Paras Medical Publishers; 2018.
5. Society of Forensic Toxicologists/American Academy of Forensic Sciences (SOFT/AAFS). (2006). SOFT/AAFS Forensic Toxicology Laboratory Guidelines: 2006 Version. [online] Available from https://www.scribd.com/doc/55945119/SOFT-AAFS-Forensic-Laboratory-Guidelines-2006-Final. [Last accessed March, 2021].
6. United Kingdom and Ireland Association of Forensic Toxicologists (UKIAFT). (2018). The United Kingdom and Ireland Association of Forensic Toxicologists forensic toxicology laboratory guidelines. [online] Available from http://www.ukiaft.co.uk/image/catalog/documents/UKIAFT%20Lab%20Guidelines%202018%20published.pdf. [Last accessed March, 2021].
7. Government of India. (2016). Biomedical Waste Management Rule, 2016. [online] Available from https://dhr.gov.in/sites/default/files/Bio-medical_Waste_Management_Rules_2016.pdf. [Last accessed March, 2021].

Chapter 17

The Indian Laws Relating to Drugs and Poisons

■ INTRODUCTION

Drugs are vital means for the prevention and cure of diseases and ailment of different nature. It has played a vital role in the health of humanity and improved its lifespan and quality of life. With the advancement of science and research, new drugs are evolving each year and the pharmaceutical companies are flourishing with business. Therefore, various acts have been passed by the government to regulate the manufacture, composition, and sale of these drugs. Besides, it has made various laws to prevent the misuse of these drugs to harm others. The physicians and the pharmacist should be aware of the various legal acts of drugs and poisons pertaining to its profession. This chapter has attempted to bring out all the relevant acts and rules pertaining to drug and poison, which is relevant to the professionals dealing with drugs and poisons such as medical practitioners, pharmacy, and pharmaceutical industry.

In India, several legal acts have been passed to regulate and control the manufacture, sale, distribution, and possession of drugs and poisons. According to the World Health Organization (WHO) (1996) definition, drug is any substance or product that is used or intended to be used to modify or explore physiological systems or pathological states for the benefit of the recipient. As per the Drugs and Cosmetics Act, drug includes all medicines for internal or external use of human beings or animals and all substances intended to be used for or in the diagnosis, treatment, mitigation, or prevention of any disease or disorder in human beings or animals including preparation applied on human body for the purpose of repelling insects such as mosquitoes. Poison is defined as any substance which when introduced into the living body or brought into contact with any part thereof will produce ill effect or death by its local or systemic action or both.

Some of the Indian laws of importance in relation to drugs and poison are as follows:
- The Poisons Act, 1919
- The Drugs Act, 1940
- The Drugs and Cosmetics Act, 1940

- The Drugs and Cosmetics Rules, 1945
- The Pharmacy Act, 1948
- The Drugs Control Act, 1950
- The Drugs and Magic Remedies (Objectionable Advertisements) Act, 1954
- The Narcotics Drugs and Psychotropic Substances (NDPS) Act, 1985
- The Drugs (Price Control) Order, 1995
- The Indian Penal Code (IPC), 1860
- The Code of Criminal Procedure (CrPC), 1973
- The Indian Evidence Act (IEA), 1872

THE POISONS ACT, 1919

This was amended in the year 1958 and repealed in 1960. It regulates the grant of licenses and sale of poisons whether wholesale or retail. It also regulates import of any specified poisons. It extends to whole of all of India.

THE DRUGS AND COSMETICS ACT, 1940

This act was amended in 1964 to include Ayurveda and Unani drugs and it regulates the drugs of articles of cleansing (except soap), beautifying and promoting attractiveness, or altering appearances. It was recently amended in 2008 and today the act is referred to as the Drugs and Cosmetics (Amendment) Act, 2008. This act also demands the fact that every patented or proprietary medicinal preparation under this act must display a label on the container mentioning the exact formula or list of ingredients in it. This act empowers the central government to form the Drugs Technical Advisory Board and to establish a central drug laboratory to help and advice both the central and states government. It controls the quality, purity, and strength of drugs for safety. It regulates the import, manufacture, distribution, and sale of these drugs. The Amended Act has enhanced the scale of punishment for various offences including sale of spurious drugs, adulteration of drugs and cosmetics, toxic contamination, etc.

THE DRUGS AND COSMETICS RULES, 1945

This is a derivative of the Drugs and Cosmetics Act, 1940 and it covers all kinds of drugs used in therapeutics under allopathic, Ayurvedic, Unani, and Siddha preparations. The rule deals mainly with the standard and quality of drugs. It also controls the drugs by specific regulation laid down for their storage, display, sale, dispensing, labeling, prescription, etc. To advise the central and state government on technical matters relating to drug control, the following boards have been setup: The Drugs Technical Advisory Board, the Ayurvedic and Unani Drugs Technical Advisory Board, and the Drugs Consultative Committee. In order to facilitate the analysis or testing of drug samples to assess their quality, the Central Drugs Laboratory was established in 1962. Stringent punishments have laid down for manufacture, stocking,

or sale of substandard or spurious drugs. Guidelines for conducting clinical trials for new drugs have been made more strict (schedule Y). The Drugs and Cosmetics Rules, 1945 have classified drugs into various schedule as follows:
- Schedule C and C1—biological and special products such as serums, vaccines, etc.
- Schedule D—substances not intended for medicinal use—condensed or powdered milk, oats, spices, condiments, etc.
- Schedule E1—lists of poisonous substances under Ayurvedic, Siddha, and Unani systems of medicine.
- Schedule G—list includes hormone preparations, hypoglycemic agents, antihistamines, and anticancer drugs.
- Schedule H and L—these are drugs or poisons, which need to be labeled as "Schedule H Drug Warning—to be sold by retail on the prescription of registered medical practitioner only". Barbiturates, amphetamines, reserpine, ergot, antibiotics, antibacterials, and some of the sulfonamides are listed under this schedule.
- Schedule J—drugs which should not be advertised for certain diseases (which cannot be announced). This covers list of drugs which are claimed to be cure of conditions such as appendicitis, blindness, cancer, cataract, epilepsy, hydrocele, etc.
- Schedule L—antibiotics, antihistaminic, and other chemotherapeutic agent of recent origin subjected to same restrictions as Schedule H drugs.
- Schedule O—standards to be followed with regard to disinfectant fluids.
- Schedule X—barbiturates and certain other sedatives, amphetamines, etc.

■ THE PHARMACY ACT, 1948

This act makes provision for regulation of the profession of pharmacy and for the purpose of constitution of Pharmacy Council of India, which regulates study of pharmacy throughout the country. Individual states have State Pharmacy Councils for registration of pharmacist. The objective of this act is to allow only registered pharmacists to compound, prepare, mix, or dispense any medicine on the prescription of a registered medical practitioner.

■ THE DRUGS CONTROL ACT, 1950

This act regulates the supply and distribution of drugs and also guides the manufacturer or dealer in fixing the maximum price fix every drug.

■ THE DRUGS AND MAGIC REMEDIES (OBJECTIONABLE ADVERTISEMENTS) ACT, 1954

The objective of this act is to ensure that ethical standards are maintained when drugs are advertised by manufacturers. This act bans the objectionable advertisements of magical remedial drugs for curing conditions such as venereal diseases, impotency, menstrual disorders, infertility, abortion, misconception, insanity, etc. Advertisements offending decency or morality can be banned under this act.

■ THE NARCOTIC DRUGS AND PSYCHOTROPIC SUBSTANCES ACT, 1985

This act consolidates and amends the law relating to narcotic drugs (the Opium Act, 1857 and 1878 and the Dangerous Drug Act, 1930, both are repealed by this act), drugs of abuse, penalties for the drug trafficking offenses, and control over psychotropic substances. Narcotic drugs under this act include opiates, cannabis, and cocaine. The psychotropic drugs under this act refer to mind-altering drugs such as lysergic acid diethylamide (LSD), phencyclidine, amphetamines, barbiturates, methaqualone, benzodiazepines, mescaline, psilocybin, and designer drugs [3,4-methylenedioxymethamphetamine (MDMA), N,N-dimethyltryptamine (DMT), etc.]. It was again amended in 1988 and 2001. It prevents trafficking in narcotic drugs and psychotropic substances. It is applicable to all citizens of India even though they may be outside the territory of India and to all persons on ships and aircrafts registered in India, wherever they may be. The NDPS act imposes complete prohibition on the cultivation of coca, poppy, and cannabis plants and the manufacture, sale, purchase, use, or transport of any narcotics drugs or psychotropic substance, except for medical or scientific purposes.

The minimum punishment for any offence committed under the act is 10 years rigorous imprisonment and fine of Rs 1 lac, while the maximum punishment is 20 years rigorous imprisonment and fine of Rs 20 lacs. To constitute an offence the first time around, the minimum quantity seized should be equal to or over 250 mg for *heroin*, 5 g for *hashish* or *charas*, 5 g for *opium*, 125 mg for *cocaine*, and 500 g for *ganja*.

The Central Government of India constituted the Narcotics Control Bureau in 1986 with its headquarter at New Delhi and zonal offices at Mumbai, Kolkata, Chennai, and Varanasi. In 1988, the central government constitutes the Narcotic Drugs and Psychotropic Substances Consultative Committee, consisting of a chairman and 18 members from various fields, who would among other functions, conduct periodic review of the NDPS act. The NDPS act prohibits cultivation of poppy, cannabis, and coca plant. But it allows restricted cultivation of these plants under strict control for scientific and medical use.

■ THE DRUGS (PRICE CONTROL) ORDER, 1995

The Drugs (Price Control) Order, 1995 was brought in by Government of India to regulate and control the manufacture and pricing of the first schedule drugs. It has the power to fix the maximum sale prices of bulk drugs in the first schedule and also the information to be furnished by the manufacturers in relation to the scheduled bulk drugs and nonscheduled bulk drugs. It can also fix the retail price of scheduled formulations. The manufacturers should maintain a proper record of drugs and production for inspection.

■ THE INDIAN PENAL CODE, 1860

- *Section 176*: Doctors must report all cases of homicidal poisoning to police, if not they are punishable
- *Section 177*: For furnishing false information
- *Section 193*: Doctor is punishable for giving false information about poisoning case
- *Section 201*: Causing disappearance of evidence of offence
- *Section 202*: Doctor is punishable for intentional concealing of facts about poisoning case treated by him
- *Section 272*: Adulteration of food or drink intended for sale
- *Section 273*: Sale of noxious food or drink
- *Section 274*: Adulteration of drugs
- *Section 275*: Sale of adulterated drugs
- *Section 276*: Sale of drugs as a different drug or preparations
- *Section 284*: Lays down penalty for any person causing harm by rash and negligent handling of a poisonous substance, so as to endanger human life or to be likely to cause hurt and injury to any person
- *Section 299*: Culpable homicide including that caused through administration of some poisonous substance
- *Section 300, 302, 306, 307, and 309*: Murder including that caused through administration of poisonous substances with the intention of causing death
- *Section 304A*: Rash and negligent act including that caused through poisoning
- *Section 320*: Causing grievous hurt
- *Section 324*: Causing hurt by dangerous weapons or means (including poison or any corrosive substance)
- *Section 326*: Causing grievous hurt by dangerous weapons or means (including poison)
- *Section 326A*: Voluntarily causing grievous hurt by use of acid (vitriolage)
- *Section 326B*: Voluntarily throwing or attempting to throw acid
- *Section 328*: Causing hurt by means of poison or stupefying intoxicating or unwholesome drug or other thing with the intent to commit an offence.

■ THE CODE OF CRIMINAL PROCEDURE, 1973

- *Section 39*: Every person aware of the commission of or of the intention of any other person to commit any offence punishable under IPC shall forthwith give information to the nearest magistrate or police officer of such commission or intention.

- *Section 40*: Every employed officers aware of the commission of or of the intention of any other person to commit any offence punishable under IPC shall forthwith give information to the nearest magistrate or police officer of such commission or intention.
- *Section 175*: Power to summon persons by police officer proceeding under Section 174.

■ THE INDIAN EVIDENCE ACT, 1872

Section 32, Clause 1, under the IEA, allows a doctor to record dying declaration when the death of the patient is imminent and arrival of magistrate is delayed.

■ RECENT AMENDMENTS OF INDIAN PENAL CODE DEALING WITH ACID ATTACK CASE, 2013

- *IPC 326A (voluntarily causing grievous hurt by use of acid, etc.)*: Whoever causes permanent or partial damage or deformity to, or burns or maims or disfigures or disables, any part or parts of the body of a person or causes grievous hurt by throwing acid on or by administering acid to that person, or by using any other means with the intention of causing or with the knowledge that he is likely to cause such injury or hurt, shall be punished with imprisonment of either description for a term which shall not be <10 years but which may extend to imprisonment for life and with fine: provided that such fine shall be just and reasonable to meet the medical expenses of the treatment of the victim: provided further that any fine imposed under this section shall be paid to the victim. The section was introduced on the basis of the recommendation of the Justice JS Verma committee.
- *IPC 326B (voluntarily throwing or attempting to throw acid)*: Whoever throws or attempts to administer acid on any person, or attempts to use any other means, with the intention of causing permanent or partial damage or deformity or burns or maiming or disfiguring or disability or grievous hurt to that person, shall be punished with imprisonment of either description for a term which shall not be <5 years but which may extend to 7 years and shall also be liable to fine.

For the purposes of Section 326A and in this section, acid includes any substance which has acidic or corrosive character or burning nature that is capable of causing bodily injury leading to scars or disfigurement or temporary or permanent disability. For the purposes of Section 326A and in this section, permanent or partial damage or deformity shall not be required to be irreversible.

Supreme court in Laxmi vs. Union of India directed the state to consider: (1) enactment of appropriate provisions for effective regulation of sale of acid in the states/union territories, (2) measures for proper treatment after care and rehabilitation of the victims of acid attack and needs of acid attack victims, and (3) compensation payable to acid attack victims by the state or creation of some separate fund for payment of compensation to acid attack victims. In a subsequent order, in the same case, the Supreme Court issued many directions to curb the menace of acid attacks.

■ SUPREME COURT GUIDELINES TO PREVENT ACID ATTACKS

1. Over the counter, sale of acid is completely prohibited unless the seller maintains a log/register recording the sale of acid which will contain the details of the person(s) to whom acid(s) is/are sold and the quantity sold. The log/register shall contain the address of the person to whom it is sold.
2. All sellers sell acid only after the buyer has shown:
   - A photo ID issued by the government which also has the address of the person
   - Specifies the reason/purpose for procuring acid
3. All stocks of acid must be declared by the seller with the concerned Sub Divisional Magistrate (SDM) within 15 days
4. No acid shall be sold to any person who is below 18 years of age
5. In case of undeclared stock of acid, it will be open to the concerned SDM to confiscate the stock and suitably impose fine on such seller up to Rs 50,000/-
6. The concerned SDM may impose fine up to Rs 50,000/- on any person who commits breach of any of the above directions

The educational institutions, research laboratories, hospitals, government departments, and the departments of public sector undertakings, who are required to keep and store acid, shall follow the following guidelines:

1. A register of usage of acid shall be maintained and the same shall be filed with the concerned SDM
2. A person shall be made accountable for possession and safe keeping of acid in their premises
3. The acid shall be stored under the supervision of this person and there shall be compulsory checking of the students/personnel leaving the laboratories/place of storage where acid is used

■ CONCLUSION

In India, there are various acts and laws to regulate drugs and poisons. It is important to know its medicolegal aspects when we prescribe and dispense these drugs in hospital or pharmacy. Its awareness can help us to avoid negligence due to our ignorance of these rules. The professionals involved in dealing with drugs and poisons and also the law enforcing agency should be aware of these laws to deal with such cases effectively and prudently.

FURTHER READINGS

1. Sarkar PC. Criminal Major Acts, 6th edition. New Delhi: Orient Law House; 1999.
2. Government of India. (1985). The Narcotic Drugs and Psychotropic Substances Act, 1985. [online] Available from https://www.indiacode.nic.in/handle/123456789/1791?view_type=browse&sam_handle=123456789/1362. [Last accessed March, 2021].
3. Thomas KT, Rashid MA. The Indian Penal Code, 34th edition. Gurugram: LexisNexis; 2014.
4. Government of India. (2013). The Criminal Law (Amendment) Act, 2013. [online] Available from https://www.iitk.ac.in/wc/data/TheCriminalLaw.pdf. [Last accessed March, 2021].
5. Laxmi vs. Union of India. (2013). Supreme Court Judgment. [online] Available from https://www.lawnn.com/laxmi-vs-union-of-india-ors/. [Last accessed March, 2021].
6. Gandhi N, Popli H. Pharmaceutical Jurisprudence, 1st edition. New Delhi: CBS Publishers & Distributors; 1997.
7. Tripathi KD. Essentials of Medical Pharmacology, 6th edition. New Delhi: Jaypee Brothers Medical Publishers (P) Ltd.; 2018.

Appendix 1

Forensic Science Laboratories in India

Central Forensic Science Laboratories

1. Director
   Central Forensic Science Laboratory
   Sector 36-A, Plot-2
   Dakshin Marg, Chandigarh,
   Punjab-160036

2. Director
   Central Forensic Science Laboratory
   Ramanthapur, Amberpet Post
   Hyderabad, Andhra Pradesh-500013

3. Director
   Central Forensic Science Laboratory
   30, Gorachand Road
   Kolkata, West Bengal-700014

4. Director
   Central Forensic Science Laboratory
   Central Bureau of Investigation
   Block No. 4, 4th Floor
   CGO complex, Lodhi Road
   New Delhi-110003

5. Coordinator
   Central Forensic Science Laboratory
   Kumeria Road, Vill-Urput
   PS-Palashbari, PO: Maniari Tiniali
   District-Kamrup Rural
   Assam-781125

6. Coordinator
   Central Forensic Science Laboratory
   Gomantika Parisar, Jawahar Chowk
   TT Nagar, Madhya Pradesh-462003

7. Coordinator
   Central Forensic Science Laboratory
   C-38/4, Krishna Complex by-Pass
   Kharadi, Pune, Maharashtra-411014

State Forensic Science Laboratories

1. Director
   Forensic Science Laboratory
   Red Hills, Opposite Niloufer Hospital
   Hyderabad, Andhra Pradesh-500004
   Ph: 040-23390398
   Fax: 040-23394449

2. Director
   State Forensic Science Laboratory
   Kahilipara
   Guwahati, Assam-781019
   Ph: 0361-2381305, 0361-2381385
   0361-2381696, Fax: 0361-2381305

3. Director
   State Forensic Science Laboratory
   Banderdewa
   Arunachal Pradesh-791123
   Ph: 0360-2218190
   Fax: 0360-2211433

4. Director
   State Forensic Science Laboratory
   JLN Marg, PO: Shastri Nagar
   Patna, Bihar-800023
   Ph: 0612-2287535
   Fax: 0612-2281273

APPENDIX 1

5. Director
   State Forensic Science Laboratory
   Police Line Campus
   Tikrapara, Raipur
   Chhattisgarh–492002
   Ph: 0771-2251258, 9425208017
   Fax: 0771-2251258

6. Director
   State Forensic Science Laboratory
   Behind Police Bhawan
   Sector 18 A,
   Gandhi Nagar, Gujarat–382308
   Ph: 079-23256250, 09978405095
   Fax: 079-23256251

7. Director
   State Forensic Science Laboratory
   Madhuban, Karnal, Haryana–132037
   Ph: 0184-2380104
   Fax: 0184-2380104

8. Director
   State Forensic Science Laboratory
   Junga, Himachal Pradesh–173216
   Ph: 0177-2752527, 9418022220
   Fax: 0177-2752527

9. Director
   J and K Forensic Science Laboratory
   Bikram Chowk
   Jammu Tawi (Winter)-180001
   Jammu and Kashmir
   J and K Forensic Science Laboratory
   Dalgate
   Srinagar (Summer)
   Jammu and Kashmir
   Ph: 0191-2435249, 0194-2473155
   Fax: 0191-2435249, 0194-2473155

10. Director
    State Forensic Science Laboratory
    Near Birsa Munda Jail, Hotwar
    Ranchi, Jharkhand–835217
    Ph: 0651-2280540, 0651-2283834
    Fax: 0651-2280540

11. Director
    State Forensic Science Laboratory
    Madiwala
    Bengaluru, Karnataka–560068
    Ph: 080-25532910, 9880933255
    Fax: 080-25532910

12. Director
    Forensic Science Laboratory
    5, Civil Lines, Sagar
    Madhya Pradesh–470001
    Ph: 07582-267707, 07582-267791
    09425030579,
    Fax: 07582-267707

13. Director
    State Forensic Science Laboratory
    Hans Bhugra Marg
    Santacruz (E), Vidyanagari
    Mumbai, Maharashtra–400098
    Ph: 022-26670760
    Fax: 022-26670844

14. Director
    State Forensic Science Laboratory
    Pangei, Manipur–795114
    Ph: 0385-2224253
    Fax: 0385-2224253

15. Director
    State Forensic Science Laboratory
    Lumshyiap, Shillong
    Meghalaya–793001
    Ph: 0364-2226801
    Fax: 0364-2226801

16. Director
    Forensic Science Laboratory
    Mualpui, Aizawal
    Mizoram–796001
    Ph: 0389-2322315
    Fax: 0389-2334310, 0389-2335578

17. Director
    Forensic Science Laboratory
    Dimapur, Nagaland–797112
    Ph: 03862-233340

18. Director
    Forensic Science Laboratory
    Government of NCT of Delhi
    Madhuban Chowk
    Rohini, New Delhi–110085
    Ph: 011-27555890, 9212038250
    Fax: 011-27555890

19. Director
    State Forensic Science Laboratory
    Rasulgarh, Bhubaneswar
    Odisha–751010
    Ph: 0674-2586187, 0674-2586417
    Fax: 0674-2586187

APPENDIX 1

20. Director
    State Forensic Science Laboratory
    Phase – IV, SAS Nagar
    Mohali, Punjab–140413

21. Director
    State Forensic Science Laboratory
    Bank House Compound
    Vellayambalam
    Thiruvananthapuram
    Kerala–695010
    Ph: 0471-2721533, 09447303935
    Fax: 0471-2721533

22. Director
    Police Forensic Science Laboratory
    Jaipur, Rajasthan–302016
    Ph: 0141-2301584
    Fax: 0141-2301584

23. Director
    Forensic Science Department
    "Forensic House", 30-A
    Kamarajar Salai
    Mylapore, Chennai
    Tamil Nadu–600004
    Ph: 044-28447767
    Fax: 044-28447767

24. Director
    State Forensic Science Laboratory
    Narsingarh, PO: Bimangarh
    Agartala, Tripura–799015
    Ph: 0381-2341266
    Fax: 0381-2341266

25. Director
    Forensic Science Laboratory
    Post Box No. 9
    PO: Mahanagar, Lucknow
    Uttar Pradesh–226006
    Ph: 0522-2371232
    Fax: 0522-2371232

26. Director
    State Forensic Science Laboratory
    Near New Basant Vihar Police Station
    Police Housing Colony
    Dehradun, Uttarakhand
    Ph: 0135-2714101

27. Director
    State Forensic Science Laboratory
    37/1/2, Belgachia Road
    Kolkata, West Bengal–700037
    Ph: 033-25565430
    Fax: 033-25565430

28. Director
    Forensic Science Laboratory
    Port Blair, Andaman and Nicobar
    Islands–744104
    Ph: 03192-232244
    Fax: 03192-232244

29. Forensic Science Laboratory
    Taj Road, Nai Basti, Khairati
    Tola, Agra, Uttar Pradesh–282001

30. Director
    VERA CENTRE Forensic Science
    Laboratory
    Rohini sector 23 Road, Rohini
    Extension, Budh Vihar
    Delhi–110099

31. Director
    State Forensic Science Laboratory
    Near Birsa Munda Jail
    Hotwar
    Jharkhand, Ranchi–835217

32. Director
    Forensic Science Laboratory
    Near Telephone Exchange
    Phase – IV, SAS Nagar
    Mohali, Punjab–140413

33. Director
    Regional Forensic Science
    Laboratory
    Ranipool, Sikkim
    Gangtok–737102

34. Director
    Forensic Science Laboratory
    Verma, Goa
    Near Verna Police Station,
    Verna, Goa–403722

35. Director/OSD
    Forensic Science Laboratory
    Kirumampakkam Police Station
    Campus
    Puducherry–607 403

36. Director
    Forensic Science Laboratory
    Tech Towers 4–5th Floor
    Mangalagiri,
    Andhra Pradesh–522503

Appendix 2

Preparation of Reagents/Solutions

1. **0.25% Sodium nitrite solution:** 500 mg of sodium nitrite is dissolved in about 80 mL distilled water and then made up to 100 mL.
2. **0.4% Xanthydrol:** 0.4 g of Xanthone is dissolved in a mixture of 10 mL methanol and 90 mL distilled water.
3. **0.50% Sodium nitroprusside:** 0.5 g of sodium nitroprusside is dissolved in 100 mL distilled water.
4. **0.5% Solution of hydroquinone acid:** 0.5 g of hydroquinone is dissolved in 100 mL of acetic acid.
5. **10% Oxalic acid:** 10 g of oxalic acid is dissolved in 100 mL distilled water.
6. **10% aqueous solution of phenyl hydrazine hydrochloride:** 10 g of phenyl hydrazine hydrochloride is dissolved in 100 mL distilled water.
7. **10% Ethanolic potassium hydroxide solution:** 10 g of potassium hydroxide is dissolved in 100 mL of ethyl alcohol.
8. **10% Methanolic potassium hydroxide solution:** 10 g of potassium hydroxide is dissolved in 100 mL of methyl alcohol.
9. **10% Potassium hydroxide solution:** 10 g of potassium hydroxide is dissolved in 100 mL of distilled water.
10. **10% Sodium hydroxide solution:** 10 g of sodium hydroxide is dissolved in 100 mL of distilled water.
11. **2% aqueous solution of ascorbic acid:** 2 g of ascorbic acid is dissolved in 100 mL distilled water.
12. **2% Cobalt thiocyanate solution:** 2% cobalt thiocyanate in water and diluted it with 96% glycerine in 1:1.
13. **32% Potassium dichromate:** 2 g of potassium dichromate is dissolved in sufficient dilute sulfuric acid to produce 100 mL.
14. **3% Potassium permanganate solution:** 3 g of potassium permanganate is dissolved in 100 mL distilled water.
15. **5% Ammonium molybdate solution:** 5 g of ammonium molybdate is dissolved in 100 mL of warm distilled water.
16. **5% Isopropylamine solution:** 5 mL isopropylamine is mixed with 95 mL of absolute methanol.
17. **5% Phosphoric acid:** 5g of phosphoric acid is dissolved in 100 mL distilled water.
18. **5% Potassium ferricyanide:** 10 g of potassium ferricyanide is dissolved in 100 mL distilled water.
19. **6% Ammonium persulfate solution:** 6 g of ammonium persulfate is dissolved in 100 mL of distilled water.
20. **Acetaldehyde and vanillin reagent:** 0.4 g of vanillin dissolved in 20 mL of 95% ethanol followed by addition of five drops of acetaldehyde.

21. **Acidified aqueous cinchonine:** 1 g of cinchonine is dissolved in 100 mL hot water containing a few drops of nitric acid, cooled, and mixed with 2 g of potassium iodide.
22. **Alizarin S reagent:** 0.1% aqueous solution of sodium alizarin sulfonate.
23. **Alizarin:** Saturated solution of alizarin is prepared in ethanol.
24. **Alkaline solution of beta-naphthol:** 4 g beta-naphthol is dissolved in 100 mL of 2N sodium hydroxide.
25. **Aluminon reagent:** A saturated solution of ammonium salt of aurine tricarboxylic acid.
26. **Ammonium acetate:** 231 g of the ammonium acetate is dissolved in 100 mL of water.
27. **Ammonium carbonate (4 N):** 160 g of ammonium carbonate is dissolved in 1 liter with water containing 140 mL concentrated ammonia.
28. **Ammonium chloride:** 169 g of the ammonium chloride is dissolved in 100 mL of water.
29. **Ammonium hydroxide:** 335 mL of concentrated solution is diluted to 1 liter of distilled water.
30. **Ammonium mercury thiocyanate:** 0.8 g of mercuric chloride and 0.9 g of ammonium thiocyanate are dissolved in 10 mL of water or proportionate amount.
31. **Ammonium molybdate reagent:** 45 g of the commercial salt or 40 g of pure molybdenum trioxide is mixed with 70 mL of concentrated ammonia solution and 140 mL of water. Add it very slowly and with vigorous stirring to a mixture of 250 mL of concentrated nitric acid and 500 mL of water, and dilute to 1 liter. Allow to stand 1–2 days and decant and use the clear solution.
32. **Ammonium molybdate-quinine sulfate:** It is prepared by dissolving 1 g of finely powdered ammonium molybdate in 5 mL of water and adding and stirring a solution of 0.025 g of quinine sulfate in 20 mL of concentrated nitric acid.
33. **Ammonium oxalate (0.5 N):** 35 g of ammonium oxalate is dissolved in 1 liter of water.
34. **Ammonium phosphate (0.5 N):** 22 g of ammonium phosphate is dissolved in 1 liter of water.
35. **Ammonium sulfate:** 132 g of ammonium sulfate is dissolved in 100 mL of water.
36. **Ammonium thiocyanate and o-Toluidine:** 0.1 g of o-toluidine and 0.5 g of ammonium thiocyanate are added in 5 mL of acetone.
37. **α-naphthylamine:** 0.3 g of α-naphthylamine is boiled with 70 mL of water, filtering or decanting from the small residue and mixing with 30 mL of glacial acetic acid.
38. **Antazoline hydrochloride solution:** Saturated solution of antazoline hydrochloride is prepared in water.
39. **Barium chloride (0.5 N):** 61 g of barium chloride is dissolved in 1 liter of water.
40. **Benedict's reagent:** (a) 1.73 g of copper sulfate is dissolved in 10 mL of water. (b) 17.3 g of trisodium citrate and 10 g of anhydrous sodium carbonate are mixed in 80 mL water with aid of heat. Solution (b) is poured into solution (a) and made up to 100 mL with water.
41. **Benzidine:** 50 g of benzidine is dissolved in 10 mL glacial acetic acid, dilute to 100 mL with water. Both the solutions are mixed together with vigorous shaking and then added 15 mL of glacial acetic acid, diluted to 250 mL and then allowed to stand and filtered.

APPENDIX 2

42. **Bromine solution:** Saturated solution of bromine is prepared in water.
43. **Bromine water:** 1.1 g sodium bromide, 10.7 mL 1 M hydrochloric acid, 7.6 mL sodium hypochlorite and 32 mL distilled water are mixed and made up to 50 mL water.
44. **Cadion 2B:** 0.02 g of cadion 2B is dissolved in 100 mL of ethanol to which 1 mL of 2 M potassium hydroxide is added.
45. **Calcium chloride:** 55 g of the hydrated calcium chloride is dissolved in 100 mL of water.
46. **Chlorine water:** 250 mL of water is saturated with chlorine gas. Preserve in a dark colored bottle.
47. **Chloroplatinic acid:** 2.6 g of hydrated chloroplatinic acid is dissolved in 10 mL of water.
48. **Chromotropic acid solution:** 50 mg of sodium salt of chromotropic acid is dissolved in 100 mL of concentrated sulfuric acid and then heated in a hot water bath at 60°C for 30 minutes, and then cooled.
49. **Cobalt nitrate:** 44 g of the cobalt nitrate is dissolved in 100 mL of water.
50. **Cobalt sulfate (0.05 N):** 125 g of cobalt sulfate is dissolved in 1 liter of water containing 3 mL of concentrated H_2SO_4.
51. **Cobalt thiocyanate solution:** 2.5 g cobalt thiocyanate is dissolved in 100 mL water.
52. **Cobaltous acetate solution:** 0.1 g of cobaltous acetate tetrahydrate is dissolved in 100 mL of absolute methanol, and finally 0.2 mL of glacial acetic acid is added.
53. **Congo red:** 0.4 g of Congo red is dissolved in 100 mL of 50% ethanol.
54. **Coniferyl alcohol reagent:** 0.1 g of coniferyl is warmed until it melts, dissolved in 3 mL of ethanol and diluted to 10 mL with ethanol.
55. **Copper sulfate solution:** 5 g $CuSO_4.5H_2O$ is dissolved in 100 mL 1N of HCl.
56. **Copper sulfate:** 125 g of copper sulfate is dissolved in 100 mL of water containing 3 mL of concentrated sulfuric acid.
57. **Dille-Koppanyi reagent:** 0.1 g cobaltous acetate tetrahydrate is dissolved in 100 mL absolute methanol and then add 0.2 mL glacial acetic acid.
58. **Dilute ferric chloride solution:** 10 g of ferric chloride is dissolved in 100 mL distilled water followed by few drops of hydrochloric acid.
59. **Dimethyl glyoxime:** 1 g of the solid salt is dissolved in 100 mL of 95% ethyl alcohol.
60. **Dinitrobenzene reagent:** 1g of 2, 4-dinitrobenzene is dissolved in 100 mL methanol.
61. **Diphenylamine solution:** 1 g of diphenylamine is dissolved in 100 mL of absolute ethanol.
62. **Diphenylcarbazide:** 0.125 g of diphenylcarbazide is dissolved in a mixture of 25 mL acetone in 25 mL water; or 0.2 g of diphenylcarbazide is dissolved in 10 mL acetic acid and dilute to 100 mL with methanol.
63. **Diphenylcarbazone:** 5 mg of diphenylcarbazone is dissolved in 100 mL of carbon tetrachloride or chloroform.
64. **Dithizone solution:** 2–5 mg of dithizone is dissolved in 100 mL chloroform.

65. **Dragendorff reagent:**
    (a) 2 g of bismuth subnitrate is dissolved in 10 mL of glacial acetic acid and made up to 100 mL water.
    (b) 40 g of potassium iodide is dissolved in 100 mL of water.

    10 mL of (a) is mixed with 10 mL of (b) and 25 mL of glacial acetic acid is added. The solution is then diluted with 100 mL of water.
66. **Duquenois-levine reagent:** 2.0% vanillin and 0.3% acetaldehyde are added in 95% ethanol.
67. **Ehrlich reagent:** 1 g of p-dimethylaminobenzaldehyde is dissolved in 10 mL methanol. Then add 10 mL concentrated ortho-phosphoric acid.
68. **Erdmann's reagent:** 1 mL of nitric acid is mixed with 30 mL of sulfuric acid.
69. **Ethylenediamine nickel reagent:** Nickel chloride solution is mixed with ethylenediamine until a violet color appears.
70. **Fast blue B reagent:** Fast blue B and anhydrous sodium sulfate in ratio of 2.5:100 are mixed in water.
71. **Ferric chloride (0.05 N):** 135 g of hydrated ferric chloride is dissolved in 1 liter of water at ready containing 20 mL of concentrated HCl.
72. **Ferric chloride solution:** 10 g of ferric chloride is dissolved in 100 mL of distilled water.
73. **Ferric salt reagent:** 1 g ferric sulfate is dissolved in 20 mL of water.
74. **Ferrous hydroxide solution:** 10 g of ferrous hydroxide is dissolved in 100 mL of distilled water.
75. **Ferrous sulfate:** 140 g of ferrous sulfate is dissolved in 100 mL of water containing 7 mL of concentrated sulfuric acid.
76. **Formaldehyde solution:** One part of commercially available 40% formaldehyde solution is mixed with seven part of water.
77. **Formaldehyde-sulfuric acid reagent:** 4 part of sulfuric acid is mixed with 6 parts of formalin.
78. **Forrest reagent:** Equal volume of 0.2% solution of potassium dichromate, 30% (v/v) solution of sulfuric acid, 20% solution of perchloric acid and 50% solution of nitric acid are mixed.
79. **FPN reagent:** 5 mL of 5% w/v, solution of ferric chloride is added 45 mL of 20% W/W perchloric acid and 50 mL of 50% w/w nitric acid in water.
80. **Froehde reagent:** 0.5 g of ammonium molybdate is dissolved in 100 mL of water.
81. **Fuchsine reagent:** 0.015 g fuchsine is dissolved in 100 mL of water.
82. **Fujiwara reagent:** Freshly prepared 20% (w/v) in sodium hydroxide solution.
83. **Furfural-H_2SO_4 reagent:** One drop of furfural is mixed with 1 mL of H_2SO_4.
84. **Furfuraldehyde reagent:** 10% solution of furfuraldehyde is prepared in ethanol.
85. **Gunzberg's reagent:** 2 g of phloroglucinol and 1 g of vanillin is dissolved in 100 mL of 95% alcohol.
86. **Hydrogen sulfide:** Iron sulfide (FeS) is heated gently with a strong acid in a Kipp's apparatus/generator.
87. **Hydroxylamine hydrochloride:** 10 g of hydroxylamine hydrochloride is dissolved in 100 mL water.

APPENDIX 2

88. **Indigo solution:** 1 g in 12 mL of concentrated H_2SO_4 is warmed and allowed to stand for 2 days. 240 mL of water is added and then the solution is filtered.
89. **Indole:** 0.15 g of indole is dissolved in 100 mL ethanol.
90. **Iodine solution (0.1 N):** 12.7 g of iodine and 20 g of potassium iodide is dissolved in 30 mL of water and diluted to 1 liter.
91. **Koppanyi-Zwikker reagent:** 1% (w/v) solution of cobalt nitrate in ethanol.
92. **Lanthanum nitrate solution:** 4.33 g of lanthanum nitrate hexahydrate is dissolved in 100 mL of water.
93. **Lead acetate solution:** 10 g of lead acetate is dissolved in 100 mL distilled water.
94. **Liebermann's reagent:** 1 g of sodium or potassium nitrite is dissolved in 10 mL of sulfuric acid with cooling and swirling to absorb the brown fumes.
95. **Litmus solution:** 10 g of the solid is powdered in a mortar. It is then dissolved in 100 mL of hot water as far as possible and kept overnight. Decanted or filtered into a stopper bottle and solution is made up to 150 mL with water.
96. **Magnesium sulfate:** 62 g of the magnesium sulfate is dissolved in 100 mL of water.
97. **Mandelin's reagent:** 1 g of ammonium vanadate is dissolved in 1.5 mL of water and diluted to 100 mL with concentrated sulfuric acid.
98. **Manganous sulfate-phosphoric acid:** Equal volumes of saturated manganous sulfate solution and concentrated phosphoric acid are mixed.
99. **Marquis reagent:** 100 mL of concentrated sulfuric acid is mixed with 1 mL of 40% (v/v) formaldehyde solution.
100. **Mayer's reagent:**
     (a) 1.355 g mercuric chloride is dissolved in 50 mL water by warming.
     (b) 5 g of potassium iodide is dissolved in 20 mL of water.
101. **Mecke's reagent:** 0.25 g of selenious acid is dissolved in 25 mL of concentrated sulfuric acid.
102. **Mercuric chloride solution:** 10 g of mercuric chloride is dissolved in 100 mL distilled water.
103. **Mercuric sulfate solution:** 5 g of mercury oxide is dissolved in 20 mL concentrated sulfuric acid and diluted with water made up to 250 mL.
104. **Mercurous nitrate reagent:** To a saturated solution of mercurous nitrate, solid sodium bicarbonate is added until effervescence ceases. This reagent should be freshly prepared, shaken immediately before use and should not be kept for more than an hour.
105. **Methanolic potassium hydroxide:** 20% (w/v) solution of potassium hydroxide in methanol.
106. **Methyl orange:** 1 g of methyl orange is dissolved in 1 liter of solution.
107. **Methylene blue solution:** 0.05 g methylene blue is dissolved in 100 mL of water.
108. **Millon's reagent:** 23.5 g of mercury is dissolved in 34 mL of cold fuming nitric acid and the solution is diluted with water up to 100 mL.
109. **N-1-naphthyl ethylenediamine dihydrochloride:** 1 g of N-1-naphthyl ethylenediamine dihydrochloride is dissolved in 100 mL of ethanol.

110. **Nessler's reagent:** (I) Dissolve 50 g of mercuric chloride and 35 g of potassium iodide are dissolved in 200 mL of water and cooled. (II) 50 g of sodium hydroxide is dissolved in 250 mL of water and cooled. Cold solution (II) and cold solution (I) are mixed and made up to 500 mL. Allow the mixture to stand and decant the clear supernatant for use. Store in dark brown bottles and keep away from light.

111. **Ninhydrin reagent:** 0.5 g of ninhydrin is dissolved in 40 mL of acetone. It should be prepared freshly always.

112. **Palladium chloride:** 0.1 g of palladium chloride is dissolved in 5 mL of 2 M hydrochloric acid by heating and dilute the solution to 100 mL with water.

113. **p-dimethylaminobenzaldehyde:** 1 g of p-dimethylaminobenzaldehyde is dissolved in 100 mL of ethanol. The solution is acidified with 10 mL of dilute hydrochloric acid.

114. **Phenolphthalein:** 5 g of phenolphthalein is dissolved in 500 mL of 50% alcohol.

115. **Phosphomolybdic acid:** 5 g of phosphomolybdic acid is dissolved in 25 mL water, filtered, and diluted to 100 mL.

116. **Picric acid:** 2% solution of picric acid is prepared in alcohol.

117. **Potassium antimonate solution:** 10.5 g of potassium antimonate is dissolved in 100 mL water and dilute the solution to 200 mL.

118. **Potassium chromate:** 49 g of the potassium chromate is dissolved in 100 mL of water.

119. **Potassium cyanide:** 10 g of potassium cyanide is dissolved in 20 mL of water containing 2 mL of NaOH solution and finally made up to 100 mL.

120. **Potassium ferricyanide solution:** 55 g of potassium ferricyanide is dissolved in 1 liter of water.

121. **Potassium ferrocyanide solution:** 53 g of potassium ferrocyanide is dissolved in 1 liter of water.

122. **Potassium iodide:** 83 g of potassium iodide is dissolved in 100 mL of water.

123. **Potassium iodide-sodium sulfite solution:** 5 g potassium iodide (KI) and 20 g sodium sulfite ($Na_2SO_3.7H_2O$) are dissolved in 100 mL of water.

124. **Potassium nitrite solution:** 10 g of potassium nitrate is dissolved in 100 mL of distilled water.

125. **Potassium thiocyanate:** 49 g of potassium thiocyanate is dissolved in 100 mL of water.

126. **Resorcinol reagent:** It is prepared by dissolving 0.2 g resorcinol and 1 g potassium bromide in 10 mL of water.

127. **Rhodamine B:** 0.01 g of Rhodamine-B is dissolved in 100 mL water or 0.05 g Rhodamine B and 15 g KCl are mixed in a solution of 15 mL concentrated HCl and 85 mL water.

128. **Rubeanic acid:** 0.05% in ethanol, a saturated ethanolic solution.

129. **Saturated caustic soda solution:** Sodium hydroxide is dissolved in water till saturation point reached.

130. **Silver nitrate (0.1 M):** 17 g of the silver nitrate is dissolved in 100 mL of water.

131. **Silver sulfate (0.05 N):** 8 g of silver sulfate is dissolved in 1 liter of water and kept in a colored bottle.

132. **Soap solution:** 20 g of soap is dissolved in 250 mL of water.
133. **Sodium acetate:** 408 g of sodium acetate is dissolved in 100 mL of water.
134. **Sodium carbonate (3 N):** 430 g of sodium carbonate is dissolved in 1 liter of water.
135. **Sodium cobalt nitrite**
    Solution I: 7.5 g of cobalt nitrate is dissolved in 30 mL of water.
    Solution II: 60 g of sodium nitrite is dissolved in 30 mL of water. Both the solutions are mixed together with vigorous shaking and then added 15 mL of glacial acetic acid, diluted to 250 mL and then allowed to stand and is filtered.
136. **Sodium hydrogen tartrate solution:** 10 g of sodium hydrogen tartrate monohydrate is dissolved in 100 mL of water. Allowed to stand for 24 hours and use the clear supernatant liquid for test.
137. **Sodium phosphate (1 N):** 120 g of sodium phosphate is dissolved in 1 liter of water.
138. **Sodium rhodizonate reagent:** 0.5 g of sodium rhodizonate is dissolved in 100 mL water.
139. **Stannous chloride solution:** 5% solution of stannous chloride dihydrate is mixed with 25% solution of hydrochloric acid.
140. **Starch solution:** 0.5 g of soluble starch is mixed with a little cold water into a thin paste and then add 25 mL of boiling water and boil it until a clear solution is obtained. This solution should be freshly prepared as required. A more stable starch solution is obtained by adding 0.5 g of potassium iodide and 2–3 drops of chloroform.
141. **Sulfanilic acid:** 1 g of sulfanilic acid is dissolved in 100 mL of warm 30% acetic acid.
142. **Sulfuric acid-fuming sulfuric acid reagent:** 7 mL of sulfuric acid is mixed with 3 mL of fuming sulfuric acid.
143. **Tartaric acid-ammonium molybdate reagent:** 0.15 mg of crystalline tartaric acid is dissolved in 1 mL of ammonium molybdate reagent.
144. **Nitrating mixture:** Equal volume of concentrated nitric and concentrated hydrochloric acid are mixed.
145. **Uranyl acetate:** 40 g of uranyl acetate is dissolved in 30 mL acetic acid and volume is made upto 500 mL by water.
146. **van-Urk reagent:** 0.125 mg para-dimethylaminobenzaldehyde is dissolved in 100 mL of sulfuric acid (65%) with 0.1 mL ferric chloride (5%).
147. **Vanadium pentoxide reagent:** 0.5 g of vanadium pentoxide is dissolved in 10 mL sulfuric acid.
148. **Vanillin reagent:** 1 g of vanillin is dissolved in 20 mL of sulfuric acid.
149. **Vanillin-H_2SO_4 reagent:** 1 pinch of vanillin is dissolved in 1 mL of H_2SO_4.
150. **Zinc nitrate:** 150 g of the zinc nitrate is dissolved in 100 mL of water.
151. **Zinc sulfate solution:** 28.8 g zinc sulfate heptahydrate is dissolved in 100 mL of water.
152. **Zinc uranyl acetate:** Uranyl zinc acetate is dissolved in water or 2 M acetic acid.
153. **Zirconyl chloride solution:** 0.1 g of solid is dissolved in 20 mL of concentrated hydrochloric acid and diluted to 100 mL.

Appendix 3

Preparation of Dilute Solutions

Acids and bases	Preparation
Dilute acetic acid (5 M)	Dilute 285 mL of concentrated acid to 1 liter with water
Dilute hydrochloric acid (5 M)	Dilute 430 mL of concentrated acid to 1 liter with water
Dilute nitric acid (5 M)	Dilute 310 mL of concentrated acid to 1 liter with water
Dilute sulfuric acid (2.5 M)	Pour carefully 140 mL of concentrated acid to about 500 mL water with constant stirring and cooling of the bottle under tap water and dilute to 1 liter with water
Ammonium solution concentrated (14.5 M)	The commercial solution of aqueous ammonia is appropriate
Ammonium solution dilute (5 M)	Dilute 335 mL of concentrated solution to 1 liter with water
Sodium hydroxide solution (5 M)	Dissolve about 220 g of the solid sticks or pellets in water and dilute to 1 liter
Potassium hydroxide solution (2 M)	Dissolve about 125 g of the solid sticks in water and dilute to 1 liter
Calcium hydroxide solution (Lime water) (0.02 M)	Shake about 3 g of solid calcium hydroxide with 1 liter of water. Filter and always stopper the bottle to protect lime water from carbon dioxide

Appendix 4

List of Periodic Table Elements Sorted by Atomic Number

Name	Symbol	Atomic No.	Atomic weight	Density (g/cm³)
Hydrogen	H	1	1.0079	0.09
Helium	He	2	4.0026	0.18
Lithium	Li	3	6.941	0.53
Beryllium	Be	4	9.0122	1.85
Boron	B	5	10.811	2.34
Carbon	C	6	12.0107	2.26
Nitrogen	N	7	14.0067	1.25
Oxygen	O	8	15.9994	1.43
Fluorine	F	9	18.9984	1.7
Neon	Ne	10	20.1797	0.9
Sodium	Na	11	22.9897	0.97
Magnesium	Mg	12	24.305	1.74
Aluminum	Al	13	26.9815	2.7
Silicon	Si	14	28.0055	2.33
Phosphorus	P	15	30.9738	1.82
Sulfur	S	16	32.065	2.07
Chlorine	Cl	17	35.453	3.21
Argon	Ar	18	39.948	1.78
Potassium	K	19	39.0983	0.86
Calcium	Ca	20	40.078	1.55
Scandium	Sc	21	44.9559	2.99
Titanium	Ti	22	47.867	4.54
Vanadium	V	23	50.9415	6.11
Chromium	Cr	24	51.9961	7.19
Manganese	Mn	25	54.938	7.43
Iron	Fe	26	55.845	7.87
Cobalt	Co	27	58.9332	8.9
Nickel	Ni	28	58.6934	8.9
Copper	Cu	29	63.546	8.96
Zinc	Zn	30	65.39	7.13
Gallium	Ga	31	69.723	5.91
Germanium	Ge	32	72.64	5.32

Continued

Continued

Name	Symbol	Atomic No.	Atomic weight	Density (g/cm³)
Arsenic	As	33	74.9216	5.72
Selenium	Se	34	78.96	4.79
Bromine	Br	35	79.904	3.12
Krypton	Kr	36	83.8	3.75
Rubidium	Rb	37	85.4678	1.63
Strontium	Sr	38	87.62	2.54
Yttrium	Y	39	88.9059	4.47
Zirconium	Zr	40	91.224	6.51
Niobium	Nb	41	92.9064	8.57
Molybdenum	Mo	42	95.94	10.22
Technetium	Tc	43	98	11.5
Ruthenium	Ru	44	101.07	12.37
Rhodium	Rh	45	102.9055	12.41
Palladium	Pd	46	106.42	12.02
Silver	Ag	47	107.8682	10.5
Cadmium	Cd	48	112.411	8.65
Indium	In	49	114.818	7.31
Tin	Sn	50	118.71	7.31
Antimony	Sb	51	121.76	6.68
Tellurium	Te	52	127.6	6.24
Iodine	I	53	126.9045	4.93
Xenon	Xe	54	131.293	5.9
Cesium	Cs	55	132.9055	1.87
Barium	Ba	56	137.327	3.59
Lanthanum	La	57	138.9055	6.15
Cerium	Ce	58	140.116	6.77
Praseodymium	Pr	59	140.9077	6.77
Neodymium	Nd	60	144.24	7.01
Promethium	Pm	61	145	7.3
Samarium	Sm	62	150.36	7.52
Europium	Eu	63	151.964	5.24
Gadolinium	Gd	64	157.25	7.9
Terbium	Tb	65	158.9253	8.23
Dysprosium	Dy	66	162.5	8.55
Holmium	Ho	67	164.9303	8.8
Erbium	Er	68	167.259	9.07
Thulium	Tm	69	168.9342	9.32
Ytterbium	Yb	70	173.04	6.9

Continued

APPENDIX 4

Continued

Name	Symbol	Atomic No.	Atomic weight	Density (g/cm³)
Lutetium	Lu	71	174.967	9.84
Hafnium	Hf	72	178.49	13.31
Tantalum	Ta	73	180.9479	16.65
Tungsten	W	74	183.84	19.35
Rhenium	Re	75	186.207	21.04
Osmium	Os	76	190.23	22.6
Iridium	Ir	77	192.217	22.4
Platinum	Pt	78	195.078	21.45
Gold	Au	79	196.9665	19.32
Mercury	Hg	80	200.59	13.55
Thallium	Tl	81	204.3833	11.85
Lead	Pb	82	207.2	11.35
Bismuth	Bi	83	208.9804	9.75
Polonium	Po	84	209	9.3
Astatine	At	85	210	-
Radon	Rn	86	222	9.73
Francium	Fr	87	223	-
Radium	Ra	88	226	5.5
Actinium	Ac	89	227	10.07
Thorium	Th	90	232.0381	11.72
Protactinium	Pa	91	231.0359	15.4
Uranium	U	92	238.0289	18.95
Neptunium	Np	93	237	20.2
Plutonium	Pu	94	244	19.84
Americium	Am	95	243	13.67
Curium	Cm	96	247	13.5
Berkelium	Bk	97	247	14.78
Californium	Cf	98	251	15.1
Einsteinium	Es	99	252	-
Fermium	Fm	100	257	-
Mendelevium	Md	101	258	-
Nobelium	No	102	259	-
Lawrencium	Lr	103	262	-
Rutherfordium	Rf	104	261	-
Dubnium	Db	105	262	-
Seaborgium	Sg	106	266	-
Bohrium	Bh	107	264	-

Continued

Continued

Name	Symbol	Atomic No.	Atomic weight	Density (g/cm³)
Hassium	Hs	108	277	-
Meitnerium	Mt	109	268	-
Darmstadtium	Ds	110	281	-
Roentgenium	Rg	111	272	-
Copernicium	Cn	112	-	-
Ununtrium	Uut	113	-	-
Flerovium	Fl	114	-	-
Ununpentium	Uup	115	-	-
Livermorium	Lv	116	-	-
Ununseptium	Uus	117	-	-
Ununoctium	Uuo	118	-	-

Appendix 5

Important Laws Related to Poisoning in India

1. The Indian Penal Code (IPC): 284, 299, 300, 304A, 306, 307, 309, 324, 326, 328
2. The Criminal Procedural Code (CrPC): 39, 40, 175, 293
3. The Indian Evidence Act (IEA)
4. The Narcotics Drugs and Psychotropic Substance Act, 1985
5. The Drugs and Magic Remedies Act, 1954
6. The Drugs Control Act, 1950
7. The Pharmacy Act, 1948
8. The Drugs and Cosmetics Rules, 1945
9. The Drugs and Cosmetics Act, 1940
10. The Drugs Act, 1940
11. The Poison Act, 1919

Appendix 6

Table 1: Therapeutic ("normal"), toxic, and comatose-fatal blood-plasma/serum concentrations (μg/mL) in man.

S. No.	Substances	Therapeutic ("normal")	Toxic (from)	Comatose-fatal (from)	t½ (hours)
1.	Acamprosate	Approximately 0.37–0.65			13–20
2.	Acebutolol	0.2–2 (0.5–1.255)		15–20	3–11
3.	N-acetylacebutolol	1–2.5		90–150	9–14
4.	Acecainide	See N-acetylprocainamide			
5.	Acecarbromal(um)	10–20 (sum)	25–30		
6.	Acemetacin	See indomethacin			
7.	Acenocoumarol	0.03–0.1	0.1–0.15		3–11
8.	Acetaldehyde	0–30	100–125		
9.	Acetaminophen	See paracetamol			
10.	Acetazolamide	(4–) 10–20	25–30		2–6
11.	Acetohexamide	20–70	500		1.3
12.	Acetone	(2–) 5–20	100–400; 2,000	550	(6–) 8–31
13.	Acetonitrile			0.77	
14.	Acetyldigoxin	0.0005–0.0008	0.0025–0.003	0.005	40–70
15.	Acetylsalicylic acid (ASS, ASA)	20–200	300–350	400–500	3–20
16.	Acitretin	Approximately 0.01–0.05			2–4
17.	Acyclovir	(0.4–0.63) 0.5–1.5			2–5

Continued

APPENDIX 6

S. No.	Substances	Blood-plasma/serum concentration (μg/mL)			t½ (hours)
		Therapeutic ("normal")	Toxic (from)	Comatose-fatal (from)	
18.	Adipiodone-meglumine	850–1,200			0.5
19.	Athanol	See ethanol			0.15 (+ and –) 0.05% per hour
20.	Ajmaline	(0.1–) 0.53–2.21		5.5	1.3–1.6, 5–6
21.	Albendazole	0.5–1.5			8–9
22.	Albuterol	See salbutamol			
23.	Alcuronium	0.3–3			3.3 ± 1.3
24.	Aldrin	–0.0015	0.0035		
25.	Alendronate	<0.005			in days
26.	Alfentanil	0.03–0.6			0.6–2.3
27.	Alfuzosin	0.003–0.06			3–9
28.	Alimemazine (trimeprazine)	0.05–0.4	0.5	1–3.2	8
29.	Alizapride	0.1–2			2–3
30.	Allobarbital	2–5	10	20	40–48
31.	Allopurinol	2–19			0.5–3
32.	Alphaprodine	0.87–1			1.6–2.6
33.	Alprazolam	0.005–0.05 (–0.008)	0.1–0.4	0.21 ug/mL	6–20
34.	Alprenolol	0.025–0.14	1–2	40–48	2–7
35.	Aluminum	<0.005	0.05–0.15	4.4	Approximately 0.5
36.	Amantadine	0.2–0.6 (–1)	1; 2.4	21	9–15
37.	Amikacin	10–25	30		2–3

Continued

APPENDIX 6

Continued

S. No.	Substances	Blood-plasma/serum concentration (µg/mL)			t½ (hours)
		Therapeutic ("normal")	Toxic (from)	Comatose-fatal (from)	
38.	Aminobenzoic acid	300–600	600		
39.	Aminoglutethimide	0.5–25			13.3 ± 2.65
40.	Aminophenazone	10–20			Approximately 2–4
41.	4-aminopyridine (fampridine)	0.025–0.075	0.14; 0.2		3–3.5
42.	5-aminosalicylic acid (5-AS, 5-ASA)	See mesalazine			
43.	Amiodarone	(0.5–) 1–2 (–2.5)	2.5–3		30–120
44.	Amisulpride	~0.4			12–18
45.	Amitriptyline	0.05–0.3	0.5–0.6	1.5–2	30–50
46.	Amlodipine	0.005–0.015 (0.003–0.011)	0.088	0.1–0.2	34–50
47.	Ammonia	0.5–1.7			
48.	Amobarbital	1–5	5–6	10	15–30
49.	Amodiaquine	~0.05			Active metabolite desethylamodiaquine 1–10 days
50.	Amoxapine	0.18–0.6	3	5	8
51.	Amoxicillin	0.5–1 (5–15)			1–2
52.	Amphetamine	0.02–0.1	0.2	0.5–1	4–8
53.	Amphotericin B	(0.1–) 0.2–3	(3–) 5–10		24–48
54.	Ampicillin	0.02–2 (2–20)			1
55.	Amrinone	1–2 (–4)			3–12
56.	Amsacrine	0.1–0.5 (0.15–5.5)			5–7

Continued

APPENDIX 6

S. No.	Substances	Blood-plasma/serum concentration (µg/mL)			t½ (hours)
		Therapeutic ("normal")	Toxic (from)	Comatose-fatal (from)	
57.	Anileridine	<0.5		0.9	
58.	Aniline	Approximately –1 (urine)		6	
59.	Antimony	~0.01	0.2		
60.	Antipyrine	See phenazone			Approximately 0.75
61.	Apomorphine	0.002–0.02			
62.	Aprindine	1–2	2–3		13–50
63.	Aprobarbital	4–20	30–40	50	14–34
64.	Arsenic	0.002–0.07	0.05–0.25	9–15	
65.	Articaine	<1.5–2			0.3 (–1)
66.	Ascorbic acid (vitamin C)	4–15			In days
67.	Astemizole	0.002–0.05	14		Approximately 20
68.	Atenolol	0.1–1 (–2)	2–3	27	4–14
69.	Atovaquone	13.9 ± 6.9 (>15)			2–3
70.	Atracurium besylate	0.1–0.5 (–5)			Approximately 0.5
71.	Atropine	0.002–0.025	0.03–0.1	0.2	2–6.5, 13–38
72.	Azapropazone (apazone)	40–80			8–24
73.	Azathioprine	~2			1–4
74.	Azelastine	0.002–0.003 (–0.01)			22–25
75.	Azithromycin	Approximately 0.04–1			50–60 (2–4)
76.	Aztreonam	1–10 (50–250)			1.5–2
77.	Baclofen	0.08–0.4 (–0.6)	1.1–3.5	6–9.6	6.8 ± 0.7

Continued

APPENDIX 6

Continued

S. No.	Substances	Blood-plasma/serum concentration (μg/mL)			t½ (hours)
		Therapeutic ("normal")	Toxic (from)	Comatose-fatal (from)	
78.	Bambuterol	See terbutaline			10
79.	Barbital	2–20	20–50	50	57–120
80.	Barium	–0.001			
81.	Bendrofluazide	0.05–0.1			Approximately 3
82.	Benoxaprofen	–50			19–39
83.	Benperidol	Approximately –0.002			4–8
84.	Benzbromarone	2–10			2–4
85.	Benzene	–0.0002		0.95	
86.	Benzphetamine	0.025–0.5	0.5	14	
87.	Benztropine	0.01–0.18	0.005	0.2–0.7	
88.	Benzyl alcohol		18		1.5 h in days after iv administration
89.	Benzylpenicillin	1.2–12			1
90.	Bepridil	0.6–2.5			33–42
91.	Beryllium	–0.0003			
92.	Beta-carotene	4–6			
93.	Betaxolol	0.005–0.05		36	14–22
94.	Bethanidine	0.02–0.5			9–10
95.	Bevantolol	0.2–2			2
96.	Bezafibrate	–15			2
97.	Bicalutamide	1.5–17.5 (–25)			(3–) 7–10

Continued

APPENDIX 6

S. No.	Substances	Blood-plasma/serum concentration (µg/mL)			t½ (hours)
		Therapeutic ("normal")	Toxic (from)	Comatose-fatal (from)	
98.	Biperiden	0.05–0.1		0.25	18–24
99.	Bismuth	<0.05 (–0.1)	0.05–0.1		In days
100.	Bisoprolol	0.01–0.1			10–12
101.	Bopindolol	0.001–0.015			4–8
102.	Borate	0–7	20	200	
103.	Boron	0.8–6	20–50	50–150	
104.	Brallobarbital (brallobarbitone)	4–8	8–10	15	20–40
105.	Bretylium	0.8–2.4			6–11
106.	Brodifacoum		0.02	0.03–0.17; acute: 3.9	20–60
107.	Bromadiolone		0.02		
108.	Bromazepam	(0.05–) 0.08–0.2	0.3–0.4	1–2	8–22
109.	Bromide	10–50	500–1,500; 3,000	2,000	12–13
110.	Bromisoval	10–20	30–40		Approximately 4
111.	Bromoxynil		20		
112.	Bromperidol	0.001–0.02			20–36
113.	Brompheniramine	0.005–0.015	0.2		2–10 (–20)
114.	Brotizolam	0.001–0.02			4–10
115.	Budipine	Approximately 0.1–0.3		10	30
116.	Buflomedil	Approximately 0.2–0.5 (–1.0)	15–25	25–50; 275	2–4
117.	Bunitrolol	0.001–0.015			2–6

Continued

APPENDIX 6

Continued

S. No.	Substances	Blood-plasma/serum concentration (µg/mL)			t½ (hours)
		Therapeutic ("normal")	Toxic (from)	Comatose-fatal (from)	
118.	Bupivacaine	(0.25–) 0.5–1.5 (–2)	2–4		0.5–3
119.	Bupranolol	Blood drug concentration following therapeutically effective doses below detection limit			2–4
120.	Buprenorphine	0.0005–0.005 (–0.01)	0.2	1.1; 4–13	3–5
121.	Bupropion (amfebutamone)	0.01–0.02; 0.05–0.1	1.2	7.3	10–20
122.	Buspirone	0.001–0.004 (–0.01)			2–3
123.	Butabarbital	See secbutabarbital			
124.	Butalbital	1–5	10–15	15–30	30–40
125.	Butanone	–10	500		
126.	Butaperazine	0.02–0.3 (–0.7)			12
127.	Butorphanol	0.0006–0.002			4–9
128.	Butriptyline	0.07–0.15	0.4–0.5		
129.	Cadmium	–0.0065	0.015–0.05		
130.	Caffeine (coffein)	(2–) 4–10	15–20	180	2–10
131.	Calcifediol	0.01–0.05			
132.	Camazepam	0.1–0.6	2		20–24
133.	Camphor		0.3–0.4	1.7	
134.	Candesartan	0.08–0.18			5–7
135.	Canrenone	See spironolactone			

Continued

APPENDIX 6

Continued

S. No.	Substances	Blood-plasma/serum concentration (µg/mL)			t½ (hours)
		Therapeutic ("normal")	Toxic (from)	Comatose-fatal (from)	
136.	Captopril	0.05–0.5 (–1)	5–6	60	1–2
137.	Carazolol	–0.015			9
138.	Carbamazepine	2–8 (4–12)	10	20	12–60 (7–35)
139.	Carbaryl		5	6	
140.	Carbenoxolone	Approximately 5–30			8–20
141.	Carbimazole	0.5–3.4			3–5
142.	Carbinoxamine	Approximately 0.02–0.04			Approximately 10–15
143.	Carbochromene	0.8–2.4			0.2–1.5
144.	Carbon monoxide	≤5% (elderly: ~15%); smoker: 8–10%)	25–30%	50–60%	
145.	Carbon tetrachloride	0.07	7.1; 20–50	100–200	2.5–6
146.	Carboplatin	Maximum 10–25			
147.	Carbromal(um)	2–10	15–20	40	7–15
148.	Carisoprodol	10–30	40	50	8
149.	β-carotene	See beta-carotene			
150.	Carteolol	0.01–0.1			3–7
151.	Carvedilol	Approximately 0.02–0.15 (–0.3)			6–10
152.	Cefaclor	13–35 (IV 900)			0.5–1
153.	Cefalexin	–65			1–1.5
154.	Cefaloridine	20–80			1.5
155.	Cefamandole	1–5 (10–40–150)			0.5–1.2

Continued

APPENDIX 6

Continued

S. No.	Substances	Blood-plasma/serum concentration (μg/mL)			t½ (hours)
		Therapeutic ("normal")	Toxic (from)	Comatose-fatal (from)	
156.	Cefazolin	~150			1.5–2
157.	Cefoperazone	~250			1–2 (–5)
158.	Cefotaxime	0.5–2 (10–50, IV 225)			1–1.5
159.	Cefotetan	65–90			3.5
160.	Cefotiam	~150[71]			0.7–1.5 (–2)
161.	Cefoxitin	~150			0.7–1
162.	Cefsulodin	20–100			1.6–1.9
163.	Ceftazidime	20–40 (50–200)			1.6–2
164.	Ceftibuten	Approximately 3–20			2–4
165.	Ceftizoxime	40–160			6–9
166.	Ceftriaxone	15–75			6.5–8.5
167.	Cefuroxime	0.5–1 (–180); 7–59			1.1–1.3
168.	Celiprolol	0.05–0.5			3–6
169.	Cephalothin (cefalotin)	~30			0.5–0.6
170.	Cerivastatin	0.002–0.04			1.5–3
171.	Cetirizine	Approximately 0.02–0.3	2–5		7–9
172.	Chinidine	See quinidine			
173.	Chinine	See quinine			
174.	Chloral hydrate	1.5–15	40–50	60–100	80–30
175.	Chlorambucil	0.15–0.3 (–1.0)			1.5–3
176.	Chloramphenicol	5–10 (–15)	25		2–6

Continued

APPENDIX 6

Continued

S. No.	Substances	Blood-plasma/serum concentration (µg/mL)			t½ (hours)
		Therapeutic ("normal")	Toxic (from)	Comatose-fatal (from)	
177.	Chlordane	~0.001	0.0025	1–7	
178.	Chlordecone		0.5		
179.	Chlordiazepoxide	0.4–3	3.5–10	20	6–24
180.	Chlormethiazole	See clomethiazole			
181.	Chlormezanone	(3–) 5–9 (–14)	Approximately 20	18; 53	20–30
182.	Chlorobutanol		75		
183.	Chloroform	20–50	70–250	390	
184.	Chlorophacinone		0.1		
185.	Chloroquine	0.02–0.5	1	3	Dose dependent
186.	Chlorothiazide	Approximately 6			0.5–2
187.	Chlorpheniramine	0.003–0.017		1.1	15–25
188.	Chlorpromazine	0.03–0.1 (0.5)	1–2	3–4	10–30
189.	Chlorpropamide	30–150	200–750		25–60
190.	Chlorprothixene	0.02–0.2	0.4	0.8	10–30
191.	Chlorpyrifos		0.2		27
192.	Chlorthalidone	0.15–0.3 (–1.4)	Approximately 2		44–48 (35–70)
193.	Chlortetracycline	1–5 (–10)	30		5–6
194.	Chromium	~0.00035		32	
195.	Cibenzoline	0.2–0.4 (–0.9)	0.5–1		7–8
196.	Cicletanine	Approximately 1–2			5–23
197.	Ciclosporin	See cyclosporine			

Continued

Continued

S. No.	Substances	Blood-plasma/serum concentration (μg/mL)			t½ (hours)
		Therapeutic ("normal")	Toxic (from)	Comatose-fatal (from)	
198.	Cidofovir	Approximately 7–43			2.5
199.	Cilazapril(-)at	0.003–0.09			30–50
200.	Cimetidine	0.25–3 (0.75–4)	30–50	110	1.5–4
201.	Cinoxacin	Approximately 15			1.5–4
202.	Ciprofloxacin	2.5–4	11.5		3–6
203.	Cisapride	0.04–0.08			6–12
204.	Citalopram	Approximately 0.01–0.02 (–0.1)		5–6	Approximately 33
205.	Cladribine	Approximately 0.006			0.1–0.2 (6.4–19.7)
206.	Clarithromycin	Approximately 0.2–2			3–7[217]
207.	Clemastine	Approximately 0.001–0.002			Approximately 8
208.	Clenbuterol	0.0003–0.0006	0.003		34–35
209.	Clindamycin	Approximately 0.5			2–3
210.	Clobazam	0.1–0.4			10–32
211.	Clobutinol	Approximately 0.05–0.2			23–34
212.	Clofibrate	50–250			10–18
213.	Clomethiazole (chlormethiazole)	0.7–2	(2.8–) 4–15	50	3–7
214.	Clomipramine	(0.02–) 0.09–0.25 (–0.4)	0.4–0.6	1–2	20–26
215.	Clonazepam	(0.004–) 0.01–0.08	0.1		20–60
216.	Clonidine	0.001–0.002 (0.004)	0.025–0.05 (0.009)	0.23	8–25
217.	Clopenthixol	0.002–0.015	0.05–0.1		15–25

Continued

APPENDIX 6

Continued

S. No.	Substances	Blood-plasma/serum concentration (μg/mL)			t½ (hours)
		Therapeutic ("normal")	Toxic (from)	Comatose-fatal (from)	
218.	Clorazepate	See nordazepam			1–2
219.	Clotiazepam	0.1–0.7			3–15
220.	Cloxacillin	5–30 (–85)			0.5–1 (0.3–2)
221.	Clozapine	(0.1–) 0.3–0.6 (>0.35)	0.6–1 (9.5)	1.2; 2; 5.2	6–14
222.	Cobalt	0.0001–0.0022			
223.	Cocaine	0.05–0.3	0.5–1	4	0.5–1
224.	Codeine	0.03–0.25	0.5–1	1.8	3–4
225.	Coffeine	See caffeine			
226.	Colchicine	0.0003–0.0025	0.005	0.024	11–32
227.	Colistin	1–5			2–5
228.	Copper	0.6–1.5	2	5	
229.	Cotrimoxazole	See sulfamethoxazole and trimethoprim			
230.	Cresol (methylphenols)		Approximately 50	120	
231.	Cromolyn (cromoglycate)	Approximately –0.01			1–1.5
232.	Cyanide	0.001–0.006, smoker: 0.005–0.012 (–0.15) ug/mL	0.5	1–3	Approximately 19
233.	Cyclizine	0.1–0.25	0.75–1	15	24
234.	Cyclobarbital	2–6	10	20	8–17
235.	Cyclobenzaprine	Approximately 0.003–0.04	0.4		18 (9–40)
236.	Cyclohexane	–0.4			

Continued

S. No.	Substances	Blood-plasma/serum concentration (μg/mL)			t½ (hours)
		Therapeutic ("normal")	Toxic (from)	Comatose-fatal (from)	
237.	Cyclophosphamide	10–25			4–8 (1.3–1.6)
238.	Cyclopropane	80–180			
239.	Cyclosporine A (CsA)	<0.1–0.15–0.25	0.3–0.4		10–27
240.	Cyproheptadine	Approximately –0.05		0.47	Approximately 16
241.	Cyproterone acetate				30–40
242.	Cytarabine	0.05–0.5			0.1–0.2 (1.9–2.5)
243.	2,4-D	See 2,4-Dichlorophenoxyacetic acid			
244.	Danazol	Approximately –0.2			4.5
245.	Dantrolene	(0.1–) 0.4–1.5 (–3)			4–12
246.	Dapsone	0.5–2	10	18	25–31
247.	Deferoxamine (desferrioxamine)	3–15			4–6
248.	Demoxepam	0.5–0.74	1	2.7	
249.	Desipramine	0.01–0.5 (0.12–0.25)	0.5–1	3	15–25
250.	Desmethyldiazepam	See nordazepam			40–80
251.	Dexamethasone	Approximately 0.05–0.256			2.5–9.5
252.	Dexfenfluramine	Approximately 0.03–0.06	0.15–0.25		Approximately 18
253.	Dextromethorphan	0.01–0.04	0.1	3	2–4
254.	Dextromoramide	0.075–0.15	0.2	0.9	0.1–1.5
255.	Dextropropoxyphene	0.05–0.3 (–0.5)	1	1–2	10–30
256.	3,4-diaminopyridine (DAP)	<0.04	0.1		0.3–2

APPENDIX 6

Continued

S. No.	Substances	Blood-plasma/serum concentration (μg/mL)			t½ (hours)
		Therapeutic ("normal")	Toxic (from)	Comatose-fatal (from)	
257.	Diazepam	0.2–2 (–2.5)	3–5		24–48
258.	Diazinon		0.05–0.1 (–0.5)		
259.	Diazoxide	10–20 (–50)	50 (–100)		20–36 (–48)
260.	Dibenzepin	0.025–0.15 (0.1–0.5)	3	18	3.5–5
261.	Dichloromethane		200	280	
262.	2,4-Dichlorophenoxyacetic acid (2,4-D)		Approximately 100	200; 392; 720	Approximately 18
263.	Dichlorvos			29	0.16
264.	Diclofenac	0.5–3	50; 60		1–2
265.	Dicoumarol	8–30	50–70		1–4
266.	Dicyclomine (dicycloverine)	–0.1	Approximately 0.2	0.5	1.8–2
267.	Didanosine	Approximately 1–30 μmol/L			1
268.	Dieldrin	–0.0015	0.15–0.3		
269.	Diethylcarbamazine	>0.8–1.0			4–15
270.	Diethylpentenamide (valdetamide)	2–10	20	45	6–7
271.	Diethylpropion	0.003–0.007 (–0.2)	2	5.4	4–8
272.	Difenacoum		0.5		
273.	Diflunisal	40–100 (–200)	300–500	600	5–12
274.	Digitoxin	0.01–0.025	0.03	0.04	140–200
275.	Digoxin	0.0005–0.0008 (–0.002)	0.0025–0.003	0.005	40–70
276.	Dihydralazine	See hydralazine			

Continued

Continued

S. No.	Substances	Blood-plasma/serum concentration (μg/mL)			t½ (hours)
		Therapeutic ("normal")	Toxic (from)	Comatose-fatal (from)	
277.	Dihydrocodeine	0.03–0.25	0.5–1	2	3–4
278.	Dihydroergotamine	0.001–0.01			7–9
279.	Diltiazem	0.03–0.13 (–0.25)	0.8–1	206; 7; 8	2–6 (4–9)
280.	Dimenhydrinate	See diphenhydramine			
281.	Dimethadione	700–1,000	1,000		
282.	Dimethindene	0.01–0.05			Approximately 6
283.	N,N-Dimethyltryptamine	0.001–0.1			
284.	4,6-Dinitro-2-methylphenol		40		
285.	Dinitro-o-cresol (DNOC)	1–5	30–60	75	4–10, 20–60
286.	Diphenhydramine	0.05–0.1 (–1)	1–2 (–4)	5–10	2–3
287.	Diphenoxylate	Approximately 0.01			
288.	Dipipanone	Approximately –0.05	0.2		
289.	Diprophylline	See dyphylline			
290.	Dipyridamole	0.1–1.5	4		11–13
291.	Dipyrone	See metamizole			
292.	Diquat	2–7	0.1–0.4		
293.	Disopyramide	0.05–0.4	8		5–8
294.	Disulfiram	Approximately 0.3	5	8	Approximately 5–7
295.	Dixyrazine	Approximately 0.01–0.1		5.5; 9.4	
296.	Domperidone				12–16

Continued

APPENDIX 6

S. No.	Substances	Blood-plasma/serum concentration (μg/mL)			t½ (hours)
		Therapeutic ("normal")	Toxic (from)	Comatose-fatal (from)	
297.	Donepezil	Approximately 0.03–0.075			70–100
298.	Dothiepin (dosulepin)	0.02–0.1	0.8	1	11–40
299.	Doxacurium	0.01–0.3			1–2
300.	Doxapram	1.5–2.5	9		2.4–9.9
301.	Doxazosin	0.01–0.15			10–22
302.	Doxepin	0.01–0.2 (0.03–0.1)	0.5–1	2–4	8–25
303.	Doxorubicin (adriamycin)	0.006–0.02			20–48
304.	Doxycycline	1–5 (–10)	30		7–20
305.	Doxylamine	0.05–0.2	1–2	5	9–11
306.	Dronabinol (delta-9-tetrahydrocannabinol, THC)	0.005–0.01 (–0.05)			50–100
307.	Droperidol	Approximately –0.05			1.5–2.5
308.	Dyphylline	6.5–14 (–20)	40		2
309.	Edrophonium	–0.15	Approximately 0.15		1.3–2.4
310.	Emetine	Approximately –0.1	0.5		
311.	Enalapril	0.01–0.05 (–0.1)			8–11
312.	Encainide	Effective plasma concentration for the 2 active metabolites: O-desmethylencainide (0.05–0.3 ug/mL) and 3- methyoxy-O-desmethylenecainide (0.06–0.28 ug/mL) during long-term treatment			1.5–3.5

Continued

APPENDIX 6

Continued

S. No.	Substances	Blood-plasma/serum concentration (μg/mL)			t½ (hours)
		Therapeutic ("normal")	*Toxic (from)*	*Comatose-fatal (from)*	
313.	Endrin	–0.003	0.01–0.03		3–6
314.	Enoxacin	1–4			4–7
315.	Enoximone	≥0.2			1.5–3.5
316.	Entacapone	0.4–1.0 (–7.0)			3–11
317.	Ephedrine	0.02–0.2	1	5	24–52
318.	Epirubicin	0.01–0.05			5–9
319.	Eprosartan	0.4–1.0 (–1.85)			1–3
320.	Erythromycin	2–6 (–8)	12–15		4–16 minutes
321.	Esmolol	0.15–2			10–24
322.	Estazolam	0.055–0.2			2.5–4
323.	Ethamsylate	15–20			1–4
324.	Ethacrynic acid	0.05–0.1			2.5–3.5
325.	Ethambutol	0.5–6	10		0.15 + or –0.05% per hour
326.	Ethanol		1,000–2,000	3,500–4,000	10–25 (–35)
327.	Ethchlorvynol	0.5–8	20	50	Approximately 2
328.	Ethinamate	1.5–10	50–100	200	30–60
329.	Ethosuximide	30–100 (40–60)	150–200	250	
330.	Ethylene glycol		200–500	2,000	
331.	Etidocaine	0.5–1.5	1.6–2		2–3
332.	Etilefrine	Approximately 0.06			2–3.5

Continued

607

APPENDIX 6

S. No.	Substances	Blood-plasma/serum concentration (µg/mL)			t½ (hours)
		Therapeutic ("normal")	Toxic (from)	Comatose-fatal (from)	
333.	Etodolac	>14			6–8
334.	Etomidate	0.1–0.5 (–1)			3.9 ± 1.1 (2–11)
335.	Etoposide	1–6			4–11
336.	Ezetimibe	>0.015			Approximately 30
337.	Famotidine	0.02–0.2	0.42		2–4.5
338.	Fampridine	See 4-aminopyridine			
339.	Felbamate	50–110	200		20–24
340.	Felbinac	Approximately 0.4–1 (topical)			10–17
341.	Felodipine	0.001-0.012	0.01		22–27
342.	Fenbufen	Approximately –60			10–12
343.	Fendiline	0.02–0.15			Approximately 20
344.	Fenfluramine	0.04–0.3	0.5–0.7	6	1–2, 18–25
345.	Fenitrothion			1.1	
346.	Fenofibrate	5–30			20–22
347.	Fenoldopam	0.003–0.06			0.1
348.	Fenoprofen	(25–) 30–60			2–3
349.	Fenoterol	(0.001–) 0.01–0.04			Approximately 7
350.	Fentanyl	0.003–0.3		0.003–0.002	1–3.5 (transdermal patch: approximately 17)
351.	Fexofenadine	Approximately –0.3			14–18
352.	Finasteride	0.008–0.01			5–7

Continued

Continued

APPENDIX 6

S. No.	Substances	Blood-plasma/serum concentration (µg/mL)			t½ (hours)
		Therapeutic ("normal")	Toxic (from)	Comatose-fatal (from)	
353.	Flecainide	(0.2–) 0.4–0.8	1–2	2.6;13	10–20
354.	Fleroxacin	1–4			8–13
355.	Flucloxacillin	3–30			0.7–1.5
356.	Fluconazole	Approximately 1–5 (–15)	20;95		22–31
357.	Flucytosine	35–70 (20–50)	100		3–5
358.	Flumazenil	(0.01–) 0.02–0.1	0.5		1–2
359.	Flunarizine	0.025–0.2	0.3		Days
360.	Flunitrazepam	0.005–0.015	0.05		10–20
361.	Fluoride	0.095–0.190	2	3	Short
362.	5-fluorouracil	0.05–0.3	0.4–0.6		<0.5
363.	Fluoxetine	Approximately 0.16–0.5	1	6	2–4
364.	Flupentixol	0.0005–0.002			19–39
365.	Fluphenazine	0.0002–0.004	0.05–0.1		10–18
366.	Flupirtine	0.5–1.5	Approximately 3–4		7–11
367.	Flurazepam	0.02–0.1	0.2–0.5	0.8;24	Approximately 2
368.	Flurbiprofen	5–15			3–4
369.	Flutamide	0.4–1.5			7–20
370.	Fluvoxamine	Approximately (0.05–) 0.15–0.25	0.65	2.8	15–22
371.	Furosemide (frusemide)	1–6			1–3
372.	Fusidic acid	30–200	25–30		4–6
373.	Gabapentin	5.9–21	85		5–8

Continued

APPENDIX 6

S. No.	Substances	Blood-plasma/serum concentration (μg/mL)			t½ (hours)
		Therapeutic ("normal")	Toxic (from)	Comatose-fatal (from)	
374.	Galanthamine	Approximately 0.03–0.14			6–8
375.	Gallopamil	0.02–0.1		8	3–8
376.	Gamma-hydroxybutyricacid (gamma-butyrolactone, GHB, liquid ecstasy)				
377.	Ganciclovir	(0.29–0.51) 0.5–5	3–5		2–4
378.	Gemcitabine	15–20 μmol/L	Metabolite 2',2'-difluorodeoxyuridine (dFdU) has minimal antitumor activity but may contribute to the toxicity of gemcitabine		0.05 (0.18–0.43)
379.	Gemfibrozil	Approximately ~25			1.5
380.	Gentamicin	(2–) 4–10	12		1.5–6
381.	Glibenclamide (glyburide)	0.05–0.2	0.6		10
382.	Glipizide	0.1–1.0 (–1.5)	2		3–7
383.	Glutethimide	0.2–5	10–30	20–50	5–20
384.	Glyburide	See glibenclamide			
385.	Glyceryl trinitrate	See nitroglycerin			
386.	Gold	3–8	10–15		
387.	Granisetron	0.009–0.017			3–14

APPENDIX 6

S. No.	Substances	Blood-plasma/serum concentration (µg/mL)			t½ (hours)
		Therapeutic ("normal")	Toxic (from)	Comatose-fatal (from)	
388.	Griseofulvin	0.3–1.3			22
389.	Guaifenesin	Approximately 0.3–1.4			Approximately 1
390.	Guanethidine	0.01			5–10
391.	Halazepam	See nordazepam			30–40
392.	Haloperidol	0.005–0.017 (0.001–0.02)	0.05–0.5	0.5; 0.18	10–35
393.	Hematin	50–100			
394.	Hemin	See hematin			
395.	Heptabarbital	0.5–4	8–15	20	6–11
396.	Heptaminol	Approximately 0.2–1 (–1.5)			2–3
397.	Hexachlorophene	0.003–0.65 (–1)		35	6–44
398.	n-hexane	–0.01			
399.	Hexapropymate	2–5	10–20		4–6
400.	Hexabarbital	1–5	10–20	50	(1–) 2.5–3
401.	Rec-hirudin	Target range of activated partial thromboplastin time (aPTT) is prolongation of 50–70 s, aPPT prolongation of >100 s sec has been associated with an increased risk of hemorrhagic events			
402.	Hydralazine	0.05–0.5 (–1.5)			2–6
403.	Hydrochlorothiazide	Approximately 0.04–2			10–12
404.	Hydrocodone	0.01–0.05	0.1	0.2	Approximately 4
405.	Hydromorphone	Approximately 0.005–0.015	0.1	0.2	2–3

APPENDIX 6

Continued

S. No.	Substances	Blood-plasma/serum concentration (μg/mL)			t½ (hours)
		Therapeutic ("normal")	Toxic (from)	Comatose-fatal (from)	
406.	4-gamma-hydroxybutyrate (GHB)	Approximately 50–120	80 (abuse)	250–280 (abuse)	0.3–0.5 (–1)
407.	Hydroxychloroquine	–0.1 (0.4)	0.5–0.8	4	Dose dependent
408.	Hydroxyzine	0.05–0.1	0.1	39	7–20
409.	Ibuprofen	15–30	200		2–3
410.	Idebenone	0.05–0.2			16–22
411.	Iloprost	Approximately 0.0001			Approximately 0.5
412.	Imatinib	0.72			Approximately 18
413.	Imipenem	0.5–5 (20–75)			1
414.	Imipramine	0.05–0.35	0.5–1	1.5–2	6–20
415.	Indinavir	At this time (March, 2003), there is insufficient evidence to recommend a general therapeutic range	0.5		1.5–2
416.	Indomethacin	0.3–1 (–3)	4–5		3–11
417.	Indoramin	Approximately 0.025–0.1			12 (3.5–15)
418.	Iproniazid	Approximately –5			
419.	Iridium	–0.02			
420.	Iron	0.5–2	6	17	
421.	Isoniazid (INH)	5–10	20	30–100	1–3
422.	Isosorbide mononitrate (ISMN)	0.1–1			2–5

Continued

APPENDIX 6

Continued

S. No.	Substances	Blood-plasma/serum concentration (μg/mL)			t½ (hours)
		Therapeutic ("normal")	Toxic (from)	Comatose-fatal (from)	
423.	Isotretinoin	Approximately 0.001–0.002 (topical)			10–20
424.	Isoxicam	5–15			20–50
425.	Isradipine	0.0005–0.002 (–0.01)	0.01	0.26	5–10
426.	Itraconazole	Approximately 0.4–2			24–36
427.	Ivermectin	Approximately 0.0551			16–28
428.	Kanamycin	1–4 (10–25)	25–30		0.5–3
429.	Ketamine	1–6	7 (abuse)	7 (abuse)	1–3
430.	Ketanserin	0.05–0.5			10–22
431.	Ketazolam[15]	0.001–0.02			1–3
432.	Ketobemidone	Approximately 0.3		0.6	2–2.5
433.	Ketoconazole	1–3 (–6)			6–10
434.	Ketoprofen	1–6 (–20)		1,100	1,5–2 (–4)
435.	Ketorolac	0.5–3	5		4–10
436.	Ketotifen	0.001–0.004	0.02	1.2	21
437.	Labetalol	0.03–0.18 (–0.65)	1		3–10
438.	Lacidipine	0.003–0.006			12–19
439.	Lamivudine	The inhibitory concentration to reduce the level of extracellular hepatitis B DNA by 50% varies from 2.3 ug/mL–1.3 ug/mL			(3–) 5–7

Continued

APPENDIX 6

S. No.	Substances	Blood-plasma/serum concentration (µg/mL)			t½ (hours)
		Therapeutic ("normal")	Toxic (from)	Comatose-fatal (from)	
440.	Lamotrigine	(1–5) 3–14	15–30	50	24–36
441.	Lead	–0.16 (–0.3)	0.4–0.6	3	Days, upto years in chemically exposed workers
442.	Leflunomide	8.8 ± 2.9, 18 ± 9.6, and 63 ± 36			11 (4–28)
443.	Levetiracetam	10–37	400		5–8
444.	Levocabastine	<0.001–0.01			33–40
445.	Levodopa (L-Dopa)	0.3–1.6		650	1–3
446.	Levomeromazine	0.005–0.025 (–0.2)	0.4	0.5	15–30
447.	Levomethadone	0.04–0.3	1	0.2	10–40
448.	Levorphanol	0.007–0.02	0.1	2.7	11–30
449.	Levothyroxine	0.045–0.14			6–8
450.	Lidocaine (lignocaine)	(1–) 1.5–5	6–7	10	1–4
451.	Lisinopril	(0.005–) 0.02–0.07	0.5		12
452.	Lithium	4–8	13	14	8–50
453.	Lofepramine	0.003–0.01			10–20
454.	Loperamide	Cmax 3–5 h after 4 mg oral loperamide hydrochloride: 1–3 ng/mL active metabolite N-desmethylclopramide			7–15
455.	Loprazolam	0.003–0.01			11–20
456.	Loratadine	0.001–0.02			8–14

Continued

APPENDIX 6

Continued

S. No.	Substances	Blood-plasma/serum concentration (μg/mL)			t½ (hours)
		Therapeutic ("normal")	Toxic (from)	Comatose-fatal (from)	
457.	Lorazepam	(0.02–) 0.08–0.25	0.3–0.5		10–40
458.	Lorcainide	(0.04–) 0.1–0.4 (–0.9)			5–10
459.	Lormetazepam	0.005–0.025 (–0.1)			10–15
460.	Losartan	<0.2			1.5–2
461.	Loxapine	0.01–0.003 (–0.1)	1	7.7	4 (1–14)
462.	Lysergide (lysergic acid diethylamide, LSD)	0.0005–0.005	0.001	0.002–0.005	Approximately 2–5
463.	Magnesium	55–75	120–140	150–180	
464.	Malathion		0.5	175	
465.	Manganese	0.0005–0.0015			
466.	Maprotiline	0.1–0.6 (0.1–0.25)	0.5–1	1–5	20–60
467.	MCPA	See 2-methyl-4-chlorophenoxyacetic acid			
468.	MCPP	See 2-methyl-4-chlorophenoxypropionic acid			
469.	Mebendazole	≥0.1	Approximately 0.6		2.8–9
470.	Medazepam	0.1–0.5 (–1)			2–5
471.	Mefenamic acid	2–10 (–20)	25		2–4
472.	Mefloquine	0.4–1	1.5–2		Approximately 21
473.	Melitracen	0.01–0.1			12–23
474.	Meloxicam	0.4–2			17–22

Continued

APPENDIX 6

Continued

S. No.	Substances	Blood-plasma/serum concentration (μg/mL)			t½ (hours)
		Therapeutic ("normal")	Toxic (from)	Comatose-fatal (from)	
475.	Melperone	<0.2		17.1	4-8
476.	Melphalan	~1.5			1.5-2
477.	Meperidine	See pethidine			
478.	Mephenesin	3-10			Approximately 2-4
479.	Mepindolol	0.007-0.07			3-6
480.	Mepivacaine	Approximately 0.4 (~4)	5-6 (~10)		1-3
481.	Meprobamate	5-10	10-25	50	6-17
482.	Meptazinol	0.025-0.25		30	2-3
483.	Mercury	Approximately 0.0015-0.002 (<0.005)	0.05-0.2	0.5	Approximately 3
484.	Mesalazine (mesalamine)	Approximately 1			0.5-2.4
485.	Mesoridazine	0.15-1	3-5	3; 4; 16	20
486.	Mesuximide	See methsuximide			1-2
487.	Metaclazepam	0.05-0.2			7-23
488.	Metamizole (dipyrone)	10	20		6-8
489.	Metformin	0.1-1 (0.6-1.3)	5-10	64, 85, 91; 166	2-4 (~10)
490.	Methadone	(0.05-) 0.1-0.5 (~0.75)	0.2	0.4	23-25 (13-55)
491.	Methamphetamine	0.01-0.05	0.2-1	10-40	6-9
492.	Methanol	Approximately ~2	200	900	
493.	Methapyrilene	Approximately 0.1	4		
494.	Methaqualone	1-3	3-5	5-10	10-40

Continued

APPENDIX 6

Continued

S. No.	Substances	Blood-plasma/serum concentration (μg/mL)			t½ (hours)
		Therapeutic ("normal")	Toxic (from)	Comatose-fatal (from)	
495.	Methemoglobin	Normal: ≤2–3% of total Hb; from 15–20%: cyanosis, headache, dizziness	25–30%	60–70%	
496.	Methimazole	0.5–2			2–28
497.	Methocarbamol	25–40 (–50)	250		0.9–2
498.	Methohexital	(0.5–) 1–6			1–3
499.	Methomyl			28 (8–57)	
500.	Methotrexate	0.04	0.4		2–10
501.	Methotrimeprazine	See levomepromazine			
502.	Methoxsalen (8-methoxypsoralen)	0.025–0.1 (–0.2)	1		
503.	Methsuximide (mesuximide)	10–40	40–50		20–40
504.	D-methamphetamine	–0.1	1		
505.	2-methyl-4-chlorophenoxyacetic acid (MCPA)		Approximately 100	Approximately 180	Dependent of urine PH, if alkaline approximately 8–10 h
506.	2-methyl-4-chlorophenox-ypropionic acid (MCPP)		Approximately 100	669; 715	17
507.	Methyldopa	1–5	9		1.5–3
508.	3,4-methylenedioxyamphetamine (MDA)	–0.4	1.5	2	
509.	3,4-methylenedioxyethylamphetamine (MDEA)	0.2		1	

Continued

APPENDIX 6

S. No.	Substances	Blood-plasma/serum concentration (µg/mL)			t½ (hours)
		Therapeutic ("normal")	Toxic (from)	Comatose-fatal (from)	
510.	3,4-methylenedioxymethylamphetamine (XTC < MDMA)	0.1–0.35	0.35–0.5	0.4	9–10
511.	Methylphenidate	0.01–0.06	0.5; 1	2.3	2–7
512.	4-methylthioamphetamine (4-MTA, p-MTA)			2; 4.2; 7.4	
513.	Methyprylon	<10–20	12–75	50 (–100)	3–6, 9–11
514.	Metiamide	0.01–0.06			
515.	Metildigoxin	0.0005–0.0008	0.0025–0.003	0.005	40–70
516.	Metipranolol	0.02–0.08			2–3.5
517.	Metoclopramide	0.05–0.15	0.2	4.4	3–6
518.	Metocurine	Approximately ~0.4			
519.	Metoprolol	0.035–0.5	0.65; 12–18	4.7; 12; 63	3–6
520.	Metrifonate	Approximately 1.4–3.6			2–5
521.	Metronidazole	3–10 (–20)	200		6–10 (–14)
522.	Mexiletine	(0.5–) 0.7–2	2.5		5–26
523.	Mianserin	0.01–0.15	0.5–5	35	8–19
524.	Miconazole	Approximately 1			24
525.	Midazolam	0.04–0.1 (–0.25)	1–1.5		1.5–3
526.	Mifepristone	Approximately 2.5 umol/L (1 ug/ml) 24 h after single dose of 100–800 mg and during daily treatment with 200 mg			24–48 (20–54)

Continued

APPENDIX 6

S. No.	Substances	Blood-plasma/serum concentration (μg/mL)			t½ (hours)
		Therapeutic ("normal")	Toxic (from)	Comatose-fatal (from)	
527.	Milrinone	0.15–0.25	0.3		1–2
528.	Minaprine	Approximately –0.1			
529.	Minoxidil	Approximately 0.02–0.25	1.4; 3.1	2.7	2.8–4.2
530.	Mirtazapine	–0.3	1–2		20–40
531.	Mizolastine	Approximately 0.2–0.8			8–17
532.	Moclobemide	Approximately 0.5–1.5 (–3)	11; 25–60		1–3
533.	Modafinil	Approximately 2–			12–15
534.	Molindone	Approximately –0.5			
535.	Molsidomine	0.002–0.01			1–2.5
536.	Molybdenum	–0.005			
537.	Montelukast	Approximately 0.05–0.3			3–6
538.	Moricizine	Approximately 0.12–1.27			6–13
539.	Morphine	0.01–0.1	0.1	0.1–4	1–4
540.	Moxonidine	0.001–0.002 (–0.004)			2–3
541.	Muromonab-CD3 (OKT 3)	Approximately 0.7–1.3			Approximately 18
542.	Mycophenolate mofetil				16–18
543.	Nabumetone				
544.	Nadolol	0.01–0.25		1.3	14–24
545.	Naftidrofuryl (nafronyl)	<0.5			1–2
546.	Nalbuphine	0.02–0.2			2.5–7
547.	Nalidixic acid	10–30	40–50		1–7

Continued

APPENDIX 6

Continued

S. No.	Substances	Blood-plasma/serum concentration (µg/mL)			t½ (hours)
		Therapeutic ("normal")	*Toxic (from)*	*Comatose-fatal (from)*	
548.	Nalmefene	~0.1			8.5–11
549.	Naloxone	0.01–0.03			1–2
550.	Naltrexone	~0.05			4–10
551.	Naproxen	20–50 (–100)	200–400; 414		10–20
552.	Naratriptan	Approximately 0.01–0.05			5–6
553.	Nebivolol	<0.02 (–0.2)	0.48		10 (8–27)
554.	Nedocromil	<0.025			1.5–3.3
555.	Nefazodone	Approximately 0.01–0.3	5.5		2–7
556.	Nefopam	0.01–0.1	4	12	3–8
557.	Neostigmine	Approximately 0.001–0.01			0.4–1.3
558.	Netilmicin	1–12			2–3
559.	Nicardipine	0.07–0.1			7–12
560.	Nickel	~0.003	0.005		
561.	Nicotine	0.005–0.02 (–0.03)	0.4 (–1)	5; 13.6	1–4
562.	Nicotinic acid	4–18			0.3–1
563.	Nifedipine	0.025–0.1	Approximately 0.15–0.2	5.4	2–5
564.	Niflumic acid	2–35			2–3
565.	Nilvadipine	<0.01			11–20
566.	Nimesulide	Approximately 1–3			2–7
567.	Nimodipine	0.01–0.05			1–2 (8–9)

Continued

APPENDIX 6

Continued

S. No.	Substances	Blood-plasma/serum concentration (μg/mL)			t½ (hours)
		Therapeutic ("normal")	Toxic (from)	Comatose-fatal (from)	
568.	Nimustine	0.0002–0.0005			
569.	Nisoldipine	0.0003–0.001			7–12
570.	Nitrazepam	0.03–0.1	0.2–3	5	20–30
571.	Nitrendipine	0.01–0.05			8–12
572.	Nitrofurantoin	1–3	3–4		1 ± 0.3
573.	Nitroglycerin (Glyceryl trinitrate)	Approximately –0.015			20–30 minutes
574.	Nitroprusside	See thiocyanate	See also cyanide		
575.	Nizatidine	0.05–0.5 (–1.0)			0.7–2.1
576.	Nomifensine	0.01–0.1	8–10		2–5
577.	Nordazepam	0.02–0.2 (–0.8)	1.5–2		40–80
578.	Norephedrine	See phenylpropanolamine			
579.	Norfenefrine	–0.4			2–3
580.	Norfloxacin	0.5–5			3–4
581.	Normesuximide	10–30	40		38
582.	Nortriptyline	0.02–0.2 (0.05–0.15)	0.5	1–3	18–56
583.	Obidoxime	1–10 (approximately 10–15 μmol/L)			
584.	Ofloxacin	Approximately 2.5–5.5	30–40		(3–) 5–8
585.	OKT 3	See Muromonab-CD3			
586.	Olanzapine	Approximately 0.02–0.03 (–0.05)	0.2	1; 4.9	33 (21–54)

Continued

APPENDIX 6

S. No.	Substances	Blood-plasma/serum concentration (μg/mL)			t½ (hours)
		Therapeutic ("normal")	Toxic (from)	Comatose-fatal (from)	
587.	Omeprazole	Plasma concentrations does not correspond with pharmacological effects			0.5–1 (–1.5)
588.	Ondansetron	0.03–0.3			3–5.5
589.	Opipramol	0.1–0.5	2–3	7–10	6–12
590.	Orphenadrine	0.1–0.2 (–0.6)	1.7	3.6; 5–7	14–18
591.	Oxatomide	0.02–0.1			14–30
592.	Oxazepam	0.2–1.5	2	3–5	6–20
593.	Oxazolam	See nordazepam			1–2
594.	Oxcarbazepine	12–24			1–2.5
595.	Oxpentifylline	See pentoxifylline			
596.	Oxprenolol	0.05–0.3 (–1.0)	2–3	10	1–4
597.	Oxycodone	(0.005–) 0.02–0.05	0.2	0.6; 5	2–5
598.	Oxyfedrine	Approximately 0.06			4.2
599.	Oxypurinol	5–15	20		18–30
600.	Oxytocin	Approximately –0.0002			3–5 minutes
601.	Paclitaxel	0.085–1			4–8 (–13)
602.	Pamidronate	Approximately 0.5–1			Approximately 2.5
603.	Pancuronium	0.1–0.6	0.4	1.6	1.5–2.5
604.	Pantoprazole	Approximately –4.6			1–2
605.	Papaverine	(0.2–) 0.6–1 (–2)			1–2, 6–7

Continued

APPENDIX 6

Continued

S. No.	Substances	Therapeutic ("normal")	Toxic (from)	Comatose-fatal (from)	t½ (hours)
		Blood-plasma/serum concentration (μg/mL)			
606.	Paracetamol	(5–) 10–25	100–150	200–300	2–4
607.	Paraldehyde	10–100	200	400–500	4–10
608.	Paraoxon		0.005		
609.	Paraquat		0.05	1–2	
610.	Parathion		0.01–0.05	0.05–0.08	
611.	Paroxetine	<0.01–0.05 (–0.1)	0.35–0.4		16–24
612.	Pefloxacin	1–10 (3–6)	25		8–15
613.	Pemoline	Approximately 1–7			7–13
614.	Penbutolol	0.01–0.3 (–1.0)			20–26
615.	Penfluridol	0.004–0.025			70
616.	D-penicillamine	1.7–5.6 (–11)			1–3
617.	Pentachlorophenol	–0.2	30	45	
618.	Pentamidine	Approximately 0.3–0.5			6–9
619.	Pentazocine	0.01–0.2	1–2	3	2–5
620.	Pentobarbital	1–10	10–19	15–25	20–40
621.	Pentoxifylline	Approximately 0.5–2			0.5–2 (4–6)
622.	Perazine	0.02–0.35	0.5 (6.1)		8–16 (–35)
623.	Periciazine	0.005–0.03	0.1		
624.	Perindopril	0.08–0.15			0.8–1.5
625.	Perphenazine	0.001–0.02 (0.0008–0.0024)	0.05		8–12 (–21)

Continued

APPENDIX 6

Continued

S. No.	Substances	Blood-plasma/serum concentration (μg/mL)			t½ (hours)
		Therapeutic ("normal")	Toxic (from)	Comatose-fatal (from)	
626.	Pethidine	0.1–0.8	1–2	2–3	3–6 (–10)
627.	Phenacetin	5–10 (–20)	50		Approximately 1
628.	Phenazone (antipyrine)	5–25	50–100		10–12
629.	Phencyclidine (PCP)		0.007–0.24	1–5	1–12
630.	Phendimetrazine	0.02–0.24 (–0.3)			2–4
631.	Phenelzine	0.001–0.002 (–0.04)	0.5	1.5	6–8
632.	Phenformin	0.03–0.1	0.6	3	4–13
633.	Pheniramine	0.01–0.27		2	16–19
634.	Phenmetrazine	0.02–0.25	0.5	4	Case report
635.	Phenobarbital	10–30 (15–40)	30–40	50–60	60–130
636.	Phenol		50	90	
637.	Phenprocoumon	0.16–3.6 (1–5)	Approximately 5		100–160
638.	Phensuximide	4–10 (–20)	80		4–12
639.	Phentermine	0.03–0.1	0.9	1	Approximately 20
640.	Phenylbutazone	50–100	120–200	400	30–175
641.	Phenylephrine	0.04–0.1			2–3
642.	Phenylpropanolamine (norephedrine)	0.1–0.5	2	48	3–7
643.	Phenytoin	5–15 (10–20)	20–25	43; 50	10–60
644.	Pholcodine	Approximately –0.2			
645.	Physostigmine	<0.001–0.005			0.4–1

Continued

APPENDIX 6

Blood-plasma/serum concentration (μg/mL)

S. No.	Substances	Therapeutic ("normal")	Toxic (from)	Comatose-fatal (from)	t½ (hours)
646.	Pimozide	Approximately 0.004–0.01 (–0.02)			24–55
647.	Pinazepam	0.01–0.05			16
648.	Pindolol	0.02–0.15	0.7–1.5		2–5
649.	Pipamperone	0.1–0.4	0.5–0.6		<4
650.	Piperacillin	1–5 (20–70)			1–2
651.	Piperazine	0.02–0.1	0.5		
652.	Pipotiazine	0.001–0.06	0.1		8–11
653.	Piracetam	Approximately 20–50			4.5–7
654.	Pirenzepine	0.03–0.45			8–20
655.	Piritramide	0.0088 ± 0.0053			4–10
656.	Pirmenol	1–4			6–18
657.	Piroxicam	2–6	14		30–70
658.	Pizotifen	0.007–0.009			26
659.	Prajmalium	0.06–0.44			5–8
660.	Pramipexole	Approximately 0.0002–0.007			8–14
661.	Pranlukast	Approximately 0.2–1.2			Approximately 2–9
662.	Prazepam	0.2–0.7	1		1–3
663.	Praziquantel	Approximately 0.2			1–2.5
664.	Prazosin	0.001–0.02	0.9		2.9 ± 0.8
665.	Prednisolone	0.5–1			2–6

Continued

APPENDIX 6

Continued

S. No.	Substances	Blood-plasma/serum concentration (µg/mL)			t½ (hours)
		Therapeutic ("normal")	Toxic (from)	Comatose-fatal (from)	
666.	Prilocaine	0.5–1.5 (–2)	5–6	Approximately 20	1–2
667.	Primaquine	Approximately 0.1–0.2			4–7
668.	Primidone	4–12 (8–15)	20–50	65	4–12, 9–22
669.	Probenecid	100–200 (20–150)			3–18
670.	Procaine	0.2–2.5 (–10)	15–20	20	–0.5
671.	Procainamide	4–10 (3–9)	10–15	20	2–5
672.	N-acetylprocainamide	5–30 (10–35, 15–40)			3–7
673.	Prochlorperazine	0.01–0.05	0.2–0.3	5	7–9 (–18)
674.	Procyclidine	0.08–0.63	1–2	7.8	7–16
675.	Proguanil	Approximately 0.04–0.15			13–24
676.	Promazine	0.01–0.05 (–0.4)	1	5	5–41 (8 ± 7)
677.	Promethazine	0.05–0.2 (–0.4)	1–2	2.4; 1.8–5.4	8–15 (–20)
678.	Propafenone	0.4–3 (0.06–1)	2–3	7.7	5–8, 2–32
679.	Propallylonal	0.3–10	>10		Approximately 3
680.	2-propanol	See isopropanol			
681.	Propantheline	Approximately –0.02			1–3
682.	Propiomazine	<0.3			8–10
683.	Propofol	Approximately 2–8			3–8
684.	Propoxyphene	See dextropropoxyphene			
685.	Propranolol	0.02–0.3	(0.5–) 1–3	4–10	2–6
686.	Propylene glycol	0.05–0.5	1,000–2,000; 4,700		

Continued

APPENDIX 6

Continued

S. No.	Substances	Blood-plasma/serum concentration (μg/mL)			t½ (hours)
		Therapeutic ("normal")	Toxic (from)	Comatose-fatal (from)	
687.	Propylhexedrine	0.01	0.5	2–3	
688.	Propyphenazone	3–12			1–1.5 (–3)
689.	Prothipendyl	Approximately 0.05–0.2	Approximately 0.5–1		2–3
690.	Protriptyline	0.0.5–0.3	0.5	1	50–200
691.	Pseudoephedrine	0.5–0.8		19–20	9–16
692.	Pyrazinamide	30–75			9–10 (–25)
693.	Pyridostigmine	<0.05–0.2			1–2.5
694.	Pyridoxine	0.003–0.018			3–6
695.	Pyrimethamine	Approximately –1.5			80–96
696.	Pyrithyldione	1–10			11–20
697.	Quazepam	0.01–0.05 (–0.15)			39 (25–41)
698.	Quetiapine	<1	1.8	12.7	Approximately 5–7
699.	Auinidine	1–5	6–10	10–15	4–12
700.	Quinine	1–7	10		4–15
701.	Rabeprazole	Approximately –0.6			1–2
702.	Ramipril	Approximately 0.001–0.001			1–5
703.	Ranitidine	0.05–1			2–4
704.	Reboxetine	C_{max} < 0.3			12–14
705.	Recainam	1.3–5.7			5–7
706.	Remoxipride	2.15 ± 0.59		41–150	5–10
707.	Retinol (vitamin A)	0.2–0.8 (0.7–2.8 μmol/L)			

Continued

APPENDIX 6

S. No.	Substances	Blood-plasma/serum concentration (μg/mL)			t½ (hours)
		Therapeutic ("normal")	Toxic (from)	Comatose-fatal (from)	
708.	Ricin		0.0005		
709.	Rifabutin	0.05–0.15			45
710.	Rifampicin (rifampin)	0.1–10		55	2.3–5
711.	Rifapentine				13.2
712.	Riluzole	Approximately 0.05–0.5 (–1.5)			9–15
713.	Risperidone	Approximately 0.006		1.8	2–4
714.	Ritonavir	Approximately 5–11 (–20)			3–5
715.	Rivastigmine				1–2
716.	Rizatriptan	Approximately –0.1			2–3
717.	Ropinirole	0.0004–0.006			6 (2–10)
718.	Ropivacaine		1–2		2
719.	Roxatidine	0.1–0.8			5–6
720.	Roxithromycin	4–12			12
721.	Salbutamol (albuterol)	<0.01–0.02	0.1–0.15	0.16	3–6
722.	Salicylamide	5–40			Approximately 1
723.	Salicylic acid	20–200	300–350	400–500	3–20
724.	Scopolamine	0.0001–0.0003 (–0.001)			Approximately 3
725.	Secbutabarbital	5–10 (–15)	20	30	34–42
726.	Secobarbital	1.5–5	7–10	10–15	15–30
727.	Selegiline	See amphetamine and methamphetamine			1.2

Continued

Continued

APPENDIX 6

S. No.	Substances	Blood-plasma/serum concentration (µg/mL)			t½ (hours)
		Therapeutic ("normal")	Toxic (from)	Comatose-fatal (from)	
728.	Selenium	0.045–0.13	0.4		24–28
729.	Sertraline	0.05–0.25 (–0.5)	0.29	1.6; 3	3–5
730.	Sildenafil	Approximately 0.05–0.5			57–63
731.	Silver	–0.005	0.06–0.6		0.1
732.	Sirolimus	0.005–0.015	0.015–0.06		
733.	Sodium nitroprusside	See thiocyanate			
734.	Sodium oxybate (GHB)	See 4-hydroxybutyrate			
735.	Sodium valproate	See valproic acid			
736.	Sotalol	0.5–3 (–4)	7.5–16	40; 43	5–13 (–17)
737.	Sparteine	0.5–1			2.6
738.	Spiramycin	Approximately –3			5–8
739.	Spironolactone	(0.05–) 0.1–0.25 (–0.5)			13–24
740.	Stiripentol	Approximately 4–22	20		13
741.	Streptomycin	1–5 (15–40)	40–50		2–4
742.	Strontium	–0.03			
743.	Strychnine		0.075–0.1	0.2–2	Approximately 10–15
744.	Sufentanil	0.0005–0.01		0.001–0.007	2–5, 22
745.	Sulbactam	–80			1–270
746.	Sulfamethoxazole	30–60	200–400		9–12
747.	Sulfasalazine	5–30 (–70)			4–10

Continued

APPENDIX 6

Continued

S. No.	Substances	Blood-plasma/serum concentration (μg/mL)			t½ (hours)
		Therapeutic ("normal")	Toxic (from)	Comatose-fatal (from)	
748.	Sulfinpyrazone	6–17			3–5
749.	Sulindac	1–5			Approximately 7
750.	Sulpiride	0.05–0.4 (0.6)			4–7
751.	Sultiame (sulthiame)	0.5–12.5 (6–10)	12–15	20–25	3–30
752.	Sumatriptan	0.018–0.06			2
753.	Suramin	>100	300		44–54
754.	2,4,5-T	See 2,4,5-trichlorophenoxyacetic acid			
755.	Tacrine	Approximately 0.01			2–4
756.	Tacrolimus (FK506)	0.005–0.015 (–0.02)	(0.015–) 0.02–0.025		9–16
757.	Talinolol	0.04–0.15		5; 20	10–14
758.	Talipexole	Approximately 0.0001–0.001			5–9
759.	Tamoxifen	0.05–0.5			5–7
760.	Taxol	See paclitaxel			
761.	Teicoplanin	(10–) 15–20 (–40)	200		10–15; 83–168
762.	Temazepam	0.02–0.15 (–0.9)	1	8.2; 14	6–25
763.	Tenoxicam	Approximately 5–10			(50–) 70–90
764.	Terazosin	Approximately 0.02–0.08			8–12
765.	Terbinafine	0.01–0.03			22–26
766.	Terbutaline	0.001–0.006 (–0.01)		0.04	16–20
767.	Terfenadine	<0.01	0.06	0.4	15–22

Continued

APPENDIX 6

S. No.	Substances	Blood-plasma/serum concentration (μg/mL)			t½ (hours)
		Therapeutic ("normal")	Toxic (from)	Comatose-fatal (from)	
768.	Tetrachloroethylene			4–5	
769.	Tetracycline	1–5 (5–10)	30		6–10
770.	Tetrazepam	0.05–0.6 (–1)			10–26
771.	Thalidomide	0.5–1.5 (–8)			5–9
772.	Thallium		0.1–0.5; 5.6	0.5–11	Days
773.	Theobromine	10–15	20		6–10
774.	Theophylline	(5–) 8–15 (–20)	20	50	6–9
775.	Thiamphenicol	0.5–3–10 (–15)	20		2–7
776.	Thiazinamium	0.05–0.15	0.3		
777.	Thiocyanate	1–2	35–50	200	3–4
778.	From nitroprusside	5–30	50–100		
779.	Thiopental	1–5		10–15	3–8
780.	Thioproperazine	Approximately 0.001–0.02	0.1		
781.	Thioridazine	0.1–2 (0.2–0.8–1.25)	2.5–5	3–10	7–13 (–36)
782.	Thiothixene	See tiotixene			
783.	Thyroxine	See levothyroxine			
784.	Tiagabine	0.05–0.2	0.5–0.6; 3.1		7–9 (4–13)
785.	Tiapride	Maximum 1–2			Approximately 3–4
786.	Tiaprofenic acid	Approximately 15–40			1.5–3
787.	Ticlopidine	<1–2			0.8
788.	Tilidine	0.05–0.12	1.7		Approximately 3

Continued

APPENDIX 6

S. No.	Substances	Blood-plasma/serum concentration (μg/mL)			t½ (hours)
		Therapeutic ("normal")	Toxic (from)	Comatose-fatal (from)	
789.	Tiludronate	0.2–1.5			65–78 (–150)
790.	Timolol	0.005–0.05 (–0.1)			2–6
791.	Tin	0.03–0.14			
792.	Tinidazole	Maximum –60			11–15
793.	Tiopronin	Approximately 2–5			23 ± 11
794.	Tiotixene	0.001–0.03 (0.002–0.014)	0.1		34–36
795.	Tizanidine	Approximately 0.015			Approximately 2.5
796.	Tobramycin	4–10	12–15		2–3
797.	Tocainide	4–12 (6–10)	13–15; 20	74; 140	8–25
798.	Tofenacine	0.025–0.1	0.5–1		4–12
799.	Tolbutamide	50–100	400–500	640	4–12
800.	Tolmetin	10–80	60		2–4
801.	Toluene			10	
802.	Topiramate	3.4–5.2 (–10)			20–30
803.	Topotecan	Approximately 0.001–0.01			2–3
804.	Tramadol	0.1–1 (>0.3)	1	2; 13; 38.3	5–10
805.	Tranexamic acid	10–50			10
806.	Tranylcypromine	–0.2	0.5	0.7; 5	1.5–3.5
807.	Trapidil	(4–) 6–10			2–6, 12
808.	Trazodone	(0.5–) 0.8–1.6	4	12–15	4–8 (6–13)

APPENDIX 6

Continued

S. No.	Substances	Blood-plasma/serum concentration (µg/mL)			t½ (hours)
		Therapeutic ("normal")	Toxic (from)	Comatose-fatal (from)	
809.	Triamterene	0.01–0.1			1.5–4
810.	Triazolam	0.002–0.02	0.04		2–5
811.	2,2,2-tribromoethanol		50	90	
812.	Trichloroethane			10–1,000	
813.	2,2,2-trichloroethanol	5–15	40–70	60–100	
814.	2,4,5-trichlorophenoxyacetic acid (2,4,5-T)		Approximately 100	200	23–33
815.	Trifluoperazine	0.001–0.01 (0.05)	0.1–0.2		7–18
816.	Triflupromazine	0.03–0.1	0.3–0.5		Approximately 6
817.	Trihexyphenidyl	Data on effective plasma concentrations for parkinson's disease not available	0.5		3–5
818.	Trimeprazine	See alimemazine			
819.	Trimethadione	20–40			
820.	Trimethobenzamide	1–2			
821.	Trimethoprim	1.5–2.5	20		8–11
822.	Trimipramine	0.01–0.25	0.5	1.7–8.2	10–20 (–40)
823.	Tripelennamine	0.02–0.06		10	5–8
824.	Triprolidine	0.004–0.045			2–5
825.	Tropisetron	Approximately 0.02–0.05			5.6–8.6
826.	Tubocurarine	(0.6–) 1–3 (–6)			2–4

Continued

APPENDIX 6

Continued

S. No.	Substances	Blood-plasma/serum concentration (μg/mL)			t½ (hours)
		Therapeutic ("normal")	Toxic (from)	Comatose-fatal (from)	
827.	Tungsten	~0.035			
828.	Urapidil	Approximately 0.1–0.2			2.7–7
829.	Valdetamide	See diethylpentenamide			
830.	Valnoctamide	5	40		
831.	Valproic acid	40–100 (50–150)	150–200	720	10–20 (7–17)
832.	Vanadium	~0.05			
833.	Vancomycin	≤5–10 (–12)	30		4–11
834.	Vecuronium	Approximately 0.2–0.37 (–0.5)			1–1.5
835.	Venlafaxine	Approximately 0.2–0.4	1–1.5	6.6	3–5
836.	Verapamil	(0.01–) 0.02–0.25 (–0.4)	1	2.5; 3.9	6–14
837.	Vigabatrin	2–9 (–15)			5–8
838.	Viloxazine	6.0–8.0			2–5
839.	Vincamine	<0.25			1–2 (8–17)
840.	Vinylbital	1–3	5	8	18–33
841.	Viquidil	Approximately 0.15–0.25			6–12
842.	Vitamin A	See retinol			
843.	Vitamin C	See ascorbic acid			
844.	Vitamin D	>50 nmol/L			Approximately 30
845.	Warfarin	1–3 (–7)	10–12	100	37–50
846.	Wismut	See bismuth			

Continued

Continued

S. No.	Substances	Blood-plasma/serum concentration (µg/mL)			t½ (hours)
		Therapeutic ("normal")	Toxic (from)	Comatose-fatal (from)	
847.	Xamoterol	Approximately 0.02–0.04 (–0.1)			7–8
848.	Xipamide	~20			5–8
849.	Xylene			3–40	
850.	Yohimbine	Approximately 0.05–0.3			1–3
851.	Zafirlukast	0.005–0.03			10
852.	Zalcitabine	Approximately 0.1 (0.5 µmol/L)			1–3
853.	Zanoterone	0.1–0.5			
854.	Zidovudine	0.1–0.3 (–1)	2–3		1–1.5
855.	Zinc	0.6–1.3	2	42	
856.	Zipeprol	0.1–0.7		5.8; 10.6	
857.	Ziprasidone	0.02–0.06			2–7
858.	Zolmitriptan	Approximately 0.007–0.01			2.5–3
859.	Zolpidem	0.08–0.15 (–0.2)	0.5	2–4	2–5
860.	Zonisamide	(15–) 20–30 (–40)	(30–) 40–70	100	50–70
861.	Zopiclone	<0.1	0.15	0.6–1.8	3.5–8
862.	Zotepine	0.01–0.15	0.15–0.2		14–16
863.	Zuclopenthixol	0.005–0.1	0.15–0.3		Approximately 20

Source: M Schulz, A Schmoldt. Therapeutic and toxic blood concentration of more than 800 drugs and other xenobiotics. Pharmazie. 2003;58(7):447–74.

Appendix 7

Specifications of the Small and Commercial Quantity of Narcotic Drug or Psychotropic Substances [SO 1055 (E), dated 19-10-2001 As Amended]

Sl. No.	Names of narcotic drug and psychotropic substance [International Nonproprietary Name (INN)]	Other nonproprietary name	Chemical names	Small quantity (in g)	Commercial quantity (in g/kg)
1	2	3	4	5	6
1.	Acetorphine		3-0-acetyltetrahydro-7-alpha-(1-hydroxy-1-methylbutyl)-6, 14-3-endoetheno-oripavine	2	50 g
2.	Acetyl-alpha-methylfentanyl		N-[1-(a pha-methylphenethyl)-4-piperidyl] acetanilide	0.005	0.1 g
3.	Acetyldihydrocodeine		Acetyl dihydrocodeine	5	100 g
4.	Acetylmethadol		3-acetoxy-6-dimethyl amino-4,4-diphenylheptane	2	50 g
5.	Alfentanil		N-[1-[2-(4-ethyl-4,5-dihydro-5-oxo-1H-tetrazol-1-yl)ethyl]-4-(methoxymethyl)-4-piperidinyl]-N-phenylpropanamide	0.005	0.1 g
6.	Allylprodine		3-allyl-1 methyl-phenyl-4-propionoxypiperidine	2	50 g
7.	Alphacetylmethadol		Alpha-3-acetoxy-6-dimethylamino-4,4-diphenylheptane	5	100 g
8.	Alphameprodine		Atpha-3-ethyl-1-methyl-4-phenyl-4-propionoxypiperidine	2	50 g
9.	Alphamethadol		Alpha-5-dimethylamino-4,4-diphenyl-3-heptanol	2	50 g
10.	Alpha-methylfentanyl		N-[1(alpha-methylphenethyl)-4-piperidyl]propionanilide	0.005	0.1 g
11.	Alpha-methylthiofentanyl		N-[1-[1-methyl-2-(2-thienyl)ethyl]-4-piperidyl]propionanilide	0.005	0.1 g
12.	Alphaprodine		Alpha-1,3-dimethyl-4-phenyl-4-propionoxypiperidine	5	100 g

Continued

APPENDIX 7

Continued

Sl. No.	Names of narcotic drug and psychotropic substance [International Nonproprietary Name (INN)]	Other nonproprietary name	Chemical names	Small quantity (in g)	Commercial quantity (in g/kg)
13.	Anileridine		1-para-aminophenethyl-4-phenylpiperidine-4-carboxylic acid ethyl ester*	2	50 g
14.	Benzethidine		1-(2-benzyloxyethyl)-4-phenylpiperidine-4-carboxylic acid ethyl ester	5	100 g
15.	Benzylmorphine		3-o-benzylmorphine	2	50 g
16.	Betacetylmethadol		Beta-3-acetoxy-6-dimethylamino-4,4-diphenylheptane	2	50 g
17.	Beta-hydroxyfentanyl		N-[1-beta-hydroxyphenethyl)-4-piperidyl]propionanilide	0.005	0.1 g
18.	Beta-hydroxy-3-methyl fentanyl		N-[1-(beta-hydroxyphenethyl)-3-methyl-4-piperidyl] propionanilide	0.005	0.1 g
19.	Betameprodine		Beta-3-ethyl-1-methyl-4-phenyl-4-propionoxypiperidine	5	100 g
20.	Betamethadol		Beta-6-dimethylamino-4,4-diphenyl-3-heptanol	2	50 g
21.	Betaprodine		Beta-1,3-dimethyl-4-phenyl-4-propinoxypiperidine	5	100 g
22.	Bezitramide		1-(3-cyano-3,3-diphenylpropyl)-4-(2-oxo-3-propionyl-1-benzimidazolinyl)-piperidine	5	100 g
23.	Cannabis and cannabis resin	Charas, Hashish	Extracts and tinctures of cannabis	100	1 kg
24.	Clonitazene		2-para-chlorbenzyl-1-diethylaminoethyl-5-nitrobenzimidazole	2	50 g
25.	Coca derivatives		(excluding cocaine) and its salts	2	50 g
26.	Coca leaf			100	2 kg
27.	Cocaine		Methyl ester of benzoylecgonine	2	100 g
28.	Codeine		3-o-methylmorphine	10	1 kg
29.	Codoxime		Dihydrocodienone-6-carboxymethyloxime	5	100 g

Continued

APPENDIX 7

Continued

Sl. No.	Names of narcotic drug and psychotropic substance [International Nonproprietary Name (INN)]	Other nonproprietary name	Chemical names	Small quantity (in g)	Commercial quantity (in g/kg)
30.	Concentrate of poppy straw		The material arising when poppy straw has entered into a process for the concentration of its alkaloids when such material is made available in trade	20	500 g
31.	Desomorphine	Permonid, scopermid	Dihydrodeoxymorphine	2	50 g
32.	Dextromoramide		(+)-4-[2-methyl-4-oxo-3,3-diphenyl-4-(1-pyrrolidinyl)butyl]-morpholine	1	20 g
33.	Dextropropoxyphene		Alpha-(+)-4-dimethylamino-1,2-diphenyl-3-methyl-2-butanol proponate	20	500 g
34.	Diampromide		N-[2-(methylphenethylamino)-propyl]propionanilide	2	50 g
35.	Diethylthiambutene	Themalon	3-diethylamino-1,1-di-(2-thienyl)-1-butene	5	100 g
36.	Difenoxin	Diphenoxylic acid	1-(3-cyano-3,3-diphenylpropyl)-4-phenylisonipecotic acid	2	50 g
37.	Dihydrocodeine		Dihydrocodeine	10	200 g
38.	Dihydromorphine	Paramorfan	Dihydroxydihydromorphinone	5	100 g
39.	-		2-dimethylaminoethyl-1-ethoxy-1,1-diphenylacetate	1	20 g
40.	Dimenoxadol		6-dimethylamino-4,4-diphenyl-3-heptanol	2	50 g
41.	Dimepheptanol		3-dimethylamino-1,1-di-(2-thienyl)-1-butene	5	100 g
42.	Dimethylthiambutene		Ethyl-4-morpholino-2,2-diphenylbutyrate	5	100 g
43.	Dioxaphetyl butyrate		1-(3-cyano-3,3-diphenylpropyl)-4-phenylpiperidine-4-carboxylic acid ethyl ester	2	50 g
44.	Diphenoxylate			2	50 g
45.	Dipipanone		4,4-diphenyl-6-piperidine-3-heptanone	5	100 g

Continued

APPENDIX 7

Continued

Sl. No.	Names of narcotic drug and psychotropic substance [International Nonproprietary Name (INN)]	Other nonproprietary name	Chemical names	Small quantity (in g)	Commercial quantity (in g/kg)
46.	Drotebanol		3,4-dimethoxy-17-methylmorphinan-6-beta-14-diol	1	20 g
47.	Ecgonine		Its esters and derivatives which are convertible to ecgonine and cocaine	2	50 g
48.	Ethylmethylthiambutene		3-ethylmethylamino-1,1-di(2-thienyl)-1-butene	2	50 g
49.	Ethylmorphine	Dionine	3-o-ethylmorphine	10	200 g
50.	Etonitazene		1-diethylaminoethyl-2-para-ethoxybenzyl-5-nitrobenzimidazole	5	50 g
51.	Etorphine		Tetrahydro-7-alpha-(1-hydroxy-1-methylbutyl)-6,14-3ndoetheno-oripavine	5	100 g
52.	Etoxeridine		1-[2-(2-hydroxyethoxy)-ethyl]-4-phenylpiperidine-4-carboxylic acid ethyl ester	2	50 g
53.	Fentanyl		1-phenethyl-4-N-propionylanilinopiperidine	0.005	0.1 g
54.	Furethidine		1-(2-tetrahydrofurfuryloxyethyl)-4-phenylpiperidine-4-carboxylic acid ethyl ester	1	20 g
55.	Ganja			1000	20 kg
56.	Heroin		Diacetylmorphine	5	250 g
57.	Hydrocodone	Dicodide, codinovo, diconone, hycodan, and multacodin nycodide	Dihydrocodeine	1	20 g
58.	Hydromorphinol		14-hydroxydihydromorphine	2	50 g

Continued

639

APPENDIX 7

Continued

Sl. No.	Names of narcotic drug and psychotropic substance [International Nonproprietary Name (INN)]	Other nonproprietary name	Chemical names	Small quantity (in g)	Commercial quantity (in g/kg)
59.	Hydromorphone	dilaudide, dimorphid, and novalaudon	Dihycromorphinone	1	20 g
60.	Hydroxypethidine		4-meta-hydroxyphenyl-1-methylpiperidine-4-carboxylic acid ethyl ester	5	100 g
61.	Isomethadone		6-dimethylamino-5-methyl-4,4-diphenyl-3-hexanone	2	50 g
62.	Ketobemidone		4-m-ta-hydroxyphenyl-1-methyl-4-propionylpiperidine	2	50 g
63.	Levomethorphan		(-)-3-methoxy-N-methylmorphinane	2	50 g
64.	Levomoramide		(-)-4-[2-methyl-4-oxo-3,3-diphenyl-4-(1-pyrrolidinyl)-butyl] morpholine	2	50 g
65.	Levophenacylmorphan		(1)-3-hydroxy-N-phenacylmorphinan	2	50 g
66.	Levorphanol	Levorphan	(-)-3-hydroxy-N-methylmorphinan	1	20 g
67.	Metazocine		2-hydroxy-2,5,9-trimethyl-6,7-benzomorphan	5	100 g
68.	Methadone		6-dimethylamino-4,4-diphenyl-3-heptanone	2	50 g
69.	Methadone intermediate		4-cyano-2-dimethylamino-4,4-diphenyl-butane	2	50 g
70.	Methyldesorphine		6-methyl-delta-6-deoxymorphine	2	50 g
71.	Methyldihydromorphine		6-methyldihydromorphine	2	50 g
72.	3-methylfentanyl		N-(3-methyl-1-phenethyl-4-piperidyl)propionanilide	0.005	0.1 g
73.	3-methylthiofentanyl		N-(3-methyl-1-[2-(2-thienyl)ethyl]-4-piperidyl)propionanilide	0.005	0.1 g
74.	Metopon		5-methyldihydromorphinone	2	50 g
75.	Moramide intermediate		2-methyl-3-morpholino-1,1-diphenylpropane carboxylic acid	5	100 g

Continued

APPENDIX 7

Continued

Sl. No.	Names of narcotic drug and psychotropic substance [International Nonproprietary Name (INN)]	Other nonproprietary name	Chemical names	Small quantity (in g)	Commercial quantity (in g/kg)
76.	Morpheridine		1-(2-morpholinoethyl)-4-phenylpiperidine-4-carboxylic acid ethyl ester	2	50 g
77.	Morphine		Morphine	5	250 g
78.	Morphine methobromide		And other pentavalent nitrogen morphine derivatives, including in particular the morphine-N-oxide derivatives, one of which is codeine-N-oxide	2	50 g
79.	Morphine-N-oxide	Genomorphine N-oxy morphine		2	50 g
80.	MPPP		1-methyl-4-phenyl-4-piperidinol propionate (ester)	2	50 g
81.	Myrophine		Myristylbenzylmorphine	5	100 g
82.	-		N-cyclopropylmethyl-7,8-dihydro-7-(1-hydroxy-1 methyl-3-ethyl) o-methyl-6-14-endoethanonormorphine	5	100 g
83.	Nicocodine		6-nicotinylcodeine	10	200 g
84.	Nicodicodine		6-nicotinyldihydrocodeine	5	100 g
85.	Nicomorphine		3,6-dinicotinylmorphine	2	50 g
86.	Noracymethadol		(±)-alpha-3-acetoxy-6-methylamino-4,4-diphenylheptane	2	50 g
87.	Norcodeine		N-demethylcodeine	5	100 g
88.	Norlevorphanol		(-)-3-hydroxymorphinan	2	50 g
89.	Normethadone		6-dimethylamino-4,4-diphenyl-3-hexanone	5	100 g
90.	Normorphine		Demethylmorphine or N-demethylated morphine	2	50 g
91.	Norpipanone		4,4-diphenyl-6-piperidino-3-hexanone	5	100 g

Continued

641

APPENDIX 7

Continued

Sl. No.	Names of narcotic drug and psychotropic substance [International Nonproprietary Name (INN)]	Other nonproprietary name	Chemical names	Small quantity (in g)	Commercial quantity (in g/kg)
92.	Opium		And any preparation containing opium	25	2.5 kg
93.	Opium derivatives		Other than diacetylmorphine (heroin), morphine, and those listed herein	5	250 g
94.	Oxycodone	Dihydroxy codeinone	14-hydroxydihydrocodeinone	2	50 g
95.	Oxymorphone		14-hydroxydihydromorphinone	2	50 g
96.	Para-fluorofentanyl		4-fluoro-N-(1-phenethyl-4-piperidyl)propionanilide	0.005	0.1 g
97.	PEPAP		1-phenethyl-4-phenyl-4-piperidinol acetate (ester)	10	50 g
98.	Pethidine		1-methyl-4-phenylpiperidine-4-carboxylic acid ethyl ester	10	200 g
99.	Pethidine intermediate A		4-cyano-1-methyl-4-phenylpiperidine	10	200 g
100.	Pethidine intermediate B		4-phenylpiperidine-4-carboxylic acid ethyl ester	10	200 g
101.	Pethidine intermediate C		1-methyl-4-phenylpiperidine-4-carboxylic acid	10	200 g
102.	Phenadoxone		6-morpholino-4,4-diphenyl-3-heptanone	5	100 g
103.	Phenampromide		N-(1-methyl-2-piperidinoethyl)-propionanilide	5	100 g
104.	Phenazocine		2-hydroxy-5,9-dimethyl-2-phenethyl-6,7-benzomorphan	1	20 g
105.	Phenomorphan		3-hydroxy-N-phenethylmorphinan	5	100 g
106.	Phenoperidine		1-(3-hydroxy-3-phenylpropyl)-4-phenylpiperidine-4-carboxlic acid ethyl ester	2	50 g
107.	Pholcodine	Nomocodeine, Hybernil	Morpholinylethylmorphine	5	100 g
108.	Piminodine		4-phenyl-1-(3-phenylaminopropyl)-piperidine-4-carboxylic acid ethyl ester	5	100 g

Continued

APPENDIX 7

Continued

Sl. No.	Names of narcotic drug and psychotropic substance [International Nonproprietary Name (INN)]	Other nonproprietary name	Chemical names	Small quantity (in g)	Commercial quantity (in g/kg)
109.	Piritramide		1-(3-cyano-3,3-diphenylpropyl)-4-(1-piperidino)-piperidine-4-carboxylic acid amide	2	50 g
110.	Poppy straw			1,000	50 kg
111.	Preparations made from the extract or tincture of Indian hemp			5	100 g
112.	Proheptazine		1,3-dimethyl-4-phenyl-4-propionoxyazacycloheptane	2	50 g
113.	Properidine		1-methyl-4-phenylpiperidine-4-carboxylic acid isopropylester	2	50 g
114.	Propiram		N-(1-methyl-2-piperidinoethyl)-N-2-pyridylpropionamide	10	200 g
115.	Racemethorphan		(±)-3-methoxy-N-methylmorphinan	2	50 g
116.	Racemoramide		(±)-4-[2-methyl-4-oxo-3,3-diphenyl-4-(1-pyrrolidinyl)-butyl]-morpholine	2	50 g
117.	Racemorphan		(±)-3-hydroxy-N-methylmorphinan	2	50 g
118.	Sufentanil		N-[4-(methoxymethyl)-1-[2-[2-thienyl-ethyl]-4-piperidyl] propionanilide	0.005	0.1 g
119.	Thebacon		Acetyldihydrocodeinone	2	50 g
120.	Thebaine		3,6-dimethoxy-4,5-epoxy-9a-methylmorphine-6,8-diene	2	100 g
121.	Thiofentanyl		N-[1-[2-(2-thienyl)ethyl]-4-piperidyl]propionanilide	0.005	0.1 g
122.	Tilidine		(±)-ethyl-trans-2-(dimethylamino)-1-phenyl-3-cyclohexene-1-carboxylate	10	200 g
123.	Trimeperidine		1,2,5-trimethyl-4-phenyl-4-propionoxypiperidine	10	200 g

Continued

APPENDIX 7

Continued

Sl. No.	Names of narcotic drug and psychotropic substance [International Nonproprietary Name (INN)]	Other nonproprietary name	Chemical names	Small quantity (in g)	Commercial quantity (in g/kg)
124.	Brolamfetamine	DOB	(±)-4-bromo-2,5-dimethoxy-alpha-methylphenethylamine	0.5	10 g
125.	Cathinone		(x)-(s)-2-aminopropiophenone	2	50 g
126.		DET	3-[2-(diethylamino) ethyl]indole, N,N, diethyltryptamine	0.1	2 g
127.		DMA	(+)-2,5-dimethoxy-alpha-methylphenethylamine	0.5	10 g
128.		DMHP	3-(1,2-dimethylheptyl)-7,8,9,10-tetrahydro-6,6,9-trimethyl-6H-dibenzo(b,d)pyran-1-ol	2	50 g
129.		DMT	3-[2-(dimethylamino)ethyl]indole,N,N Dimethyltryptamine	0.1	2 g
130.		DOET	(+)-4-ethyl-2,5-dimethoxy-alpha-phenethylamine	0.5	10 g
131.	Eticyclidine	PCE	N-ethyl-1-phenylcyclohexylamine	2	50 g
132.	Ethryptamine		3-(2-aminobutyl)indole	2	50 g
133.	(+) Lysergide	LDS, LSD-25	9,10-didehydro-N,N-diethyl-6-methylergoline-8Beta-carboxamide	0.002	0.1 g
134.		MDMA, ecstasy	(+)-N-alpha-dimethyl-3,4-(methylenedioxy)phenethylamine	0.5	10 g
135.	Mescaline		3,4,5-trimethoxyphenethylamine	5	100 g
136.	Methcathinone		2-(methylamino)-1-phenylpropan-1-one	2	50 g
137.		4-methylaminorex	(+)-cis-2-amino-4-methyl-5-phenyl-2-oxazoline	0.5	10 g
138.		MMDA, ecstasy	2-methoxy-alpha-methoxy-alpha-methyl-4,5-(methylenedioxy) pher ethylamine	0.5	10 g
139.	4-MTA		Alpha-Methyl-4-Methylthiophenethylamine	0.5	10 g
140.	N-ethyl MDA		(±)-N-ethyl-alpha-methyl-3,4-(methylenedioxy) phenethylamine	0.5	10 g

Continued

APPENDIX 7

Sl. No.	Names of narcotic drug and psychotropic substance [International Nonproprietary Name (INN)]	Other nonproprietary name	Chemical names	Small quantity (in g)	Commercial quantity (in g/kg)
141.		N-hydroxy MDA	(±)-N-[alpha-methyl-3,4-(methylenedioxy)phenethyl] hydroxylamine	0.5	10 g
142.		Parahyxyl	3-hexyl-7,8,9,10-tetrahydro-6,6,9-trimethyl-6H-dibenzo(b,d) pyran-1-01	2	50 g
143.		PMA	p-methoxy-alpha-methylphenethylamine	0.5	10 g
144.		Psilocin, psilotsin	3-[2-(dimethylamine)ethyl]indol-4-ol	2	50 g
145.	Psilocybine		3-[2-(dimethylamino)ethyl]indol-4-yl dihydrogen phosphate	2	50 g
146.	Rolicyclidine	PHP, PCPY	1-(1-phenylcycohexyl)pyrrolidine	2	50 g
147.		STP, DOM	2,5-dimethoxy-alpha, 4-dimethylphenethylamine	0.5	10 g
148.	Tenamfetamine	MDA	Alpha-methyl-3,4-(methylenedioxy) phenethylamine	0.5	10 g
149.	Tenocyclidine	TCP	1-[1-(2-thienyl)cyclohexyl]piperidine	2	50 g
150.		Tetrahydrocannabinol	The following isomers and their stereochemical variants: • 7,8,9,10-tetrahydro-6,6,9-trimethyl-3-pentyl-6H-dibenzo(b, d)pyran-1-ol • (9R,10aR)-8,9,10,10a-tetrahydro-6,6,9-trimethyl-3-pentyl-6H-dibenzo(b,d)pyran-l-ol • (6aR,9R,10aR)-6a,9,10,10a-tetrahydro-6,6,9-trimethyl-3-pentyl-6H-dibenzo(b,d)pyran-1-ol • (6aR,10aR)-6a,7,10,10a-tetrahydro-6,6,9-trimethyl-3-pentyl-6H-dibenzo(b,d)pyran-l-ol • 6a,7,8,9-tetrahydro-6,6,9-trimethyl-3-pentyl-6H-dibenzo(b,d)pyran-1-ol • (6aR,10aR)-6a,7,8,9,10,10a-hexahydro-6,6-dimethyl-9-methylene 3-pentyl-6H-dibenzo(b,d)pyran-1-ol	2	50 g

Continued

APPENDIX 7

Continued

Sl. No.	Names of narcotic drug and psychotropic substance [International Nonproprietary Name (INN)]	Other nonproprietary name	Chemical names	Small quantity (in g)	Commercial quantity (in g/kg)
151.		TMA	(+)-3,4,5-trimethoxy-alpha-methylphenethylamine	0.5	10 g
152.	Amfetamine	Amphetamine	(±)-alpha-methylphenethylamine	2	50 g
153.		2 C-B	4-bromo-2,5-dimethoxyphenethylamine	0.5	10 g
154.	Dexamfetamine	Dexamphetamine	(+)-alpha-methylphenethylamine	2	50 g
155.	Fenetylline		7-[2-[(alpha-methylphenethyl)amino]ethyl] theophylline	0.5	10 g
156.	Levamfetamine	Levamfetamine	(x)-(R)-alpha-methylphenethylamine	2	50 g
157.		Levomethamphetamine	(x)-N,alpha-dimethylphenethylamine	2	50 g
158.	Mecloqualone		3-(o-chlorophenyl)-2-methyl-4(3H)-quinazolinone	20	500 g
159.	Metamfetamine	Methamphetamine	(±)-(S)-N, alpha-dimethylphenethylamine, (+)2 methylamino-1-phenylpropane	2	50 g
160.	Metamfetamine racemate	Methamphetamine racemate	(±)-N,alpha-dimethylphenethylamine	2	50 g
161.	Methaqualone		2-methyl-3-O-tolyl-4(3H)-quinazolinone	20	500 g
162.	Methylphenidate		Methyl alpha-phenyl-2-piperidineacetate	2	50 g
163.	Phencyclidine	PCP	1-(1-phenylcyclohexyl)piperidine	2	50 g
164.	Phenmetrazine		3-methyl-2-phenylmorpholine	5	100 g
165.	Secobarbital		5-allyl-5-(1-methylbutyl)barbituric acid	20	500 g
166.	Dronabinol	Delta-9-tetrahydrocannabinol and its stereochemical variants	(6aR,10aR)-6a,7,8,10a-tetrahydro-6,6,9-trimethyl-3-pentyl-6H-dibenzo(b,d)pyran-1-ol	2	50 g
167.	Zipeprol		Alpha-(alpha-methoxybenzyl)-4-(beta-methoxyphenethyl)-1-piperazineethanol	5	100 g

Continued

APPENDIX 7

Continued

Sl. No.	Names of narcotic drug and psychotropic substance [International Nonproprietary Name (INN)]	Other nonproprietary name	Chemical names	Small quantity (in g)	Commercial quantity (in g/kg)
168.	Amobarbital		5-ethyl-5-isopentylbarbituric acid	20	500 g
169.	Buprenorphine		21-cyctopropyl-7-alpha-[(S)-1-hydroxy-1,2,2-trimethylpropyl]-6,14,endo-ethano-6,7,8,14-tetrahydrooripavine	1	20 g
170.	Butalbital		5-allyl-5-isobutylbarbituric acid	20	500 g
171.	Cathine	(+)-norpseudoephedrine	(+)-(R)alpha-[(R)-1-aminoethyl]benzylalcohol	2	50 g
172.	Cylobarbital		5-(1-cyclohexen-1-yl)-5-ethylbarbituric acid	20	500 g
173.	Flunitrazepam		5-(o-fluorophenyl)-1,3-dihydro-1-methyl-7-Nitro-2H-1,4-benzodiazepin-2-one	5	100 g
174.	Glutethimide		2-ethyl-2-phenylglutarioide	20	500 g
175.	Pentazocine		(2R,6R,11R)-1,2,3,4,5,6-hexahydro-6,11-dimethyl-3-(3-methyl-2-butenyl)-2,6-methano-3-benzazocin-8-ol	20	500 g
176.	Pentobarbital		5-ethyl-5-(1-methylbutyl)barbituric acid	20	500 g
177.	Allobarbital		5,5-diallylbarbituric acid	20	500 g
178.	Alprazolam		8-chloro-1-methyl-6-phenyl-4H-s-triazolo(4,3-a) (1,4) benzodiazepine	5	100 g
179.	Amfepramone	Diethylpropion	2-(diethylamino)propiophenone	10	250 g
180.	Aminorex		2-amino-5-phenyl-2-oxazoline	5	100 g
181.	Barbital		5,5-diathylbarbituric acid	20	500 g
182.	Benzphetamine	Benzphetamine	N-benzyl-N,alpha-dimethylphenethylamine	20	500 g
183.	Bromazepam		7-bromo-1,3-dihydro-5-(2-pyridyl)-2H-1,4-benodiazepin-2-one	20	500 g
184.	Butobarbital	Butobarbital	5-butyl-5-ethylbarbituric acid	20	500 g

Continued

APPENDIX 7

Continued

Sl. No.	Names of narcotic drug and psychotropic substance [International Nonproprietary Name (INN)]	Other nonproprietary name	Chemical names	Small quantity (in g)	Commercial quantity (in g/kg)
185.	Brotizolam		2-bromo-4-(o-chlorophenyl)-9-methyl-6H-thieno(3,2-f)-s-triazolo(4,3-a)(1,4)diazepine	5	100 g
186.	Camazepam		7-cholor-1,3-dihydro-3-hydroxy-1-methyl-5-phenyl-2H-1,4-benzo-Iiazepin-2-one dimethylcarbamate (ester)	20	500 g
187.	Chlordiazepoxide		7-chloro-2-(methylamino)-5-phenyl-3H-1,4-benzodiazepine-4-oxide	20	500 g
188.	Clobazam		7-chloro-1-methyl-5-phenyl-1H-1,5-benzodiazepine-2,4(3I-,5H)-dione	10	250 g
189.	Clonazepam		5-(O-chlorophnyl)-1,3-dihydro-7-nitro-2H-1,4-benzodiazepin-2-one	5	100 g
190.	Clorazepate		7-chloro-2,3-dihydro-2-oxo-5-phenyl-1H-1,4-benzodiazepine-3-carboxylic acid	10	250 g
191.	Clotiazepam		5-(O-chlorophenyl)-7-ethyl-1,3-dihydro-1-methyl-2H-thieno(2,3-e)-1,4-diazepin-2-one	10	250 g
192.	Cloxazolam		10-chloro-1 lb-(O-chlorophenyl)-2,3,7,1lb-tetrahydroxazolo-(3,2-d) (1,4)benzodiazepine-6(5H)-one	5	100 g
193.	Delorazepam		7-chloro-5-(O-chlorophenyl)-1,3-dihydro-2H-1,4-benzodiazepin-2-one	5	100 g
194.	Diazepam		7-chloro-1,3-dihydro-1-methyl-5-phenyl-2H-1,4-benzodiazepin-2-one	20	500 g
195.	Estazolam		8-chloro-6-phenyl-4H-s-triazolo(4,3-a)(1,4)benzodiazepine	5	100 g
196.	Ethchlorvynol		1-chloro-3-ethyl-1-penten-4-yn-3-ol	20	500 g

Continued

APPENDIX 7

Continued

Sl. No.	Names of narcotic drug and psychotropic substance [International Nonproprietary Name (INN)]	Other nonproprietary name	Chemical names	Small quantity (in g)	Commercial quantity (in g/kg)
197.	Ethinamate		1-ethynylcyclohexanol carbamate	20	500 g
198.	Ethyl loflazepate		Ethyl7-chloro-5-(O-fluorophenyl)-2,3-dihydro-2-oxo-1H-1,4-benzodiazepine-3-carboxylate	10	250 g
199.	Etilamfetamine	N-ethylamphetamine	N-ethyl-alpha-methylphenethylamine	2	50 g
200.	Fencamfamin		N-ethyl-3-phenyl-2-norboranamine	2	50 g
201.	Fenproporex		(±)-3-[(alpha-methylphenethyl)amino]propionitrile	2	50 g
202.	Fludiazepam		7-chloro-5-(o-flurophenyl)-1,3-dihydro-1-methyl-2H-1,4-benzodiazepin-2-one	5	100 g
203.	Flurazepam		7-chloro-1-[2-diethylamino)ethyl]-5-(o-flurophenyl)-1,3-dihydro-2H-1,4-benzodiazepin-2-one	5	100 g
204.		GHB	γ-hydroxybutyric acid	10	250 g
205.	Halazepam		7-chloro-1,3-dihydro-5-phenyl-1-(2,2,2-trifluroethyl)-2H-1,4-benzodiazepin-2-one	20	500 g
206.	Haloxazolam		10-bromo-11b-(o-flurophenyl)-2,3,7,11b-tetrahydrooazolo(3,2-d)(1,4)benzodiazepine-6(5H)-one	20	500 g
207.	Ketazolam		11-chloro-8,12b-dihydro-2,8-dimethyl-12b-phenyl-4H-(1,3)oxazino(3,2-d)(1,4) benzodiazepine-4,7(6H)-dione	10	250 g
208.	Lefetamine	SPA	(x)-N,N-dimethyl-1,2-diphenylethylamine	10	250 g
209.	Loprazolam		6-(o-chlorophenyl)-2,4-dihydro-2-[(4-methyl-1-piperazinyl)methylene]-8-nirtro-1H-imidazo (1,2-1)(1,4) benzodiazepine-1-one	5	100 g

Continued

APPENDIX 7

Sl. No.	Names of narcotic drug and psychotropic substance [International Nonproprietary Name (INN)]	Other nonproprietary name	Chemical names	Small quantity (in g)	Commercial quantity (in g/kg)
210.	Lorazepam		7-chloro-5-(o-chlorophenyl)-1,3-dihydro-3-hydroxy-2H-1,4-benzodiazepin-2-one	10	250 g
211.	Lormetazepam		7-chloro-5-(o-chlorophenyl)-1,3-dihydro-3-hydroxy-1-methyl-2H-1,4-benzodiazepin-2-one	10	250 g
212.	Mazindol		5-(p-chlorophenyl)-2,5-dihydro-3H-imidazo[2,1-a]isindol-5-ol	10	250 g
213.	Medazepam		7-chloro-2,3-dihydro-1-methyl-5-phenyl-1H-1,4-benzodiazepine	20	500 g
214.	Mefenorex		N-(3-chloropropyl)-alpha-methylphenethylamine	2	50 g
215.	Meprobamate		2-methyl-2propyl-1-,3-propanedio dicarbamate	20	500 g
216.	Mesocarb		3-(alpha-methylphenethyl)-N-(phenylcarbamoyl)sydnone imine	5	100 g
217.	Methylphenobarbital		5-etyl-1-methyl-5-phenylbarbituric acid	20	500 g
218.	Methyprylon		3,3-diethyl 1-5-methyl-2,4-piperidinedione	20	500 g
219.	Midazolam		8-chloro-6-(O-fluorophenyl)-1-methyl-4H-imidazo (1,5-a](1,4) benzodiazepine	20	500 g
220.	Nimetazepam		1,3-dihydro-1-methyl-7-nitro-5-phenyl-2H-1,4-benzodiazepin-2-one	10	250 g
221.	Nitrazepam		1,3-dihydro-7-nitro-5-phenyl-2H-1,4-benzodiazepin-2-one	20	500 g
222.	Nordazepam		7-chloro-1,3-dihydro-5-phenyl-2H-1,4-benzodiazepin-2-one	20	500 g
223.	Oxazepam		7-chloro-1,3-dihydro-3-hydroxy-5-phenyl-2H-1,4-berzodiazepin-2-one	20	500 g

Continued

Continued

APPENDIX 7

Sl. No.	Names of narcotic drug and psychotropic substance [International Nonproprietary Name (INN)]	Other nonproprietary name	Chemical names	Small quantity (in g)	Commercial quantity (in g/kg)
224.	Oxazolam		10-chloro-2,3,7,1 lb-tetrahydro-2-methyl-1 lb-phenyloxazolo (3,2-d)(1,4) benzodiazepine-6(5H)-one	20	500 g
225.	Pemoline		2-amino-5-phenyl-2-oxazolin-4-one(-2-imino-5-phenyl-4-oxazolidinone)	2	50 g
226.	Phendimetrazine		(+)-(2S,3S)-3,4-dimethyl-2-phenylmorpholine	20	500 g
227.	Phenobarbital		5-ethyl-5-phenylbarbituric acid	20	500 g
228.	Phentermine		Alpha,alpha-dimethylphenethylamine	20	500 g
229.	Pinazepam		7-chloro-1,3-dihydro-5-phenyl-1(2-propynyl)-2H-1,4-benzodiazepin-2-one	10	250 g
230.	Pipradrol		1,1-diphenyl-1-(2piperidyl)-methanol	20	500 g
231.	Prazepam		7-chloro-1(cyclopropytmethyl)-1,3-dihydro-5-phenyl-2H-1,4-benzodiazepin-2-one	20	500 g
232.	Pyrovalerone		4-methyl-2-(1-pynrolidinyl) valerophenone	2	50 g
233.	Secbutabarbital		5-sec-butyl-5-ethylbarbituric acid	20	500 g
234.	Temazepam		7-chloro-1,3-dihydro-3-hydroxy-1-methyl-5-phenyl-2H-1,4-benzodiazepin-2-one	20	500 g
235.	Tetrazepam		7-chloro-5(1-cyclohexen-1-yl)-1,3 dihydro-1-methyl-2H, 1,4-benzodiazepin-2-one	20	500 g
236.	Triazolam		8-chloro-6(o-chlorophenyl)-1 methyl-4H-s-triazolo(4,3-a)(1,4) benzodiazepine	5	100 g
237.	Vinylbital		5-(1-methylbutyl)-5-vinylbarbituric acid	20	500 g

Continued

APPENDIX 7

Sl. No.	Names of narcotic drug and psychotropic substance [International Nonproprietary Name (INN)]	Other nonproprietary name	Chemical names	Small quantity (in g)	Commercial quantity (in g/kg)
238.	Zolpidem		N,N,6-trimethyl-2-p-tolylimidazo (1,2-alpha) pyridine-3-acetanide	10	250 g
1238A.	Dihydroetorphine		7,8-dihydro-7a-[1-(R)-hydroxy-1-methylbutyl]-6,14-endo-ethar otetrahydrooripavine	0.01	0.5 g
238B.	Oripavine			2	100 g
238C.	Remifentanil		1-(2-methoxy carbonylethyl)-4-(phenylpropionylamino) piperidine-4-carboxylic acid methyl ester	0.004	0.2 g
238D.	Amineptine		7-[1C,11-dihydro-5H-dibenzo (a,d) cyclohepten-5-yl) amino] heptanoic acid	20	1 kg
238E.	Ketamine		2-(2-chlorphenyl)-2-(methylamino)cyclohexanone	10	500 g
2238F.	Mephedrone	4-methylmethcathinone (4-MMC) 4-methylephedrone	(RS)-2-methylamino-1-(4-methylphenyl)propan-1-one	2	50 g
3238G.	AH-7921		3,4-dichloro-N-[(1-dimethylamino)cyclohexylmethyl] benzamide	4	200 g
238H.	25B-NBOMe	2C-B-NBOMe	2-(4-bromo-2,5-dimethoxyphenyl)N-(2-methoxybenzyl) ethanamine	0.8	40 g
238I.	25C-NBOMe	2C-C-NBOMe	2-(4-chloro-25-dimethoxyphenyl)-N-(2-methoxybenzyl) ethanamine	0.005	0.25 g
238J.	25I-NBOMe	2C-I-NBOMe	2-(4-iodo-2,5-dimethoxyphenyl)-N-(2-methoxybenzyl) ethanamine	0.05	2.5 g

APPENDIX 7

Continued

Sl. No.	Names of narcotic drug and psychotropic substance [International Nonproprietary Name (INN)]	Other nonproprietary name	Chemical names	Small quantity (in g)	Commercial quantity (in g/kg)
238K.	n-benzylpiperazine	Benzylpiperazine, BZP	1-benzylpiperazine	5	250 g
238L.	JWH-018	AM-678	Naphthalene-1-yl(1-pentyl-1H-indol-3-yl) methanone	0.25	12.5 g
238M.	AM-2201	JWH-2201	[1-(5-fluoropentyl)-1H-indol-3-yl] (naphthalene-1-yl) methanone	0.25	12.5 g
238N.	MDPV	3,4-Methylene-dioxypyrovalerone	(R/S)-1-[Benzo(d)(1,3)dioxol-5-yl]-2-(pyrrolidin-1-yl)pentan-1-one	0.5	25 g
238O.	Methylone	Beta-keto-MDMA	(RS)-2-methylamino-1-(3,4-methylenedioxyphenyl)propan-1-one	7.5	375 g
[4]238P.	-	Acetylfentanyl	N-phenyl-N-[1-(2-phenylethyl)-4-piperidinyl] acetanimide	1.0	50 g
238Q.	-	MT-45	1-cyclohexyl-4-(1,2-diphenylethyl) piperazine	2.0	100 g
238R.	-	Para-methoxymethyl-amphetamine, PMMA	1-(4-methoxyphenyl)-N-methylpropan-2-amine	1.0	50 g
238S.	-	α-pyrrolidinovalerophenone, α-PVP	1-phenyl-2-(pyrrolidin-1-yl)pentan-1-one	0.1	5 g
238T.	-	Para-methyl-4-methylaminorex, 4,4'-DMAR	4-methyl-5-(4-methylphenyl)-4,5-dihydro-1, 3-oxazol-2-amine	1.0	50 g
238U.	-	Methoxetamine, MXE	2-ethylamino-2-(3-methoxyphenyl) cyclohexanone	5.0	250 g
238V.	-	Phenazepam	7-bromo-5-(2-chlorophenyl)-1,3-dihydro-2H-1, 4-benzodiazepin-2-one	0.5	25 g

Continued

APPENDIX 7

Continued

Sl. No.	Names of narcotic drug and psychotropic substance [International Nonproprietary Name (INN)]	Other nonproprietary name	Chemical names	Small quantity (in g)	Commercial quantity (in g/kg)
239.	Any mixture of preparation that of with or without a neutral material of any of the above drugs			*	**

[1] Inserted vide GSR 1430 (E), dated 21-6-2011,

[2] Inserted vide GSR 375 (E), dated 5-2-2015,

[3] Inserted vide GSR 2375 (E), dated 12-7-2016, and

[4] Inserted vide GSR 1384 (E), dated 2-5-2017

* Lesser of the small quantity between the quantities given against the respective narcotic drugs or psychotropic substances mentioned above forming part of the mixture.

**Lesser of the commercial quantity between the quantities given against the respective narcotic drugs or psychotropic substances mentioned above forming part of the mixture.

Note:

1. The small quantity and the commercial quantity given against the respective drugs listed above apply to isomers, within specific chemical designation, the esters, ethers, and salts of these drugs, including salts of esters, ethers, and isomers, whenever existence of such substance is possible.
2. The quantities shown against the respective drugs listed above also apply to the preparations of the drug and the preparations of substances of note 1 above.
3. "Small quantity" and "commercial quantity" with respect to cultivation of opium poppy is not specified separately as the offence in this regard is covered under clause (c) of Section 18 of the Narcotic Drugs and Psychotropic Substances Act, 1985.
4. The quantities shown in column 5 and column 6 of the table relating to the respective drugs shown in column 2 shall apply to the entire mixture or any solution or any one or more narcotic drugs or psychotropic substances of that particular drug in dosage form or isomers, esters, ethers, and salts of these drugs, including salts of esters, ethers, and isomers, wherever existence of such substance is possible and not just of its pure drug content.

Source: The Narcotic Drug Psychotropic Substance Act, 1985 (As amended vide SO 1383 (E), dt. 2-5-2017) along with subsequent amendments in 2018. BARE ACT, 2019 with short comments, Commercial Law Publishers (India) Pvt. Ltd., Delhi.

Index

Page numbers followed by *f* refer to figure, *fc* refer to flowchart, and *t* refer to table.

A

Abdominal pain 86
Abortion 568
Abrus precatorius 174, 175
Absorbance accuracy 372
Absorption bands, designation of 346
Absorption burner system, parts of 390
Absorption cell 389
Abuse, drug of 46, 47
Accidents 494
Accreditation 514, 515
  benefits of 515
  body 515
  history of 503
  process 516
Acepromazine 106, 274
Acetaldehyde 57, 100, 578
Acetic acid 155, 158, 181, 204, 335, 336
Acetone 57, 101
Acetonitrile 54, 295, 316
Acetophenazine 106, 107
Acetophos 52, 90
Acetylated cellulose 197
Acetylene flame 392
Acidic drug 296, 338
Acidic silica gel plates 197
Acidified aqueous cinchonine 579
Acids 155
  and bases
    classification of 155*t*
    color tests for 155
  attacks, prevent 572
  classification of 155
  test for 156
Acne 139
Aconitine 120
  analysis of 380
Aconitum napellus 174, 178
Acute barbiturate intoxication, symptoms of 65
Acyl benzenes, derivatives of 361
Acylation 257
Adsorption chromatography 186

Adsorptive stripping voltammetry 407, 408
Aerodrome management 498
Agent, preparation of reducing 434
Agglutination test 176
Agitation 335
Agricultural samples, different elements in 398
Air-acetylene
  elements 390
  flame 391
Alcohol 296, 494
  consumption of 494
  metabolism 501
  peak of 271*f*
  postsampling formation of 499
  use of 499
Alcometer testing 496
Aldosteronism, primary 397
Aldrin 97
  endosulfan 90
Alicyclic dienes 354
Alizarin 579
  reagent 579
  test 136
Alkaline
  distillation 59
  fast blue B salt 204
  solution of beta-naphthol 579
Alkaloids 69, 88, 120, 336
  color tests for 120
  extraction for 69
  isolation methods for 69
Alkaly 161
  test for 161
Alkyl substituents 354
Allobarbital 117, 271
Allobarbitone 65, 116
Alpha-naphthylamine test 164, 172
Alprazolam 272
Alumina 186, 188
  plates 197
Aluminium 128, 136
  analysis of 438

INDEX

Aluminon reagent 579
  test 136
Aluminum chloride 204
  test 96
Aluminum foil-lined lids 46
Aluminum nitrate, amount of 438
Aluminum phosphide 98
Aluminum silicate 188
Alvarez reaction test 121, 178
Amanita
  muscaria 83
  phalloides 83
Amethocaine 274
Amino acid 315
Amitriptyline 272, 273, 532
Ammonia 155, 162, 425
Ammonium
  acetate 579
    buffer, preparation of 426, 431
  carbonate 579
  chloride 579
  hydroxide 162, 336, 579
    test 101
  mercury thiocyanate 133, 579
  oxalate 579
    test 162
  peroxydisulfate test 138
  persulfate solution 578
  phosphate 579
  sulfate 579
  sulfide solution test 139
  thiocyanate 134, 579
Ammonium molybdate 204
  quinine sulfate 579
    test 172
  reagent 579
  solution 578
  test 90, 92, 93, 95, 129, 172
Amobarbital 271
Amobarbitone 65, 116
Amperometric detector 312
  functions 312
Amphetamine 147, 151, 273, 333, 532, 540
Ampicillin 140
Analytical column, regeneration of 316
Analytical toxicology, forensic application of 1
Anemia 86
Anesthetic gases 48
Aniline 57
  E- and b-bands of 347*f*
  isolation of 87

Anisidine phthalate 204
Anodic stripping voltammetry 405, 407
Antazoline hydrochloride
  solution 579
  test 157
Antemortem ingestion 540
Anthrax 139
Antiallergens 334
Antibiotics 78
  color tests for 139
  isolation of 84
Antidepressants 272, 334
  identification of 272
  quantification of 272
  second-generation 334
Antihistamines 274, 334
  identification of 274
  quantification of 274
Antimony 128, 130
  chloride 204
  pentachloride test 176
Apiezon grease 234, 240
Apoatropine 69
Appetite, loss of 87
Aprobarbitone 65
Apron 557*f*
Aprotic solvents 316
Aqueous layer 74
Arecoline 69
Argemone mexicana 174, 181
Argon ionization detector 241, 246, 246*f*
Arsenic 128, 129
  analysis of 433, 435*t*
  bulletin of 420
Ascorbic acid, aqueous solution of 578
Assessor role 518
Asynchronous noise 328
Atomic absorption 311
  burner system 390*f*
  instruments, types of 386
  process 384, 385*f*
  technique 384
Atomic absorption spectrometry 383, 399, 403
  advantages of 384
  applications of 396
  disadvantages of 384
  principle of 383
Atomic emission 311
  process 385*f*
  spectroscopy 36
Atomic fluorescence 311
Atomic spectroscopic detector 311

INDEX

Atrocin 69
Atropa belladonna 147, 153
Atropine 69, 147, 153
Audit 505
   criteria 505
   evidence 505
   findings 505
   first-party 509
   principles of 509
   second-party 509
   third-party 509
   types 509
Audit program 505, 512
   objectives, establishing 511
   parts of 512
   records, managing and maintaining 513
Automatic thin-layer chromatography sprayer 195f
Autopsy 39
   report 554
Auxiliary electrode 411, 412f, 419
Auxochrome 351
   increment 358t
Avenin 52, 90
Azacyclonol 61, 107, 274

B

Bacillus anthracis 139
Bacterial infections 139
   types of 139
Balanced pressure system 264, 264f
Bam Ford's test 175
Bandwidth, determination of 369f
Barbitone 65, 116
Barbiturate 88, 117, 147, 150, 198, 201, 532
   analysis of 221, 222t
   color tests for 116
   extraction methods for 65
   identification of 271
   isolation methods for 65
   quantification of 271
   test for 117
Barium 128, 137, 399
   chloride 171, 579
      test 158, 167, 173
   hydroxide 155, 162
   sulfate test 171
Baseline flatness, test for 368f
Basic drugs, analysis of 221, 273
Bauxite 188

B-bands 346
Beer's law 343, 346f
   graphical representation of 386f
Beer–Lambert law 343
Benactyzine 61
Benedict's reagent 579
Benedict's test 141, 145
Benzene 57, 102, 199, 335
   hexachloride 268
Benzidine 579
   solution test 164
Benzocaine 274
Benzoctamine 106, 108
Benzodiazepine 42, 61, 116, 147, 150, 335, 379, 532, 569
   analysis of 272
   drugs of 379
   derivatives, absorption of 379t
Benzoinoxime test 134
Benzphetamine 273
Benzyl alcohol 57
Berberine 69, 120, 122
Beta-naphthol test 102
Bettendorf's test 130
Bhang, test for 180
Bial's reagent 211
Bicarbonate test 134
Bidrin 90
Bifenthrin 90, 269, 333
Biological fluid 39, 55
   bile 42
   blood 39
   body fluids 43
   cerebrospinal fluid 43
   urine 40
   vitreous humor 41
Biological hazard 556
Biological material, waste disposal procedures for 29, 560
Biological tissues 44
Biomedical waste 560
   classification of 562t
Biomedical Waste (Management and Handling) Rules 560, 561
Birlane 90
Bismuth 128, 131
Blank analysis 417
Blood 55, 59, 61, 64
   alcohol
      concentration 498, 540
      level 496
   and urine 441
      heavy metal in 434

INDEX

chemicals in 1
during collection, dilution of 500
level, actual 500
microwave digestion of 488
serum, magnesium in 397
Blood-to-breadth ratio 500
Bonded stationary phase 304
Bone
  and muscle tissue 46
  marrow samples 47
Borate 163, 165
Boric acid 146, 434, 436
Brain tissue 403
Breath alcohol 501
  analyzer 494
  concentration 500
  testing
    device 495, 501
    principle of 495
Breathalyzer 494, 496f, 501
  calibration of 496
  operators 497
  types of 494
  using photocell 497f
Bridged ethylene hybrid 322
Bromate 163, 167
Bromazepam 106, 108, 272
Bromide 163, 165, 205, 212, 312
Bromine solution 580
Bromine water 580
Bromocresol green 204
Bromophenol blue 205
Bromophos 52, 90
Brompheniramine 274
Bronchopneumonia 88
Brown sugar 147
Brucine 120, 121, 174, 179
  test 157, 172
Buffer preparation 436, 438, 441, 443
Bulk property detectors 306
Burner heads 390, 401
Burns 564
Butacaine 274
Butaperazine 106, 108
Butobarbitone 65, 116
Butriptyline 272

C

Cadmium 128, 135
  acetate 211
Caffeine 273

Calatropis
  gigantean 174
  procera 174
Calcium
  analysis of 397
  hydroxide 162, 188
  oxalate 188
  silicate 188
  sulphate 188
Calcium carbonate 188
  test 158
Calcium chloride 580
  test 160, 166, 172
Calculate column's efficiency 290
Calibration method 397f
Calotropis gigantica 78, 82, 174
  isolation of 82
Calotropis procera 78, 82, 174
  isolation of 82
Camazepam 272
Cannabis sativa 174, 179
Capillary column 233, 234f, 237
Carbamates 52, 90, 199, 223, 535
  pesticides 91, 269, 315, 333
Carbaryl 90
Carbofuran 90
Carbon
  disulfide 57, 103
  monoxide 46, 532
Carbon tetrachloride 57, 205, 478
  carbon disulfide test 93
  test 93, 97
Carbowax 240
Cardiac drugs, applied for 337
Cardiac glycosides 85
Cardiotoxic poisons 85
Carfenazine 106, 108, 274
Carrier gas 229
  arrangement of 232f
Castiglioni's test 104
Catecholamines 311
Cathodic stripping voltammetry 407
Cause-and-effect relationships 508
Caustic potash test 101
Caustic soda test 138, 157
Cefaloridine 139, 140
Cell, type of 366
Cellulose plates 197
Central drugs laboratory 567
Central nervous system 46, 146
Ceramic materials 478
Cerebera thevetia 85

INDEX

Cerebrospinal fluid 43
Cetirizine 334
Charas, test for 180
Chelating resins 303
Chelidonine 120, 122
Chemical 23f
  criminology 338
  hazard 556
  interferences 395
  list of 17t
  substance 381
Chemiluminescent nitrogen detector 307, 313
Chiral detector 314
Chlamydia 139
  psittaci 140
  trachomatis 140
Chloral hydrate 57, 103, 378
Chloramphenicol 140
Chloranil reagent 206
Chlorate 163, 164
Chlordiazepoxide 106, 109, 380
  azacyclonol 106
Chloride 165, 209
Chlorine water 580
  test 165, 166
Chlorodiazepoxide 379
Chloroform 57, 102, 199
Chloroform-pyridine test 169
Chloroplatinic acid 580
  test 161
Chloroprocaine 274
Chloropromazine hydrochloride 380
Chlorothion 90, 332
Chlorphenamine 334
Chlorpheniramine 273
Chlorpromazine 61, 106, 109, 274, 540
Chlorpyrifos 52, 90, 332
Chlortetracycline 141
Chlorthion 52
Chopper 389
Chromate 173
Chromatogram 251, 251f, 252f, 255f, 256f, 290f
  development of 202, 203f, 218
Chromatographic column, types of 302
Chromatography 186
Chromic acid test 149
Chromium 128, 136
Chromophore 350, 351t
Chromosulfuric acid 213
Chromotropic acid 580
  test 100, 136

Cinchona succirubra 336
Cinchonine 69
Cis and trans isomers 378
Claviceps purpurea 82, 336
Cleistanthus collinus 78, 81
Clindamycin 141
Clinical toxicology 219
Clobazam 106, 109, 272
Clofenotane 94
Clomipramine 272
Clomocycline 139, 141
Clonazepam 379, 539
Clopenthiol 106, 109
Clorazepate 379
Clorazepic acid 272
Coating efficiency 255
Cobalt acetate test 169
Cobalt acetate-o-toluidine reagent 205
Cobalt nitrate 580
  test 138, 168, 169
Cobalt sulfate 580
Cobalt thiocyanate 205
  solution 578, 580
  test 151
Cobalt-acetate test 117
Cobaltous acetate solution 580
Cocaine 42, 69, 147, 149, 222, 274, 539
Code of criminal procedure 535, 567, 570
Codeine 120, 122, 148
Coiled column, packing of 238f
Cold start 419
Colocynth, isolation of 82
Column chromatography 186, 186f
Column coating 237
Column injection 300
Column lifetime and performance, maintenance of 303
Column packing 237, 305
Coma 86
Combined audit 510
Common biomedical waste treatment facility 561
Common drugs, identification of 333
Common solvents 240t
Complete toxicological analysis 40
Complexing reagent 439
Compressed air 391
Concentrated formic acid 152
Concentrated hydrochloric acid test 174
Concentrated sulfuric acid test 174
Conducting closing meeting, procedure for 523

INDEX

Conductivity detector 312
Congo red 580
  paper test 156
Coniferyl alcohol
  reagent 580
  test 145
Coniine 69
Conjugated compound 378
Control unit 267
Copper 128, 133
  turning test 158
Copper sulfate 206, 580
  pyridine test 168
  solution 580
  test 133, 144, 166, 169
Coramine 69
Corona detector 314, 314f
Corrected retention time 252
Cough syrups 499
Cresol 58
  isolation of 86
Crime
  examining scene of 547
  investigation, field of 35
Croton tiglium 78, 174, 175
  isolation of 79
Crotonic acid 79
Crystal test 105, 121, 179
Cupric acetate test 182
Cuprous iodide test 131
Customer focus 506
Cyanate 163, 168
Cyanide 46, 60, 104, 163, 168, 532, 534
  analysis of 434, 437t
  extraction method for 60
  isolation method for 60
  sulphide 312
  voltammogram of 436
Cyanosis 86
Cyclizine 274
Cyclobarbital 118
Cyclobarbitone 65
Cyclohexane 199
Cyclopentobarbital 118
Cycloserine 142
Cyfluthrin 90, 269, 333
Cyolane 52, 90
Cypermethrin 269

D

Dasanit 52, 90
Datura fastuosa 174, 179

DDQ reagent 206
Delorazepam 272
Deltamethrin 90, 269, 333
Demeclocycline 139, 142
Demeton 52, 90
Denigès–Oliver's test 125, 181
Deoxyribonucleic acid 39
Derivatization 257
  techniques 319
  types of 319
Desflurane 335
Desipramine 272
Detection limit 394
Detectors, type of 245
Deuterium lamp 363
  test 371, 371f
Developing solvent system 199t
Dextromethorphan 540
Diabetes 397
Diacetylmorphine 147
Diamorphine 536, 539
Diarrhea, causes of 84
Diazepam 106, 110, 379
Diazinon 52, 90, 94
Diazotization test 163
Diazotized 215
Dicalcium phosphate 188
Dicapthon 52, 90
Dichlorodiphenyltrichloroethane 95, 268
  analysis of 380
Dichlorofluorescein 206
Dichlorovinyl 333
Dichlorvos 90, 332
Dichromate 163, 173
  test 98
Dieldrin 90, 97
Dielectric loss factor 478
Diethylene glycol succinate 241
Digestors, closed 486t
Digitalin test 176
Digitalis purpurea 174, 176
Digitoxin 174
  test 176
Dille-Koppanyi
  reagent 580
  test 150
Dilute ferric chloride solution 580
Dilute solutions, preparation of 585
Dimefox 52, 90
Dimethoate 52, 90, 94, 332
Dimethothiazine 274

INDEX

Dimethyl glyoxime 580
  reagent test 136
Dimethylamphetamine 273
Dinitrobenzene 379
  potassium hydroxide reagent test 150
  reagent 580
Dinitro-p-diphenyl carbazide test 135
Dinitrophenyl hydrazine test 94
Dinitrotoluene 379
Dionine 69
Diphenhydramine 274
Diphenyl
  carbazide tests 136
  oxalate tablets 540
Diphenylamine 206
  solution 580
  test 156, 157
Diphenylcarbazide 580
Diphenylcarbazone 206, 580
  test 131
Diphenylpyraline 274
Dipole rotation 478
Dipole-dipole interaction 287
Diquinolyl test 134
Direct gas-pressure system 300
Dispatch and forwarding samples 551
Disposables, use of 48
Disyston 52
Dithizone 207, 209
  solution 580
  test 135
Dizziness 86
  loss of 87
Double-beam
  atomic absorption spectrophotometer 387f
  spectrophotometer 362
  ultraviolet-visible spectrophotometer, technical specifications of 375
Doxepin 272
Doxycycline 139, 142
Dragendorff's reagent 206, 581
  test 177
Dragendorff's test 126
Drinking after offence 499
Driving belt 413, 413f
Dropping mercury electrode 410
Drug
  (price control) order 567, 569
  abuse, analysis of 316
  alcohol interactions 499
  analysis of 45

  and poisons, laws relating to 566
  basic 296
  designer 569
  identification 47
  of abuse, color tests for 146
  standard, list of 30t
  synergistic effect of 536
Drugs Act 566
Drugs and Cosmetics (Amendment) Act 566, 567
Drugs and Cosmetics Rules 567
Drugs and Magic Remedies (Objectionable Advertisements) Act 567, 568
Drugs Control Act 567, 568
Drugs Technical Advisory Board 567
Drunken driving 498
Dry ashing method 77
Dummy stopper 414, 414f
Duquenois–Levine
  reagent 581
  test 180
Dursban 52
Dynamic coating 238

E

E-bands 346
Ecgonine 69
Eddy diffusion 292, 293f
Edifenphos 52, 332
Effective theoretical plates 253
Ehrlich's reagent 154, 581
  test 153
Ekatin 52
Electrochemical detector 311, 312f
Electrochemical stripping analysis techniques 406
Electrode 410, 436, 439
  less discharge lamp 388, 389
  test 416
  washing of 417
Electrolyte 478
Electromagnetic spectrum 340, 340f
Electron capture detector 241, 243, 243f, 266, 282
Electron spin resonance spectroscopy 341
Electronic energy levels 348f
Electronic transitions, types of 347, 348f
Elixir 499
Emerson reagent 207

INDEX

Encyclopedia britannica 481f
Endocyclic conjugated 354
Endosulfan 268
Endrin 90, 96
Enzymatic processes, disruptive of 75
Ephedrine 273
   HCl 69
Equipment,
   list of major 25t
   list of minor 27t
Erdmann's reagent 581
Ergometrine 82, 120, 122
Ergot 174, 182
   isolation of 82
Ergotamine 82, 120, 123
Ergotoxin 82
Erythromycin 139, 142
Erythroxylum coca 146
Estazolam 272
Ester test 99, 174
Ethanol 48, 204, 211
   production 42
   test 91
   vapors, inhalation of 499
Ethanolic potassium hydroxide solution 578
Ether 335
Ethion 52
Ethomoxane 106, 110
Ethopropazine 61, 274
Ethyl
   alcohol 58, 98, 534
   benzoate test 149
   methyl ketone reagent test 103
Ethylene
   diamine nickel test 171
   glycol polymer 240f
Ethylenediamine nickel reagent 581
Ethylenediaminetetraacetic acid 441
Ethylmethyl ketone test 97
Euphoria, inducing 334
Evaporative light scattering detector 314
Evidential breath alcohol testing 500
E-waste rules 561
Exocyclic conjugated 354
Explosive 337
   analysis of 275, 378
   compounds, chromatogram of 275f
Expressing report, ways of 533
Eye 86
   accident 564
   witnesses, statements of 547

F

Facial paralysis 86
False-negative report, causes of 538
False-positive
   breath 500
   report, causes of 540
Faraday's law 312
Fast blue B
   potassium hydroxide test 175
   reagent 581
   test 179
Fatigue 86
Feigl's test 133
Femur ring 46
Fenitrothion 52, 90
Fenpropathrin 90, 333
Fenthion 52, 90
Fenvalerate 90, 333
Ferric chloride 207, 581
   acid test 183
   solution 581
   test 145, 158, 159, 169, 170, 176, 177, 182
Ferric salt reagent 581
Ferric salt test 181
Ferric thiocyanate test 168
Ferrous hydroxide
   paper test 105
   solution 581
Ferrous sulfate 581
   test 157, 169, 170
Fertilizer, microwave digestion of 490
Filtration method, coating by 236
First aid box 563, 563f
   contents of 563f
First aid emergency treatment 562
Fischer–Morris test 152
Flame 390
   function of 390
   ionization detector 241, 242f, 266, 282
   photometric detector 241, 245, 245f, 266, 282
   process 391f
   system 401
   test 132, 137, 161, 162
Flavone reagent 207
Flaxedil 69
Flow-metering stem 391
Fluanisone 106, 110
Fluorescein sodium salt 206
Fluorescence
   index 307
   test 183

INDEX

Fluorescent plates 197
Fluoride 163, 166
Fluorimetric detector 311, 311*f*
Fluphenazine 61
Flurazepam 272, 379
Forensic application 221
Forensic chemistry 403
Forensic sample 333
   barium in 399
   lead in 399
   tin in 399
Forensic science 398
   laboratories 575
Forensic scientists 2
Forensic toxicology 35
   laboratory, layout of 36*f*
   reporting 532
Formaldehyde 58, 100, 207
   solution 581
Formaldehyde-sulfuric acid 207
   reagent 581
      test 151, 154
      test 108-116, 146
Formic acid 155, 158, 336
Formothion 52
Forrest reagent 208, 581
   test 154
Forrest test 107, 108, 111, 113, 115, 116
Fourier-transform infrared spectroscopy 36
FPN reagent 581
   test 154
FPN test 107, 113, 114
Froehde's reagent 581
   test 152-154, 182
Froehde's test 124, 125, 148, 174, 180
Fuchsin test 170
Fuchsine reagent 581
Fujiwara test 102, 103, 140
Fume hood 191, 192*f*
Fuming nitric acid 125
Functional group, detection of 376
Functionalized silica materials 303
Furfural acid 207
Furfuraldehyde 111, 112
   reagent 581
Furfural-sulfuric acid test 184

G

Ganja, test for 180
Gardona 52, 90, 199
Gas chromatographic conditions
   with derivatization 272

   without derivatization 272
Gas chromatography 228, 249
   derivatization 257
   headspace technique 263*f*
   mass spectroscopy 36
   troubleshooting in 276
Gas density balance detector 241, 247, 247*f*
Gas-liquid chromatography 229, 229*f*, 241, 251, 258, 259*f*, 262, 265, 270, 276, 276*t*, 277, 277*t*, 282, 331
   forensic applications of 267
   solid support for 235
   techniques of 229
Gelsemium 69
General drug screening 533
Generate microwave energy 481
Gentamicin 139, 143
Gentian violet-bromine 208
Gerrard's test 154
Gibb's reagent 208
Glacial acetic acid 183, 211
Glass capillaries 193, 194*f*
Glass carbon electrodes 406
Glass indicating oxygen traps 261
Glass thin-layer chromatography
   sprayer 194*f*
Glasswares 12, 16*f*
   list of 13*t*
Glassy carbon electrode 411, 412*f*
Glassy materials 478
Glucuronic acid 42
Glutaraldehyde 539
Glutathione 42
Glycoprotein 311
Glymidine 275
Gold chloride test 149, 178
Gonorrhea 139
Gradient device 299
Gradient separation 295
Graphite furnace
   atomic absorption 479
   system 401
Griess reagent 208
Group test 133
Guaiacum copper sulfate test 105, 159
Guard column 258, 303
Gum disease 139
Gunzberg's reagent 581
Gunzberg's test 157
Guthion 52
Gutzeit test 129

663

H

Haemophilus influenzae 140
Hair 403
  and nail 47
  microwave digestion of 489
Halogen containing pyrethroids 269
Handling microwave digestor 484
Handmade plates 195
Handmade thin-layer chromatography plates 196*f*
Hanging mercury drop electrode 411, 427, 432, 435, 437, 439, 442
Hard plastics, use of 48
Hazardous chemical 560
Hazardous wastes 561
Headache 86
  loss of 87
Headspace
  gas chromatography 263
  sampler 267
Heart damage 86
Heavy metal 47
  monitoring of 405
Helium ionization detector 241, 247, 248*f*
Henry's law 496
Hepatic metabolism 147
Hepatic portal system 44
Heptabarbitone 65, 116
Herbicides 296
  drug 338
Heroin 42, 120, 123, 147, 222, 536, 539
  brown 338
Heteroannular diene 354, 356
Heterocyclic compounds 147
Hexacyanoferrate 163, 169, 170
Hexamethyldisilazane 235
Hexane 199
Hexylcaine 274
High capacity oxygen traps 260
High strength silica 322
High-performance liquid chromatography 36, 276*t*, 287, 288, 295*fc*, 296*f*, 297*f*, 309, 314, 317, 323, 328*t*
  column 301, 301*f*
  detectors 306, 307*t*
  elution techniques in 295
  forensic applications of 332
  guard column 304*f*
  instrument setup 325*fc*
  normal-phase 294*fc*
  pumps, types of 300
  relevance of 331
  solvents 29, 34*f*
    list of 33*t*
  system, technical specifications for 317
  theory of 288
  types of 294
High-pressure liquid chromatography 299
Hollow cathode lamp 388, 388*f*
  process 388*f*
Holmium perchlorate solution 371*f*
  test 370
Homatropine 69
Homicidal poisoning deaths 547
Homicides 494
Homoannular dienes 354
Human resource 1
Husemann's test 125, 180
Hydrastine 120, 123
Hydrastinine 120, 123
Hydride generation system 400
Hydrobromic acid 155-157, 238, 336, 482, 483
Hydrocarbons 495
Hydrochloric acid 155, 215, 336
  test 91, 106, 134, 138, 150, 181, 184
Hydrocyanic acid 58, 60, 98, 155, 159, 336, 478, 481, 483
Hydrogen
  discharge lamps 363
  peroxide 213, 398, 478, 482, 483
    test 173
  sulfide 581
    test 132, 135
Hydroiodic acid 155, 156, 336
Hydrophobic interactions 287
Hydroquinine 120, 124
  acid, solution of 578
  test 95
Hydroxyamphetamine 273
Hydroxylamine 208
  hydrochloride 581
Hydroxylapatite 188
Hydroxyzine 61, 274
Hygroscopic alkaloid 83
Hyoscine 69
Hyoscyamine 69
Hyperchromic effect 352
Hypochlorites 163, 168
Hypochromic effect 352

INDEX

I

Ibogaine 120, 124
Illicit drug 316
Imidan 52
Imipramine 61, 380
Implementing Audit Program 512
Impotency 568
Indian Evidence Act 567, 571
Indian Penal Code 567, 570
Indigo solution 582
Indigo test 164
Indole 582
   test 164
Infertility 568
Infrared
   photometric system 496f
   radiation 340
Injection port 231
Injection sites 47
Injector septa 258
Insecticides 296
   color tests for 90
   drug 338
   isolation methods for 52
Insomnia 335
Iodate 163, 167
Iodide 163, 166
   nitrite 312
Iodine
   solution 582
   vapor 208
Iodoform test 98, 102
Iodoplatinate solution 209
Ion-exchange chromatography 287
Ionic conductance 478
Ionization 395
   nature of 316
Iproniazid 272
Iron 208
Isocratic separation 295
Isoflurane 335
Isoniazid 539
Isopropanol 316
Isopropyl alcohol 58
Isopropylamine solution 578

J

Jamalgota 78, 79
Jumping baseline 331

K

Kaner, isolation of 85
K-bands 346
Keller's test 183
Kerosene 58
   oil, isolation of 87
Ketones 495
Kidney 86
Kinetic function 375
Koppanyi–Zwikker
   reagent 209, 582
   test 117, 118, 143, 146

L

Laboratory accidents, emergency
   management of 564t
Laced drinks 499
Lambert's law 343
Lambert–Beer law 343, 345
   application of 345
Lamp current optimization 396
Lanthanum chloride 399
Lanthanum nitrate solution 582
Lanthanum nitrate test 158
Laser light scattering detector 313
Lead 128, 134, 399
   acetate
      solution 582
      test 103, 166, 173
   assessor, role of 519
   nitrate test 168, 170
Lead Acid Batteries [Batteries
   (Management and Handling) Rules
   561
Leaves, microwave digestion of 489
Legal defense 498
Legal status 497
Legal's test 101
Levomepromazine 106, 110
Liebermann's reagent 582
Liebermann's test 94, 97, 106, 107,
   110-115, 119, 123, 124, 126, 128, 140,
   141, 152
Light sources 388
Lime water test 160
Lindane 268
Lipophilic drugs 46
Liquid chromatography 228
   mass spectroscopy 315
Liquid phase 240

665

INDEX

Liquid-liquid chromatography 288
Lisdexamfetamine 333
Litmus
  paper test 155, 161
  solution 582
Liver 44, 86, 403
Local anesthetics 274
  identification of 274
  quantification of 274
Longitudinal diffusion 293
Loprazolam 272
Lorazepam 106, 111, 379
Loxapine 106, 111
Lymecycline 139, 143
Lysergic acid diethylamide 147, 338, 569
Lysergide 147, 154

M

Macrolide antibiotic 139
Mafenide 139, 143
Maggots 47
Magnesia 188
Magnesium 128, 138
  peroxide test 156
  silicate 188
  sulfate 582
Magnetron 481
Malaria 139
Malathion 52, 90, 93, 332
Malonic acid 65
Mammalian toxicity 269
Management system 503
Managing audit program 510
Mandelin's test 148
Mandelin's reagent 209, 582
  test 182
Mandelin's test 107, 110, 114, 116, 124, 128, 140, 143, 148
Mandrax 146
Manganese 128, 137
  dioxide test 127
Manganous sulfate test 167
Manganous sulfate-phosphoric acid 582
  test 164
Marquis reagent 151, 210, 582
  test 151, 154
Marquis test 106-116, 122-124, 126-128, 140-143, 147, 148, 152, 153, 175, 180
Mask 557f
Mass detector 250

Mass transfer coefficient 293
Matrix interferences 395
Mayer's reagent 582
  test 177
Mayer's test 126
Mebutamate 106, 111
Mecke's reagent 582
  test 152, 153, 155
Mecke's test 125, 148
Meconic acid 181
Medazepam 106, 111
Menazon 52
Menstrual disorders 568
Mepazine 61
Meprobamate 106, 112
Mercuric chloride solution 582
Mercuric nitrate test 156
Mercuric oxide 441
Mercuric sulphate
  solution 582
  test 117, 118, 119
Mercuric sulfate-diphenylcarbazone
  test 150
Mercurous nitrate
  reagent 210, 582
  test 117, 119, 145, 162
Mercury 128, 131, 209
  analysis of 441
  arc lamps 364
  drop catcher 414
  electrode
    capillary for 419
    needles for 419
Mescaline 146, 147, 152, 273, 569
Metal in foodstuffs, drinks and
  beverages, analysis of 398
Metal ions, analysis of 415
Metallic elements, analysis of 396
Metallic poisons 88, 128, 534
  color tests for 128
  extraction methods for 75
  isolation methods for 75
Metallic standard, list of 31t
Metals, analysis of different 416
Methacycline 139, 143
Methadone 539
Methamphetamine 147, 151, 333
Methanol 295, 316, 320, 336
Methanolic potassium hydroxide 582
  solution 578
Methaqualone 146, 147, 151, 569
Methenamine 139, 143

Methohexital 118
Methoxyamphetamine 273
Methoxychlor 97
Methoxypromazine 61
Methyl
  alcohol 58, 99, 534
  chloride 478
  orange 582
  parathion 52, 90, 332
  violet test 158
  yellow 210
Methylamine 155
Methylcrotonic acid 79
Methyldemeton 52
Methylene
  blue solution 582
  blue test 156, 171
  chloride 316
Methylenedioxyamphetamine 273
Methylephedrine 273
Methylphenidate 273
Methylphenobarbitone 65
Metrohm trace metal analyzer 409f
Mevinphos 90
Micro test 130
Microargon detector 249
Microbial cells, death of 84
Microdetector 250f
Microscopic test 179
Microwave
  characteristics of 477
  digester 425, 426t
  material behavior of 477
Microwave digestion 476
  method 77, 492
  system 476
Microwave technology
  over thermal convection, advantages of 479
  principles of 477
Milk powder, microwave digestion of 490
Millon's reagent 582
Mipafox 52, 90
Miscellaneous poisons, extraction methods for 78
Mix dimethyl sulfoxide 316
Mixture, separation of 256
Mobile phase, miscibility chart of 298f
Modern liquid chromatograph 298f
Modern toxicology laboratory 1
  area 3

case opening room 5
document record room 4
engineering specifications 10
equipment and machinery 24
extraction and isolation unit 8
human resource 1
physical facility 3
reference material 25
requirements 12
sample analysis 8
screening test unit 9
security 29
space requirement 3
toxicology museum 5
washing room 10
Modes for quantitative analysis 419
Moisture traps 260
Molar absorptivity 344
Molar extinction coefficient 344
Molybdatophosphoric acid 210
Monitoring audit program 513
Monoamine oxidase inhibitors 334
Monochromator 364, 392, 393f, 401
Monocrotaline 120, 124
Monohydroxy phenol 80
Morphine 69, 120, 124, 146, 147, 222, 336, 539
  analysis of 380
Morphothion 52, 90, 332
Motor Vehicle Act 498
Mouth alcohol 501
M-phenylenediamine 212
Multi-mode electrode 410, 410f, 427, 432, 435, 437, 439, 442
Municipal solid wastes 561
Muscle tissue 403
Mushrooms 78
  isolation of 83
Mycoplasma pneumoniae 140

N

N-1-naphthyl ethylenediamine dihydrochloride 582
Nails, microwave digestion of 489
Naphthalene 58, 78
  isolation of 79
Naphthylethylenediamine
  dihydrochloride test 92
  hydrochloride test 94
Narceine 120, 126
Narcotic 198, 296

analysis of 222, 222t
drug 222, 636
  identification of 270
  quantification of 270
Narcotic Drugs and Psychotropic
  Substances Act 567, 569
National AIDS Control Organization
  561
Nausea 86
Nealbarbitone 65
Nebulizer 401
Neisseria gonorrhoeae 140
Neopine 120, 126
Nerium odorum 85
Nessler's reagent 583
  test 102, 103, 162, 176
Nessler's test 111, 112, 141-143
Neurotransmitters 311
Neutral and acid distillation 59
Neutral hexane extract 535
Nickel 128, 136
  amine reagent 210
Nicotiana tabacum 174, 177
Nicotine 69, 78, 120, 126
  isolation of 83
Ninhydrin 211
  reagent 151, 583
  test 143
Nitrate 163
Nitrating mixture 584
  reagent test 102
Nitrazepam 106, 112, 272, 539
Nitric acid 155, 157, 187, 211, 336, 478,
  482, 483
  test 121, 125, 148, 181
Nitric oxide 487
Nitrite 163
Nitrobenzene 58, 87
  isolation of 86
Nitrofurantoin 144
Nitrofurazone 139, 144
Nitrogen
  gas, bubbling of 409
  phosphorus detector 266, 282
Nitrohydrochloric acid 482, 483
Nitronaphthalene test 135
Nitroprusside test 104
Nitrous acid 155, 160, 336, 392
Nitroxoline 144
Noisy baseline 328
Nonconformity, classification of 520
Nonoxidizing acid 483

Nonpolar stationary phase 305f
Nonsilanized capillary 413f
Nortriptyline 272
Novocaine 69
Nuclear magnetic resonance
  detector 313

O

O-cresol test 92
Odihydroxy 80
Oduvan, isolation of 81
Oleander 174
Open digestors 486t
Open tubular column 232
  dynamic coating of 238f
O-phenylenediamine-trichloroacetic
  acid 212
O-phthalaldehyde 315
Opiates and narcotics 532
Opioid 47
Opium alkaloids 174, 180
Optics 375, 401
Optimization, techniques for 396
Orcinol 211
Organic compounds, basis of color in
  353
Organic molecules
  absorption by 347
  electrons present in 347
Organochlorated insecticides 46
Organochlorine
  compound 52, 535
  insecticides 53, 268
Organochloro compound 90, 200, 223
Organochloro insecticides 91
Organophosphorus 199, 223
  compound 52, 90, 535
  insecticides 90, 268, 332
  pesticides 90
Otitis media 139
O-toluidine 134, 215, 579
Oven and pneumatic control system
  265
Oxalate 163, 172
Oxalic acid 99, 155, 160, 336, 578
Oxazepam 272, 379
Oxethazaine 274
Oxidation reaction 495
Oxidizing agents 398
Oxybuprocaine 274
Oxygen traps 260
Oxypertine 106, 112

P

Packed column 232, 233f, 237
Packing samples 550
Palet's reaction test 120, 178
Palladium chloride 583
  solution 211
  test 92, 93, 120, 141
Panchnama 552
P-anisaldehyde 204
P-anisidine hydrochloride 204
Papaver somniferum linn, capsules of 69
Paraffin oil 211
Paraldehyde 58
Paraoxon 52, 90, 332
Parathion 90, 92, 332
  analysis of 380
Particular ion 313
P-dimethylaminobenzaldehyde 206, 583
  test 122, 178
Pecazine 106, 112
Penicillin 84
Penicillium 84
Pentobarbitone 65, 116
Perchloric acid 155, 156, 187, 487
  test 161
Perfluoroalkoxy 476, 478, 482, 487
Pericyazine 106, 113, 274
Periodic table elements, list of 586
Periodontitis 139
Permanganate
  crystal test 149
  test 172
Permethrin 90, 333
Perphenazine 61, 106, 113
Pertussis 139
Pesticide 198, 296, 332
  analysis of 223, 223t
  color tests for 90
  drug 338
  identification of 332
  isolation methods for 52
  poisoning 332
  standard, list of 30t
  test for 92
Pethidine 69
Petrabenazine 106
Petroleum ether 199
Petroleum products
  analysis of 275
  chromatogram of 276f

Pharmacy Act 567, 568
Phenethylamine 146
Pheniramine 274
Phenmetrazine 273
Phenobarbital 119
Phenobarbitone 65
Phenol 58
Phenol-barbitone 116
Phenolphthalein 583
Phenothiazine 147, 274, 335, 380, 532
  analysis of 274
  drugs 154
Phentermine 273
Phenyl azide-sulfanilic acid test 96
Phenyl hydrazine
  hydrochloric reagent 211
  hydrochloride, aqueous solution of 578
Phenylhydrazine sulfonate 212
Phenylhydrazine-potassium ferricyanide test 100
Phenylhydrazine-sodium nitroprusside test 100
Phosalone 52, 332
Phosdrin 90
Phosphamidon 90, 332
Phosphate 163, 172
  reduction of 540
Phosphide 532, 534
Phosphinon 90
Phosphomolybdic acid 212, 583
  test 177
Phosphomolybdic test 126
Phosphoric acid 52, 99, 206, 207, 212, 215, 578
  test 184
Phosphotungstic acid 212
Photocathode 392
Photocell 366, 366f
Photodiode array 307
  detector 309, 310f, 318
Photoionization detector 241, 248, 249f
Photometric accuracy 372
  test of 373f
Photomultiplier tube 365, 365f, 392
Photovoltaic cell 365, 366f
Phthalylsulfacetamide 144
Phthalylsulfathiazole 144
Physical hazard 556
Physostigmine 69
Picric acid 583
  paper test 105
  test 159

INDEX

Pinacryptol yellow 212
Piperacetazine 106, 114
Plant poisons
  applied for 336
  color tests for 174
Plasma 316, 403
  inductively coupled 36
Plastic containers 49f
Plasticware 22, 25f
  list of 23t
Plates
  after coating, treatment of 198
  coating of 198
Platinum electrode 411
Pneumatic intensifier pumps 300
Poisoning
  accidental 268
  case of 1
Poisoning deaths
  crime investigation of 547
  investigation of 547
Poisons 316, 537, 564
  act 566, 567
  anions 532
  chronic 47, 82
  classification of 532
  color tests for different 90
  common 533
  deaths 532
  drugs 532
  gases 532
  isolation methods for 78
  metals 532
  miscellaneous substances 532
  pesticides 532
  presence of 1
  samples, list of 5t
  volatile substances 532
Polar stationary phase 304, 304f
Polarographic trace metal analyser,
    application of 445t
Polarographic vessel 409
Police investigating officers 552
Polyethylene 478, 481
Polypropylene 48
Polytetrafluoroethylene 46, 48, 250, 476, 478, 481, 487
Polyvinyl chloride 478
Porous layer
  beds 305
  open tubular 282
  columns 234

Porous polymeric beds 305
Porphyroxine test 125
Portable breath analyzer 495f
Positive ion spectra 315
Postmortem 532
  drug redistribution 537
Potasan 52, 90
Potassium
  chloride 427, 432, 435, 439, 442
  ferricyanide 578
  fluoride 48
  iodate starch reagent 211
  oxalate 48
  perchlorate 398
  thiocyanate 583
Potassium antimonite
  solution 583
  test 161
Potassium chromate 583
  solution test 138
Potassium cyanide 434, 583
  test 135, 170
Potassium dichromate 213, 373f, 495, 578
  solution test 372
  sulfuric acid test 128
  test 137
Potassium ferrocyanide
  solution 583
  test 132, 139
Potassium hydroxide 155, 161, 215, 434, 436
  solution 578
  test 91, 94-96, 102, 144, 183
Potassium iodide 583
  cinchonine test 132
  sodium sulfite solution 583
  starch paper test 168
  test 134
Potassium nitrate 137, 373f
  solution 583
  test 373
Potassium permanganate 99, 171, 213, 495
  chromotropic acid test 99
  solution 578
  test 160
Potentiometric detector 313
P-phenylenediamine test 134
Pramoxine 274
Prazepam 272, 379
Precoated plates 195

Precoated thin-layer chromatography
  plates 196*f*
Premixed burner 389
Pressurized loop system 265, 265*f*
Prilocaine 274
Procaine 69, 274
Prochlorperazine 61
Program for microwave digestion of
  blood 488*t*
  dried leaves 490
  fertilizer 491*t*
  hair 489*t*
  milk powder 490*t*
  nails 489*t*
  sauce 492*t*
  soil 491*t*
  tissue 488*t*
  urine 489*t*
Promazine 61, 274
  hydrochloride 380
Promethazine 61, 274, 334
Proper biological samples, collection
  of 39
Propiomazine 274
Propoxycaine 274
Protriptyline 272
Proxymetacaine 274
Prussian blue test 104, 159, 168
Pseudoephedrine 273, 540
Psilocin 147, 153
Psilocybin 153, 569
Psychostimulant drug 333
Psychotropic drugs 272
Psychotropic substances 636
P-toluenesulfonic acid 215
Pulmonary edema 88
Pulse, differential 437
Pump
  quaternary gradient 317
  types of 295
Pyrazinamide 144
Pyrethroid 52, 90, 91, 200, 224, 269, 333, 535
Pyridine 155, 211
Pyrimidone test 163

Q

Quaaludes 146
Qualitative analysis 320, 377

Quality 504
  assurance 504
  audit 509
  control 504
  manager 504
  manual 504
  planning 504
Quality management
  principles 506
  system 504, 506
  tool for 503
Quantitative analysis 320, 321, 377
Quartz glass 476
Quinine 69

R

Radiation sources 363
Radioactive wastes 560
Radiometric detector 314, 315*f*
R-bands 346
Readout system 393
Reagents 23*f*, 425, 482
  detection 202
  list of 17*t*
  preparation of 578
Reciprocating pumps 300
Reference electrode 411, 412*f*, 419
Refractive index 307
  detector 310, 310*f*, 318
Reinsch's test 129, 130, 131
Relationship management 508
Reserpine 61
Resins ion exchangers, silica-based 303
Resolution power 369
Resorcinol
  reagent 583
  test 103, 163
Respiratory expression 88
Retention factor 203
Retention time 251
Retention volume 251
Rheodyne injector 300
Rhodamine B 583
  solution 213
  test reagent 130
Rifamycin 145
Ring test 150
Rolitetracycline 145
Root cause analysis 517

INDEX

Rotating disk electrode 411f
Rotation information, sign of 314
Round-the-clock pain 146
Roussin's test 178
Rubeanic acid 583
   test 133

S

Safety goggles 557f
Salicylates 532
Salicylic acid 143
Saliva 403
Sample cells 364
Sample injection system 231f, 300
Sample preparation 425
Sample preservation and storage 48
Saturated caustic soda solution 583
Scene of crime 551
Schiff's reagent test 99, 100
Schindel Misser's test 177
Scopolamine 69
Scott test 149
Sealed viscera bottles 49f
Secbutabarbital 119
Secobarbital 271
Secobarbitone 65
Seizures 335
Selective serotonin reuptake inhibitors 334
Semecarpus anacardium 78
   isolation of 80
Sensitivity 393, 394
Septum injectors 300
Serotonin-norepinephrine reuptake inhibitors 334
Serum 316
Silanized capillary 413f
Silanizing agent 236f
Silica gel 186, 188, 188f, 189f, 197
   G plates 197
      testing of 198
   plates, basic 197
   with starch 197
Silicon
   oil 240
   polymer 240f
   rubber gun 240
Silicotungstic acid test 177
Silver chloride 427, 432, 435, 439, 442, 443
Silver nitrate 92, 94, 213, 583
   solution test 129
   test 156, 157, 160, 165, 167, 170, 173
Silver sulfate 583
Silyl derivatives 257
Silylation 257
Simon's method 151
Simultaneous analysis, voltammogram of 442f
Single-beam atomic absorption spectrophotometer 386f
Single-beam ultraviolet 363f
Skin 86
   disinfection 499
Slurry method, coating by 237
Snakebite 47
Soap bubble meter 231f
Soap solution 584
Sodium 48
   acetate 584
   azide 213
   bicarbonate solution 74
   bismuthate test 137
   bisulfate test 101
   carbonate 137, 584
   chloride 441
   cobalt nitrite 584
   hydrogen
      phosphate test 138
      tartrate solution 584
      tartrate test 162
   hydroxide 103, 155, 161, 425
      solution 578
      test 93, 162, 175
   nitrite solution 578
   nitroprusside test 93, 101, 141, 142, 144, 171, 578
   phosphate 584
      test 138
   rhodizonate
      reagent 584
      test 171
Software 402
   and data station 375
Soil, microwave digestion of 491
Solanidine 120, 127
Solanine 69, 120, 127
Solid support, treatment of 236f
Solid tissues, scarcity of 46
Solvent 23f, 48, 198
   list of 17t
   peak, tailing on 330
   reservoir 297
Sophisticated analytical instrumental unit 9

Sparteine 69
Special test 176
Spectral bandwidth 345
Spectral interferences 394
Spectroscopy 341, 381
  atomic 341
  molecular 341
Spectrum bandwidth 369
Spray chamber 401
Spraying reagents, different 204t
Squalane 234
Stained soil 64
Stainless steel unions 259
Standard addition
  method 397f
  technique 433f, 436f, 438f, 440f, 444f
Standard column hardware 302f
Standard solution, preparation of 434
Stannic chloride 213
Stannous chloride
  aniline test 131
  solution 584
Starch
  iodide test 160, 163
  paper test 167
  solution 584
  test 164
State Forensic Science Laboratories 575
Static coating 239
  method 239f
Static mercury drop electrode 410
Stirrer 412f
Stomach
  contents 44, 45
  infections 140
  wash 55, 63, 67, 72
Stop flow injectors 300
Stray light interference 372f
  test 371
Streptococcus pneumoniae 140
Streptomyces 84
  mediterranei 140
Streptomycin 84, 140, 145
Stripping methods 406
Stripping voltammetric
  method, types of 407
  techniques 405
Strychnine 120, 127, 174, 179, 336
  analysis of 380
Substance
  dipole moments of 478t
  dopamine 147
Suicides 494

Sulfacetamide 275
Sulfadiazine 145, 275
Sulfadimidine 275
Sulfafurazole 275
Sulfamerazine 146, 275
Sulfamethizole 275
Sulfamethoxazole 275
Sulfamethoxydiazine 275
Sulfamethoxypyridazine 275
Sulfamoxole 275
Sulfanilic acid 164, 172, 584
  test 161
Sulfaphenazole 275
Sulfapyridine 275
Sulfate 42, 163, 171
Sulfathiazole 275
Sulfide 163, 171
Sulfites 170
Sulfocyanate test 105, 160
Sulfonamide 78, 139
Sulfuric acid 143, 155, 158, 184, 187,
    207, 213, 214, 336, 478, 482, 483, 487,
    584
  test 91, 96, 97, 106, 110, 111, 114, 115,
    122, 142, 143, 158, 165, 183
Sulphite 163, 312
Sulphonamides
  analysis of 275
  isolation of 79
Sumithion 90, 93
Surgical gloves 557f
Suspensions, preparation of 197
Synchronous noise 328
Synthesize heroin 69
Syringe injection system 263, 264f
Syringe-type pumps 300
Systematic errors 476

T

Talbutal 65
Tartaric acid-ammonium molybdate
  reagent 584
Technical assessor, role of 519
Teflon 46, 48
Temperature, advantages of increase
  in 317
Tetrabenazine 114
Tetracycline 84, 139, 146
  antibiotic 139
Tetrahydrofuran 295
Tetranitrodiphenyl 214
Tetrathion 52, 332

INDEX

Tetrazolium blue 214
Thalleioquin test 124
Thallium 128, 138
    analysis of 432t
    determination of 429
Thebaine 120, 128
Theoretical plate 253, 290, 291f, 291t
    calculation 291f
Therapeutic drug monitoring 316
Thermal conductivity detector 241, 244, 244f, 266, 282
Thermostated column compartment 317
Thialbarbital 120
Thimet 52
hin layer chromatography 186, 187, 216, 220
    advantages of 216
    chamber 189, 190f
    glass plates 189f
    spray cabinet 192
    sprayer 194
Thin layer chromatography plate 187, 191f, 218f, 219f
    heater 190
    holder 190f
    preparation of 197, 217f
    substance on 201
    types of 195
    visualization of 219f
Thin-film membrane-polytetrafluoroethylene 482
Thin-layer plates, preparation of 217
Thiocyanate 163, 169
    test 104
Thiopental 120
Thiopentone 65
Thiophos ME 52
Thiophosphoric acid 52
Thiopropazate 61
Thioproperazine 106, 116
Thioridazine 61, 106, 115, 274, 380
Thiosulfate 163, 170, 312
Third-party attestation 504
Thymol 214
Tin 128, 132
Tiotixene 106, 115
Tissue 46, 53, 61, 62, 66, 70
    microwave digestion of 488
Tollen's reagent 214
    test 100, 101

Toluene in hexane, resolution of 370f
Total consumption burner 389
Toxic
    anions 163
        color tests for 163
    drug 316
    effects 79
    elements
        in wine analysis, determination of 398
        monitoring of 398
    symptoms 83
Toxicological analysis 39, 44
Toxicological emergencies 320
Toxicological examination, steps in 533
Toxicology 398, 403
    analysis, sample for 42
    museum 5t
    report 532, 554
        legal standing of 535
        objectives of 533
Toxins 320
Trace metal analyser 405
    principle of 405
    technical specifications of 419
Trace metal analysis 444
Tranquilizers 88, 198, 201
    analysis of 221, 222t, 380
    color tests for 106
    isolation methods for 61
    specific absorption of 380t
Treating anxiety 335
Tricalcium phosphate 188
Trichlorfon 332
Tricyclic antidepressants 42
Trifluoperazine 61, 274
Triflupromazine 61
Trimeprazine 61, 274
Trimerazine 274
Trimethoxyamphetamine 273
Trimethylsilyl 257
    radical 235
Trimetozim 106, 115
Trimipramine 272
Trinitrobenzene 379
Trinitrotoluene 379
Tropine 69
Tungstophosphoric acid 215
Turmeric paper test 165
Turpentine oil 78, 106
    isolation of 78

INDEX

U

Ultra-performance liquid chromatography 322, 323
Ultrapure water 425, 434, 438, 443
Ultraviolet
  absorption spectra 342
  detector 308, 308f, 318
Ultraviolet visible
  region 383
  spectrophotometer 344, 374
    calibration of 368
    forensic applications of 379
  spectroscopy 340, 342, 379
    solvents for 376
Unconjugated compound 378
Uranyl acetate 138, 584
Urea 215
Urinary tract infections 139, 140
Urine 55, 59, 63, 67, 72, 403
  microwave digestion of 489
  specimen 40
Urotropine test 181

V

Vacuum degasser 318
Valve injection 300
Vamidothion 52
van Deemter plot 292f
Vanadium pentoxide 398
  reagent 584
Vanadium reagent test 96
Vanillin 215
  reagent 578, 584
  test 117-120
Vanilline-sulfuric acid test 184
Van-Urk's
  reagent 584
  test 175
Vapour generation accessory system 401
Venereal diseases 568
Vesparex 65
Vibrational spectroscopy 341
Vinylbital 271
Viscera 59, 550
Visualizing chromatogram 218
  spraying reagents for 202
Vitali's test 121, 153, 179, 182
Vitamins 410
Vitreous humor 41
  and urine 540
  disadvantage of 42

Volatile poisons 48, 57, 88
  color tests for 98
  isolation methods for 57
Voltammetric conditions 432t, 435t, 437t
Voltammetric trace metal analyser
  advantages of 418
  characteristics of 415
  detection limit of 417
  limitations of 418
Voltammetric trace metal analysis 415, 419
Voltammetric vessel 409, 436
Voltammogram 437f, 444f
Vomit 55, 63, 67, 72, 86
  stained garments 64, 68
Vortman's test 104, 159

W

Wall-coated open tubular columns 234
Warfarin, applied for 337
Water 295
Wavelength accuracy 370
  test of 371f
Weakness 86
Whether drug 537
Woodward–Fieser rules 355, 357
Working electrode 410, 419

X

Xanthydrol 578
  test 95
Xenobiotics 39
Xenon 335
  discharge lamps 364

Y

Yersinia pestis 139
Yohimbine 69, 120, 128

Z

Zinc 128, 132
  chloride diphenylamine reagent 215
  nitrate 584
  phosphide 98
  sulfate solution 584
  uranyl acetate 584
    test 156, 162
Zirconium-alizarin test 166
Zirconyl chloride solution 584
Zwikker's reagent 215